An Aid to the MRCP PACES
VOLUME 3
STATION 5

'MRCP; Member of the Royal College of Physicians. . .
They only give that to crowned heads of Europe'.
From *The Citadel* by A.J. Cronin

Dear Reader of *An Aid to the MRCP PACES*,

Please help us with the next edition of these books by filling in the survey on our website for every sitting of PACES that you attend. It does not matter if you pass or fail or pass well or fail badly. We need information from all these situations. These books are only as they are because of candidates in the past who filled in the surveys. Please do your bit for the candidates of the future. The website where you can fill in the survey is **www.ryder-mrcp.org.uk**
Good luck on the day.

Best wishes,
*Bob Ryder*
*Afzal Mir*
*Anne Freeman*
*Edward Fogden*

# An Aid to the MRCP PACES

## FOURTH EDITION
## VOLUME 3
## STATION 5

### R.E.J. Ryder, M.A. Mir,
### E.A. Freeman and E.N. Fogden

*Departments of Medicine, City Hospital, Birmingham,*
*University Hospital of Wales and*
*University of Wales College of Medicine, Cardiff*
*and Department of Integrated Medicine,*
*Royal Gwent Hospital, Newport*

WILEY-BLACKWELL

A John Wiley & Sons, Ltd., Publication

This edition first published 2013 © 1986, 1999, 2003 by Blackwell Publishing Ltd, 2013 by John Wiley & Sons Ltd.

Wiley-Blackwell is an imprint of John Wiley & Sons, formed by the merger of Wiley's global Scientific, Technical and Medical business with Blackwell Publishing.

*Registered office:*   John Wiley & Sons, Ltd, The Atrium, Southern Gate, Chichester, West Sussex, PO19 8SQ, UK

*Editorial offices:*   9600 Garsington Road, Oxford, OX4 2DQ, UK
The Atrium, Southern Gate, Chichester, West Sussex, PO19 8SQ, UK
111 River Street, Hoboken, NJ 07030-5774, USA

For details of our global editorial offices, for customer services and for information about how to apply for permission to reuse the copyright material in this book please see our website at www.wiley.com/wiley-blackwell.

*Library of Congress cataloging-in-publication data*

An aid to the MRCP PACES. – 4th ed. p. ; cm. Aid to the Membership of the Royal College of Physicians Practical Assessment of Clinical Examination Skills includes bibliographical references and index. Summary: "The first volume in this revised suite of the best-selling MRCP PACES revision guides is now fully updated. It reflects both feedback from PACES candidates as to which cases frequently appear in each station. Also taken into account is the new marking system introduced in which the former four-point marking scale has been changed to a three-point scale and candidates are now marked explicitly on between four and seven separate clinical skills"–Provided by publisher. ISBN 978-0-470-65509-2 (v. 1 : pbk. : alk. paper) – ISBN 978-0-470-65518-4 (v. 2 : pbk. : alk. paper) – ISBN 978-1-118-34805-5 (v. 3 : pbk. : alk. paper) I. Wiley-Blackwell (Firm) II. Title: Aid to the Membership of the Royal College of Physicians Practical Assessment of Clinical Examination Skills. [DNLM: 1. Physical Examination–Great Britain–Examination Questions. 2. Ethics, Clinical–Great Britain–Examination Quest

A catalogue record for this book is available from the British Library.

Wiley also publishes its books in a variety of electronic formats. Some content that appears in print may not be available in electronic books.

Cover image: © Wiley-Blackwell
Cover design by Sarah Dickinson

Set in 8.75/11.5 pt Minion by Toppan Best-set Premedia Limited
Printed and bound in Malaysia by Vivar Printing Sdn Bhd

1   2013

# Contents

# Preface

'MRCP; Member of the Royal College of Physicians . . . They only give that to crowned heads of Europe.'*

## A short history of *An Aid to the MRCP PACES*

*'Remember when you were young, you shone like the sun . . .'†*

At the beginning of the 1980s, Bob Ryder, an SHO working in South Wales, failed the MRCP short cases three times (an SHO in modern parlance is a core medical trainee [CMT]).‡ On each occasion I passed the long case and the viva which constituted the other parts of the MRCP clinical exam in those days but each time failed the short cases. Colleagues from the year below who had been house physicians, with me the SHO, came through and passed§ while I was left humiliated and without this essential qualification for progression in hospital medicine.

The battle to overcome this obstacle became a two or more year epic that took over my life. I transformed from green and inexperienced¶ to complete expert in everything to do with the MRCP short cases as viewed from the point of view of the candidate. I experienced every manifestation of disaster (and eventually triumph) recorded by others in Volume 2, Section F. By the time of the third attempt, I was so knowledgeable that I was out of tune with the examiner on a neurology case simply because I was thinking so widely on the case concerned.‖ I believed at the time that I came close to passing at that attempt, although one never really knows and it was, after all, the occasion where I failed to feel for a collapsing pulse!** This was an important moment in the story because it was from this failure, along with the experience in the neurology case in my second attempt¶, that the examination *routines* and *checklists*, which are so central to this book, emerged. I finally passed on the fourth attempt whilst working as a registrar.†† During the journey, various consultants, senior registrars and colleague registrars tried to help in their various ways and amongst these, one of the consultants in my hospital, Afzal Mir, offered the advice that I should make a list of all the likely short cases and make notes on each and learn them off by heart. His exact advice was to 'put them on your shaving mirror'. An important point should be made at this juncture. In order to be able to achieve this, one needed to attain the insight that it was indeed possible to do this. In those days there was no textbook for the exam, like the one you are reading, and there was no syllabus. Things had perhaps improved a little since the quote at the top of this Preface from A.J. Cronin* but nevertheless, the MRCP did carry with it an awe, a high failure rate and an aura that the exam was indeed one consisting of cases you had not seen before and questions you did not know the answer to. Indeed, many of us sitting it at the time would have found this a reasonable definition of the MRCP short cases.

A crucial part of my two or more years, four-attempt, journey that formed the seed that eventually grew into the first edition of this book was the realization that, in fact, behind the mystique, the reality was that the same old cases were indeed appearing in the exam over and over again, that there was a finite list and, indeed, from that list some cases occurred very frequently indeed.‡‡ The realization of this led me to do exactly what Afzal Mir had advised (without the shaving mirror bit!). At the time there was a free, monthly journal that we all received called *Hospital Update* and it had a regular feature dedicated to helping candidates with the MRCP. In one issue the writer listed 70 cases which he reckoned were the likely short cases to appear in the exam and an eye-balling of this suggested it was fairly comprehensive.

And so I studied each of these 70 cases in the textbooks and made notes which were distilled into their classic features and other things that seemed important to remember and I wrote out an index card for each of the 70. Thus, the original drafts of the main short case *records* were penned whilst I was still sitting the MRCP.

Another major contributor to my final success with the exam was junior doctor colleague Anne Freeman. She had been on the Whipps Cross MRCP course with me prior to our first sittings of the exam and she passed where I had failed. Until that point, I think we would have considered ourselves equals in knowledge, ability and likelihood of passing.‡ I would describe Anne as being like Hermione Granger.§§ In her highly organized manner, she had written down the likely instructions that might be given in the short cases exam and under each had recorded exactly what she would do and in what order, should she get that instruction. She then practised over and over again on her spouse (Dr Peter Williams, to whom she is especially grateful) until she could do it perfectly, without thought or mistake or missing something out, even in the stress of the exam.** I, on the other hand, was not like Hermione Granger. I could examine a whole patient perfectly in ordinary clinical life but had not actually thought through exactly what I would do, and in what order, when confronted with an instruction such as 'examine this patient's legs' until it actually occurred in the exam.¶ And so eventually I did what Anne Freeman had done and the first versions of the *checklists* (for which I am especially grateful to my wife, Anne Ryder, who wrote them out tidily and then ticked off each point as I practised the examining, pointing out whenever I missed something out!) and primitive versions of the examination *routines* were born, again whilst I was still sitting the MRCP.

Having finally passed the exam, it seemed a shame to waste all the insights into the exam and the experience I had gained, and all the work creating the 70 short case index cards and the examination *routine checklists* I had created and practised and honed so laboriously – and so I conceived the idea of putting them in a book for others to have the benefit without having to do so much of the work or, perhaps, to go through the ordeal of failing through poor preparation as I had done. I shortlisted what seemed to be the four major publishers of the moment and on a day in 1982 was sitting in the library of the University Hospital of Wales penning a draft letter to them. At a certain moment I got stuck over something – I have long since forgotten what – and on an impulse went down to Afzal Mir's office to ask him something to do with whatever it was I was stuck over. It was a defining moment in the history of these volumes. When I left Afzal Mir's office, the project had changed irrevocably. I was a registrar, he was a consultant. He was extremely interested in the subject himself and my consultation with him ended up with the project being one with both of us involved and me with a list of instructions (consultant to registrar!) as to what to do next!

And so an extremely forceful and creative relationship began, which led to *An Aid to the MRCP Short Cases*. It was not that we worked as a peaceful collaborative team – rather the thing came into existence through creativity on a battleground occupied by two equally creative and forceful (in very different ways) people

with very different talents and approaches. There are famous examples of this type of creative force, e.g. Lennon and McCartney or Waters and Gilmour.¶¶ Looking back, there is no doubt that without the involvement of myself and Afzal working together, an entirely different and inferior book would have emerged (probably the short 100-page pocket book desired by Churchill Livingstone – see below) but at the time I did not realize this and only thought that I was losing control of my project through the consultant–registrar hierarchy! My response was to bring in Anne Freeman, who I am sure would be very happy to be thought of as the Harrison/Starr or the Wright/Mason of the band!¶¶

Anne and I, in fact, also became a highly creative force through the development of the idea of surveying successful MRCP candidates to find out exactly what happened in the exam. It started off with me interviewing colleagues and this led to the development of a questionnaire to find out what instruction they had been given, what their findings were, what they thought the diagnosis was and their confidence in this, what supplementary questions they were asked, and their comments on the experience of that sitting. I distributed it to everyone I could find in my own and neighbouring hospitals, whilst Anne took on, with tremendous response, the immense task of tracking down every successful candidate at one MRCP sitting and getting a questionnaire to them! We asked all to report on both their pass and previous fail experiences.

Our overture to the publishers resulted in offers to publish from Churchill Livingstone (now owned by Elsevier Ltd) and Blackwell Scientific Publications (now owned by John Wiley & Sons) with the former coming in first and so we signed up with them. They were thinking of a 100-page small pocket book (70 brief short cases, a few examination routines, hardly any illustrations) sold at a price that would mean the purchaser would buy without thinking. The actual book, however, created itself once we got down to it and its size could not be controlled by our initial thoughts or the publisher's aspirations. We based the book on the, by now, extensive surveys of candidates who had sat the exam and told us exactly what happened in it – the length and the breadth. This information turned the list of 70 cases into 150 and from the surveys also emerged the 20 examination *routines* required to cover most of the short cases which occurred. As to what should be included with each short case, that was determined by ensuring that we gave everything that the candidate might need to know according to what they told us in the surveys. We were determined to cover everything that the surveys dictated might occur or be asked. It was also clear that pictures would help. We battled obsessively over every word and checked and polished it until it was as near perfect as possible. By the time it was finished three years later, the 100-page pocket book had turned into a monster manuscript full of pictures.

I took it to Churchill Livingstone who demanded that it be shrunk down to the size in the original agreement or at least some sort of compromise size. We were absolutely certain that what we had created was what the MRCP short case-sitting candidates wanted and we refused to be persuaded. And so we were rejected by Churchill Livingstone. This was a very depressing eventuality! I resurrected the original three-year-old offer letter from Blackwell Scientific Publications and made an appointment to see the Editorial Director – Peter Saugman. I turned up at his office carrying the massive manuscript and told him the tale. Wearing his very experienced publisher hat, he instantly and completely understood the Churchill Livingstone reaction but also understood something from my passion and certainty about the market for the book. He explained that he was breaking every publishing rule but that he was senior enough to do that and that he would go ahead and publish it in full on a hunch. In 1986, he was rewarded by the appearance of a 400-page textbook-sized book, which rapidly became one bought and studied by almost every MRCP candidate. Indeed, that original red and blue edition can be found on the bookshelves either at home or in the offices of nearly every medical specialty consultant in the UK.

After this, our first and best, we all pursued solo careers, with Afzal making clinical videos of patients depicting how to examine them, and writing other books such as *An Atlas of Clinical Diagnosis* (Saunders Ltd, second edition, 2003), Anne developing services for the elderly and people with stroke in Gwent, and me pursuing diabetes clinical research in various areas. Meanwhile, Anne in particular continued to accumulate survey data and in the second half of the 1990s we came together again to make the second, blue and yellow, edition of the book (1999). The surveys (which by this stage were very extensive indeed) had uncovered a further 50 short cases that needed to be included and the original material all needed updating.

Then, in 2001, the Royal Colleges changed the clinical exam to PACES. Until then the short cases exam had been a room full of patients of all different kinds with the candidate being led round them at random – according to the examiner's whim – for exactly 30 minutes. Anything from four to 11 patients might be seen. This was now transformed into Stations 1, 3 and 5 of the PACES exam, each 20 minutes long, thus doubling the time spent with short cases and ensuring that patients from all the main medical specialty areas were seen by every candidate. Hence, *An Aid to the MRCP Short Cases* was transformed into *An Aid to the MRCP PACES Volume 1*, with the short cases divided into sections according to the Stations. Specialists helped us more than ever with the updating and by now surveys had revealed that there were 20 respiratory cases that might occur, 19 abdominal cases, 27 cardiovascular cases, 52 central nervous system cases, 51 skin cases, 19 locomotor cases, 18 endocrine cases, 21 eye cases and eight 'other' cases. The long case and viva sections of the old clinical exam were replaced by Stations 2 (History taking) and 4 (Communications and ethics). To help us with these we recruited new blood – a bright and enthusiastic young physician who had recently passed the MRCP – Dev Banerjee, and he led on the Volume 2 project. Dev now confesses that 'one of the hardest aspects of writing Volume 2 back then before 2003 was coming up with enough surnames. You cannot believe how hard it was. Should I refer to the Bible? Should I refer to the Domesday Book? I decided in the end, as I had grown up in Leeds and supported Leeds United all my life, to use the 1970s Leeds United team sheet for surnames. It's not obvious, but if you look carefully, it is there!'. Finally, in 2003, the third edition was published in silver and gold.

After many years intending to do this, we also created a medical student version of the short cases book on the grounds that medical student short cases exams are essentially the same as the MRCP in that it is the same pool of patients and the examiners are all MRCP trained so that is how they think. However, whilst most MRCP candidates continue to use our books, most medical students have not discovered their version – it has the wrong title because medical students no longer have short cases exams – they have OSCEs! Those who have discovered it report that they have found it useful for their OSCEs.

And now the Royal Colleges have changed the exam again. And so *An Aid to the MRCP PACES* has become a trilogy. Stations 1 and 3 remain roughly the same and hence Volume 1 covers Stations 1 and 3 and Volume 3 has been created to deal with the new style of Station 5. Each short case has been checked and updated by one or more specialist(s) and these are now acknowledged at the start of the station concerned against the short case they have taken responsibility for. The same applies to the short cases in Station 5. Nevertheless, I have personally checked every suggestion and update and took final editorial responsibility, changing and amending as I thought fit. The order of short cases was again changed according to new surveys (now done online) and yet again a few more new short cases were found from surveys: only four for Volume 1 – kyphoscoliosis and collapsed lung for Respiratory, PEG tube for Abdominal and Ebstein's anomaly for Cardiovascular. New young blood has again been recruited – a further two bright, young and enthusiastic physicians. The updating of Volume 2 covering Stations 2 (History taking) and 4 (Communications and ethics) has been led by Nithya Sukumar. For Volume 3, covering the new Station 5, Ed Fogden has created the new Section H (Integrated clinical assessment).

We are grateful to Julie Elliott from Wiley Blackwell for collecting, in person, the manuscripts edited by the specialists to ensure no possibility of them being lost, for the initial processing of these manuscripts and for overseeing the production of all three volumes; and we are especially grateful to Helen Harvey, freelance project manager for Wiley Blackwell, for working with us painstakingly on every word, and every page of the trilogy which is now the fourth edition. Throughout this process she had maintained her calm, cheerful efficiency and kept us all in line with her enduring support, patience and understanding.

We are grateful to the specialists, now listed in the appropriate sections, who have checked and updated the short cases in their specialties in Volumes 1 and 3, and who helped Ed Fogden with the scenarios in Section H, Volume 3; and we are especially grateful for the enthusiasm with which they have done this despite the considerable workload involved. We are grateful to

Mrs Jane Price, Lead Nurse for Patient Experience, Aneurin Bevan Health Board, for her significant input to the section on Station 4. Her knowledge/experience in communication skills and medical ethics and her years of experience in dealing with these situations in clinical practice and guiding doctors in real-life scenarios have given great insight into the needs of PACES candidates. She has, therefore, contributed significantly to the development of the new cases included in this edition, and she also updated and enhanced the Introduction to Section E, Volume 2. Our surveys have always dictated the content of the books and so we are especially grateful to all the PACES candidates who have taken the trouble to fill in the online MRCP PACES survey at www.ryder-mrcp.org.uk. Finally, we are particularly grateful to our colleagues for their support in the ongoing project, which is a considerable undertaking, and we reiterate the deep thanks to our families expressed in the previous prefaces to Volume 1.

'Life is what happens to you while you're busy making other plans.'‖‖
The above, my all time favourite quote, of course can be applied to the candidate who passes when he should have failed and even more so perhaps to the one who fails when he should have passed; especially when this happens more than once as in the case of the SHO working in South Wales mentioned at the the start of this Preface. More so, it seems to me, it is really quite staggering the extent to which this quote seems to apply to life in general.

*Bob Ryder*
2013

---

*From *The Citadel* by A.J. Cronin.
†From the song *Shine on You Crazy Diamond* by Pink Floyd from the album *Wish You Were Here* (1975).
‡'The result comes as a particular shock when you have been sitting exams for many years *without* failing them.' Vol. 2, Section F, Quotation 374.
§Vol. 2, Section F, Experience 108.
¶Vol. 2, Section F, Experience 109.
‖Vol. 2, Section F, Experience 145.
**Vol. 2, Section F, Experience 144.
††Vol. 2, Section F, Experience 175. I measured my pulse just before going in to start this, my final attempt at the MRCP clinical, and the rate I remember is 140 beats/minute, but in retrospect I feel it must have magnified in my mind through the years – nevertheless whatever it was, it was very high. It is clear, though, that stress remains a major component of the exam – see Vol. 2, Section F, Experience 15.

‡‡Vol. 2, Section F, Useful tip 328 and Quotations 349 and 411–415.
§§A prominent character in the Harry Potter books by J.K. Rowling. Highly organized; expert at preparing for and passing exams.
¶¶Lennon and McCartney were the writing partnership of the Beatles with Harrison and Starr as the other members of the band. Similarly Waters and Gilmore for Pink Floyd with Wright and Mason as the other band members. In both cases it is believed that there was a special creativity through the coming together of the different talents of the individuals concerned, though the relationship was sometimes adversarial.
‖‖John Lennon, from the song, 'Beautiful Boy (Darling Boy)' from the album *Double Fantasy* (1980). It is particularly poignant that this quote should come from John Lennon, considering what happened to him later in the year of the quote.

# Introduction

*'My Station 5 was a complete nightmare.'*[*]

The MRCP PACES (Practical Assessment of Clinical Examination Skills) exam in general is discussed in the introduction to Volume 1 of *An Aid to the MRCP PACES*, and Volumes 1 and 2 deal with Stations 1–4 of the PACES exam. The volume you are now reading devotes itself entirely to Station 5. In the autumn of 2009, Station 5 changed. Prior to that Station 5 concerned itself with the clinical cases that were not addressed by Station 1 (respiratory and abdominal) and Station 3 (cardiovascular and neurological). These came under the headings Skin, Locomotor, Endocrine, Eyes and Miscellaneous. With the change in format of Station 5, we felt it important to establish what the Colleges' aspirations and intentions were with regard to these groups of clinical cases. We therefore communicated with the Station 5 group of the MRCP (UK) Clinical Examining Board. The following are quotes from those communications we received from the Colleges:

'. . . there is no plan to remove skin, locomotor, endocrine, and eye problems from the clinical issues that may be assessed in the new Station 5. Candidates must prepare to be examined in these areas as they do now.'

'New Station 5 opens the opportunity to test integrated clinical thinking about a range of clinical problems from the curriculum in a way that junior doctors practise every day – including skin, locomotor, endocrine, and eye problems as well as others. It also offers the opportunity to assess communication skills in a further two encounters and so the new PACES exam is capable of assessing these crucial skills explicitly.'

'. . . trainees will then need to think on their feet about real issues relevant to everyday medicine, including the traditional disciplines of old Station 5.'

'. . . the existing components of Station 5 can feature in new Station 5 – and so candidates must learn and prepare

for these cases. The difference is that the cases will be presented as clinical problems – so the candidate can take a relevant history and examine appropriately and not just look.'

'There is no intention to replace real patients in Station 5 with actors. It is possible to use surrogate patients in the new Station 5 for particular scenarios – and many real patients do not have physical signs. These are often a good test for the candidate provided they do not know they are facing a surrogate patient. Surrogate patients will form a small minority of encounters – just as we allow at Stations 1 and 3 in the exam now. They are a safety net for the host centre to ensure delivery of candidate assessments when there are problems sourcing patients.'

'Ophthalmoscopy is specifically included as a skill that candidates may have to demonstrate in the exam – in Station 3 or new Station 5. Additionally, recognition of fundal abnormalities on photographs will continue to feature in the Part 2 written paper.'

Thus, the Colleges made it clear that there was no intention to reduce the requirement for candidates to be skilled in the disciplines of the old Station 5.

If you look through the Station 5 experiences in the 17 recent PACES experiences in Volume 2, Section F, of *An Aid to the MRCP PACES*, you will see that the Colleges' aspirations have indeed come to pass. The old Station 5 cases are continuing to occur – goitre, exophthalmos, Graves' disease, hyperthyroidism, acromegaly, psoriatic arthropathy, systemic sclerosis, mixed connective tissue disease, arthropathy associated with inflammatory bowel disease, Marfan's, swollen knee, psoriasis, rash of uncertain cause, Raynaud's, pemphigoid, yellow nail syndrome and diabetic retinopathy all being reported and ophthalmoscopy still being called upon to be undertaken.

In view of this we have in this volume, in Section I, provided all the clinical cases from the old Station 5

---

[*]Vol. 2, Section F, Experience 10.

disciplines that have occurred in the MRCP over the years and have had them updated by specialists in the same way as we did for Stations 1 and 3.

Reading the 17 experiences in Volume 2, there were old Station 5 short cases but with a twist – a diabetic with vision problems that turned out to be due to homonymous hemianopia, a patient with ankylosing spondylitis and a dense hemiplegia, a diabetic with visual problems and diabetic maculopathy, but also possibly amaurosis fugax and a patient with heartburn, dysphagia and breathlessness but only debatable sclerodactyly as evidence of systemic sclerosis.

The Colleges have also achieved their aspirations in that, reading the 17 experiences in Volume 2, it is clear that Station 5 now has further new challenges, as well as the old ones. Cases such as dementia, polymyalgia rheumatica, migrainous headaches requiring the use of an ophthalmoscope, mononeuritis multiplex, falls in a patient with lots of potential causes, headache followed by diplopia, a patient with a pansystolic murmur and SBE, TIA, vasovagal attack, palpitations after cocaine use, watery diarrhoea (an actor), diabetic with collapse with several possible causes and upper motor neurone facial palsy. It is clear that many of these represent the challenges faced in the medical assessment unit (MAU) and we are sure this is the intention of the Colleges in supporting them.

Thus, in Section H, we have addressed the new Station 5. As is clear from the above, from more survey information and from discussions with examiners, whilst the disciplines in the old Station 5 are indeed addressed in the new Station 5, cases can occur from all disciplines. Thus we have, in Section H, provided examples addressing the new exam format, not only from the old Station 5 disciplines but also from other disciplines that have turned up in the exam. Indeed, as the old Station 5 disciplines are addressed so comprehensively in Section I, we have concentrated especially on examples from the other disciplines in Section H. With the possibility of clinical examination skills from any discipline being required in the new Station 5, we have reproduced our examination *routines* from Volume 1 in Section G of this volume.

The marking system for PACES is subject to change and you should study it at www.mrcpuk.org. At the time of writing, marking was being done in the skills of:

- Physical examination
- Identifying physical signs
- Clinical communication
- Differential diagnosis
- Clinical judgement
- Managing patient concerns
- Managing patient welfare.

The following table shows, at the time of writing, the stations at which each of these skills are tested, with Station 5 in particular highlighted.

| Skill | Station 1: Respiratory | Station 1: Abdominal | Station 2 | Station 3: Cardiovascular | Station 3: Neurological | Station 4 | Station 5: Brief clinical consultation 1 | Station 5: Brief clinical consultation 2 |
|---|---|---|---|---|---|---|---|---|
| Physical examination | ✓ | ✓ | ✗ | ✓ | ✓ | ✗ | ✓ | ✓ |
| Identifying physical signs | ✓ | ✓ | ✗ | ✓ | ✓ | ✗ | ✓ | ✓ |
| Clinical communication | ✗ | ✗ | ✓ | ✗ | ✗ | ✓ | ✓ | ✓ |
| Differential diagnosis | ✓ | ✓ | ✓ | ✓ | ✓ | ✗ | ✓ | ✓ |
| Clinical judgement | ✓ | ✓ | ✓ | ✓ | ✓ | ✓ | ✓ | ✓ |
| Managing patient concerns | ✗ | ✗ | ✓ | ✗ | ✗ | ✓ | ✓ | ✓ |
| Managing patient welfare | ✓ | ✓ | ✓ | ✓ | ✓ | ✓ | ✓ | ✓ |

At the time of writing the system is that, on the mark-sheet, the examiner in the station concerned gives for each skill being tested in that station one of the following marks:

Satisfactory mark = 2
Borderline mark = 1
Unsatisfactory mark = 0.

If you study the marking system, and you can be bothered to do the analysis, you will be able to work out the minimum number of scores of 2 that you need assuming all other scores are 1. However, in practice, this is probably of limited use because undoubtedly you will be trying to get a score of 2 in everything regardless. Two things are important, however.

1. At the time of writing the College states on its website that: *'The onus is on the candidate to demonstrate each of the skills noted on the marksheet for each encounter (see above table) and, in the event that any one examiner decides that a skill was not demonstrated by a candidate in any one particular task, an unsatisfactory mark (score = 0) will be awarded for this skill'*. Thus, it is important to always be aware of the station that you are in and to be proactive, as far as you can, in ensuring that you attempt to demonstrate your abilities in each of the headings concerned – the ones that are relevant to that station according to the above table. With regard to Station 5, it is especially noteworthy that it is the only station where all seven skills are being marked simulta-neously. Thus in Station 5 more than any other station, you must be very aware of the seven skills and ensure that during the 10 minutes of the Station 5 case, a deliberate effort is made to demonstrate the skills under all seven headings. The marking system with regard to Station 5 is considered further in Section G.

2. It is essential to remember as you move from station to station that all 10 examiners mark independently and as you go into the next station, the examiners have no idea how you did in the station you have just left so essentially you start with a blank sheet with them. If you have done badly in a station and fear you have scored some zeros, these can be compensated for by scoring more 2s in other stations. In the 5 minutes between stations it is crucial to recharge yourself psychologically, forget what has just happened in the station you have left and give yourself a complete fresh start – see 'Getting psyched up' in Section A, Volume 1.*

As emphasized above, you should read the first 17 experiences in Volume 2, Section F, of *An Aid to the MRCP PACES* to find actual accounts of the new Station 5 – please also, whenever you sit the MRCP, whether you pass or fail, fill in our survey at www.ryder-mrcp.org.uk for all the cases you meet, but especially the ones in the new Station 5. It is only because of the candidates in the past who have filled in our surveys that we have the information that we pass on to you. If you find our books useful, please in your own turn do the same – for the candidates of the future.

*See also introductory comment to Station 5, and overall comment on the exam in Vol. 2, Section F, Experiences 1 and 16.

# Section G
# Examination *Routines*

*'Work out the best method for examination and
practise it until it is second nature to you.'*[*]

*Vol. 2, Section F, Quotation 348.

These books exist as they are because of many previous candidates who, over the years, have completed our surveys and given us invaluable insight into the candidate experience. Please give something back by doing the same for the candidates of the future. For all of your sittings, whether they be a triumphant pass or a disastrous fail . . .

**Remember to fill in the survey at www.ryder-mrcp.org.uk**

THANK YOU

'*The outpatient department layout was very odd and I felt like I was being spun in circles in between stations and literally being herded through doors by the exam staff. This resulted in me attempting to exit my cardiovascular station via a cleaner's cupboard, much to the examiners' amusement. Fortunately, my sense of direction was not being assessed and they passed me anyway.*'[*]

In this chapter *routines* are suggested for the clinical assessment of various subsystems. These are readily adaptable to your individual methods. The subsystems are arranged according to the examiners' standard instructions (e.g. examine the heart, abdomen, hands, etc.). We have retained the original choice of subsystems, which was governed by our first edition surveys, except for the addition of 'Examine this patient's knee' and 'Examine this patient's hip', when PACES was first introduced. Examples of variations of the instruction are given both from our original survey and from our original PACES survey. Even though Stations 1 and 3 are in Volume 1 and Station 5 is now covered in Volume 3, we have kept all the examination *routines* together as we believe they represent 'a whole' and we present them in both Volume 1 and Volume 3. They have, in more or less unchanged form, prepared candidates for the MRCP for over a quarter of a century and, on the grounds that '*if it ain't broke, don't fix it*',[†] we have left them relatively undisturbed. It is accepted that with the new Station 5, spot diagnosis *routines* (e.g. 'What is the diagnosis?') are likely to be overtly called upon less often. Nevertheless, the conditions lending themselves to spot diagnosis will undoubtedly continue to appear and although the instruction from the examiner may be different, you will still be expected to 'spot' the diagnostic clues in your *visual survey*. Indeed, as is pointed out in the Introduction to Section I, examples of cases in the new Station 5 where spotting the diagnosis early in the new station (where time is so precious) conferred advantage to the candidate, have already been reported to us. The *routines* as a whole prepare you for the challenge of being able to examine anything wherever that challenge comes in PACES. Under each subsystem a list of the possible short cases is presented in order of their occurrence based on our surveys that led up to the third edition. We have not felt any merit in making any changes for the fourth edition. The percentages given represent our estimate of your chances of each diagnosis being present when you hear the particular instruction.[‡] These lists of diagnoses have guided our suggested *routines*. The latter are broken down into numbered constituents to aid memory and *checklists* are given in Appendix 1 which match up to the numbered points in the examination *routine*. The *checklists* are to help your practice with each subsystem.

The idea is to develop a controlled, spontaneous and flawless technique of examination for each subsystem, so that you do not have to keep pausing and thinking what to do next and so that you do not miss out important steps (see Vol. 2, Section

[*]Vol. 2, Section F, Experience 3, final comment.
[†]Accredited to Bert Lance, American businessman, 1977.
[‡]As with all our survey analyses, we graded the confidence of each candidate in his retrospective diagnosis of each short case seen. The percentages are not meant to add up to 100% because: (i) there are always missing percentages representing those short cases we could not be certain about; (ii) sometimes more than one diagnosis was considered worth counting for one instruction (for example, in order to give you the percentage of 'heart' cases with clubbing, when clubbing was present it was counted as well as the underlying cardiac condition). The figures are best used to give an index of the *relative importance* of the different conditions in terms of frequency of occurrence when you hear a given instruction.

F, Experience 144). Often you will not need the complete sequence in the examination (for example, with regard to the 'Examine this patient's chest' *routine*, often the examiner will ask you to only examine 'the back of this patient's chest') but it will certainly increase your confidence if you enter the examination armed with the complete *routines* so that you can adapt them as necessary. The examination methods are supplemented with appropriate hints to avoid common pitfalls and to simplify the diagnostic maze.

The *routines* are presented in a single section without necessarily being associated with a particular station because our PACES survey has confirmed that many of the routines may be called upon in more than one station. For example, assessment of visual fields may be required in Station 3 for a patient with a hemiplegia who might have homonymous hemianopia, or Station 5 for a patient with acromegaly who might have a bitemporal hemianopia. It is essential that you bear in mind the station you are in when you are given the particular instruction and adapt it accordingly, but you also need to be wary of jumping to conclusions. For example, we are aware of the anecdote from a PACES pilot, hosted by Dr Ryder at City Hospital for the Royal Colleges, of a patient with acromegaly who had had a cerebrovascular accident secondary to acromegalic hypertension; her visual fields were required to be examined in Station 5 and showed homonymous hemianopia! Similarly, the only radial nerve palsy patient to occur in any of our surveys since the 1980s turned up in Station 5, Locomotor, of a PACES sitting. In Vol. 2, Section F, Experience 27 and Anecdote 88, accounts are given of patients with Marfan's syndrome appearing in Station 1, Respiratory, so it is important to remain open to many possibilities whilst taking into account the station you are in. Finally, as is clear from the cases that have been reported to us as occurring in the new Station 5, the variety of which is discussed in the Introduction to this volume, in the new Station 5 you can be called upon to examine just about any system.

Before dealing with the individual subsystems, we would make some general points. You should avoid repeating the instruction or echoing the last part of it. Refrain from asking questions like: 'Would you like me to give you a running commentary or give the findings at the end?'. Such a response wastes invaluable seconds which could be used running through the *checklist* and completing your *visual survey*. It is like a batsman asking a bowler in a cricket match whether he would like his ball hit for a six or played defensively! You must do what you are best at and hope that the examiner does not ask you to do otherwise. As suggested below, a well-rehearsed procedure suited to each subsystem should make it possible for you to start purposefully without delay.

Your approach to the patient is of great importance. You should introduce yourself to him and ask his permission to examine him.* Permission should also be sought for various manoeuvres, such as adjusting the backrest when examining the heart or before removing any clothing. These polite exchanges will not only please most examiners and patients, but will also provide you with an opportunity to calm your nerves, collect your thoughts and recall the appropriate *checklist*.

---

*Throughout the book we often use him/his for brevity when we
are talking about patients, examiners or candidates, when of
course we mean him/her or his/hers.

Although we have continually emphasized the value of looking for signs peripheral to the examiner's instruction (e.g. examine this patient's heart, abdomen, chest), we would also like to emphasize that *dithering* may be counterproductive. In the *visual survey*, you should be scanning the patient rapidly and purposefully with a trained eye, not gazing helplessly at him for a long period while you try to decide what to do next. While you are feeling the pulse (heart) or settling the patient lying flat (abdomen), a quick look at the hands should establish whether there are any abnormalities or not. Pondering over normal hands from all angles at great length looks as unprofessional as, indeed, it is. It is of paramount importance to be gentle with the patient. Rough handling (e.g. roughly and abruptly digging deep into the patient's abdomen so that he winces with pain) has always been a behaviour which will bring you instantly to the pass/fail borderline or below it (see Vol. 2, Section F, Experience 192). The new PACES marking system is now formally seeking to confirm that all the candidates who pass achieve near perfection under the heading 'Managing Patient Welfare'. At the time of writing, the marking system requires a score of at least 90% under this heading to ensure a pass. Make sure that you cover the patient up when you have finished examining him, and thank him.

# 1 | 'Examine this patient's pulse'

*Variations of instruction from our original survey*
Feel this pulse
Examine this patient's pulse – look for the cause
Examine this patient's pulses

*Diagnoses from our original survey in order of frequency*
1 Irregular pulse (Vol. 1, Station 3, Cardiovascular, Case 8) 44%
2 Slow pulse (Vol. 1, Station 3, Cardiovascular, Case 31) 12%
3 Graves' disease (Station 5, Endocrine, Case 3) 12%
4 Aortic stenosis (Vol. 1, Station 3, Cardiovascular, Case 5) 9%
5 Complete heart block (Vol. 1, Station 3, Cardiovascular, Case 31) 9%
6 Brachial artery aneurysm 9%
7 Impalpable radial pulses due to low output cardiac failure 9%
8 Tachycardia 6%
9 Takayasu's disease (Station 5, Other, Case 3) 3%
10 Hypothyroidism (Station 5, Endocrine, Case 5) 3%
11 Fallot's tetralogy with a Blalock shunt 3 (Vol. 1, Station 3, Cardiovascular, Case 23) 3%

## Examination *routine*

As you approach the patient from the right and ask for his permission to examine him you should:

1 look at his **face** for a *malar flush* (mitral stenosis, myxoedema) or for any signs of *hyper-* or *hypothyroidism*. As you take the arm to examine the right radial pulse, continue the *survey* of the patient by looking at

2 the **neck** (Corrigan's pulse, raised JVP, thyroidectomy scar, goitre) and then the *chest* (thoracotomy scar). Quickly run your eyes down the body to complete the *survey* (ascites, clubbing, pretibial myxoedema, ankle oedema, etc.) and then concentrate on

3 the **pulse** and note

4 its **rate** (count for at least 15 sec), volume and

5 its **rhythm**. A common diagnostic problem is presented by *slow atrial fibrillation* which may be mistaken for a regular pulse. To avoid this, concentrate on the *length of the pause* from one beat to another and see if each pause is equal to the succeeding one (see also Vol. 1, Station 3, Cardiovascular, Case 8). This method will reveal that the pauses are variable from beat to beat in controlled slow atrial fibrillation.

6 Assess whether the **character** (waveform) of the pulse (information to be gained from radial, brachial and carotid) is normal, *collapsing*, *slow rising* or jerky. To determine whether there is a collapsing quality, put the palmar aspect of the four fingers of your left hand on the patient's wrist just below where you can easily feel the radial pulse. Press gently with your palm, lift the patient's hand above his head and then place your right palm over the patient's axillary artery. If the pulse has a *water-hammer* character you will experience a flick (a sharp and tall upstroke and an abrupt downstroke) which will *run* across all four fingers and at the same time you may also feel a flick of the axillary artery against your right palm. The pulse does not merely become palpable when the hand is lifted but its character changes and it imparts a

sharp knock. This is classic of the pulse that is present in haemodynamically signifi-cant aortic incompetence and in patent ductus arteriosus. If the pulse has a collapsing character but is not of a frank water-hammer type then the flick runs across only two or three fingers (moderate degree of aortic incompetence or patent ductus arteriosus, thyrotoxicosis, fever, pregnancy, moderately severe mitral incompetence, anaemia, atherosclerosis). A *slow rising* pulse can best be assessed by palpating the brachial pulse with your left thumb and, as you press *gently*, you may feel the anacrotic notch (you will need practice to appreciate this) on the upstroke against the pulp of your thumb. In mixed aortic valve disease, the combination of plateau and collapsing effects can produce a bisferiens pulse. Whilst feeling the brachial pulse, look for any catheterization *scars* (indicating valvular or ischaemic heart disease).

**7** Proceed to feel the **carotid** where either a slow rising or a collapsing pulse can be confirmed.

**8** Feel the **opposite radial pulse** and determine if both radials are the same (e.g. Fallot's with a Blalock shunt; see Vol. 1, Station 3, Cardiovascular, Case 23), and then feel

**9** the **right femoral pulse** checking for any *radiofemoral delay* (coarctation of the aorta). If you are asked to examine the pulses (as opposed to the pulse), you should continue to examine

**10** all the other **peripheral pulses**. It is unlikely that the examiner will allow you to continue beyond what he thinks is a reasonable time to spot the diagnosis that he has in mind. However, should he not interrupt, continue to look for

**11** **additional diagnostic clues.** Thus, in a patient with atrial fibrillation and features suggestive of thyrotoxicosis, you should examine the thyroid and/or eyes. In a patient with atrial fibrillation and hemiplegia or atrial fibrillation and a mitral valvotomy scar, proceed to examine the heart.

See Appendix 1, Checklist 1, Pulse.


# 2 | 'Examine this patient's heart'


*Variations of instruction in initial PACES survey (resultant diagnoses in brackets)*
Examine this patient's heart (mitral stenosis)
Examine this patient's cardiovascular system (mitral valve disease and aortic regurgi-tation; mitral valve disease; mixed aortic valve disease; prosthetic valves; aortic stenosis; atrial fibrillation and prosthetic mitral valve; corrected Fallot's tetralogy)
Examine this gentleman's heart. He has been complaining of palpitations (atrial fibrillation and mitral stenosis)
The GP has referred this 72-year-old lady with a murmur. Please examine her (mitral regurgitation)
This patient has been having palpitations – can you find a cause? (atrial fibrillation and mitral stenosis)
This patient is short of breath. Please examine the heart (mixed aortic valve disease)
You are seeing this elderly lady in the cardiology clinic which she has been attending for some time (prosthetic valve)

This young lady presented with increasing shortness of breath on exertion. Examine the cardiovascular system (aortic incompetence)

This lady has a heart murmur. Please examine her cardiovascular system (mitral stenosis and cerebrovascular accident)

This patient had a myocardial infarct 1 year ago. Please examine the cardiovascular system (aortic stenosis)

This man has been complaining of chest pain and palpitations. Please examine the cardiovascular system (aortic stenosis)

This patient has had an acute episode of breathlessness. Please examine the cardiovascular system (aortic stenosis)

This patient presented with shortness of breath. Please examine the cardiovascular system (mixed mitral valve disease and atrial fibrillation; aortic incompetence)

This gentleman came in on the take 2 days ago and he was breathless. Examine his cardiovascular system (atrial fibrillation and mitral regurgitation)

This man has just returned from the ITU. Please examine his cardiovascular system (prosthetic valves)

This woman, who is about 60 years of age, is becoming increasingly breathless. Can you examine her cardiovascular system and see if you can find a reason? (atrial fibrillation and mitral stenosis)

Look at this patient and describe what you see. Then listen to the heart (Marfan's syndrome and prosthetic aortic valve)

The GP has noted a murmur – can you tell me what you think? (mixed aortic valve disease)

This man has a heart murmur. Please examine him (mitral regurgitation)

Examine the cardiovascular system (hypertrophic cardiomyopathy)

### *Diagnoses from survey in order of frequency*

   1  Prosthetic valves (Vol. 1, Station 3, Cardiovascular, Case 1) 17%
   2  Mitral incompetence (lone) (Vol. 1, Station 3, Cardiovascular, Case 2) 13%
   3  Mixed aortic valve disease (Vol. 1, Station 3, Cardiovascular, Case 6) 9%
   4  Mixed mitral valve disease (Vol. 1, Station 3, Cardiovascular, Case 3) 9%
   5  Other combinations of mitral and aortic valve disease (Vol. 1, Station 3, Cardiovascular, Case 9) 8%
   6  Mitral stenosis (lone) (Vol. 1, Station 3, Cardiovascular, Case 7) 7%
   7  Aortic stenosis (lone) (Vol. 1, Station 3, Cardiovascular, Case 5) 7%
   8  Aortic incompetence (lone) (Vol. 1, Station 3, Cardiovascular, Case 4) 5%
   9  Ventricular septal defect (Vol. 1, Station 3, Cardiovascular, Case 12) 3%
  10  Irregular pulse (Vol. 1, Station 3, Cardiovascular, Case 8) 2%
  11  HOCM (Vol. 1, Station 3, Cardiovascular, Case 20) 2%
  12  Marfan's syndrome (Station 5, Locomotor, Case 9) 2%
  13  Eisenmenger's syndrome (Vol. 1, Station 3, Cardiovascular, Case 27) 2%
  14  Mitral valve prolapse (Vol. 1, Station 3, Cardiovascular, Case 10) 2%
  15  Patent ductus arteriosus (Vol. 1, Station 3, Cardiovascular, Case 29) 2%
  16  Tricuspid incompetence (Vol. 1, Station 3, Cardiovascular, Case 11) 2%
  17  Fallot's tetralogy/Blalock shunt (Vol. 1, Station 3, Cardiovascular, Case 23) 0.9%
  18  Raised jugular venous pressure (Vol. 1, Station 3, Cardiovascular, Case 18) 0.9%
  19  Coarctation of the aorta (Vol. 1, Station 3, Cardiovascular, Case 26) 0.9%

20 Slow pulse (Vol. 1, Station 3, Cardiovascular, Case 31) 0.9%

21 Dextrocardia (Vol. 1, Station 3, Cardiovascular, Case 21) 0.5%

22 Pulmonary stenosis (Vol. 1, Station 3, Cardiovascular, Case 14) 0.5%

23 Cannon waves (Vol. 1, Station 3, Cardiovascular, Case 25) 0.5%

24 Subclavian-steal syndrome (Vol. 1, Station 3, Central Nervous System, Case 49) 0.3%

25 Pulmonary incompetence (Vol. 1, Station 3, Cardiovascular, Case 30) 0.3%

26 Infective endocarditis (Vol. 1, Station 3, Cardiovascular, Case 28) 0.3%

27 Atrial septal defect (Vol. 1, Station 3, Cardiovascular, Case 16) 0.1%

Other diagnoses were: chronic liver disease due to tricuspid incompetence (<1%), pulmonary stenosis (<1%), cor pulmonale (<1%), complete heart block (<1%), transposition of the great vessels (<1%), repaired thoracic aortic aneurysm (<1%) and left ventricular aneurysm (<1%).

## Examination *routine*

When asked to 'examine this patient's heart', candidates are often uncertain as to whether they should start with the pulse or go straight to look at the heart. On the one hand, it would be absurd to feel all the pulses in the body and leave the object of the examiner's interest to the last minute, whilst on the other hand it would be impetuous to palpate the praecordium straight away. Repeating the examiner's question in the hope that he might clarify it, or asking for a clarification, does nothing but communicate your dilemma to the examiner. You should not waste any time. Bear in mind that our survey has confirmed that the diagnosis is usually mitral and/ or aortic valve disease. Approach the right-hand side of the patient and adjust the backrest so that he reclines at 45° to the mattress. If the patient is wearing a shirt, you should ask him to remove it so that the chest and neck are exposed. *Meanwhile*, you should complete a *quick*:

  1 *visual survey*. Observe whether the patient is
    (a) breathless,
    (b) *cyanosed*,
    (c) pale, or
    (d) whether he has a *malar flush* (mitral stenosis).
    Look briefly at the earlobes for creases* and then at the *neck* for *pulsations*:
    (e) forceful carotid pulsations (Corrigan's sign in aortic incompetence; vigorous pulsation in coarctation of the aorta), or
    (f) tall, sinuous venous pulsations (congestive cardiac failure, tricuspid incompetence, pulmonary hypertension, etc.).
    Run your eyes down onto the chest looking for:
    (g) a *left thoracotomy scar* (mitral stenosis†) or a *midline sternal scar* (valve replacement‡), and then down to the feet looking for:

---

*Frank's sign: a diagonal crease in the lobule of the auricle: grade 3 = a deep cleft across the whole earlobe; grade 2A = crease more than halfway across the lobe; grade 2B = crease across the whole lobe but superficial; grade 1 = lesser degrees of wrinkling. Earlobe creases are associated statistically with coronary artery disease in most population groups.

†NB: Vol. 2, Section F, Experiences 111 and 114.
‡Other scars may also be noted during your *visual survey* – those of previous cardiac catheterizations may be visible over the brachial arteries.

(**h**) ankle oedema. As you take the arm to feel the pulse, complete your *visual survey* by looking at the hands (a quick look; don't be ponderous) for

(**i**) clubbing of the fingers (cyanotic congenital heart disease, subacute bacterial endocarditis) and splinter haemorrhages (infective endocarditis).

If the examiner does not want you to feel the pulse he may intervene at this stage – otherwise you should proceed to

**2** note the *rate* and *rhythm* of the **pulse**.

**3** Quickly ascertain whether the pulse is **collapsing** (particularly if it is a large-volume pulse) or not (make sure you are seen lifting the arm up; see Vol. 2, Section F, Experience 144).

Next may be an opportune time to look for

**4 radiofemoral delay** (coarctation of the aorta), though this can be left until after auscultation if you prefer and if you are sure you will not forget it (see Vol. 2, Section F, Experience 108).

**5** Feel the brachial pulse followed by the carotid pulses to see if the pulse is a **slow rising** one, especially if the volume (the upstroke) is small.

If the pulsations in the neck present any interesting features you may have already noted these during your initial *visual survey*. You should now proceed to confirm some of these impressions. The Corrigan's sign in the neck (forceful rise and quick fall of the carotid pulsation) may already have been reinforced by the discovery of a collapsing radial pulse. The individual waves of a large venous pulse can now be timed by palpating the opposite carotid. A large *v* wave, which sometimes oscillates the earlobe, suggests tricuspid incompetence and you should later on demonstrate peripheral oedema and the pulsatile liver using the bimanual technique. If the venous wave comes before the carotid pulsation, it is an *a* wave suggestive of pulmonary hypertension (mitral valve disease, cor pulmonale) or pulmonary stenosis (rare). After

**6** assessing the height of the **venous pressure** in centimetres vertically above the sternal angle, you should move to the praecordium* and

**7** localize the **apex beat** with respect to the mid-clavicular line and ribspaces, firstly by inspection for visible pulsation and secondly by *palpation*. If the apex beat is vigorous you should stand the index finger on it, to localize the point of maximum impulse, and *assess* the extent of its thrust. The impulse can be graded as just palpable, lifting (diastolic overload, i.e. mitral or aortic incompetence), thrusting (stronger than lifting) or heaving (outflow obstruction).

**8** Palpation with your hand placed from the lower left sternal edge to the apex will detect a tapping impulse (left atrial 'knock' in mitral stenosis) or *thrills* over the mitral area (mitral valve disease), if present.

**9** Continue palpation by feeling the **right ventricular lift** (left parasternal heave). To do this, place the flat of your right palm parasternally over the right ventricular area and apply *sustained* and gentle pressure. If right ventricular hypertrophy is present, you will feel the heel of your hand lifted by its force (pulmonary hypertension).

**10** Next, you should **palpate** the pulmonary area for a *palpable second sound* (pulmonary hypertension), and the aortic area for a palpable *thrill* (aortic stenosis).†

---

*The *visual survey* and the examination steps 2–6 should be completed *quickly* and efficiently, particularly if you have been asked to examine the *heart*.

†The thrill of aortic stenosis is best felt if the patient leans forwards with his breath held after expiration.

If you feel a strong right ventricular lift, quickly recall, and sometimes recheck, whether there is a giant *a* wave (pulmonary hypertension, pulmonary stenosis) or *v* wave (tricuspid incompetence, congestive cardiac failure) in the neck. A palpable thrill over the mitral area (mitral valve disease) or palpable pulmonary second sound over the pulmonary area (pulmonary hypertension) should make you think of, and check for, the other complementary signs. You should by now have a fair idea of what you will hear on auscultation of the heart but you should keep an open mind for any unexpected discovery.

**11** The next step will be **auscultation** and you should only stray away from the heart (examiner's command) if you have a strong expectation of being able to demonstrate an interesting and relevant sign (such as a pulsatile liver to underpin the diagnosis of tricuspid incompetence). *Time* the first heart sound with either the apex beat, if this is palpable, or by feeling the carotid pulse (see Vol. 2, Section F, Experience 188). It is important to listen to the expected murmurs in the most favourable positions. For example, mitral diastolic murmurs are best heard by turning the patient *onto the left side*, and the early diastolic murmur of aortic incompetence is made more prominent by asking the patient to *lean forwards* with his breath held after expiration.* For low-pitched sounds (mid-diastolic murmur of mitral stenosis, heart sounds), use the bell of your chest-piece but do not press hard or else you will be listening through a diaphragm formed by the stretched skin! The high-pitched early diastolic murmur of aortic incompetence is very easily missed (see Vol. 2, Section F, Anecdote 276). Make sure you specifically listen for it.

If the venous pressure is raised you should check for

**12 sacral oedema** and, if covered, expose the feet to demonstrate any *ankle oedema*. Auscultation over

**13** the **lung bases** for inspiratory crepitations (left ventricular failure), though an essential part of the routine assessment of the cardiovascular system, is seldom required in the examination. You may make a special effort to do this in certain relevant situations such as a breathless patient, aortic stenosis with a displaced point of maximum impulse or if there are any signs of left heart failure (orthopnoea, pulsus alternans, gallop rhythm, etc.). Similarly, after examination of the heart itself it may (on rare occasions only) be necessary to

**14** palpate the **liver**, especially if you have seen a large *v* wave and heard a pansystolic murmur over the tricuspid area. In such cases you may be able to demonstrate a *pulsatile* liver by placing your left palm posteriorly and the right palm anteriorly over the enlarged liver.† Finally, you should offer to

**15** measure the **blood pressure**. This is particularly relevant in patients with aortic stenosis (low systolic and narrow pulse pressure), and aortic incompetence (wide pulse pressure).

See Appendix 1, Checklist 2, Heart.

---

*With the diaphragm of your chest-piece *ready* in position: 'Take a deep breath in; now out; hold it'. Listen intently for the absence of silence in early diastole. Ask the patient to repeat the exercise if necessary.

†An alternative and useful way of demonstrating a pulsatile liver is to place the knuckles of your closed right fist against the inferior border of the liver in the right hypochondrium (warn the patient beforehand!). Your fist will oscillate with each pulsation of the liver.

# 3 | 'Examine this patient's chest'

***Variations of instruction in initial PACES survey (resultant diagnoses in brackets)***

Examine this patient's chest (bronchiectasis; pleural effusion with chest drain; pleural effusion; bilateral lower lobectomy and fibrosis)

This gentleman is breathless on climbing stairs. Examine his respiratory system (chronic obstructive pulmonary disease)

Examine this patient's respiratory system (lung transplant and bronchiolitis obliterans; lung cancer)

This gentleman presented with a cough and shortness of breath. Please examine his respiratory system (pleural effusion)

This is a 56-year-old lady who has been dyspnoeic for a long time. Examine her respiratory system (Marfan's syndrome and pulmonary fibrosis)

This patient is complaining of shortness of breath. Please examine the chest (pleural effusion)

Examine this man's chest from the back (reduced expansion with reduced breath sounds and increased vocal resonance)

This patient presented with worsening shortness of breath. Please examine his chest (pulmonary fibrosis)

This lady is short of breath, please examine her respiratory system (pulmonary fibrosis)

This man has a long history of breathlessness. Please examine his respiratory system (pulmonary fibrosis)

Examine this lady's respiratory system from the front. About half a minute later I was asked to examine her chest from the back (carcinoma of the lung)

This gentleman has been getting more breathless in recent months. Please examine his chest (thoracotomy)

This lady is breathless. Please examine her chest (emphysema)

This man has noisy breathing. Please examine his chest to find out why (upper airways obstruction)

This man has developed a productive cough. Please examine his chest and suggest a cause (aspergillosis and old tuberculosis)

Examine this patient's respiratory system and comment on positive findings as you go (pulmonary fibrosis)

This young man is breathless. Please examine his chest (chronic obstructive pulmonary disease and α1-antitrypsin deficiency)

This man has a cough. Please examine his chest (bronchiectasis)

This man has been becoming increasingly breathless over the past 2 years. He is a non-smoker. Please examine his respiratory system to determine a cause (no diagnosis reached)

This man complains of shortness of breath. Examine him and find out why (no diagnosis reached)

***Diagnoses from survey in order of frequency***

**1** Interstitial lung disease (fibrosing alveolitis) (Vol. 1, Station 3, Respiratory, Case 1) 21%

2 Pneumonectomy/lobectomy (Vol. 1, Station 3, Respiratory, Case 2) 16%

3 Bronchiectasis (Vol. 1, Station 3, Respiratory, Case 4) 12%

4 Dullness at the lung bases (Vol. 1, Station 3, Respiratory, Case 5) 10%

5 Chronic bronchitis and emphysema (Vol. 1, Station 3, Respiratory, Case 3) 8%

6 Rheumatoid lung (Vol. 1, Station 3, Respiratory, Case 6) 8%

7 Old tuberculosis (Vol. 1, Station 3, Respiratory, Case 7) 6%

8 Stridor (Vol. 1, Station 3, Respiratory, Case 11) 4%

9 Superior vena cava obstruction (Vol. 1, Station 3, Respiratory, Case 22) 3%

10 Kartagener's syndrome (Vol. 1, Station 3, Respiratory, Case 15) 2%

11 Marfan's syndrome (Station 5, Locomotor, Case 9) 2%

12 Lung transplant (Vol. 1, Station 3, Respiratory, Case 16) 2%

13 Cor pulmonale (Vol. 1, Station 3, Respiratory, Case 20) 2%

14 Chest infection/consolidation/pneumonia (Vol. 1, Station 3, Respiratory, Case 8) 1%

15 Obesity/Pickwickian syndrome (Vol. 1, Station 3, Respiratory, Case 18) 1%

16 Tuberculosis/apical consolidation (Vol. 1, Station 3, Respiratory, Case 23) 1%

17 Carcinoma of the bronchus (Vol. 1, Station 3, Respiratory, Case 13) <1%

18 Pneumothorax (Vol. 1, Station 3, Respiratory, Case 19) <1%

19 Cystic fibrosis (Vol. 1, Station 3, Respiratory, Case 17) <1%

## Examination *routine*

While approaching the patient, asking for his permission to examine him and settling him reclining at 45° to the bed with his chest bare, you should observe from the end of the bed

1 his **general appearance**. Note any evidence of *weight loss*. The features of conditions such as superior vena cava obstruction (see Vol. 1, Station 1, Respiratory, Case 22), systemic sclerosis (see Station 5, Locomotor, Case 3) and lupus pernio (see Station 5, Skin, Case 9) may be readily apparent as should be severe kyphoscoliosis. However, *ankylosing spondylitis* is easily missed with the patient lying down (see Vol. 2, Section F, Experiences 110 and 139). Observe specifically whether the patient

2 is **breathless** at rest or from the effort of removing his clothes,

3 **purses** his lips (chronic small airways obstruction), or

4 has central **cyanosis**\* (cor pulmonale, fibrosing alveolitis, bronchiectasis). Central cyanosis may be difficult to recognize; it is always preferable to look at the oral mucous membranes (see below). Observe

5 if the **accessory muscles** are being used during breathing (chronic small airways obstruction, pleural effusion, pneumothorax, etc.),

6 if there is generalized **indrawing** of the intercostal muscles or supraclavicular fossae (hyperinflation) or if there is indrawing of the lower ribs on inspiration (due to low, flat diaphragms in emphysema). Localized indrawing of the intercostal muscles suggests bronchial obstruction.

---

\*Occurs with mean capillary concentration of $\geq 4\,g\,dL^{-1}$ of deoxygenated haemoglobin (or $0.5\,g\,dL^{-1}$ methaemoglobin). Alternatively, the presence of cyanosis may be supported by demonstrating a low arterial oxygen saturation (<85%) noninvasively with an ear oximeter applied to the antihelix of the ear. Central cyanosis is more readily detected in patients with polycythaemia than in those with anaemia – because of the low haemoglobin, patients with anaemia require a much lower oxygen saturation to have $4\,g\,dL^{-1}$ of unsaturated haemoglobin in capillary blood.

*Listen* to the breathing with unaided ears whilst you observe the chest wall and hands (but do not dither). This will allow a dual input whereby a combination of what you hear and what you see may help you form a diagnostic impression. You should listen to whether *expiration* is more *prolonged* than inspiration (normally the reverse), and difficult (chronic airways obstruction), whether it is *noisy* (breathlessness) and if there are any additional noises such as *wheezes* or *clicks*. Difficult and noisy inspiration is usually caused by obstruction in the major bronchi (mediastinal masses, retrosternal thyroid, bronchial carcinoma, etc.) while the more prolonged, noisy and often wheezy expiration is caused by chronic small airways obstruction (asthma, chronic bronchitis). Note the character of any cough, whether it is productive (?bronchiectasis) or dry. While you are listening, observe

**7** the *movement* of the **chest wall**. It may be mainly *upwards* (emphysema) or *asymmetrical* (fibrosis, collapse, pneumonectomy, pleural effusion, pneumothorax). In the context of the examination, it is particularly important to look for localized *apical flattening* suggestive of underlying fibrosis due to old tuberculosis (see Vol. 1, Station 1, Respiratory, Case 7) or pneumonectomy (see Vol. 1, Station 1, Respiratory, Case 2). You may also note a thoracotomy or thoracoplasty *scar* (see Vol. 1, Station 1, Respiratory, Case 2 and 7) or the presence of *radiotherapy field markings* (Indian ink marks) or radiation *burns* on the chest (intrathoracic malignancy; see Station 5, Skin, Case 31).

Before touching the patient, ensure that you have looked for any peripheral clues, such as sputum pots for haemoptysis or purulent sputum, nebulizer therapy, inhaler therapy, oxygen (what rate per minute?), temperature chart, peak flow chart or transplant pagers.

Check the hands for

**8 clubbing** (see Station 5, Skin, Case 17), *tobacco staining*, coal dust tattoos or other conditions which affect the hands and may be associated with lung disease such as rheumatoid arthritis (nodules; see Station 5, Locomotor, Case 1) or systemic sclerosis (see Station 5, Locomotor, Case 3).

**9** Feel the **pulse** and if it is bounding, or if the patient is cyanosed, check for a *flapping tremor* of the hands ($CO_2$ retention) or a fine tremor due to β-agonist therapy (salbutamol or terbutaline). If there is doubt about the presence of cyanosis, you could at this point check the tongue and the buccal mucous membranes over the premolar teeth before moving to the neck to look for

**10 raised venous pressure** (cor pulmonale) or fixed distension of the neck veins (superior vena cava obstruction). Next examine

**11** the **trachea**. Place the index and ring fingers on the manubrium sternae over the prominent points on either side. Use the middle finger as the exploring finger to gently feel the tracheal rings to detect either *deviation* or a *tracheal tug* (i.e. the middle finger being pushed upwards against the trachea by the upward movement of the chest wall). Check the *notch–cricoid* distance.*

**12** Feel for **lymphadenopathy** (carcinoma, tuberculosis, lymphoma, sarcoidosis) in the cervical region and axillae. As the right hand returns from the left axilla, look for

---

*The length of trachea from the suprasternal notch to the cricoid cartilage is normally three or more finger breadths. Shortening of this distance is a sign of hyperinflation.

**13** the **apex beat** (difficult to localize if the chest is hyperinflated) which in conjunction with tracheal deviation may give you evidence of mediastinal displacement (collapse, fibrosis, pneumonectomy, effusion, scoliosis).

**14** To look for **asymmetry**, rest one hand lightly on either side of the front of the chest to see if there is any diminution of movement (effusion, fibrosis, pneumonectomy, collapse, pneumothorax). Next grip the chest symmetrically with the fingertips in the ribspaces on either side and approximate the thumbs to meet in the middle in a straight horizontal line in order to

**15** assess **expansion** first in the inframammary and then in the supramammary regions. Note the distance between each thumb and the midline (may give further information about asymmetry of movement) and between both thumbs and try to express the expansion in centimetres (it is better to produce a tape measure for a more accurate assessment of the expansion in centimetres). Comparing both sides at each level,

**16** **percuss** the chest from above downwards starting with the supraclavicular fossae and over the clavicles* and do not forget to percuss over the axillae. Few clinicians now regularly map out the area of cardiac dullness. In healthy people there is dullness behind the lower left quarter of the sternum which is lost together with normal liver dullness in hyperinflation. Complete palpation by checking for

**17** **tactile vocal fremitus** with the ulnar aspect of the hand applied to the chest.

**18** Auscultation of the **breath sounds** should start *high* at the apices and you should remember to listen in the *axillae*. You are advised to cover both lung fields first with the bell† before using the diaphragm (if for no other reason than that this allows you a chance to check the findings without appearing to backtrack!). In the nervousness of the examination, harsh breathing heard with the diaphragm near a major bronchus (over the second intercostal space anteriorly or below the scapula near the mid-line posteriorly) may give an impression of bronchial breathing, particularly in thin people. Compare corresponding points on opposite sides of the chest. Ensure that the patient breathes with the mouth open, regularly and deeply, but not noisily (see Vol. 2, Section F, Experience 162). Auscultation is completed by checking

**19** **vocal resonance**‡ in all areas; **if** you have found an area of bronchial breathing (the sounds may resound close to your ears – aegophony), check also for whispering pectoriloquy. The classic timings of crackles/crepitations of various origins are:

    **(a)** *early inspiratory*: chronic bronchitis, asthma,

    **(b)** *early and mid-inspiratory and recurring in expiration*: bronchiectasis (altered by coughing),

    **(c)** *mid/late inspiratory*: restrictive lung disease (e.g. fibrosing alveolitis§) and pulmonary oedema.

**20** **To examine the back** of the chest, sit the patient forward (it may help to cross the arms in front of the patient to pull the scapulae further apart) and repeat steps 14–19. You may wish to start the examination of the back by palpating for cervical

---

*Percussion on the bare clavicle may cause discomfort to the patient.

†Many physicians prefer to use the diaphragm in their routine examination of the chest, though purists believe that as the respiratory auscultatory sounds are usually of low pitch, the bell is preferable.

‡See Footnote, Vol. 1, Station 1, Respiratory, Case 21.

§In fibrosing alveolitis, late inspiratory crackles may become reduced if the patient is made to lean forward; thereby the compressed dependent alveoli (which crackle open in late inspiration) are relieved of the pressure of the lungs.

nodes from behind (particularly the scalene nodes between the two heads of the sternomastoid).

Though with sufficient practice this whole procedure can be performed rapidly without loss of efficiency, often in the examination you will only be asked to perform some of it – usually 'examine the back of the chest'. As always when forced to perform only part of the complete *routine*, be sure that the partial examination is no less thorough and professional. Be prepared to put on your 'wide-angled lenses' so as not to miss other related signs (see Vol. 2, Section F, Experience 108 and Anecdotes 254 and 255).

Though by now you will usually have sufficient information to present your findings, occasionally you will wish to check other features on the basis of the findings so far. Commonly, you will wish to inspect the ankles for oedema and, if relevant and available, the peak flow chart and temperature chart. Further purposeful examination gives an impression of confidence but it should not be overdone. For example, looking for evidence of Horner's syndrome or wasting of the muscles of one hand* in a patient with apical dullness and a deviated trachea will suggest professional keenness whereas routinely looking at the eyes and hands after completion of the examination may only suggest to the examiner that you do not have the diagnosis and are hoping for inspiration! If you suspect airways obstruction, the examiner may be impressed if you perform a bedside respiratory function test – the *forced expiratory time* (FET).†

See Appendix 1, Checklist 3, Chest.

# 4 | 'Examine this patient's abdomen'

*Variations of instruction in initial PACES survey (resultant diagnoses in brackets)*

Examine this patient's abdomen (transplanted kidney; hepatomegaly and lymph nodes; ascites and chronic liver disease; ascites and hepatosplenomegaly)

This gentleman was found collapsed. Examine his abdomen and give a differential as to the cause of his collapse (alcoholic liver disease)

This gentleman has lost weight and is experiencing fullness in his abdomen. Please examine the abdomen (hepatosplenomegaly and axillary lymph nodes)

---

*A good *visual survey* may reveal such signs at the beginning.
†Ask the patient to take a deep breath in and then, on your command (timed with the second hand of your watch), to breathe out as hard and as fast as he can until his lungs are completely empty. A normal person will empty his lungs in less than 6 sec (1 sec for every decade of age, e.g. a normal 30-year-old will do it in 3 seconds). An FET of >6 sec is evidence of airways obstruction. You need to practise this test with patients if it is to be slick. As with peak flow rate (PFR) and forced expiratory volume in 1 second (FEV 1), etc., it is important to make sure that certain patients, particularly females, *are* blowing as hard and as fast as they can ('don't worry about what you look like – give it everything you've got – like this' and give a demonstration) and empty their lungs completely ('keep going, keep going . . . keep going, well done!').

This lady has thrombocytopenia. Examine her abdomen and come up with a likely diagnosis (splenomegaly)

This patient is complaining of tiredness, examine his abdomen (hepatosplenomegaly and rheumatoid hands)

Examine this gentleman's abdomen (alcoholic liver disease, tender hepatomegaly and encephalopathy)

This man has pain on walking. Please examine his abdomen (hepatosplenomegaly and polycythaemia rubra vera)

This patient's abdomen has shown intermittent swelling – what could one cause be? (alcoholic liver disease)

Examine this abdomen (jaundice, parotid swelling and palpable liver; hepatosplenomegaly and ascites; hepatosplenomegaly and Dupuytren's contracture)

This patient has been referred from the cardiology clinic with sweats and a mass in the abdomen. Please examine (infective endocarditis)

Please examine this gentleman's abdominal system and comment on the findings (alcoholic liver disease)

I was given some haematology results which were suggestive that the patient might have a spleen palpable. Examine the abdomen (splenomegaly)

This patient attends the renal clinic with hypertension. Please examine his abdominal system (transplanted kidney)

This 62-year-old man has a lymphocytosis. Please examine his abdomen (splenomegaly)

This lady has been having abdominal pain. Please examine and suggest a cause (polycystic kidneys and polycystic liver)

Examine this man's abdomen, commenting on what you are doing (hepatosplenomegaly)

Please examine the abdomen of this man who is complaining of pruritus (polycystic kidneys)

This man has high blood pressure. Please examine his abdomen (heart transplant and dialysis fistula)

This 43-year-old man failed a routine medical examination for insurance purposes. Please examine the abdomen and suggest if you can find a reason why (hepatomegaly)

Examine this man's abdomen and tell me what you find (chronic liver disease)

### Diagnoses from survey in order of frequency
 1  Chronic liver disease (Vol. 1, Station 1, Abdominal, Case 3) 21%
 2  Hepatosplenomegaly (Vol. 1, Station 1, Abdominal, Case 4) 17%
 3  Polycystic kidneys (Vol. 1, Station 1, Abdominal, Case 2) 14%
 4  Splenomegaly (without hepatomegaly) (Vol. 1, Station 1, Abdominal, Case 6) 13%
 5  Transplanted kidney (Vol. 1, Station 1, Abdominal, Case 1) 9%
 6  Hepatomegaly (without splenomegaly) (Vol. 1, Station 1, Abdominal, Case 5) 5%
 7  Ascites (Vol. 1, Station 1, Abdominal, Case 7) 4%
 8  Polycythaemia rubra vera (Vol. 1, Station 1, Abdominal, Case 10) 4%
 9  Abdominal mass (Vol. 1, Station 1, Abdominal, Case 9) 2%
 10 Carcinoid syndrome (Vol. 1, Station 1, Abdominal, Case 18) 2%

11  Crohn's disease (Vol. 1, Station 1, Abdominal, Case 9) 1%

12  Idiopathic haemochromatosis (Vol. 1, Station 1, Abdominal, Case 16) 1%

13  Nephrotic syndrome (Vol. 1, Station 1, Abdominal, Case 20) <1%

14  Hereditary spherocytosis (Vol. 1, Station 1, Abdominal, Case 15) <1%

15  Felty's syndrome (Vol. 1, Station 1, Abdominal, Case 23) <1%

16  Generalized lymphadenopathy (Vol. 1, Station 1, Abdominal, Case 14) <1%

17  Single palpable kidney (Vol. 1, Station 1, Abdominal, Case 13) <1%

18  Primary biliary cirrhosis (Vol. 1, Station 1, Abdominal, Case 17) <1%

Other diagnoses were: aortic aneurysm (1%), haemochromatosis (<1%), polycystic kidneys and a transplanted kidney (<1%), splenomegaly and generalized lymphadenopathy (<1%), abdominal lymphadenopathy (<1%), postsplenectomy (<1%) and normal abdomen (<1%).

**Examination *routine***

Analysis of the above list reveals that in over 80% of cases, the findings in the abdomen relate to a palpable spleen, liver or kidneys. Bearing this in mind, you should approach the right-hand side of the patient and position him so that he is lying supine on one pillow (if comfortable), with the whole abdomen and chest in full view. Ideally, the genitalia should also be exposed but to avoid embarrassment to patients, who are volunteers and whose genitals are usually normal, we suggest that you ask the patient to lower his garments and ensure that these are pulled down to a level about halfway between the iliac crest and the symphysis pubis. While these preparations are being made you should be performing

  1  a *visual survey* of the patient. Amongst the many relevant physical signs that you may observe in these few seconds are pallor, pigmentation, jaundice, spider naevi, xanthelasma, parotid swelling, gynaecomastia, scratch marks, tattoos, abdominal distension, distended abdominal veins, an abdominal swelling, herniae and decreased body hair. If you use the following *routine* most of these will also be noted during your subsequent examination but at this stage you should particularly note any

  2  **pigmentation**. As the patient is being correctly positioned,

  3  *quickly* **examine the hands**\* for:

    (a)  Dupuytren's contracture,

    (b)  clubbing,

    (c)  leuconychia,

    (d)  palmar erythema, and

    (e)  a flapping tremor (if relevant).

After asking you to examine the abdomen, many examiners would like, and *expect*, you to concentrate on the abdomen itself without delay, and yet they will not forgive you for missing an abnormal physical sign elsewhere. This emphasizes the importance of a good *visual survey*; a trained eye will miss nothing important on the face or in the hands while the patient is being properly positioned with the hands by his side. Thus, steps 1–3 need not occupy you for more than a few seconds; you may wish to omit steps 5 and 6 if there is no visible abnormality, and steps 7–11 can be completed as part of the *visual survey*.

---

\*For a full list of the signs that may be visible in the hands in chronic liver disease, see Vol. 1, Station 1, Abdominal, Case 3.

**4** Pull down the lower eyelid to look for *anaemia*. At the same time check the sclerae for *icterus* and look for *xanthelasma*. The guttering between the eyeball and the lower lid is the best place to look for pallor or for any discoloration (e.g. cyanosis, jaundice, etc.).

**5** Look at the lips for cyanosis (cirrhosis of the liver) and shine your pen torch into the mouth* looking for swollen lips (Crohn's), telangiectasis (Osler–Weber–Rendu), patches of pigmentation (Peutz–Jeghers) and mouth ulcers (Crohn's).

**6 Palpate the neck** and supraclavicular fossae for *cervical lymph nodes*.† If you do find lymph nodes you should then proceed to examine the axillae and groins for evidence of generalized lymphadenopathy (lymphoma, chronic lymphatic leukaemia). As you move from the neck to the chest, check for

**7 gynaecomastia** (palpate for glandular breast tissue in obese subjects),

**8 spider naevi** (may have been noted already on hands, arms and face and may also be present on the back), and

**9 scratch marks** (may have been noted on the arms, and may also be found on the back and elsewhere). Next,

**10** look at the chest (in the male) and in the axillae for **paucity of hair** (if diminished, note facial hair in the male; pubic hair, if not visible, may be noted later).

**11 Observe the abdomen in** *three segments* (epigastric, umbilical and suprapubic) for any visible signs such as *pulsations*, generalized *distension* (ascites) or a *swelling* in one particular area. Note any scars or fistulae (previous surgery; Crohn's). Look for distended *abdominal* veins (the flow is away from the umbilicus in portal hypertension but upwards from the groin in inferior vena cava obstruction).

With practice, the examination to this point can be completed very rapidly and will provide valuable information which may be overlooked if proceeding carelessly straight to palpation of the abdomen (see Vol. 2, Section F, Experience 109). If the examiner insists that you start with abdominal palpation‡ it suggests that there is little to be found elsewhere, but you should nevertheless be prepared to use your 'wide-angled lenses' in order not to miss any of the above features.

**12 Palpation** of the abdomen should be performed in an orthodox manner; any temptation to go straight for a visible swelling should be resisted. Put your palm gently over the abdomen and ask the patient if he has any tenderness and to let you know if you hurt him. First systematically examine the whole of the abdomen with *light palpation*. Palpation should be done with the *pulps* of the fingers rather than the tips, the best movement being a gentle flexion at the metacarpophalangeal joints with the hand flat on the abdominal wall. Next, examine specifically for the *internal organs*. For both liver and spleen, start in the right iliac fossa (you cannot be frowned

---

*Though a brief examination of the mouth is usefully included as part of the full 'examine the abdomen' *routine*, it is worth noting that in our survey when there were the findings mentioned, the candidates were given a more specific instruction such as 'Look at this patient's mouth'.

†The supraclavicular lymph nodes, particularly on the left side, may be enlarged with carcinoma of the stomach (*Troisier's sign*; NB: *Virchow's node* behind the left sternoclavicular joint) or

carcinoma of any other abdominal organ or with carcinoma of the bronchus.

‡Some examiners admit to being irritated at seeing candidates examine normal hands for a long time after being asked to examine the abdomen. They argue that the information obtainable from the face, mouth and hands can be gathered without delay during the inspection part of the examination (see Vol. 2, Section F, Anecdote 265).

upon for following this orthodox procedure*), working upwards to the right hypochondrium in the case of the *liver* and diagonally across the abdomen to the left hypochondrium in the case of the *spleen*. The organs are felt against the radial border of the index finger and the pulps of the index and middle fingers as they descend on inspiration, at which time you can gently press and move your hand upwards to meet them. The *kidneys* are then sought by bimanual palpation of each lateral region. The lower pole of the normal right kidney can sometimes be felt, especially in thin women. Palpation of the internal organs may be difficult if there is ascites. In this case, the technique is to press quickly, flexing at the wrist joint, to displace the fluid and palpate the enlarged organ ('dipping' or 'ballotting'). In a patient well chosen for the examination, a mass in the left hypochondrium may present a problem of identification (see Vol. 2, Section F, Experiences 131 and 245, and Anecdotes 269 and 270); the examiner (testing your confidence) may ask you if you are sure that it is a spleen and not a kidney or vice versa. Do not forget to establish whether you can *get above* the mass and *separate* it from the costal edge, whether you can *bimanually* palpate it and whether the percussion note over it is *resonant* (all features of an enlarged kidney; see also Vol. 1, Station 1, Abdominal, Case 6 for the features of a spleen). Palpate *deeply* with the pulps to look for the *ascending* and *descending colons* in the flanks, and use *gentle* palpation to feel for an *aortic aneurysm* in the mid-line. Complete palpation by feeling for *inguinal lymph nodes*, noting obvious herniae and, at the same time, adding information about the distribution and thickness of pubic hair to that already gained about the rest of the body hair.

**13 Percussion** must be used from the nipple downwards on both sides to locate the upper edge of the liver on the right and the spleen on the left (NB: the left lower lateral chest wall may become dull to percussion before an enlarged spleen is palpable). The lower palpable edges of the spleen and liver should be defined by percussion in an orthodox manner, proceeding from the resonant to dull areas. If you suspect free fluid in the peritoneum, you must establish its presence by demonstrating

**14 shifting dullness.** Initially check for *stony dullness* in the flanks. There is no need to continue with the procedure of demonstrating shifting dullness if this is not present. By asking the patient with ascites to turn on his side, you can shift the dullness from the upper to the lower flank.

Before you conclude the palpation and percussion of the abdomen, ask yourself whether you have found anything abnormal. If there are no abnormal physical signs, make sure that you have not missed a polycystic kidney or a palpable splenic edge (or occasionally a mass in the epigastrium or iliac fossae). During your auscultation listen carefully for a bruit over the aorta and renal vessels. Generally speaking,

**15 auscultation** has very little to contribute in the examination setting, but as part of the full *routine* you should listen to the bowel sounds, check for renal artery bruits and for any other sounds such as a rub over the spleen or kidney or a venous hum (both excessively rare).

Examination of the

---

*Even though it is the time-honoured, orthodox procedure, many clinicians these days are opposed to this practice. They argue that a grossly enlarged spleen will be picked up on the initial light palpation which makes the approach from the right iliac fossa unnecessary. If they do not feel a mass in the left hypochondrium on initial palpation, they start deep palpation a few centimetres below the left costal edge.

**16 external genitalia** is not usually required in the examination for the reasons given above, and we have never heard of a case where

**17 a rectal examination** was required. You should, however, comment that you would like to complete your examination of the abdomen by examining the external genitalia (especially in the male with chronic liver disease – small testes; or cervical lymphadenopathy – drainage of testes to paraaortic and cervical lymph nodes) and rectum. You may of course never get this far since the examiner may interrupt you at an appropriate stage to ask for your findings. If you are allowed to conclude the examination and you have found nothing abnormal despite your careful search, on rare occasions the diagnosis of a normal abdomen will be accepted (see Vol. 1, Station 1, Abdominal, Case 11).

See Appendix 1, Checklist 4, Abdomen.

# 5 | 'Examine this patient's visual fields'

**Variations of instruction from our original survey**
Examine this patient's visual fields and fundi*

**Diagnoses from our original survey in order of frequency**
**1** Homonymous hemianopia (Vol. 1, Station 3, CNS, Case 13) 25%
**2** Optic atrophy (Station 5, Eyes, Case 3) 21%
**3** Bitemporal hemianopia (Vol. 1, Station 3, CNS, Case 13) 21%
**4** Unilateral hemianopia (Vol. 1, Station 3, CNS, Case 13) 7%
**5** Partial field defect in one eye due to retinal artery branch occlusion (Station 5, Eyes, Case 16) 7%
**6** Bilateral homonymous quadrantic field defect (Vol. 1, Station 3, CNS, Case 13) 4%
**7** Acromegaly (Station 5, Endocrine, Case 2) 4%

**Examination *routine***
Ask the patient to sit upright on the side of the bed while you position yourself in visual confrontation about a metre away. This apposition will help you to test the visual fields of his left and right eyes against those of your right and left respectively. As he is doing this, perform

**1** a *visual survey* (acromegaly, hemiparesis, cerebellar signs in multiple sclerosis) of the patient. Test both temporal fields together so that you do not miss any *visual inattention*. Ask the patient to look at your eyes while you place your index fingers just inside the outer limits of your temporal fields. Then move your fingers in turn and then both at the same time, and ask him: 'Point to the finger which moves'. If there is visual inattention, the patient will only point to one finger when you move both at the same time. Next test each eye individually and ask him to cover his right eye with his right hand, and close your left eye: 'Keep looking at my eye'.

*See also Introduction to Volume 1.

**2** Examine his **peripheral visual fields**. Test his left temporal vision against your right temporal by moving your wagging finger from the periphery towards the centre: 'Tell me when you see my finger move'.* The temporal field should be tested in the horizontal plane and by moving your finger through the upper and lower temporal quadrants. Change hands and repeat on the nasal side. By comparing his visual field with your own, any areas of field defect are thus mapped out. The visual fields of his right eye are similarly tested.

**3** **A central scotoma** is tested for with a red-headed hat pin. If you have already found a field defect which does not require further examination, or if the examiner does not wish you to continue, he will soon stop you. Otherwise, comparing your right eye with the patient's left, as before, move the red-headed pin from the temporal periphery through the central field to the nasal periphery, asking the patient: 'Can you see the head of the pin? What colour is it? Tell me if it disappears or changes colour'.

Patients with optic neuropathy may report altered colour vision even if there is no absolute central loss of vision. If there is no scotoma, find his blind spot and compare it with your own. The blind spot may be enlarged in chronic papilloedema or consecutive optic atrophy.

Having found the field defect, look for

**4** **additional features** (e.g. acromegaly, hemiparesis, nystagmus and cerebellar signs) if appropriate. Recall the possible causes for each type of field defect as this question, at the end of the case, is inevitable (see Vol. 1, Station 3, CNS, Case 13).

See Appendix 1, Checklist 5, Visual fields.

# 6 | 'Examine this patient's cranial nerves'

*Variations of instruction in initial PACES survey (resultant diagnoses in brackets)*
Examine this patient's cranial nerves (right homonymous hemianopia)
Examine this patient's cranial nerves and check the reflexes in the lower limbs as this
   patient has had a noticeable weakness of both legs (multiple sclerosis)

*Diagnoses from our MRCP surveys*
**1** Right homonymous hemianopia with macula sparing
**2** Bulbar palsy
**3** Internuclear ophthalmoplegia – multiple sclerosis
**4** Cerebellopontine angle syndrome
**5** Myasthenia gravis

*This will pick up most gross visual field defects rapidly. Moving objects are more easily detected and therefore your moving finger will be immediately noticed by the patient as it moves out of the blind area into his field of vision. Remember that his area of blindness to a stationary object may be greater than that to a moving object. In the dysphasic patient, you should ask him to point at the moving finger when he sees it rather than telling you he sees it.

**6** Ocular palsy and dysarthria

**7** Unilateral VIth, VIIth nerve palsies and nystagmus and possibly a XIIth nerve palsy*

**8** Unilateral IXth, Xth, XIth and XIIth nerve lesions (suggesting jugular foramen syndrome†)

### Examination *routine*

Perhaps surprisingly, this instruction was comparatively rare in our surveys before PACES, but seems to have experienced a slight increase in popularity in the PACES era, appearing in 4% of the PACES survey reports we have received (see Vol. 2, Section F, Experiences 26 and 30). It is one of the most feared instructions but at the same time it can provide an opportunity to score highly. More than in any other system, the well-rehearsed candidate can appear competent and professional compared with the unrehearsed. Detailed examination of the individual nerves is not usually required but rather a quick and efficient screen like that used by neurologists at the bedside or in outpatients (it is well worth attending neurology outpatients to watch quick and efficient examination techniques, if for nothing else). Not only can you look good but also the abnormalities are usually easy to detect. Although it is to be hoped that your practised *routine* will not miss out any nerves, it is preferable to perform a smooth, professional examination, which accidentally misses out a nerve, than to test your examiner's patience through a hesitant and meditative examination which takes a long time to start and may never finish! Since the examination is most easily carried out face to face with the patient, it is best, if possible, to get him to sit on the edge of the bed facing you. First

**1** take a good general and *quick* **look** at the patient, in particular his face, for any obvious abnormality. Next ask him about

**2** his sense of **smell** and **taste**: 'Do you have any difficulty with your sense of smell?' (I). Although you should have the ability to examine taste (VII, IX) and smell formally if equipment is provided, usually questioning (or possibly the judicious use of a bedside orange) is all that is required. All the examination referable to the eyes is best performed next. Unless there is a Snellen chart available, ask the patient to look at the clock on the wall or some newspaper print to give you a good idea of his

**3** **visual acuity:**
'Do you have any difficulty with your vision?'
'Can you see the clock on the wall?' (if he has glasses for long sight he should put them on)
'Can you tell me what time it says?' (II).
A portable Snellen chart will enable you to perform a more formal test.
Now test the

**4** **visual fields** (see Examination *Routine* 5 above), including for *central scotoma*, with a red-headed hat pin. Follow this by examining

**5** **eye movements** (move your finger in the shape of a cross, from side to side then up and down): 'Look at my finger; follow it with your eyes' (III, IV, VI), asking the

---

*The candidate diagnosed a XIIth nerve palsy and passed (see Vol. 2, Section F, Experience 108), but see footnote * on the opposite page.

†This diagnosis was not made by the candidate.

patient at the extremes of gaze whether he sees one or two fingers. If he has diplopia, establish the extent and ask him to describe the 'false' image. As you test eye movements, note at the same time any

**6 nystagmus** (VIII, cerebellum or cerebellar connections; see Vol. 1, Fig. C3.21, Station 3, CNS, Case 32, or

**7 ptosis** (III, sympathetic).

Remember that either extreme abduction of the eyes or gazing at a finger that is too near can cause nystagmus in normal eyes (optokinetic). Now examine

**8** the **pupils** for the direct and consensual *light reflex* (II → optic tract → lateral geniculate ganglion → Edinger–Westphal nucleus of III → fibres to ciliary muscle) and for the *accommodation–convergence* reflex (cortex → III) with your finger just in front of his nose:

'Look into the distance'

'Now look at my finger' (see also Footnote, Examination *Routine* 13).

Finally examine the optic discs (II) by

**9 fundoscopy** (this can be left until last if you prefer). Having finished examining the eyes, examine

**10 facial movements:**

'Raise your eyebrows'
'Screw your eyes up tight'
'Puff your cheeks out' } VII
'Whistle'
'Show me your teeth'

'Clench your teeth' – feel masseters
and temporalis } motor V
'Open your mouth; stop me
closing it'

**11** then **palatal movement:**

'Keep your mouth open; say aah' (IX, X)

**12** and **gag reflex**\* – touch the back of the pharynx on both sides with an orange stick (IX, X). Look at

**13** the **tongue** as it lies in the floor of the mouth for *wasting* or *fasciculation* (XII):

'Open your mouth again'

then get the patient to:

'Put your tongue out' – note any deviation† – 'waggle it from side to side' (XII).

**14** Test the **accessory nerve:**‡

'Shrug your shoulders; keep them shrugged' – push down on the shoulders (XI).
'Turn your head to the left side, now to the right' – feel for the sternomastoid muscle on the side opposite to the turned head (XI).

Finally test

\*This can be unpleasant, so ask the examiner's permission, explain to the patient and ask for his permission as well.
†In unilateral facial paralysis, the protruded tongue, though otherwise normal, may deviate so that unilateral hypoglossal paralysis is suspected (see Vol. 1, Station 3, CNS, Case 35). In unilateral lower motor neurone XIIth nerve palsy there is wasting (?fasciculation) on the side of the lesion and the tongue curves to that side.

‡Painless neck weakness has only four causes: myasthenia gravis (see Vol. 1, Station 3, CNS, Case 27), myotonic dystrophy (see Vol. 1, Station 3, CNS, Case 2), polymyositis (see Vol. 1, Station 3, CNS, Case 45) and motor neurone disease (see Vol. 1, Station 3, CNS, Case 11).

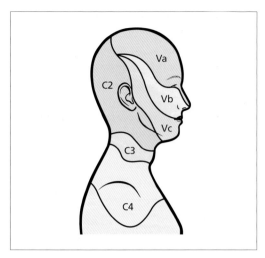

**Figure G.1** Dermatomes in the head and neck.

15  **hearing**:
    'Any problem with the hearing in either ear?'
    'Can you hear that?' – rub finger and thumb together in front of each ear in turn
        (VIII – proceed to the Rinné and Weber tests* if there is any abnormality, and
        look in the ear if you suspect disease of the external ear, perforated drum, wax,
        etc.), and
16  test **facial sensation** including *corneal reflex* (sensory V; see Fig. G.1).

See Appendix 1, Checklist 6, Cranial nerves.


# 7 | 'Examine this patient's arms'


***Variations of instruction in initial PACES survey (resultant diagnoses in brackets)***
This elderly lady has had some falls and difficulty with mobility. Please examine her
    upper limbs (drug-induced dystonia)
This patient has a worsening tremor of his upper limbs. Please give some reasons
    (intention tremor and patchy peripheral sensory neuropathy)
This patient has a 20-year history of weakness in the right arm and shoulder (C5
    radiculopathy)

---

*Weber test*: sound from a vibrating tuning fork held on the centre of the forehead is conducted towards the ear if it has a conductive defect (e.g. wax or otitis media) and away from the ear if it has a nerve deafness. *Rinné test*: a positive test (normal) is when the sound of the tuning fork is louder by air conduction (prongs by external auditory meatus) than by bone conduction (base of fork on mastoid process). Negative is abnormal.

Examine this patient's upper limbs. There has been a weakness for about the last 5
  years (motor neurone disease)

This lady has difficulty doing the housework, especially taking things out of cup-
  boards. Look at her face and examine her hands (myotonic dystrophy)

This man had an operation which is unrelated to the case, then woke with a weak
  left arm. Why? (radial nerve palsy)

This 50-year-old lady has problems driving. Examine her arms to find out why
  (arthritis secondary to ulcerative colitis)

### Diagnoses from our original survey in order of frequency

1  Wasting of the small muscles of the hand (Vol. 1, Station 3, CNS, Case 52) 26%
2  Motor neurone disease (Vol. 1, Station 3, CNS, Case 11) 19%
3  Hemiplegia (Vol. 1, Station 3, CNS, Case 8) 7%
4  Cerebellar syndrome (Vol. 1, Station 3, CNS, Case 7) 6%
5  Cervical myelopathy (Vol. 1, Station 3, CNS, Case 26) 6%
6  Neurofibromatosis (Station 5, Skin, Case 2) 4%
7  Muscular dystrophy (Vol. 1, Station 3, CNS, Case 9) 4%
8  Psoriasis (Station 5, Skin, Case 4) 4%
9  Purpura due to steroids (Station 5, Skin, Case 25) 4%
10 Parkinson's disease (Vol. 1, Station 3, CNS, Case 3) 3%
11 Syringomyelia (Vol. 1, Station 3, CNS, Case 29) 3%
12 Hemiballismus (Vol. 1, Station 3, CNS, Case 20) 3%
13 Lichen planus (Station 5, Skin, Case 11) 3%
14 Pseudoxanthoma elasticum (Station 5, Skin, Case 10) 3%
15 Old polio (Vol. 1, Station 3, CNS, Case 15) 3%
16 Rheumatoid arthritis (Station 5, Locomotor, Case 1) 3%
17 Axillary vein thrombosis 3%
18 Contracture of the elbow in a case of haemophilia 3%
19 Ulnar nerve palsy (Vol. 1, Station 3, CNS, Case 14) 1%
20 Pancoast's syndrome (Vol. 1, Station 1, Respiratory, Case 13) 1%
21 Herpes zoster (Station 5, Skin, Case 32) 1%
22 Mycosis fungoides (Station 5, Skin, Case 34) 1%
23 Polymyositis (Vol. 1, Station 3, CNS, Case 45) 1%

## Examination *routine*

Consideration of the above list from the survey reveals that the vast majority (over
80%) of conditions behind this instruction are neurological with a handful of spot
diagnoses which will usually be obvious. If the diagnosis is not an obvious 'spot' (and
you should make sure that you would recognize each on the list – see individual
short cases in this book and in Volume 1), your *routine* should commence in the
usual way by scanning the whole patient but in particular looking at

  1  the **face** for obvious abnormalities such as *asymmetry* (hemiplegia), *nystagmus*
(cerebellar syndrome), *wasting* (muscular dystrophy), sad, immobile, unblinking
facies (*Parkinson's* disease) or *Horner's* syndrome (syringomyelia, Pancoast's syndrome). You may return to seek a less obvious Horner's or nystagmus later, if necessary. In search of obvious abnormalities, run your eyes down to

**2** the **neck** (pseudoxanthoma elasticum, lymph nodes), and then scan down the arms looking in particular at

**3** the **elbows** which should be particularly inspected for *psoriasis, rheumatoid nodules* and *scars* or *deformity* underlying an ulnar nerve palsy. Before picking up the hands look for

**4** a **tremor** (Parkinson's disease), then briefly inspect

**5** the **hands** in the same way as you have practised under 'Examine this patient's hands' (see Examination *Routine* 15), looking at

  **(a)** the joints (swelling, deformity),

  **(b)** nail changes (pitting, onycholysis, clubbing, nail-fold infarcts), and

  **(c)** skin changes (colour, consistency, lesions).

If you have not already been led towards a diagnosis requiring specific action, start a full neurological examination by studying first

**6** the **muscle bulk** in the upper arms, lower arms and hands, bearing in mind that in about one-quarter of cases there will be wasting of the small muscles of the hands (see Vol. 1, Station 3, CNS, Case 52), and in one-fifth of cases there will be motor neurone disease which means wasting and

**7 fasciculation**.

**8** Test the **tone** in the arms by passively bending the arm (with the patient relaxed) to and fro in an irregular and unexpected fashion, and in the hands by flexing and extending all the joints, including the wrist in the classic 'rolling wave' fashion used to detect cog-wheel rigidity (Parkinson's disease).

**9** Ask the patient: '**Hold your arms out in front of you**' (look for *winging* of the scapulae, involuntary movements or the *myelopathy hand sign*\*); 'Now close your eyes' (look for *sensory wandering* – parietal drift or pseudoathetosis (see Vol. 1, Fig. C3.17c, Station 3, CNS, Case 26).

Next test

**10 power**:

  **(a)** 'Put your arms out to the side' (demonstrate this to the patient yourself – arms at 90° to your body with elbows flexed); 'Stop me pushing them down' (deltoid – C5),

  **(b)** 'Bend your elbow; stop me straightening it' (biceps – C5, 6),

  **(c)** 'Push your arm out straight' – resist elbow extension (triceps – C7),

  **(d)** 'Squeeze my fingers' – offer two fingers (C8, T1),†

  **(e)** 'Hold your fingers out straight' (demonstrate); 'Stop me bending them' (if the patient can do this there is nothing wrong with motor C7 or the radial nerve),

  **(f)** 'Spread your fingers apart' (demonstrate); 'Stop me pushing them together' (dorsal interossei – ulnar nerve),

---

\*With the hands outstretched and supinated, passive abduction of the little finger indicates a pyramidal lesion or ulnar nerve palsy (sensory testing should distinguish). The sign is common in, but not specific for, cervical pyramidal lesions – as the lesion becomes more severe, adjacent fingers also passively abduct.

†See Footnote, Examination *Routine* 15.

(g) 'Hold this piece of paper between your fingers; stop me pulling it out' (palmar interossei – ulnar nerve),

(h) 'Point your thumb at the ceiling; stop me pushing it down' (abductor pollicis brevis – median nerve),

(i) 'Put your thumb and little finger together; stop me pulling them apart' (opponens pollicis – median nerve).

11 **Test coordination**

(a) 'Can you do this?' – demonstrate by flexing your elbows at right angles and then pronating and supinating your forearms as rapidly as possible,

(b) 'Tap quickly on the back of your hand' (demonstrate),

(c) 'Touch my finger; touch your nose; backwards and forwards quickly and neatly' (demonstrate if necessary – vary the target).

12 Check the biceps (C5, 6), triceps (C7), supinator (C5, 6) and finger (C8) **reflexes**.

13 Finally perform a **sensory screen** with *light touch* and *pinprick*, bearing in mind the dermatomes shown in Fig. G.2 and the areas of sensation covered by the ulnar, median and radial nerves in the hand (see Fig. G.4, Examination *Routine* 15). Finally, check *vibration* and *joint position* sense.

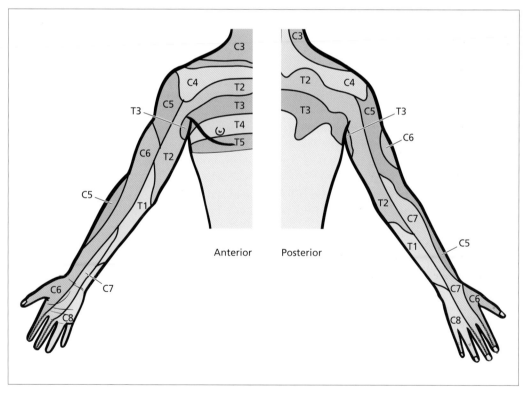

**Figure G.2** Dermatomes in the upper limb. (After Foerster, 1933, Oxford University Press, *Brain* 56: 1.) There is considerable variation and overlap between the cutaneous areas supplied by each spinal root so that an isolated root lesion results in a much smaller area of sensory impairment than the diagram indicates.

We leave you to consider where else you could look with each of the conditions given on the list in order to find additional information (see individual short cases). For example, you could look for nystagmus should you find cerebellar signs, or for Horner's syndrome should you suspect syringomyelia or Pancoast's syndrome.

See Appendix 1, Checklist 7, Arms.

# 8 | 'Examine this patient's legs'

**Variations of instruction in initial PACES survey (resultant diagnoses in brackets)**

Examine this patient's legs (subarachnoid haemorrhage; hereditary sensory and motor neuropathy; mixed upper and lower motor neurone disorders)

Examine this lady's nervous system but concentrate on the legs (Charcot–Marie–Tooth disease)

This man is unable to walk. Examine his legs (?cauda equina lesion)

This 84-year-old lady has been having difficulty walking and with her balance. Would you examine her neurologically to find out why? (peripheral neuropathy)

This lady has difficulty walking. Please examine her legs (?cervical myelopathy and diabetes)

Examine the legs but omit looking at the gait (subacute combined degeneration of the cord)

This patient has had weakness of the legs for 3 years. Please examine the legs and find out why (spastic paraparesis)

Examine this lady's lower limbs (Friedreich's ataxia)

Examine this foot (diabetic foot ulcer)

Look at, and examine, this man's legs (proximal myopathy secondary to polymyositis)

Please look at this patient's ankles and feet (Charcot's joint and foot ulcer)

This patient has diabetes. Please look at the feet (sensory loss, absent pulse and Charcot's joint)

Examine this man's legs (necrobiosis lipoidica diabeticorum).

**Diagnoses from our original survey in order of frequency**

*Group 1 (spot)*
1 Paget's disease 13%
2 Erythema nodosum 4%
3 Pretibial myxoedema 4%
4 Diabetic foot 3%
5 Necrobiosis lipoidica diabeticorum 3%
6 Erythema ab igne 2%
7 Vasculitis 2%
8 Swollen knee 1%

*Group 2 (neurological)*
1 Spastic paraparesis 13%
2 Peripheral neuropathy 12%
3 Hemiplegia 5%
4 Cerebellar syndrome 4%
5 Cervical myelopathy 4%
6 Diabetic foot 3%
7 Motor neurone disease 3%
8 Old polio 3%

9 Pemphigoid/pemphigus <1%
10 Deep venous thrombosis/ruptured Baker's cyst <1%
11 Multiple thigh abscesses <1%
12 Vasculitic leg ulcers <1%
13 Pyoderma gangrenosum <1%
14 Stigmata of sickle cell disease <1%
15 Mycosis fungoides <1%
16 Diabetic ischaemia <1%
17 Ehlers–Danlos syndrome <1%
18 Bilateral below-knee amputation <1%

9 Absent leg reflexes and extensor plantars 3%
10 Friedreich's ataxia 2%
11 Subacute combined degeneration of the cord 2%
12 Charcot–Marie–Tooth disease 1%
13 Polymyositis <1%
14 Lateral popliteal (common peroneal) nerve palsy <1%
15 Tabes <1%
16 Diabetic amyotrophy <1%

**Examination *routine***

An analysis of the conditions in our survey shows that they roughly fall into the two broad groups shown above:

*Group 1*: a spot diagnosis (these cases are covered in this volume)

*Group 2*: a neurological diagnosis (i.e. Station 3 in Volume 1).

Either way initial clues may be gained by first performing a brief

1 ***visual survey*** of the patient as a whole. Look at the head and face for signs such as *enlargement* (Paget's disease), *asymmetry* (hemiparesis), *exophthalmos* with or without *myxoedematous facies* (pretibial myxoedema) or obvious *nystagmus* (cerebellar syndrome). Run your eyes over the patient for other significant signs such as thyroid *acropachy* (pretibial myxoedema), *rheumatoid hands* (swollen knee), nicotine-stained fingers (leg amputations), *wasted hands* (motor neurone disease, Charcot–Marie–Tooth disease, syringomyelia) and for muscle *fasciculation* (usually motor neurone disease).

Turning to the legs, look at the skin, joints and general shape and for any

2 **obvious lesion**, especially from the list of disorders in group 1. If such a lesion is visible a further full examination of the legs will not be required in most cases. You will be able to begin your description and/or diagnosis immediately (see individual short cases). If there is no obvious lesion look again specifically for

3 **bowing** of the tibia (see Vol. 2, Section F, Experience 182), with or without enlargement of the skull. Though the changes of vascular insufficiency (absence of hair, shiny skin, cold pulseless feet, peripheral cyanosis, digital gangrene, painful ulcers) barely occurred in our survey, these should be *briefly* looked for (because they will direct you to examine the pulses, etc. rather than the neurological system).

Observing the legs from the neurological point of view, note whether there is

4 **pes cavus** (Friedreich's ataxia, Charcot–Marie–Tooth disease) or

5 **one leg smaller** than the other (old polio, infantile hemiplegia). Next note

6 **muscle bulk**. Bear in mind that some generalized disuse atrophy may occur even in a limb with upper motor neurone weakness (e.g. severe spastic paraparesis; see Vol. 2, Section F, Experience 109). There may be unilateral loss of muscle bulk (old

polio), muscle wasting that stops part of the way up the leg (Charcot–Marie–Tooth disease), isolated anterior thigh wasting (e.g. diabetic amyotrophy) or generalized proximal muscle wasting (polymyositis) or muscle wasting confined to one peroneal region (lateral popliteal nerve palsy). Look specifically for

**7 fasciculation** (nearly always motor neurone disease).

**8** Examine the **muscle tone** in each leg by passively moving it at the hip and knee joints (with the patient relaxed, roll the leg sideways, backwards and forwards on the bed; lift the knee and let it drop, or bend the knee and partially straighten in an irregular and unexpected rhythm).

**9** Test **power:**\*
  (a) 'Lift your leg up; stop me pushing it down' (L1,2),
  (b) 'Bend your knee; don't let me straighten it' (L5, S1,2),
  (c) (Knee still bent) 'Push out straight against my hand' (L3,4),
  (d) 'Bend your foot down; push my hand away' (S1),
  (e) 'Cock up your foot; point your toes at the ceiling. Stop me pushing your foot down' (L4,5).

Moving smoothly into testing

**10 coordination**, take your hand off the foot and run your finger down the patient's shin below the knee, saying
  (f) 'Put your heel just below your knee then run it smoothly down your shin; now up your shin, now down . . .' etc.†

**11** Check the knee (L3,4) and ankle (S1,2) **jerks**‡ and by forced dorsiflexion with the leg held in slight knee flexion. Check for *ankle clonus* (and patellar clonus if there may be pyramidal disease).

**12** Test the **plantar response**, remembering that in slight pyramidal lesions an extensor plantar is more easily elicited on the outer part of the sole than the inner.§

**13** Turning to **sensation**, dermatomes L2 to S1 on the leg (see Fig. G.3) are tested if you examine *light touch* (dab cotton wool lightly) and *pinprick* once each on the outer thigh (L2), inner thigh (L3), inner calf (L4), outer calf (L5), medial foot (L5) and lateral foot (S1). The most common sensory defect is a peripheral neuropathy with stocking distribution loss. Demonstrate this with light touch (usually the most sensitive indicator) and pinprick.

Test somewhere above the suspected sensory level:
  'Does the pin feel sharp and prickly?' – 'Yes'.

Test on the feet:

---

\*The screen of instructions from (a) to (e) will identify most legs in which there are abnormalities of motor function. You may wish to embellish these, where necessary, with instructions to test hip extension, hip adduction, hip abduction and hip rotation.

†If there is possible or definite cerebellar disease, you may wish to demonstrate dysdiadochokinesis in the foot by asking the patient to tap his foot quickly on your hand.

‡One study has suggested that the plantar strike technique for examining ankle jerks may be more reliable than the better-known tendon strike technique, especially in the elderly (*Lancet* 1994. **344**: 1619–20).

§In slight pyramidal disease the extensor plantar is first elicited on the dorsilateral part of the foot (*Chaddock's manoeuvre*). As the degree of pyramidal involvement increases, the area in which a *Babinski's sign* may be elicited first increases to cover the whole sole and then spreads beyond the foot until *Oppenheim's sign* (extensor response when the inner border of the tibia is pressed heavily; see Vol. 1, Fig. C3.17b, Station 3, CNS, Case 26) or *Gordon's reflex* (extensor response on pinching the Achilles tendon) can be elicited. In such cases the big toe may be seen to go up as the patient takes his socks off.

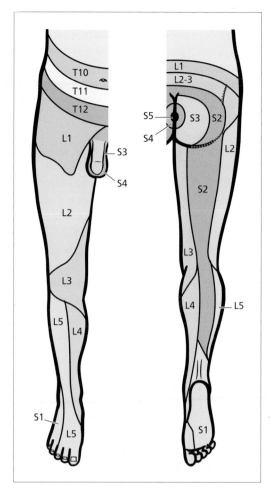

**Figure G.3** Dermatomes in the lower limb. (After Foerster, 1933, Oxford University Press, *Brain* **56**: 1.) There is considerable variation and overlap between the cutaneous areas supplied by each spinal root so that an isolated root lesion results in a much smaller area of sensory impairment than the diagram indicates.

'Does the pin feel sharp and prickly?' – 'No'.

'Tell me when it changes'.

Work up the leg to the sensory level and confirm afterwards by demonstrating the same level medially and laterally.* The level of the peripheral neuropathy may be different on the two legs. *Vibration* should be tested on the medial malleoli (and

---

*The same method can be used for rapid demonstration of a higher sensory level: normal sensation is demonstrated above the lesion, e.g. on the shoulder or chest. The pin is then rapidly moved up the whole body from the foot until the patient announces that the sensation is changing to normal. That area is then worked over rapidly to detect the actual sensory level.

knee, iliac crest, etc., if it is impaired), and *joint position* sense in the great toes (remember to explain to the patient what you mean by 'up' and 'down' in his toes before you get him to close his eyes; whilst testing the position sense hold the toe by the lateral aspects).

Sometimes the examiner will stop you before you get this far. If the lesion is predominantly motor, he may break in before you have tested sensation, and if predominantly sensory, he may lead you to test sensation earlier or stop you at this point. You should, however, be sufficiently deft to perform the full examination described above quickly and efficiently, and be prepared to complete it by examining the patient's

**14 gait** (check the patient can walk by asking for either his or the examiner's permission to examine the gait). First, watch his *ordinary walk* to a defined point and back (see Vol. 1, Station 3, CNS, Case 5) and then watch him walk *heel-to-toe* (ataxia), on his *toes* and on his *heels* (foot-drop). Finally perform

**15 Romberg's test** with the feet together and the arms outstretched. You must be ready to catch the patient if there is any possibility of ataxia. Romberg's test is only positive (sensory ataxia, e.g. subacute combined degeneration, tabes dorsalis) if the patient is more unsteady (tends to fall) with the eyes closed than open.

See Appendix 1, Checklist 8, Legs.

# 9 | 'Examine this patient's legs and arms'

***Variations of instruction in initial PACES survey (resultant diagnoses in brackets)***
This man has had a collapse – can you examine his limbs? (left hemiplegia and atrial fibrillation)

***Diagnoses from our original survey in order of frequency***
1 Motor neurone disease (Vol. 1, Station 3, CNS, Case 11) 29%
2 Cervical myelopathy (Vol. 1, Station 3, CNS, Case 26) 14%
3 Syringomyelia (Vol. 1, Station 3, CNS, Case 29) 14%
4 Friedreich's ataxia (Vol. 1, Station 3, CNS, Case 12) 14%
5 Parkinson's disease (Vol. 1, Station 3, CNS, Case 3) 7%

**Examination *routine***
As appropriate from 'Examine this patient's arms' (see Examination *Routine* 7) and 'Examine this patient's legs' (see Examination *Routine* 8).

# 10 | 'Examine this patient's gait'

## Variations of instruction in initial PACES survey (resultant diagnoses in brackets)

Examine this patient's gait (ankylosing spondylitis)

This man has difficulty walking and falls especially at night. Examine his gait and then his legs (cerebellar signs and sensory neuropathy)

This patient has difficulty in walking. Please examine him (cerebellar signs)

Examine the gait and anything else which is relevant (no diagnosis reached)

## Diagnoses from our surveys in order of frequency

1  Ataxia (Vol. 1, Station 3, CNS, Case 5) 50%

2  Spastic paraparesis (Vol. 1, Station 3, CNS, Case 6) 20%

3  Parkinson's disease (Vol. 1, Station 3, CNS, Case 3) 10%

4  Charcot–Marie–Tooth disease (Vol. 1, Station 3, CNS, Case 4) 5%

5  Ankylosing spondylitis (Vol. 1, Station 3, Cardiovascular, Case 15) 5%

6  A nightmare (see Vol. 2, Section F, Experience 42) 5%

## Examination *routine*

As you approach the patient, perform

1  a *quick **visual survey***, noting any *cerebellar signs* (nystagmus, intention tremor) or obvious signs of conditions such as *Parkinson's* disease (facies, tremor), *Charcot–Marie–Tooth* disease (peroneal wasting, pes cavus, etc.) or *ankylosing spondylitis*. Introduce yourself to the patient and ask him

2  **whether he can walk** without help (*cerebellar dysarthria* heard during his reply may be a useful clue). If he reports difficulty, reassure him that you will stay with him in case of any problems.

3  **Ask him to walk** to a defined point and back whilst you look for any of the classic abnormal gaits (see Vol. 1, Station 3, CNS, Case 5), particularly ataxic (cerebellar or sensory), spastic, steppage (Charcot–Marie–Tooth) or parkinsonian (?pill-rolling tremor). As the patient walks, make sure you note specifically

4  the **arm swing** (Parkinson's) and

5  any *clumsiness* on **the turns** (ataxia, Parkinson's) or 'sticky feet' with gait apraxia (slow, shuffling, short steps) or marche à petit pas (small, quick steps – also known as senile gait). Next test

6  **heel-to-toe** gait (demonstrate as you ask the patient to do this) which will *exacerbate* ataxia (note the side to which the patient tends to fall). Ask the patient to walk

7  **on his toes** (S1) and then

8  **on his heels** (L5; foot-drop – lateral popliteal nerve palsy, Charcot–Marie–Tooth disease). If he has a spastic gait or a hemiparesis he may find both these tests difficult to perform.

9  Now ask him to stand with his *feet together, arms out* in front; when you are satisfied with the degree of steadiness with the eyes open, ask him to *close his eyes* (you should be standing nearby to catch him if he shows a tendency to fall). **Romberg's**

**test** is only positive (*sensory ataxia*) if the patient is more unsteady (tends to fall) with the eyes closed than with them open (dorsal column disease, e.g. subacute combined degeneration, tabes dorsalis, etc.).

10 If you suspect sensory ataxia, a further test is to ask the patient to **close his eyes while walking** (he will become *more* ataxic). Again you should be ready to catch the patient should he fall. As always, be ready to look for

11 **additional features** of the conditions on the list if appropriate (see individual short cases, and consider what you would do with each).

See Appendix 1, Checklist 10, Gait.


# 11 | 'Ask this patient some questions'

*Variations of instruction from our original survey*
Talk to this patient
Examine this patient's speech
Converse with this patient

*Diagnoses from our original survey in order of frequency*
1 Dysphasia (Vol. 1, Station 3, CNS, Case 40) 24%
2 Cerebellar dysarthria (Vol. 1, Station 3, CNS, Case 7) 16%
3 Raynaud's phenomenon (Station 5, Skin, Case 22) 11%
4 Systemic sclerosis/CREST (Station 5, Locomotor, Case 3) 8%
5 Pseudobulbar palsy (Vol. 1, Station 3, CNS, Case 46) 8%
6 Myxoedema (Station 5, Endocrine, Case 9) 5%
7 Graves' disease (Station 5, Endocrine, Case 3) 5%
8 Crohn's disease (Vol. 1, Station 1, Abdominal, Case 9) 5%
9 Ankle oedema due to nephrotic syndrome (Vol. 1, Station 1, Abdominal, Case 20) 5%
10 Senile dementia 5%
11 Parkinson's disease (Vol. 1, Station 3, CNS, Case 3) 3%

**Examination** *routine*
Inspection of the list of cases in our survey which provoked this instruction reveals that they fall into four groups, each with a very different reason for the instruction:
*Group 1*: to spot the diagnosis and confirm it by eliciting *revealing answers* 39%
*Group 2*: to demonstrate and diagnose the type of a dysarthria 32%
*Group 3*: to diagnose a dysphasia 24%
*Group 4*: to assess higher mental function 5%.
With the group 1 patients you may have been given a lead such as 'Look at the hands' (Raynaud's) or 'Look at the face' (systemic sclerosis, myxoedema, etc.) before the instruction 'Ask this patient some questions'. At any rate you should start your examination as usual with

**1** a *visual survey* of the patient from head to foot, particularly looking for evidence of: (i) the spot diagnosis in group 1 patients (Raynaud's, systemic sclerosis/CREST, hypo- or hyperthyroidism, Crohn's, nephrotic syndrome); (ii) a *hemiplegia* which may be associated with dysphasia; or (iii) any of the conditions associated with dysarthria (see Vol. 1, Station 3, CNS, Case 36), especially *nystagmus* or *intention tremor* (which may be revealed by even minor movements) in cerebellar disease, *pes cavus* in Friedreich's ataxia and the *facies/tremor* of Parkinson's disease.

In the group 1 patients, once you are on to the diagnosis, the sort of

**2** **specific questions** the examiners are looking for (see also the individual short cases in Volume 1) are:

*Raynaud's* (see also Vol. 2, Section F, Anecdote 262):

'Do your fingers change colour in the cold?'

'What colour do they go?' ('Is there a particular sequence of colours?')

'How long have you had the trouble?'

'What is your job?' (vibrating tools, etc.)

and if there is any possibility of connective tissue disease:

'Do you have any difficulty with swallowing?' etc.

*Systemic sclerosis*:

'Do you have any difficulty with swallowing?'

'Do your fingers change colour in the cold?'

'Do you get short of breath?' (on hills? on flat? etc.)

We leave you to work out the straightforward questions you would ask the slow, croaking patient with *myxoedematous facies*, the patient with *exophthalmos*, or the one who has *lid retraction* and is *fidgety*, or the patient who has *multiple scars* and *sinuses* on his abdomen. In the young patient who may have nephrotic syndrome, you would be looking for the history of a sore throat.

If there are no features suggesting a group 1 patient, it is likely that the problem is either a dysarthria or dysphasia and, as already mentioned, there may be clues pointing to one of these. You need to ask the patient

**3** some **general questions** to get him *talking*:

'My name is . . . Please could you tell me your name?'

'What is your address?'

If you still need to hear a patient speak further ask

**4** **more questions** which require *long answers* such as: 'Please could you tell me all the things you ate for breakfast/lunch'.

To test

**5** **articulation**, ask the patient to repeat traditional words and phrases such as 'British Constitution', 'West Register Street', 'biblical criticism' and 'artillery'. As well as testing articulation, such

**6** **repetition** is useful for assessing speech when the patient only gives one-word answers to questions. If necessary ask the patient to repeat long sentences after you. Information gained from repetition may also be useful in your assessment of dysphasia (see below).

If the problem is *dysarthria*, it is really a spot diagnosis to test your ability to recognize and demonstrate the features of the different types (see Vol. 1, Station 3, CNS, Case 36). It is recommended that you find as many patients as possible with the conditions causing the various types of dysarthria and listen to them speak so that, as with murmurs, the diagnosis is a question of instant recognition. This is particularly true of the ataxic dysarthria of cerebellar disease. When you have heard enough to make the diagnosis, you should either describe the speech (see Vol. 1, Station 3, CNS, Case 36) and, with supporting signs seen on inspection, give the diagnosis, or proceed to look for

**7  additional signs** (in the same way as you might do after the 'What is the diagnosis?' instruction).

If the patient has a *dysphasia* (see Vol. 1, Station 3, CNS, Case 40), you may wish to demonstrate that

**8  comprehension** is good (expressive dysphasia) or impaired (receptive dysphasia). Perform a few simple commands *without gesturing*, e.g.

'Please put your tongue out'

'Shut your eyes'

'Touch your nose', etc.

Assuming these are performed adequately, proceed to look for expressive dysphasia by asking the patient to name some everyday items, e.g. a comb, pen, coins. If the patient is unable to name the objects, test for

**9  nominal dysphasia**. Hold up your keys:

'What is this?' – patient does not answer.

'Is this a spoon?' – 'No'.

'Is it a pen?' – 'No'.

'Is it keys?' – 'Yes'.

If the patient is able to name objects, test the ability to form sentences by asking the patient to describe something in more detail, e.g.

'Could you tell me where you live and how you would get home from here?'

'Could you tell me the name of as many objects in this room as possible?'

If there are expressive problems you should check to see if the problem is true expressive dysphasia or whether there is

**10  orofacial dyspraxia.**\* Ask the patient to perform various orofacial movements (assuming there is no receptive dysphasia). These should be tested first by command *without gesture*, e.g.

'Please show me your teeth'

'Move your tongue from side to side'.

Subsequently ask the patient to obey the same commands but *with gesture*, i.e. so the patient can mimic. This should give some idea as to whether the patient has either ideational or ideomotor dyspraxia.†

Our survey showed that it is extremely rare for candidates to be asked to assess

---

\*It is important to make this distinction so that the type of speech therapy is appropriate. In orofacial dyspraxia the therapist needs to work on mouth movements rather than concentrating only on linguistic problems. It has recently been established that the lesion which leads to orofacial dyspraxia is in the operculum.

†Again it is relevant to therapy to establish if the patient can make movements when aided by gesture.

**11 higher mental functions.**\* This is, however, an assessment which every Membership candidate should be equipped to make. The following is the 'abbreviated mental test' – more than four of the questions wrong suggests a well-established dementia:

1 Age

2 Time (to nearest hour)

3 Address for recall at end of test – this should be repeated by the patient to ensure it has been heard correctly: 42 West Street

4 Year

5 Name of this place

6 Recognition of two persons (doctor, nurse, etc.)

7 Date of birth (day and month sufficient)

8 Year of First World War

9 Name of present monarch

10 Count backwards from 20 to 1.

Agnosia, apraxia, dyslexia, dysgraphia and dyscalculia are considered in Vol. 1, Station 3, CNS, Case 8.

See Appendix 1, Checklist 11, Ask some questions.

# 12 | 'Examine this patient's fundi'

***Variations of instruction in initial PACES survey (resultant diagnoses in brackets)***

Examine this patient's fundi (diabetic retinopathy – many cases, all stages; unilateral optic atrophy and angioid streaks)

Look at the fundi (diabetic retinopathy – many cases, all stages)

Examine the eyes of this patient with diabetes (panretinal photocoagulation and exudates near macula)

This patient feels as if he is walking on cotton wool and has had recurrent Bell's palsies. Please examine his eyes (it turned out to be preproliferative diabetic retinopathy)

This patient is blind. Examine his fundi (retinitis pigmentosa and cataracts)

This man had sudden-onset blindness. Please look at the fundi and suggest why (glaucoma and retinal artery occlusion)

\*Traditionally this has been rarely assessed in previous versions of MRCP (see Vol. 2, Section F, Anecdote 286), though it has already occurred in the new Station 5 (see Vol. 2, Section F, Experience 1, Station 5).

This patient has visual loss. Please examine the fundi (diabetic maculopathy)

Your house officer has examined this lady's fundi. She is a 23-year-old nurse. He is worried and has asked for your opinion (myelinated nerve fibres)

Examine this man's fundus – just the right one (diabetic retinopathy)

Look at the fundi and describe what you find (cataracts and diabetic retinopathy)

This man has trouble with his vision. Examine the fundi (retinitis pigmentosa)

Examine the fundi. The patient has a central scotoma (retinitis pigmentosa and diabetic maculopathy)

This elderly man has had sudden onset of blindness in the right eye. Please examine him and tell me why (optic atrophy)


*Diagnoses from our survey in order of frequency*
 1 Diabetic retinopathy (Station 5, Eyes, Case 1) 41%
 2 Retinitis pigmentosa (Station 5, Eyes, Case 2) 16%
 3 Optic atrophy (Station 5, Eyes, Case 3) 6%
 4 Papilloedema (Station 5, Eyes, Case 8) 4%
 5 Retinal vein thrombosis (Station 5, Eyes, Case 6) 2%
 6 Old choroiditis (Station 5, Eyes, Case 7) 2%
 7 Cataracts (Station 5, Eyes, Case 9) 2%
 8 Albinism (Station 5, Eyes, Case 11) 2%
 9 Myelinated nerve fibres (Station 5, Eyes, Case 13) 1%
10 Hypertensive retinopathy (Station 5, Eyes, Case 14) 1%
11 Glaucoma (Station 5, Eyes, Case 15) 1%
12 Laurence–Moon–Bardet–Biedl (Station 5, Eyes, Case 19) <1%
13 Asteroid hyalosis (Station 5, Eyes, Case 17) <1%
14 Retinal artery occlusion (Station 5, Eyes, Case 16) <1%
15 Drusen (Station 5, Eyes, Case 18) <1%
16 Cytomegalovirus choroidoretinitis (AIDS) (Station 5, Eyes, Case 20) <1%
17 Normal (Station 5, Eyes, Case 21) <1%


*Special note*
Although, with the new Station 5, a fundus case is no longer mandatory, the College has made it clear that fundoscopy continues to be a skill that all MRCP candidates should be competent in. Though there are only a limited number of possibilities, it is clear from our surveys that a lot of candidates experience more difficulty with a fundus than with any other short case. On our questionnaire, a considerable number of candidates reported 'I said optic atrophy . . .' or 'I said diabetic retinopathy . . . but I hadn't got a clue what it was' (see Vol. 2, Section F, Experiences 158–160). Clearly, there is not a lot that a book like this can do to help other than to warn you in advance of the problem, to provide you with a list of the likely conditions and to describe them (see individual short cases). Other than this, the art of fundoscopy and fundal diagnoses can only be acquired with practice. With a moderate degree of clinical expertise and common sense, most candidates ought to be able to overcome this hurdle.

## Examination *routine*

Almost invariably, if you are asked to look at the fundus the diagnosis must be in the fundus. However, it is good practice to precede fundoscopy with

**1** a **quick general look** at the patient (this will rarely help but the occasional person with diabetes in the examination may also have *foot ulcers* or *necrobiosis lipoidica* or may be wearing a *Medic-Alert* bracelet or neck chain), at his eyes (*arcus lipidus* at an inappropriately young age may suggest diabetes), and at his pupils (usually, but not always, dilated for the examination).

Turning to ophthalmoscopy, it may be your practice to focus immediately on the fundus and, in the vast majority of cases, this will provide the diagnosis. However, it would be preferable to cultivate the habit (if you can gain sufficient expertise to do it quickly and efficiently) of looking first at

**2** the structures in front of the fundus, particularly the **lens** (people with diabetes will often reward you with early *cataract* formation; your examiner will sometimes not have noticed it, but as long as you are right when he checks, you may increase your score). Adjust the lenses of the ophthalmoscope so that you move down through

**3** the **vitreous**, noting any *opacities* (e.g. asteroid hyalinosis; see Station 5, Eyes, Case 17), *haemorrhages, fibrous tissue* or *new vessel formation* (diabetes) until you get to

**4** the **fundus**. Localize the disc and examine it and its margins for *optic atrophy*,* *papillitis* (see Station 5, Eyes, Case 3) or *papilloedema* (see Station 5, Eyes, Case 8) and for *myelinated nerve fibres* (see Station 5, Eyes, Case 13). Trace the

**5** **arterioles** and **venules** out from the disc, noting particularly their calibre, light reflex (*silver wiring*) and AV crossing points (*AV nipping*; see Station 5, Eyes, Case 14).

**6** Examine **each quadrant** of the fundus and especially the **macular area** and its temporal aspect.† You are looking particularly for *haemorrhages* (dot, blot, flame-shaped), *microaneurysms, exudates* both hard (well-defined edges; increased light reflex) and soft (fluffy with ill-defined edges; *cotton-wool spots*). If hard exudates are present see if these form a ring (*circinates* in diabetes).

If you see haemorrhages you must look specifically for

   **(a)** dot haemorrhages/microaneurysms,

   **(b)** new vessel formation, and

   **(c)** photocoagulation scars.

If you diagnose diabetic retinopathy, your examiner will expect you to be able to comment on the presence or absence of all of these (see Vol. 2, Section F, Experience 160). If you cannot find these diagnostic clues, you may have noted the features that suggest hypertensive rather than diabetic retinopathy (silver wiring, AV nipping,

---

*There are normal variations in disc colour; in both infancy and old age it is naturally pale, as is the enlarged disc of a myopic eye. The advice of a well-known neurologist and experienced MRCP teacher to his MRCP candidates was: 'Don't diagnose optic atrophy unless it is a "barn door" optic atrophy'. It is well worth bearing this advice in mind (see Vol. 2, Section F, Experience 159). Temporal pallor of the disc due to a lesion in

the papillomacular bundle is often seen in multiple sclerosis. However, temporal pallor is not always pathological.
†The macula will come into view if you ask the patient with a dilated pupil to look at the ophthalmoscopic light. Ideally, you should use the dot light for this, if it is available in your ophthalmoscope.

more soft exudates than hard, haemorrhages which are mainly flame-shaped, early disc swelling with loss of venous pulsation* or frank papilloedema).

In the patient with diabetic retinopathy, it is of particular clinical significance to assess whether lesions (especially hard exudates) involve or threaten (i.e. are near to) the centre of the fovea.†

It would be useful if you knew that the patient has diabetes (see Vol. 2, Section F, Experience 204 and Quotation 379) but if you remain in doubt, remember that diabetes and hypertension often coexist in a patient, and that it is more important that you have checked comprehensively for the above features, and report your findings honestly (mentioning the features in favour of one diagnosis or the other), than to guess or make up findings. In PACES, the College is keen that the instruction tells you the patient has diabetes if he/she does. In general, this does not help as many of the patients with different types of retinal pathologies in the exam have diabetes, because patients with diabetes are the one group having regular fundal checks which may turn up pathologies other than diabetic retinopathy, e.g. drusen, old choroiditis, myelinated nerve fibres, etc. However, in the patient with haemorrhages and exudates it is of great value to know if the patient has diabetes.

We leave you to master the findings of the other fundal short cases and to ensure that you would recognize each (see individual short cases in this book and in Volume 1). The final point in this important *routine* is to

7 **keep examining until** you have finished and are **ready** to present your findings. Do not be put off by the impatient words or mumblings of your examiner; these will be forgotten when you present accurate findings and get the diagnosis right. Conversely, it is too late to go back and check if the examiner asks whether you saw a . . . and you are not sure (Vol. 2, Section F, Experience 160). You need to be able to give a clear and unequivocal 'yes' or 'no'. Thus, the best tip we can offer as you look around the fundus is to stop at the disc, the macula and in each quadrant of each eye and ask yourself the question: 'Are there any abnormalities? What are they?' before moving on to the next area.

See Appendix 1, Checklist 12, Fundi.

---

*Observation of venous pulsation is an expertise which comes with much practice of looking at normal as well as abnormal fundi. Though it could be useful if you have acquired this expertise before the examination, do not get bogged down studying the venous pulsation for too long if you are not used to it. See also Station 5, Eyes, Case 8.

†The UK National Screening Committee diabetic retinopathy screening guidelines suggest that patients with hard exudates within one disc diameter of the centre of the fovea should be referred to an ophthalmologist (see Station 5, Eyes, Case 1).

# 13 | 'Examine this patient's eyes'

## Variations of instruction in initial PACES survey (resultant diagnoses in brackets)

Examine this patient's eyes (retinitis pigmentosa; Graves' disease; complete IIIrd nerve palsy; IIIrd, IVth, VIth nerve palsy)

Examine the eyes and anything else appropriate (Graves' eye disease and signs of hyperthyroidism)

Look at this patient's eyes (exophthalmos; IIIrd nerve palsy)

This woman presents with painful eyes. Please examine her (chemosis and goitre)

Examine this lady's eye movements (partial IIIrd nerve palsy)

This lady has had neurosurgery. Please examine her eyes (right upper homonymous hemianopia)

This man is followed up in the eye clinic. Have a look at him and tell me why (exophthalmos and lid lag)

## Diagnoses from our original survey in order of frequency

 1 Exophthalmos (Station 5, Eyes, Case 12) 27%
 2 Ocular palsy (Station 5, Eyes, Case 4) 23%
 3 Nystagmus (Vol. 1, Station 3, CNS, Case 32) 11%
 4 Diabetic retinopathy (Station 5, Eyes, Case 1) 8%
 5 Optic atrophy (Station 5, Eyes, Case 3) 7%
 6 Myasthenia gravis (Vol. 1, Station 3, CNS, Case 27) 4%
 7 Visual field defects (Vol. 1, Station 3, CNS, Case 13) 3%
 8 Ptosis (Vol. 1, Station 3, CNS, Case 18) 3%
 9 Retinitis pigmentosa (Station 5, Eyes, Case 2) 2%
10 Horner's syndrome (Vol. 1, Station 3, CNS, Case 41) 2%
11 Holmes–Adie pupil (Vol. 1, Station 3, CNS, Case 31) 1%
12 Argyll Robertson pupils (Vol. 1, Station 3, CNS, Case 38) 1%
13 Cataracts (Station 5, Eyes, Case 9) 1%
14 Papilloedema (Station 5, Eyes, Case 8) 1%

Other diagnoses were: buphthalmos in a patient with Sturge–Weber syndrome (1%), normal eyes in a patient who was supposed to have internuclear ophthalmoplegia (1%) and retinal detachment (<1%).

## Examination *routine*

A study of the above list maps out your examination steps when you hear this instruction. It is basically going to be a part of your cranial nerves *routine* (see Examination *Routine* 6) but carried out in slightly more detail. It should be your habit to commence all examination *routines* by *scanning* the whole patient. The patient with nystagmus due to cerebellar disease (see Vol. 1, Station 3, CNS, Case 7) may have an *intention tremor* which will occasionally be noticeable even with minor movements. The patient with exophthalmos may have *pretibial myxoedema* or *thyroid acropachy*. A number of other conditions with stigmata elsewhere on the body may cause eye signs. Though these conditions were not prominent in our survey, they should be borne in mind as you complete this *visual survey*: face and hands of acromegaly, foot ulcers in diabetes, pes cavus in Friedreich's ataxia, the long, lean look of myotonic dystrophy, etc. As you finish your *visual survey* briefly look again at

1 the **face** (e.g. myasthenic facies, tabetic facies, facial asymmetry in hemiparesis), and then concentrate on

2 the **eyes**. Ask yourself if there is

   **(a)** exophthalmos,

   **(b)** strabismus,

   **(c)** ptosis, or

   **(d)** other abnormalities such as xanthelasma or arcus senilis.

Look at

3 the **pupils** for inequality of size and shape; whether one or both are small (Argyll Robertson, Horner's) or large (Holmes–Adie, IIIrd nerve palsy). Remember it may be necessary to use subdued light to elicit anisocuria, particularly due to unilateral Horner's syndrome. Also check for iris abnormalities such as Lisch nodules in neurofibromatosis. Next, it is traditional to check

4 the **visual acuity** by asking the patient to read a newspaper or other print which you hold up, and by asking him to look at the clock on the wall (see Examination *Routine* 6); alternatively it would be preferable to pull out a pocket-sized Snellen chart.* In the traditional *routine* you should next test

5 **visual fields** (see Examination *Routine* 5). However, in the majority of cases the important findings are on testing

6 **eye movements** (see Examination *Routine* 6). We leave you to decide if you wish to follow the traditional *routine* or check eye movements before acuity and visual fields (see Vol. 2, Section F, Experience 145 and Quotation 388). You are looking for

   **(a)** ocular palsy (see Vol. 1, Station 3, CNS, Case 16),

   **(b)** diplopia,

   **(c)** nystagmus, or

   **(d)** lid lag.

In order to test

7 the **pupillary light reflex**, take out your pen torch and shine the light twice (*direct* and *consensual*) in each eye. Then test

8 the **accommodation–convergence reflex** – hold your finger close to the patient's nose:

   'Look into the distance',

then suddenly

   'Now look at my finger'.†

Finally, examine

9 the **fundi** (see Examination *Routine* 12).

---

*We advise you to take a pocket-sized Snellen chart. It will enable you to put an approximate value on the patient's visual acuity while taking no extra time.

†Some neurologists believe that as this traditional method of examining the accommodation–convergence reflex may involve a change in optical axis and luminance, it is better to get the patient to follow a target down the optical axis over 2 m.

As usual, when you have the diagnosis, think what else you could look for (e.g. cerebellar signs in a patient with nystagmus; sympathectomy scar over the clavicle in a patient with Horner's syndrome; absent limb reflexes in Holmes–Adie pupil) before shouting out the diagnosis even if it is obvious (e.g. exophthalmos).

See Appendix 1, Checklist 13, Eyes.

# 14 | 'Examine this patient's face'

***Variations of instruction in initial PACES survey (resultant diagnoses in brackets)***
Look at the face (hereditary haemorrhagic telangiectasia)
Look at this patient's face (lupus pernio)
Look at this man's face and examine whatever else you think is necessary

***Diagnoses from our original survey in order of frequency***
1 Lower motor neurone VIIth nerve lesion (Vol. 1, Station 3, CNS, Case 35) 12%
2 Lupus pernio (Station 5, Skin, Case 19) 8%
3 Ptosis (Vol. 1, Station 3, CNS, Case 18) 7%
4 Sturge–Weber syndrome (Station 5, Skin, Case 24) 7%
5 Hypothyroidism (Station 5, Endocrine, Case 5) 7%
6 Osler–Weber–Rendu syndrome (Station 5, Skin, Case 3) 7%
7 Myotonic dystrophy (Vol. 1, Station 3, CNS, Case 2) 4%
8 Jaundice (Vol. 1, Station 1, Abdominal, Cases 3 and 15–17) 4%
9 Horner's syndrome (Vol. 1, Station 3, CNS, Case 41) 4%
10 Systemic sclerosis/CREST (Station 5, Locomotor, Case 3) 3%
11 Peutz–Jeghers syndrome (Station 5, Skin, Case 26) 3%
12 Upper motor neurone facial weakness (Vol.1, Station 3, CNS, Case 8) 3%
13 Systemic lupus erythematosus (Station 5, Locomotor, Case 16) 3%
14 Parkinson's disease (Vol. 1, Station 3, CNS, Case 3) 3%
15 Cushing's syndrome (Station 5, Endocrine, Case 6) 2%
16 Neurofibromatosis (Station 5, Skin, Case 2) 2%
17 Superior vena cava obstruction (Vol. 1, Station 1, Respiratory, Case 22) 2%
18 Plethora (polycythaemia rubra vera) (Vol. 1, Station 1, Abdominal, Case 10) 2%
19 Hypopituitarism (Station 5, Endocrine, Case 8) 2%
20 Vitiligo and a goitre (Station 5, Skin, Case 8 and Endocrine, Case 4) 2%
21 Cyanosis (see Footnote, Examination *Routine* 3) 2%
22 Paget's disease (Station 5, Locomotor, Case 7) 1%
23 Bilateral parotid enlargement (Station 5, Other, Case 1) 1%
24 Exophthalmos (Station 5, Eyes, Case 12) 1%
25 Acromegaly (Station 5, Endocrine, Case 2) 1%
26 Dermatomyositis (hands and face) (Station 5, Skin, Case 6) 1%
27 Xanthelasma and arcus senilis (Station 5, Skin, Case 7) 1%

**28** Acne rosacea 1%

**29** Dermatitis herpetiformis (Station 5, Skin, Case 39) 1%

**30** Malar flush (Vol. 1, Station 3, Cardiovascular, Case 7 and Station 5, Skin, Case 5) 1%

## Examination *routine*

This instruction is really just a variation on the 'spot diagnosis' theme (see Examination *Routine* 22), only easier because you are told where the abnormalities lie. In a way similar to that described in the 'What is the diagnosis?' *routine*,

**1** *survey* the patient from head to foot and then

**2 scan the face** and skull. The abnormality will usually be obvious (see above list) but if you find none then proceed to

**3 break down the parts** of the face into their constituents and scrutinize each, asking yourself the question: 'Is it normal?'. Thus, if you have scanned the eyes and have not been struck by any obvious abnormality (e.g. ptosis or an abnormal pupil), you should look at all the structures such as the *eyelids* (mild degree of ptosis, heliotrope rash on the upper lid in dermatomyositis), *eyelashes* (sparse in alopecia*), *cornea* (arcus senilis, ground-glass appearance in congenital syphilis), *sclerae* (icteric, congested in superior vena cava obstruction and polycythaemia), *pupils* (small, large, irregular, dislocated lens in Marfan's, cataract in myotonic dystrophy) and *iris* ('muddy iris' in iritis)† on both sides. Look at the *face* for any erythema or infiltrates (lupus pernio, SLE, dermatomyositis, malar flush), around the *mouth* for tight, shiny, adherent skin (systemic sclerosis) or pigmented macules (Peutz–Jeghers) and, if indicated, in the mouth for telangiectases (Osler–Weber–Rendu), cyanosis or pigmentation (Addison's). The whole face can be rapidly covered in this manner. Having spotted the abnormality and, you hope, made the diagnosis, you should, if appropriate, try to score extra points by demonstrating

**4 additional features** in the same way as described under 'What is the diagnosis?'. Go through each diagnosis on the list and work out what additional features you would see elsewhere. Thus, if you find a lower motor neurone VIIth nerve lesion, demonstrate the weakness in the upper as well as the lower part of the face (see Vol. 1, Station 3, CNS, Case 35), then be seen to examine the ears for evidence of herpes zoster (Ramsay Hunt syndrome).

If despite carrying out the above routine there is still no apparent abnormality then examine the facial musculature (see 'Examine this patient's cranial nerves') for evidence of a VIIth nerve lesion which is not obvious.

See Appendix 1, Checklist 14, Face.

---

*May be associated with the organ-specific autoimmune diseases (see Station 5, Skin, Cases 8 and 14).

†Another uncommon but important sign which may occur in the iris is neovascularization in diabetes (rubeosis iridis).

However, it is unlikely that this would occur in the context of 'Examine this patient's face' at the examination.

# 15 | 'Examine this patient's hands'

*Variations of instruction in initial PACES survey (resultant diagnoses in brackets)*

Examine this patient's hands (rheumatoid hands and nodules; rheumatoid hands and cervical collar; osteoarthritis; psoriasis; rheumatoid arthritis)

Examine these hands (psoriasis; scleroderma; neurofibromatosis; deforming arthropathy, ?type)

Please examine this patient's hands. He is a 15-year-old boy who presented with carpopedal spasm as a child (pseudohypoparathyroidism?)

This man has a painful knee. Please examine his hands and suggest why (gout)

This man has had painful hands. Please examine him (rheumatoid hands)

Look at this patient's hands (rheumatoid arthritis)

This is a lady of about 80 years. Please look at her hands (osteoarthritis and gout)

Examine the hands and any other relevant joints (CREST)

Examine these hands (chronic tophaceous gout)

This patient has rheumatoid arthritis. Please check the functional status (rheumatoid arthritis)

Have a look at this lady's hand and talk me through your examination (rheumatoid hands)


*Diagnoses from our original survey in order of frequency*

1 Rheumatoid hands (Station 5, Locomotor, Case 1) 22%
2 Systemic sclerosis/CREST (Station 5, Locomotor, Case 3) 13%
3 Wasting of the small muscles of the hand (Vol. 1, Station 3, CNS, Case 52) 12%
4 Psoriatic arthropathy/psoriasis (Station 5, Locomotor, Case 2) 11%
5 Ulnar nerve palsy (Vol. 1, Station 3, CNS, Case 14) 9%
6 Clubbing (Station 5, Skin, Case 17) 7%
7 Raynaud's (Station 5, Skin, Case 22) 3%
8 Vasculitis (Station 5, Locomotor, Case 10) 3%
9 Steroid changes (especially purpura) (Station 5, Skin, Case 25) 3%
10 Acromegaly (Station 5, Endocrine, Case 2) 2%
11 Motor neurone disease (Vol. 1, Station 3, CNS, Case 11) 2%
12 Xanthomata (Station 5, Skin, Case 7) 2%
13 Cyanosis (central – see Footnote, Examination *Routine* 3; peripheral – Station 5, Skin, Case 22) 2%
14 Chronic liver disease (Vol. 1, Station 1, Abdominal, Case 3) 2%
15 Thyroid acropachy (Station 5, Endocrine, Case 12) 2%
16 Carpal tunnel syndrome (Vol. 1, Station 3, CNS, Case 33) 2%
17 Osteoarthrosis (Station 5, Locomotor, Case 8) 2%
18 Osler–Weber–Rendu syndrome (Station 5, Skin, Case 3) 1%
19 Tophaceous gout (Station 5, Locomotor, Case 5) 1%

Other diagnoses were: neurofibromatosis (<1%), systemic lupus erythematosus (<1%), cervical myelopathy (<1%), dermatomyositis ('examine hands and face', <1%), nail–patella syndrome ('examine hands and knees', <1%), Charcot–Marie–

Tooth disease (<1%), superior vena cava obstruction (<1%), facioscapulohumeral muscular dystrophy (<1%), Addison's disease (<1%) and Marfan's syndrome (<1%).

**Examination *routine***

Analysis of the list given above suggests that when you hear this instruction, rheumatoid arthritis is likely to be present in about a quarter of the cases, and scleroderma, wasting of the small muscles of the hand, psoriasis, ulnar nerve palsy or clubbing in about a further half. As you approach the patient you should bear this in mind and look specifically at

1 the **face** for typical expressionless facies, with adherent shiny skin, sometimes with telangiectasia (*systemic sclerosis*). It is clear from the survey list that a variety of other conditions may show signs in either the face or in the general appearance, particularly *cushingoid* facies (steroid changes in a patient with rheumatoid arthritis), *acromegalic* facies, *arcus senilis* or *xanthelasma* (xanthomata), *icterus* and *spider naevi* (chronic liver disease) or *exophthalmos* (thyroid acropathy). We leave you to consider the changes you may note as you approach the patient with any of the other conditions on the list (see individual short cases in this book and in Volume 1). Even if the diagnosis is not immediately clear on looking at the face, it is likely that in many cases it will become rapidly apparent as you

2 **inspect the hands**. Run quickly through the six main conditions that make up 75% of cases

(**a**) *rheumatoid arthritis* (proximal joint swelling, spindling of the fingers, ulnar deviation, nodules),

(**b**) *systemic sclerosis* (sclerodactyly with tapering of the fingers, sometimes with gangrene of the fingertips, tight, shiny, adherent skin, calcified nodules, etc.),

(**c**) generalized *wasting* of the small muscles of the hand, perhaps with dorsal guttering,

(**d**) *psoriasis* (pitting of the nails, terminal interphalangeal arthropathy, scaly rash),

(**e**) *ulnar nerve palsy* (may be a typical claw hand or may be muscle wasting which spares the thenar eminence; often this diagnosis will only become apparent when you have made a sensory examination), and

(**f**) *clubbing*.

The changes that you may see in the other conditions in the list are dealt with under the individual short cases in this book and in Volume 1, but if in these first few seconds you have not made a rapid spot diagnosis, study first the dorsal and then the palmar aspects of the hands, looking specifically at

3 the **joints** for swelling, deformity or Heberden's nodes,

4 the **nails** for pitting, onycholysis, clubbing, nail-fold infarcts (vasculitis – usually rheumatoid) or splinter haemorrhages (unlikely),

5 the **skin** for *colour* (pigmentation, icterus, palmar erythema), for *consistency* (tight and shiny in scleroderma; papery thin, perhaps with purpuric patches in steroid therapy; thick in acromegaly), and for *lesions* (psoriasis, vasculitis, purpura, xanthomata, spider naevi, telangiectasis in Osler–Weber–Rendu and systemic sclerosis, tophi, neurofibromata, other rashes),

6 the **muscles** for isolated *wasting* of the thenar eminence (median nerve lesion), for generalized wasting especially of the first dorsal interosseous but sparing the

thenar eminence (ulnar nerve lesion), for generalized wasting from a T1 lesion or other cause (see Vol. 1, Station 3, CNS, Case 52) or for *fasciculation* which usually indicates motor neurone disease, though occasionally it can occur in other conditions such as syringomyelia, old polio or Charcot–Marie–Tooth disease.

Before leaving the inspection it is worth looking specifically for *skin crease pigmentation* (see Vol. 2, Section F, Experience 186) before moving to

**7 palpation** of the hands for Dupuytren's contracture, nodules (may be palpable in the palms in rheumatoid arthritis), calcinosis (scleroderma/CREST), xanthomata, Heberden's nodes or tophi. In the vast majority of cases you will have, by now, some findings demanding either specific further action (see below) or a report with a diagnosis. Nonetheless, you should be prepared to continue with a full neurological examination of the hands to confirm a suspected neurological lesion, or if you have still made no diagnosis. If the hands appear normal it may be that there is a sensory defect. In these cases, it is more efficient, therefore, to commence the examination by testing

**8 sensation.** Ask the patient if there has been any numbness or tingling in his hands and if so, when (?worse at night – carpal tunnel syndrome) and where. Bearing in mind the classic patterns of sensory defect in ulnar and median nerve lesions (see Fig. G.4) and the dermatomes (see Fig. G.2), seek and define an area of deficit to *pinprick* and *light touch* (dab cotton wool lightly), and check the *vibration* and *joint position* sense. With incomplete sensory loss due to either an ulnar or a median nerve defect, if you stroke the medial border of the little finger and the lateral border of the index finger with your fingers simultaneously, the patient may sense that the one side feels different from the other.

**9** Check the **tone** of the muscles in the hand by flexing and extending all the joints including the wrist in a 'rolling wave' fashion.

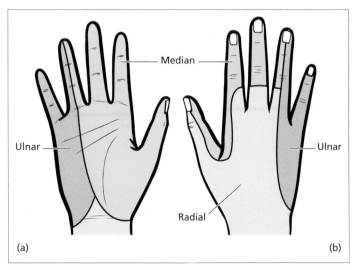

**Figure G.4** Dermatomes in the hand.

**10** The **motor** system of the hands can be tested with the instructions

(**a**) 'Open your hands; now close them; now open and close them quickly' (myotonic dystrophy)*

(**b**) 'Squeeze my fingers' – offer two fingers (C8, T1)†

(**c**) 'Hold your fingers out straight' (demonstrate); 'stop me bending them' (C7)

(**d**) 'Spread your fingers apart' (demonstrate); 'stop me pushing them together' (dorsal‡ interossei – ulnar nerve)

(**e**) 'Hold this piece of paper between your fingers; stop me pulling it out' (palmar‡ interossei – ulnar nerve)

(**f**) 'Point your thumb at the ceiling; stop me pushing it down' (abductor pollicis brevis – median nerve)

(**g**) 'Put your thumb and little finger together; stop me pulling them apart' (opponens pollicis – median nerve).

Finally, for the sake of completeness, check the

**11 radial pulses**.

The action you take after finding an abnormality at any stage during the above *routine* will depend on what you find. Most commonly, an abnormality found during the inspection will lead to most of the above being skipped in favour of a search for other evidence of the condition you suspect. It is worth emphasizing that there may be clues at

**12 the elbows** in several of the common conditions: rheumatoid arthritis (nodules), psoriatic arthropathy (psoriatic plaques), ulnar nerve palsy (scar, filling of the ulnar groove, restriction of range of movement at the elbow or evidence of fracture) and xanthomata. On the evidence of our survey, you will need to examine the elbows in over 40% of cases (do not be put off by rolled-down sleeves). It is worth considering where else you would look, what for and what other tests you would do with the other conditions on the list (see individual short cases in this book and in Volume 1), but in particular remember to look for *tophi* on the ears if you suspect gout, and if you have diagnosed acromegaly seek an associated *carpal tunnel syndrome* (see Vol. 2, Section F, Experience 116). If on inspection you suspect a neurological deficit in the hand, you may wish to confirm it by performing only that part of the above *routine* relevant to that lesion, e.g. testing abduction and opposition of the thumb and seeking the classic sensory pattern if you see lone wasting of the thenar eminence and suspect carpal tunnel syndrome.

See Appendix 1, Checklist 15, Hands.

---

*Alternatively, you could miss this step out and go straight to step (b), but then issue the instruction 'Let go' and if there is any suspicion of myotonic dystrophy move to step (a).

†Some neurologists prefer to test the deep finger flexors by trying to extend flexed fingers, whilst steadying the wrist (flexor digitorum profundus, C8).

‡Remember DAB and PAD: DAB = dorsal abduct, PAD = palmar adduct.

# 16 | 'Examine this patient's skin'

## Variations of instruction in initial PACES survey (resultant diagnoses in brackets)

Examine this patient's skin (psoriasis; neurofibromatosis)

Look at this patient's skin (psoriasis)

Examine this lady's skin (neurofibromatosis)

This man has itchy skin. Please examine (eczema)

## Diagnoses from our original survey in order of frequency*

1 Psoriasis (Station 5, Skin, Case 4) 15%

2 Vitiligo (Station 5, Skin, Case 8) 10%

3 Systemic sclerosis/CREST (Station 5, Locomotor, Case 3) 10%

4 Radiation burn on the chest (Station 5, Skin, Case 31) 10%

5 Epidermolysis bullosa dystrophica (Station 5, Skin, Case 30) 10%

6 Purpura (Station 5, Skin, Case 25) 5%

7 Pseudoxanthoma elasticum (Station 5, Skin, Case 10) 5%

8 Localized scleroderma (Station 5, Skin, Case 35) 5%

## Examination *routine*

This instruction is a rather more specific variation of the 'spot diagnosis' *routine* (see Examination *Routine* 22). You should

1 perform a *visual survey* of the patient, from scalp to sole, with regard to the fact that most dermatological lesions have a predilection for certain areas. It is as well to remember some of the regional associations as you *survey* the patient.

| | |
|---|---|
| *Scalp* | Psoriasis (look especially at the hairline for redness, scaling, etc.), alopecia,† ringworm (very uncommon) |
| *Face* | Systemic sclerosis (tight, shiny skin, pseudorhagades, beaked nose, telangiectasis), discoid lupus erythematosus (raised, red, scaly lesions with telangiectasis, scarring and altered pigmentation), xanthelasma, dermatomyositis (heliotrope colour to eyelids), Sturge–Weber, rodent ulcer (usually below the eye or on the side of the nose, raised lesion with central ulcer, the edges being rolled and having telangiectatic blood vessels) |
| *Mouth* | Osler–Weber–Rendu, Peutz–Jeghers, lichen planus (white lace-like network on mucosal surface), pemphigus, candidiasis (white exudate inside the mouth usually associated with a disease requiring multiple antimicrobial therapy or an immunosuppressive disorder, e.g. leukaemia, AIDS, etc.), herpes simplex, Behçet's |

*You may be asked to 'Examine this patient's skin'. However, it may be 'Examine this patient's hands, face or rash' or just 'Look at this patient'. The figures here apply only to when the instruction was to examine the skin.

†Some causes of alopecia:

1 Diffuse – male pattern baldness, cytotoxic drugs, hypothyroidism, hyperthyroidism, iron deficiency

2 Patchy – alopecia areata, ringworm; with scarring – discoid lupus erythematosus, lichen planus.

| | |
|---|---|
| *Neck* | Pseudoxanthoma elasticum, tuberculous adenitis with sinus formation (?ethnic origin) |
| *Trunk* | Radiotherapy stigmata, morphoea, neurofibromatosis, dermatitis herpetiformis (itching blisters over scapulae, buttocks, elbows, knees), herpes zoster along the intercostal nerves, pityriasis rosea, Addison's (areolar and scar pigmentation), pemphigus (trunk and limbs) |
| *Axillae* | Vitiligo, acanthosis nigricans (pigmentation and velvety thickening of axillary skin, perianal, areolar and lateral abdominal skin, 'tripe palms', mucous membranes involved, may be underlying insulin resistance or malignancy) |
| *Elbows* | Psoriasis (extensor), pseudoxanthoma elasticum (flexor), xanthomata (extensor), rheumatoid nodules (extensor), atopic dermatitis (flexor), olecranon bursitis, gouty tophi |
| *Hands* | Systemic sclerosis (sclerodactyly, infarcts of finger pulps, prominent capillaries at nail-folds), lichen planus (wrists), dermatomyositis (heliotrope lesions – Gottron's papules – on the joints of the dorsum of the fingers/hands, nail-fold capillary dilation and infarction), Addison's (skin crease pigmentation), granuloma annulare, erythema multiforme (polymorphic eruption, 'target' lesions, mucous membrane involvement, macules, vesicles, bullae, etc.), SLE (erythematous patches over the dorsal surface of the phalanges), scabies (not in MRCP PACES!) |
| *Nails* | Psoriasis (pitting, onycholysis), iron deficiency (koilonychia), fungal dystrophy, tuberous sclerosis (periungal fibromata) |
| *Genitalia* | Behçet's (iridocyclitis, uveitis, pyodermas, ulcers, etc.), lichen sclerosus (white plaques), candidiasis |
| *Legs* | Leg ulcer (diabetic, venous, ischaemic, pyoderma gangrenosum), necrobiosis lipoidica diabeticorum, pretibial myxoedema, erythema nodosum, Henoch–Schönlein purpura, tendon xanthomata in Achilles, erythema ab igne, pemphigoid (legs and arms), lipoatrophy |
| *Feet* | Pustular psoriasis, eczema, verrucae, keratoderma blenorrhagica (?eyes, joints, etc.) |

During this *survey* you should consider

**2** the **distribution** of the lesions (psoriasis on extensor areas, lichen planus in flexor areas, candidiasis on mucous membranes, tuberous sclerosis on nails and face, necrobiosis lipoidica diabeticorum usually bilateral, gouty tophi in the joints of hands, elbows and on the ears, etc.). Then after the *survey* (which should take a few seconds)

**3** examine the **lesions** (see Examination *Routine* 17, 'Examine this patient's rash'), looking in particular for the *characteristic* features, e.g. scaling in psoriasis, shiny purple polygonal papules with Wickham's striae in lichen planus, etc. If you have made a diagnosis, consider whether you need to look for any

**4 associated lesions** (arthropathy and nail changes with psoriasis, evidence of associated autoimmune disease with vitiligo, etc.). Go through the skin conditions which our survey has suggested occur in the exam and make sure that you would recognize each, would know what else to look for, and what to say in your presentation.

See Appendix 1, Checklist 16, Skin.

# 17 | 'Examine this patient's rash'

***Variations of instruction in initial PACES survey (resultant diagnoses in brackets)***

Take a look at this lady's rash (?examiners didn't know either – rash of uncertain cause)

This lady has a rash. Examine it (mixed connective tissue disease)

***Diagnoses from our original survey in order of frequency****

1 Psoriasis (Station 5, Skin, Case 4) 20%
2 Purpura (Station 5, Skin, Case 25) 10%
3 Vasculitis (Station 5, Locomotor, Case 10) 10%
4 Neurofibromatosis (Station 5, Skin, Case 2) 10%
5 Juvenile chronic arthritis (Still's disease) (Station 5, Locomotor, Case 18) 10%
6 Xanthomata (Station 5, Skin, Case 7) 5%
7 Necrobiosis lipoidica diabeticorum (Station 5, Skin, Case 18) 5%
8 Radiation burn on the chest (Station 5, Skin, Case 31) 5%

## Examination *routine*

This *routine* is generally the same as that discussed under 'Examine this patient's skin' (see Examination *Routine* 16).

1 You should quickly conduct a *visual survey* as described under 'skin' and note if there are any similar or related lesions elsewhere. Look at the

2 **distribution** of the lesions, whether confined to a single area (morphoea, erythema nodosum, rodent ulcer, melanoma, alopecia areata, etc.) or present in other areas such as psoriasis, neurofibromatosis, acanthosis nigricans, dermatomyositis, etc. While concentrating on the lesion in question, it is important to look at the

3 **surrounding skin** for any helpful clues such as *scratch marks* as evidence of itching,† *radiotherapy field markings* on the skin in the vicinity of a radiation burn, or *paper-thin skin* with purpura (corticosteroid therapy), etc. You should now

4 **examine the lesion** in detail. To determine the *extent* of the lesion, you may have to ask the patient to undress, a procedure which will provide you with a little more time to survey other areas. Decide if the rash is *pleomorphic* or *monomorphic* (all the lesions are similar). If so, examine one typical lesion carefully in terms of:

   (a) *colour*, e.g. erythematous or pigmented,
   (b) *size*,
   (c) *shape*, e.g. oval, circular, annular, etc.,
   (d) *surface*, e.g. scaling or eroded,
   (e) *character*, e.g. macule, papule, vesicle, pustule, ulcer, etc.,
   (f) *secondary features*, e.g. crusting, lichenification, etc.

---

*See Footnote, Examination *Routine* 16. The same sentiment applies here.
†Some causes of itching:
1 Dermatological – scabies, dermatitis herpetiformis, lichen planus, eczema

2 Medical – cholestasis, chronic renal failure, lymphoma, polycythaemia rubra vera.

It is advisable to be familiar with the correct use of the terms to describe rashes (especially if you do not recognize the lesion!). To say 'skin lesion' or 'skin rash' conveys no diagnostic meaning. In your presentation, you should be able to describe the lesion with respect to the above six features, especially if you do not know the diagnosis. The following are some of the useful terms employed in describing skin lesions:

*Macules*: flat, circumscribed lesions, not raised above the skin – size and shape vary

*Papules*: raised, circumscribed, firm lesions up to 1cm in size

*Nodules*: like papules but larger; usually lie deeper in skin

*Tumours*: larger than nodules, elevated or very deeply placed in the skin

*Weals*: circumscribed elevations associated with itching and tingling

*Vesicles*: small well-defined collections of fluid

*Bullae*: large vesicles

*Pustules*: circumscribed elevations containing purulent fluid which may, in some cases, be sterile (e.g. Behçet's)

*Scales*: dead tissue from the horny layer which may be dry (e.g. psoriasis) or greasy (e.g. seborrhoeic dermatitis)

*Crusts*: these consist of dried exudate

*Ulcers*: excavations in the skin of irregular shape; remember that every ulcer has a shape, an edge, a floor, a base and a secretion, and it forms a scar on healing

*Scars*: the result of healing of a damaged dermis.

5  Finally, if indicated, look for **additional features** (arthropathy in psoriasis or Still's disease, cushingoid facies if purpura is due to steroids, clubbing with radiation burns on the chest, etc.).

See Appendix 1, Checklist 17, Rash.

# 18 | 'Examine this patient's neck'

*Variations of instruction in initial PACES survey (resultant diagnoses in brackets)*

Examine this patient's neck (goitre; pseudoxanthoma elasticum; multinodular goitre)

This patient has noticed a swelling in his neck – please examine (goitre)

This patient has a goitre. Please examine her (exophthalmos and non-nodular goitre)

*Diagnoses from our original survey in order of frequency*

1  Goitre (Station 5, Endocrine, Case 4) 46%

2  Generalized lymphadenopathy (Vol. 1, Station 1, Abdominal, Case 14) 17%

3  Graves' disease (Station 5, Endocrine, Case 3) 12%

4  Jugular vein pulse abnormality (Vol. 1, Station 3, CNS, Cases 11, 18 and 25) 6%

5 Bilateral parotid enlargement/Mikulicz's syndrome (Station 5, Other, Case 1) 4%

6 Supraclavicular mass with Horner's syndrome (Vol.1, Station 3, CNS, Case 41) 4%

7 Facioscapulohumeral muscular dystrophy (Vol.1, Station 3, CNS, Case 9) 4%

8 Ankylosing spondylitis (Station 5, Locomotor, Case 6) 2%

9 Hypothyroidism (Station 5, Locomotor, Case 5) 2%

10 Acanthosis nigricans (Station 5, Skin, Case 48) <1%

## Examination *routine*

As usual, the first step is to

1 *survey* the patient quickly from head to foot (exophthalmos, myxoedematous facies, ankle oedema, etc.) and then to

2 **look at the neck**. According to the survey, the reason for the instruction in half of the cases will be a *goitre*. If another abnormality is visible, your further action will be dictated by what you see and we suggest you go through the list and establish a sequence of actions for each abnormality (e.g. if you see giant *v* waves you would wish to examine the heart and liver; see Vol. 1, Station 3, Cardiovascular, Case 11). If you do see a goitre, offer a drink to the patient:

'Take a sip of water and hold it in your mouth';

look at the neck:

'Now swallow'.

Watch the movement of the goitre, or the *appearance* of a *nodule* not visible before swallowing (behind sternomastoid; see Fig. I5.64c2, Station 5, Endocrine, Case 4). Next ask the patient's permission to feel the neck, and then approach him from behind. If there has been no evidence of a goitre so far you may wish to palpate the neck for lymph nodes *before* feeling for a goitre. Otherwise

3 **palpate** the thyroid. With the right index and middle fingers, feel below the thyroid cartilage where the isthmus of the thyroid gland lies over the trachea. Then palpate the two lobes of the thyroid gland which extend laterally behind the sterno-mastoid muscle. Ask the patient to swallow again while you continue to palpate the thyroid, ensuring that the neck is slightly flexed to ease palpation. Remember that if there is a goitre, when you give your presentation you are going to want to comment on its *size*, whether it is *soft* or *firm*, whether it is *nodular* or *diffusely enlarged*, whether it *moves* readily on swallowing, whether there are *lymph nodes* (see below) and whether there is a vascular *murmur* (see below). Extend palpation upwards along the medial edge of the sternomastoid muscle on either side to look for a *pyramidal lobe* which may be present. Apologize for any discomfort you may cause because the deep palpation necessary to feel the thyroid gland causes pain,* particularly in patients with Graves' disease. *Percussion* over the upper sternum is used to assess any retrosternal extension of goitre. Next palpate laterally to examine for

4 **lymph nodes**. If you find lymph node enlargement, check not only in the *supraclavicular fossae* and right up the neck but also in the *submandibular*, *post-auricular* and *suboccipital* areas, ensuring that the head is slightly flexed on the side

---

*In viral thyroiditis (rare) the patient may complain of a painful thyroid and the thyroid may be overtly tender on light palpation.

under palpation to allow access and scrutiny of slightly enlarged lymph nodes. Ascertain whether the lymph nodes are *separate* (reactive hyperplasia, infectious mononucleosis, lymphoma, etc.) or *matted* together (neoplastic, tuberculous), *mobile* or *fixed* to the skin or deep tissues (neoplastic), or whether they are *soft*, *fleshy*, *rubbery* (Hodgkin's disease) or *hard* (neoplastic). Particularly if you find lymph nodes without a goitre, examine for lymph nodes in the axillae and groins (lymphoma, chronic lymphatic leukaemia, etc.) and, if allowed, feel for the spleen.

**5 Auscultate** over the thyroid for evidence of increased vascularity. You may need to occlude venous return to rule out a venous hum, and listen over the aortic area to ensure that the thyroid bruit you hear is not, in fact, an outflow obstruction murmur conducted to the root of the neck.

**6** If there is any evidence of thyroid disease, consider beginning an assessment of **thyroid status** (see Examination *Routine* 19, 'Assess this patient's thyroid status') by feeling and counting the pulse (NB: do not miss *atrial fibrillation*, whether slow or fast). The examiner will soon stop you if he wishes to hear your description of a multinodular goitre in a euthyroid patient.

See Appendix 1, Checklist 18, Neck.


# 19 | 'Assess this patient's thyroid status'


***Variations of instruction in initial PACES survey (resultant diagnoses in brackets)***
Examine this lady's thyroid status (euthyroid)
This lady has had previous problems with her thyroid. Examine her to determine her thyroid status (euthyroid)

***Diagnoses from original survey in order of frequency***
**1** Euthyroid Graves' disease (Station 5, Endocrine, Case 3) 42%
**2** Hyperthyroidism (Station 5, Endocrine, Case 3) 17%
**3** Euthyroid simple goitre (Station 5, Endocrine, Case 4) 8%

## Examination *routine*
Although the patient usually has signs of thyroid disease (exophthalmos, goitre), you are not being asked to examine these but rather to assess whether the patient is clinically hypo-, eu- or hyperthyroid. Perform a speedy
**1** *visual survey*, looking specifically for *signs of thyroid disease* (exophthalmos, goitre, thyroid acropachy, pretibial myxoedema – all can occur in association with *any* thyroid status), and ask yourself if the facies are in any way myxoedematous. Observe the patient's

**2 composure**, whether *hyperactive, fidgety* and *restless* (hyperthyroid); normal, composed demeanour (euthyroid); or if she is somewhat *immobile* and *uninterested* in the people around her (hypothyroid).

**3 Take the pulse** and *count* it for 15 seconds, noting the presence or absence of *atrial fibrillation* (slow, normal rate or fast). If the pulse is slow (less than 60) or if you suspect hypothyroidism, proceed immediately to test for

**4 slow relaxation** of the ankle,* supinator or other jerks. To test the reflexes, you will require the patient's cooperation and the ensuing conversation may provide you with helpful clues (slow hesitant speech, slow movements, etc.). Otherwise,

**5** feel the **palms**, whether *warm* and *sweaty* or cold and sweaty (anxiety) and then

**6** ask the patient to stretch out his hands to full extension of the wrist and elbow. If the **tremor** is not obvious, place your palm against his outstretched fingers to feel for it. Alternatively, you can place a piece of paper on the dorsum of his outstretched hands – it will oscillate if a fine tremor is present.

**7** Look at the **eyes**, noting exophthalmos (sclera visible above the lower lid, a sign not related to thyroid status) but looking specifically for *lid retraction* (sclera visible above the cornea). Test for lid lag (lid lag and retraction may diminish as the hyperthyroid patient becomes euthyroid).

**8** Examine the **thyroid** as described under 'Examine this patient's neck' (see Examination *Routine* 18), remembering the steps are (i) look, (ii) palpate and (iii) auscultate.†

Putting the above findings together, it should be possible to provide a definite conclusion about thyroid status; this is considered a very basic skill and it will not be taken lightly if, in your state of nerves, you make fundamental errors. Though the examiner may put you under pressure to test your confidence, keep calm and be particularly wary of being led to diagnose hypo- or hyperthyroidism in the presence of a normal pulse rate (see Vol. 2, Section F, Experience 191).

**9** Be prepared with the **standard questions** for assessment of thyroid status (temperature preference, weight change, appetite, bowel habits, palpitations, change of temper, etc; see Station 5, Endocrine, Case 5) if there is any doubt about the thyroid status after the above examination.

See Appendix 1, Checklist 19, Thyroid status.

---

*The slow relaxing ankle jerk in hypothyroidism is best demonstrated with the patient kneeling on a chair or bed with the feet hanging over the edge, and the examiner standing behind the patient. This manoeuvre is useful for the dressed patient in the outpatient department and may be useful in the PACES exam if the patient is dressed and sitting on a chair.

†A thyroid bruit is good evidence of thyroid overactivity; if present, it can be heard over the isthmus and lateral lobe of the thyroid; it will not be obliterated by occluding the internal jugular vein (venous hum) or by rotation of the head and it will not be influenced by pressure of the stethoscope (use light pressure to avoid causing non-thyroid bruits).

# 20 | 'Examine this patient's knee'

***Possible diagnoses***
Rheumatoid arthritis
Seronegative spondyloarthropathy
   Psoriatic arthritis
   Ankylosing spondylitis
   Inflammatory bowel disease
   Reactive arthritis
Gout
Pseudogout
Septic arthritis
Osteoarthritis
Haemarthrosis
Prepatellar bursitis
Baker's cyst
Charcot's joint

## Examination *routine*
If asked to examine a patient's knees, you should bear the following in mind:
   **(a)** is it an *inflammatory* or *non-inflammatory* problem?
   **(b)** is it *a monoarthritis* or part of a more widespread arthropathy (*oligo-* or *polyarthropathy* or *spondyloarthropathy*)?
   **(c)** is the pain (if any) referred from elsewhere (i.e. hip)?
   **(d)** are there any extraarticular features?
   **(e)** what is the functional impairment?

 **1** On approaching the patient, **observe** for any other obvious features of joint disease (e.g. symmetrical deforming polyarthritis in the hands of *rheumatoid arthritis*, an asymmetrical arthritis and skin plaques of *psoriatic arthritis*, or podagra of the first MTP joint as seen in gout).

 **2 Ask** the patient if he has any pain and expose the leg from the upper thigh to the foot.

 **3 Inspect** the leg. Is there any obvious deformity (*valgus* or *varus* deformity or *flexion* deformity)? Are there any scars or wounds to suggest entry for infection? Is there any muscle wasting (*quadriceps*)? Is the knee swollen or erythematous? Look for loss of the medial and lateral dimples around the knees to suggest the presence of an effusion. Compare one side with the other as you progress through the examination.

 **4 Palpate** the joint. Is it warm? Place your whole hand gently over the patient's knee and rest it there for a few seconds. Compare the temperature of this knee with the mid calf and mid thigh on the same side as well as the opposite knee. Do not be too quick to move your hands as you may miss subtle differences in temperature. Watch the patient's face for any sign that you are causing him discomfort. Ask if the knee is tender on palpation.

   By this stage you should have an idea of whether this is an inflammatory or non-inflammatory problem and how active it is.

5 Examine for an **effusion**. For a small effusion look for the *bulge sign*. With your index finger, firmly wipe any fluid from the medial joint recess (moving from distal to proximal) into the lateral joint recess. Now apply a similar wiping motion from distal to proximal in the lateral joint recess. A distinct bulge will be seen to appear back in the medial compartment as the fluid moves back to this side of the joint. For larger effusions the bulge sign is absent and the presence of fluid needs to be assessed by the *patellar tap*. Firm pressure is applied over the suprapatellar pouch with the flat of one hand, using the thumb and index finger to push any fluid from the medial and lateral joint compartments into the retropatellar space. With the index finger or thumb of the other hand, apply a short jerky movement to the patella. The presence of significant fluid is indicated by a spongy feel followed by a 'tap' as the patella hits the anterior aspect of the lower end of the femur.

6 Assess **movement**. Ask the patient to flex the knee as far as possible. Observe the degree of flexion (and any discomfort). Normal flexion is 135°.

7 Palpate for any **crepitus** over the joint as flexion occurs and feel behind the knee for a

8 **Baker's cyst**.

9 Assess for joint **instability**. Examine for *cruciate* instability (anterior and posterior draw test*) and medial and lateral ligament instability. *McMurray's sign* can be used to examine for cartilage tears. The knee is fully flexed and then internally rotated before being straightened by the examiner. Pain, or a clunking feeling, over the knee joint suggests a cartilage tear. The test is repeated with external rotation of the knee.

10 Ask to examine the **other joints**. Do not forget to ask about examining the other knee and spine (for associated inflammatory spondylitis). Are there any features of *psoriasis, inflammatory bowel disease, reactive arthritis* (enthesitis, keratoderma blenorrhagica, conjunctivitis, balanitis) or tophi to suggest *gout*?

Finally, think of relevant *investigations* such as X-rays for changes of rheumatoid arthritis, osteoarthrosis or pseudogout; synovial fluid analysis for crystals (negative or positive birefringence on polarized microscopy, gram stain and culture for infection).

See Appendix 1, Checklist 20, Knee.

---

*With the patient supine, flex the knee to 90 degrees, place your hands around the upper calf and gently pull forward or push backward looking for significant anterior or posterior movement of the tibia plateau. Compare with the other side.

# 21 | 'Examine this patient's hip'

***Possible diagnoses***

Osteoarthrosis

Rheumatoid arthritis

Seronegative spondyloarthritis

   Ankylosing spondylitis

   Psoriatic arthritis

   Inflammatory bowel disease

   Reactive arthritis (chronic)

Septic arthritis

Avascular necrosis

Paget's

Iliopsoas bursitis

Sciatica

## Examination *routine*

**1 Inspect** the leg. Is the hip held in a flexed position? Is there any shortening of the leg? Is the leg externally rotated? Look for any scars. Are there any other obvious stigmata of rheumatic disease (e.g. rheumatoid arthritis, psoriatic arthropathy, ankylosing spondylitis, osteoarthritis)? Look for any walking aids.

**2 Ask** the patient if they have any pain. Ask them to show the location of the pain. Pain in the groin is more suggestive of hip disease.

**3** Assess **movement**. With the patient lying flat and with his knee bent, ask him to flex his hip to the chest. Then, assess the degree of internal and external rotation. With both the knee and hip flexed to 90°, rotate the hip joint internally and externally using the foot as a pointer and the knee as a pivot. Estimate the degree of rotation. Next, assess hip abduction and adduction by placing one hand on the opposite iliac crest (to keep the pelvis stationary); then, place your other hand under the ankle of the leg being examined and abduct and adduct the hip. The normal range of movement is flexion 120°, internal rotation 30°, external rotation 45°, abduction 60°, adduction 30°. A hip flexion deformity may be masked by an increased spinal lordosis. Flex the opposite hip (with knee bent) to flatten out the lumbar lordosis (feel with your hand under the patient's spine). Any fixed flexion deformity of the opposite hip will be brought out by the flattening of the lumbar spine (*Thomas's test*).

**4** If no abnormality is detected then consider whether the pain may be coming from the patient's spine. Carry out a **straight leg raise**. Slowly raise the patient's leg by taking hold of his heel and lifting the leg slowly. Stop if pain occurs. Pain in the leg to the foot is indicative of pain originating in the *spine* – nerve root entrapment. You may need to undertake a *neurological assessment* to test for abnormalities in muscle strength (particularly of ankle plantarflexion), sensation or reflexes (be prepared to differentiate a nerve root from a peripheral nerve lesion).

**5** Check for **tenderness** over the greater trochanter (trochanteric bursitis).

**6** You may need to check for **leg length** inequality* (measure from the anterior superior iliac crest to the medial malleolus on the same side, compare with other leg).

**7** Ask the patient to **walk**. An antalgic gait occurs when there is pain in one hip and the patient leans to the other side to avoid putting weight on the affected side. A waddling gait is indicative of hip muscle weakness (e.g. osteomalacia, myositis).

You would be interested to see X-rays of the pelvis. Consider what other investigations you would request for the conditions on the list above.

See Appendix 1, Checklist 21, Hip.

# 22 | 'What is the diagnosis?'

*Variations of instruction in initial PACES survey (resultant diagnoses in brackets)*
What is the diagnosis? (psoriasis)
This lady has had multiple fractures. What is your diagnosis? (?Turner's syndrome)
Examine this gentleman. What do you notice? (cushingoid due to steroids)
Examine this patient (peripheral and central cyanosis)
Look at this patient (acromegaly; scleroderma; drug eruption)
This woman has glycosuria. Look at her and examine anything that is relevant (acromegaly and xanthelasma)
This patient is tired all the time. Why is that? (koilonychia)
Examine this patient's spine (ankylosing spondylitis and aortic incompetence)
This lady has been having headaches. Please examine the appropriate systems (acromegaly)
Describe this lady's abnormalities (systemic sclerosis)
Look at this man and examine the patient as you feel appropriate (acromegaly)
This lady has had headaches. Please examine her (acromegaly)
You must know the diagnosis of this patient (neurofibromatosis)
This lady complains of some abnormalities in her gums. Please examine her (lichen planus)
This lady has uncontrolled hypertension. Please examine her (pituitary tumour)

*The reasons to examine for a shorter leg are: (i) for protrusio acetabulum, which occurs mainly in rheumatoid arthritis when the femoral head migrates through the acetabulum because of regional osteoporosis. (ii) Where there has been a fracture which has gone undetected at the neck of femur. (iii) When a patient has had a joint replacement (mainly hip, but knee also) where there has been a need to shorten the bone a bit more than the prosthesis allows. (iv) Where a Girdlestone procedure is carried out – when no hip joint prosthesis is placed (or removed) because of sepsis or patient's general health does not allow a major operation and, basically, the neck of the femur and femoral head are excised and the femur is held in place by the joint capsule, but migrates upwards. (v) Where there is apparent leg shortening which occurs due to pelvic tilt secondary to spinal disease – in this case the leg is not actually shortened, hence the need to measure both leg lengths.

This middle-aged man complains of headaches. Would you like to assess him and tell me why? (acromegaly)

Have a look at this lady who presented to the A & E department with acute shortness of breath and tell me why (spontaneous pneumothorax due to tuberous sclerosis)

Look at the hands, look at the face and give the diagnosis (hypertrophic pulmonary osteoarthropathy)

What do you think of this lady? (cushingoid due to steroids)

*Diagnoses from our original survey in order of frequency*

 1 Acromegaly (Station 5, Endocrine, Case 2) 11%
 2 Parkinson's disease (Vol. 1, Station 3, CNS, Case 3) 5%
 3 Hemiplegia (Vol. 1, Station 3, CNS, Case 8) 5%
 4 Goitre (Station 5, Endocrine, Case 4) 5%
 5 Jaundice (Vol.1, Station 1, Abdominal, Cases 3 and 15–17) 5%
 6 Myotonic dystrophy (Vol. 1, Station 3, CNS, Case 2) 4%
 7 Pigmentation (Station 5, Endocrine, Case 7) 4%
 8 Graves' disease (Station 5, Endocrine, Case 3) 4%
 9 Exophthalmos (Station 5, Endocrine, Case 1) 4%
10 Paget's disease (Station 5, Locomotor, Case 7) 3%
11 Ptosis (Vol. 1, Station 3, CNS, Case 18) 3%
12 Choreoathetosis (Vol. 1, Station 3, CNS, Case 20) 3%
13 Drug-induced parkinsonism (Vol.1, Station 3, CNS, Case 34) 3%
14 Breathlessness 2%
15 Purpura (Station 5, Skin, Case 25) 2%
16 Hypopituitarism (Station 5, Endocrine, Case 8) 2%
17 Addison's/Nelson's (Station 5, Endocrine, Case 7) 2%
18 Cushing's syndrome (Station 5, Endocrine, Case 6) 2%
19 Psoriasis (Station 5, Skin, Case 4) 2%
20 Hypothyroidism (Station 5, Endocrine, Case 5) 2%
21 Systemic sclerosis/CREST (Station 5, Locomotor, Case 3) 2%
22 Sturge–Weber syndrome (Station 5, Skin, Case 24) 2%
23 Spider naevi and ascites (Vol.1, Station 1, Abdominal, Case 7) 1%
24 Marfan's syndrome (Station 5, Locomotor, Case 9) 1%
25 Neurofibromatosis (Station 5, Skin, Case 2) 1%
26 Cyanotic congenital heart disease (Vol.1, Station 3, CNS, Case 27) 1%
27 Pretibial myxoedema (Station 5, Endocrine, Case 9) 1%
28 Uraemia and dialysis scars (Vol. 1, Station 1, Abdominal, Case 2) 1%
29 Horner's syndrome (Vol. 1, Station 3, CNS, Case 41) 1%
30 Cachexia (Vol. 1, Station 1, Respiratory, Case 13 and Station 1, Abdominal, Cases 5 and 8) 1%
31 Osler–Weber–Rendu syndrome (Station 5, Skin, Case 3) 1%
32 Ankylosing spondylitis (Station 5, Locomotor, Case 6) 1%
33 Ulnar nerve palsy (Vol. 1, Station 3, CNS, Case 14) 1%
34 Turner's syndrome (Station 5, Endocrine, Case 11) 1%
35 Down's syndrome (Station 5, Other, Case 5) 1%

**36** Bilateral parotid enlargement/Mikulicz's syndrome (Station 5, Other, Case 1) 1%

**37** Old rickets (Station 5, Locomotor, Case 17) 1%

**38** Torticollis 1%

**39** Congenital syphilis (Vol. 1, Station 3, CNS, Case 39) 1%

**40** Syringomyelia (Vol. 1, Station 3, CNS, Case 29) <1%

**41** Herpes zoster (Station 5, Skin, Case 32) <1%

**42** Pemphigoid/pemphigus (Station 5, Skin, Case 30) <1%

**43** Bell's palsy (Vol.1, Station 3, CNS, Case 35) <1%

**44** Necrobiosis lipoidica diabeticorum (Station 5, Skin, Case 18) <1%

**45** Primary biliary cirrhosis (Vol. 1, Station 1, Abdominal, Case 17) <1%

## Examination *routine*

Advice commonly given by the candidates in our survey as a result of their Membership experiences was to 'keep calm'. When you stand before a patient with a condition from the above list and hear the instruction under consideration, you are being asked to do what you do every day of your medical life. There are two differences, however, between everyday medical life and the examination: (i) the patients in the examination usually have classic, often florid, signs and should be easier to diagnose than most patients seen in the clinic; and (ii) in the examination, you may be overwhelmed by nerves and, as a result, make the most fundamental errors. You must indeed try to keep calm and remind yourself that this is likely to be an easy case, and that you will not only make a diagnosis (as you would with ease in the clinic), but will also find a way of scoring some extra marks. Unlike some of the instructions requiring long examination *routines*, the 'spot diagnosis' may be solved in seconds leaving time for something extra which you may be able to dictate, rather than leaving it to the examiner to lead. You should start with

**1** *a visual survey* of the patient, running your eyes from the head via the neck, trunk, arms and legs to the feet, seeking the areas of abnormality, and thereby the diagnosis. We would suggest that you rehearse presenting the *records* for the various possibilities on the list (see individual short cases in this book and in Volume 1). If you are well prepared with the features of these short cases, then in the majority of instances you should be able to make a diagnosis, or likely diagnosis, which you can confirm or highlight by demonstrating additional features (see below). If you have scanned the patient briefly and not found any obvious abnormality, then

**2 retrace** the same ground, scrutinizing each part more thoroughly and asking yourself at each stage, 'Is the head normal?', 'Is the face normal?', etc. If it is not normal, describe the abnormality to yourself in the mind, trying to match it up with one of the short case *records*. In this way, cover the

   **(a)** head (think especially of *Paget's* and *myotonic dystrophy* with frontal balding),

   **(b)** face (think especially of *acromegaly*, *Parkinson's*, the facial asymmetry of *hemiplegia*, the long lean look of myotonic dystrophy, tardive dyskinesia, hypopituitarism, Cushing's, hypothyroidism, systemic sclerosis),

   **(c)** eyes (*jaundice, exophthalmos*, ptosis, Horner's, xanthelasma),

   **(d)** neck (*goitre*, Turner's, ankylosing spondylitis, torticollis),

   **(e)** trunk (pigmentation, ascites, purpuric spots, spider naevi, wasting, pemphigus, etc.),

   **(f)** arms (choreoathetosis, psoriasis, Addison's, spider naevi, syringomyelia), (**g**) hands (acromegaly, *tremor*, clubbing, sclerodactyly, arachnodactyly, claw hand, etc.),

(**h**) legs (bowing, purpura, pretibial myxoedema, necrobiosis lipoidica diabeticorum), and

(**i**) feet (pes cavus).

If you still do not have the diagnosis

**3** specifically consider **abnormal colouring** such as *pigmentation, icterus* or pallor, and then cover the same ground again but in even more detail,

**4 breaking down each part into its constituents**, scrutinizing them, and continually asking yourself the question: 'Is it normal?'. This procedure is most profitable on the face (Examination *Routine* 14).

Once you have the diagnosis, the natural impulse for most people is to give it in one word, and then stand back and wait for the applause. However, it is worth remembering that the majority of the candidates, who have all worked hard and prepared for the examination, are likely to 'spot' the diagnosis and yet only a few end up with the diploma. Do not let this opportunity pass you by; try to make more of the case yourself by proceeding to

**5** look for **additional** and **associated features**, and then by making your presentation more elaborate. Describe the findings in detail (see individual short cases in this book and in Volume 1) and highlight the key features to support your diagnosis (lenticular abnormalities in myotonic dystrophy and Marfan's; thyroid bruit in Graves' disease; webbed neck in Turner's syndrome, and so on). It is worth going through the diagnoses on the list yourself, and considering what additional features you would look for, and how you could really go to town on an easy case. For example, if you diagnose acromegaly you could demonstrate the massive sweaty palms, commenting on the increased skin thickening and on the presence or absence of thenar wasting (carpal tunnel syndrome; see Vol. 2, Section F, Experience 116), and then proceed to test the visual fields. If you suspect Parkinson's disease, take the hands and test for cog-wheel rigidity at the wrist, demonstrate the glabellar tap sign (despite its unreliability) and then ask the patient to walk. If you diagnose hemiplegia, confirm that any facial weakness is upper motor neurone (see Vol. 1, Station 3, CNS, Case 8), and then check for atrial fibrillation. If you see a goitre, examine it and then assess the thyroid status.

See Appendix 1, Checklist 22, 'Spot' diagnosis.

# Section H
# Station 5, Integrated Clinical Assessment

*'Tis not in mortals to command success,*
*But we'll do more, Sempronius; we'll deserve it.'\**

\**Cato*, Act I, Scene II. Joseph Addison, 1712.

These books exist as they are because of many previous candidates who, over the years, have completed our surveys and given us invaluable insight into the candidate experience. Please give something back by doing the same for the candidates of the future. For all of your sittings, whether they be a triumphant pass or a disastrous fail . . .
**Remember to fill in the survey at www.ryder-mrcp.org.uk**

THANK YOU

## Acknowledgements
Thank you to all of our colleagues who generously gave their time to review their specialty's cases, and for the extra material they contributed.

Dr Steve Sturman, Consultant Neurologist, Sandwell and West Birmingham Hospitals NHS Trust (SWBH)

Dr Sherrini Bazir Ahmad, Specialist Registrar, Neurology, University Hospitals Birmingham Foundation Trust

Dr David Carruthers, Consultant Rheumatologist, SWBH (and author of additional rheumatology material)

Dr Teri Millane, Consultant Cardiologist, SWBH

Dr Parijat De (with some input from Dr Bob Ryder), Consultant Diabetologists/ Endocrinologists, SWBH

Dr Shivan Pancham, Consultant Haematologist, SWBH

Dr Omer Khair, Consultant Respiratory Physician, SWBH

Dr Shireen Velangi, Consultant Dermatologist, SWBH

Mr Matthew Edmunds, Wellcome Trust Clinical Research Fellow and Specialty Registrar in Ophthalmology, Centre for Translational Inflammation Research, University of Birmingham

Dr Sarah Moon, Consultant Medical Oncologist, University Hospitals of Morecambe Bay NHS Foundation Trust

Thank you to all the PACES candidates over the past few years who have contacted me with their experiences of the new Station 5, and to Dr Nidhi Sagar for her cases.

Thank you to Bob Ryder for the invitation to write this section, a little editing of the introduction, and for sprinkling the introduction with quotes from the survey; to Dr Brian Cooper for help and guidance with the introduction and for his support throughout; to Helen Harvey for all her help and support throughout the publication process, and to Anne Freeman for proof-reading this volume.

And

A big thank you to my wife, Steph, for her patience and support throughout, and to my son, Thomas, who made his entrance during the proof-reading.

*Edward Fogden*
2013

*'Once again I tried to compose myself as much as possible between stations so as to think clearly for the dreaded Station 5.'**

The new format for PACES Station 5, called 'integrated clinical assessment', was introduced in the third diet of 2009. This section has been written in response to these changes, and has been informed by the results of surveys of candidates and discussions with examiners past and present.

This 'integrated clinical assessment' consists of two brief clinical consultations during which the candidate combines focused history taking and clinical examination, followed by an explanation to the patient of the diagnosis, plan and discussion of any concerns they have, before discussing any abnormal physical signs, diagnoses and management plan (if not already covered) with the examiners.

The new Station 5 now makes up a significant part of the exam (37% of the total marks) on account of the current marking scheme. It tests all seven of the clinical skills assessed in the PACES examination (marking parameters), whereas other stations only test 4–5. The two scenarios from the new Station 5 therefore make up a third of the PACES overall mark.

## Format of the new Station 5

*'The examiners were friendly and the chief examiner came out to tell us all that it was going to be fun and not too difficult!'†*

There are two 10-minute brief clinical consultations. You receive information on both cases outside prior to the start of the station. You are given a short paragraph for each of the clinical scenarios which sets the scene (e.g. a referral letter/situation facing the senior house officer [SHO] in the medical assessment unit [MAU]) and you have 5 minutes to read them both. You are allowed to make notes and rough paper will be provided for this. You are allowed to take the scenario instructions and your rough notes into the exam station.

Each of the cases takes 10 minutes in total. You have 8 minutes to take a focused history and carry out a focused examination (which can be carried out at the same time) to define the clinical problem, explain the diagnosis and plan to the patient, and to answer any questions and directly address their concerns. The patient or surrogate will have been briefed to ask two specific questions. You will get a warning from one of the examiners after 6 minutes have passed.

The last 2 minutes of the station are for discussion with the examiners: one examiner will ask you to report on any abnormal physical signs elicited, your diagnosis or differential diagnoses, and your plan for management (if not already clear from your discussion with the patient).

In the unlikely event that you have finished before the 8 minutes are up, the examiner will tell you that there is more time and ask if there is anything further that you wish to do; if not, the short viva will start.

You then move onto the next case. You are allowed to briefly look at your second scenario, and your notes, to refresh your memory.

---

*Vol. 2, Section F, Experience 1, Station 5.                    †Vol. 2, Section F, Experience 9.

## Cases involved

*'For the first case I had a patient with atypical psoriatic arthropathy and I was fairly sure that there was some rheumatoid overlap here.'\**

*'I had a quick look at her neck when I introduced myself and it was clear that it was the thyroid.'†*

*'On examination, he had yellow nails(!) and coarse crackles throughout the chest.'‡*

*'The next patient was a 50-year-old lady with polymyalgia rheumatica and giant cell arteritis.'§*

*'My second case involved interviewing a gentleman in his 70s about his memory loss.'¶*

*'I was given a referral letter asking me to see a patient who had watery diarrhoea.'\*\**

The emphasis for the new Station 5 scenarios is that the cases should be 'active' clinical problems such as might be seen in a new patient clinic, in an acute admissions unit or on the wards.

At present, the scenarios are generated by the local host examiner and vetted by a senior examiner who will not be examining at the host's centre. This explains the variation seen in cases between centres on our survey, and increases the possibility of some eccentric scenarios (e.g. loss of libido!) as a result of the organizers' interpretation of the station and the local availability of suitable patients. Quite a lot of the submitted scenarios are rejected because they are 'old' Station 5 cases with no active features. The College is now re-vetting all Station 5 scenarios used in the exam so far, to try to collect a pool of scenarios which can be used at any centre. This may be a problem because there will be practical issues for hosts who have to find a patient with the necessary signs for the exam. This is likely to be overcome to some degree by the increased use of scenarios suitable for actors.

Although the aim will be to try and discourage old-style Station 5 cases with stable long-standing inactive pathology, reported cases in the new Station 5 have included a combination of acute medical cases (e.g. transient ischaemic attack [TIA], chest pain), often with surrogates (actors), or old Station 5 patients (eye signs, etc.) recycled into the new Station 5 scenarios by adding an acute presenting complaint.

Another aim is that specialties such as dermatology, rheumatology, endocrinology and medical ophthalmology should still be represented in the exam. On a local level, the content of the scenarios in Station 5 should not revisit areas that have been covered in the other stations. For example, if Station 2 is a new case of arthritis, Station 5 should not include a case of rheumatoid arthritis. The way that these issues are being dealt with is that eventually Station 5 scenarios will be issued from the College as is currently the case for scenarios in Stations 2 and 4.

The viva is only 2 minutes long so the examiners have very little time. The priority for the examiner is to get the candidate to give the diagnosis and/or differential diagnosis and identify any abnormal physical signs. The candidate will be expected to explain the management plan to the patient in the first 8 minutes. If the patient has not asked the specific questions of the candidate, the examiner will attempt to raise them if there is time.

\*Vol. 2, Section F, Experience 2, Station 5.
†Vol. 2, Section F, Experience 13, Station 5.
‡Vol. 2, Section F, Experience 12, Station 5.

§Vol. 2, Section F, Experience 2, Station 5.
¶Vol. 2, Section F, Experience 1, Station 5.
\*\*Vol. 2, Section F, Experience 15, Station 5.

Speed is essential and practice will be required to complete the required steps and tasks in less than 8 minutes. This chapter aims to provide a framework with which candidates can approach scenarios, and ensure that all the requirements for each and every one of the marking domains are met.

### Approach to Station 5

*'The patient smiled and gave me a thumbs-up at the end.'*\*

In the 5 minutes prior to the start of the station, read the scenarios very carefully, identify key information present in the scene-setting summary and make notes of this. Use the time allowed to build a differential diagnosis list which will help you think which questions you need to ask. It will also identify areas you will want to cover with both the patient and examiners. It is also important to remember to keep an open mind and not get drawn into following only the differential diagnoses you've considered after reading the summary.

The information on the sheet will also report background medical conditions (e.g. hypertension), and these also need to be addressed even though they may not be the primary presenting complaint.

The mark sheet (outlined below and available on the Royal College of Physicians [RCP] website) can help to remind you of the areas to cover, and it is worth having a mental checklist of all the areas that need to be covered (e.g. to help you remember to check that all the examiners' concerns have been addressed).

### The scenario

*'Time goes very quickly in Station 5 as I think everybody has experienced so far!'*†

*'It felt very rushed and the examiner expected me to have asked a bit more about the past medical history than I did.'*‡

What follows is a suggested breakdown of your time in each scenario.

### History and examination: 6½ minutes

It is important to start the history as soon as possible. Keep introductions brief. Do not spend (too much) time enquiring if the patient is comfortable, etc., provided the patient looks comfortable. Practise taking a history and starting the examination whilst still taking the history. Examination of face, skin, joints, pulse can occur whilst taking the history. History must be focused but complete with regard to the system involved, e.g. if a patient has chest pain don't forget to ask about other cardiorespiratory symptoms, smoking, drug history, family history.

### Discussion with patient: 1½ minutes

Explain the diagnosis and plan, including investigations required and treatment planned; answer questions; address concerns. It is vital to do this in plain English, avoiding medical abbreviations and technical terms if possible. The patient/surrogate will have been briefed to challenge and question candidates who use technical jargon. Remember that communication skills are being tested.

\*Vol. 2, Section F, Experience 14, Station 5.                    ‡Vol. 2, Section F, Experience 9, Station 5.
†Vol. 2, Section F, Experience 12, Comment 5.

## Discussion with examiners: 2 minutes

Explain the diagnosis (have a clear list of differential diagnoses) and examination findings. The management plan should have been explained to the patient in the 8 minutes but the examiner will ask about the management plan if it was not clear from your discussions with the patient. Answer the examiner's questions.

Outside the United Kingdom, it is possible that there will be a higher rate of proxies being used, e.g. non-speaking 'patients' with clinical signs, with a 'relative' who provides the history and asks the questions. It is important to develop an approach for these, including asking the patient's permission to speak to their 'relative' and remembering to involve both the patient and their 'relative' in discussions, answering their questions and concerns.

Don't be surprised if a patient has no physical signs on examination; surrogates/actors may well be used to try to provide a reliable, consistent history in history-dependent scenarios which include 'normal' clinical examinations. Remember that patients with significant presentations, e.g. TIA, often arrive in the MAU with little to find once they arrive.

Remember to ask for and use all of the available resources including medication lists, drug charts, observation charts (temperature, blood pressure, pulse, blood glucose), blood results, urinalysis, ECGs, chest X-rays, etc.

## Example cases

*'Minimal questioning revealed that she had established retinopathy but the new visual disturbance was like a "curtain falling over the eye".'\**

The Royal College of Physicians has published several example cases on its website http://www.mrcpuk.org/paces/pages/pacesformat.aspx which are presented in the format of real cases used in the exam, accessed January 2013. This includes:

- The information given to the candidate prior to the station
- Instructions on what to expect in terms of timings
- The case summary/referral letter or clinical setting
- The scenario given to the patient or actor (including which questions to ask the candidate)
- The examiners' instructions and requirements for pass/fail.

The new Station 5 cases in this book have been written in a similar format to allow interactive practice, and provide realistic, fully fleshed-out cases to help candidates work through example cases and develop their own strategy for approaching Station 5.

## The mark sheet

*'I scored full marks with 28 out of 28.'†*

It's important to look carefully at the mark sheet for each of the clinical skills being assessed to ensure that you satisfy the examiners on each count. The mark

---

*Vol. 2, Section F, Experience 11, Station 5.    †Vol. 2, Section F, Experience 2, Station 5.

sheet illustrates the key requirements that you need to satisfy and the areas that can't be missed.

The clinical skills being assessed are listed below in bold, followed by the 'satisfactory performance' criteria for each skill (information as per the Station 5 mark sheet, publicly available on the RCP website at http://www.mrcpuk.org/Examiners/PACESExaminers/Pages/PacesMarkSheets.aspx, accessed January 2013).

- **Clinical communication skills:** elicits history relevant to the complaint and explains information to the patient in a focused, fluent and professional manner
- **Physical examination:** correct, appropriate, practised, professional
- **Clinical judgement:** selects sensible and appropriate investigations and treatment
- **Managing patients' concerns:** detects, acknowledges and attempts to address patient's concerns; listens; empathic
- **Identifying physical signs:** identifies correct physical signs, does not find signs that are not present
- **Differential diagnosis:** constructs a sensible differential diagnosis, including the correct diagnosis
- **Maintaining patient welfare:** treats patient respectfully and sensitively and ensures comfort, safety and dignity

## How to prepare

*'On reflection, I think it helped me to try and imagine that I was on MAU. In that way I kept my focus on the patient and always tried to be confident and relaxed with the patient if not the examiners!'\**

Candidates will need lots of practice against the clock in small group teaching sessions, using these scenarios (with actors and/or fellow candidates) and whilst working on medical admissions units, clinics and the wards.

Although it often feels artificial, candidates will need to practise taking the history and examining together as encouraged by the RCP.

Communication skills need to be developed as part of the preparation for PACES. They will be tested throughout Station 5 with the need for focused history taking, explanation of the differential diagnosis and plan to patients, and eliciting and discussing patients' concerns in these short scenarios.

Candidates should think about how to get the most information out of the 'patient' in the limited time available. Extensive research has been undertaken in general practice into consultation styles and models, and these models can yield useful methods for eliciting patients' concerns, etc. Early open questions can bring out a lot of information quickly and allow more focused questions to narrow things down later in the consultation.

Candidates need to find out the patient's ideas, concerns and expectations (ICE), using questions such as 'Have you had any thoughts yourself about what's happening?', 'Is there anything in particular that you are worried about?' and 'Do you have any other questions?'.

---

*Vol. 2, Section F, Experience 1, Comment.

Time yourself during your practice consultations so that you get a feel for the speed required and it is important to have a checklist in your head, or perhaps on the notes you take into the scenario, to ensure you cover everything in each scenario. It is also essential to explain, in plain English, the differential diagnoses, planned investigations and treatments to the patient and then to answer their questions and concerns. This means avoiding medical terminology and abbreviations.

On the wards, get feedback from colleagues on your communication skills, practise explaining diagnoses and management plans in clear plain English, avoiding jargon and technical language, and use the ICE questions above to elicit and address your patients' concerns.

The cases in this book illustrate scenarios that have occurred already in the new Station 5, or those that could occur based on common presentations to acute medical assessment units, on the wards and in clinics. The information provided in the 'Discussion with patient' and 'Discussion with examiners' sections details investigation and management in a concise form; the level of detail may be greater than a candidate could expect to cover in 2 minutes. The key is to explain this management plan to the patient during the 8 minutes, address their concerns and answer their questions, and, during their 2 minutes, the examiners will clarify areas in the management plan and ask specific questions to clarify examination findings (there will be no time for a detailed discussion of investigations and treatment with the examiners).

## Conclusion

*'It was so hard to judge how I had done, especially with the severest-looking examiner, and quite a history-based station. I began to hope that I hadn't done too badly though, after the patient chirped "well done" to me as the bell tolled! Overall, it was just like being on MAU!'*

As discussed in the Introduction to this volume, you should read the first 17 experiences in Volume 2, Section F, of *An Aid to the MRCP PACES* to find actual accounts of the new Station 5. When you do this you will see, as pointed out in the Introduction, that the cases occurring in the exam divide into:
- the old Station 5 subjects which the Colleges still wish to be included and you can study these in Section I of this volume
- a wide variety of new types of Station 5 cases such as dementia, polymyalgia rheumatica, migrainous headaches requiring the use of an ophthalmoscope, mononeuritis multiplex, falls in a patient with lots of possible reasons, headache followed by diplopia, a patient with a pansystolic murmur and subacute bacterial endocarditis (SBE), TIA, vasovagal attack, palpitations after cocaine use, watery diarrhoea (an actor), diabetic with collapse with several possible causes, and upper motor neurone facial palsy. These cases represent those which you meet on the emergency take, on ward rounds and in clinics. Thus your day-to-day work is your practice and preparation and you should make sure you read up on the conditions of the patients you meet.

The new Station 5 is a challenging part of the PACES examination but is founded on clinical practice on the wards, medical admissions units, A&E and clinics. Use

*Vol. 2, Section F, Experience 1, Station 5.

your day-to-day work to prepare and practise with colleagues particularly round timings and getting used to examining whilst taking a history.

Finally please, whenever you sit the MRCP, whether you pass or fail, fill in our survey at www.ryder-mrcp.org.uk for all the cases you meet but especially the ones in the new Station 5. It is only because of past candidates who have filled in our surveys that we have the information that we pass on to you. If you find our books useful, please in your turn do the same for the candidates of the future.

# Station 5
# Scenarios by specialty

# Scenario 1 | Non-resolving leg ulcer: pyoderma gangrenosum

## Candidate's information

**Your role:** you are the senior house officer (SHO) in the medical admissions unit. A 55-year-old man is referred by his GP for non-resolving cellulitis and leg ulceration. The man has been seeing the district nurse for regular dressings but the ulceration is not improving. Culture of a swab from the ulcer was negative a week ago and the ulceration has not improved with flucloxacillin.

**Your task:** to assess the patient's problems and address any questions or concerns raised by the patient.

## Patient's information

**You are:** Bill Vine, a 55-year-old man.

**Your problem:** you have a 6-week history of raised tender lumps on your lower legs. You saw your GP who gave you antibiotics but you're not sure of the name. The lumps did not get any better; instead they've become rather enlarged and more painful and ulcerated. Your GP took a swab and asked the district nurses to do daily dressings for the ulcers. You are not improving and you had another course of antibiotics last week. Again, you're not sure what they were but you have the box with you if you're asked. You have no pain in your legs when walking.

You've lost 1 stone in weight over the past 3 months and you've noticed a change in your bowels. You're now opening your bowels three times a day, with a soft stool, compared to once a day, with formed stool, up to about 3 months ago. You have no particular abdominal pains, just occasional cramps. Occasionally you see blood on wiping and rarely you see blood in the pan, which you always put down to piles. No mucus in the stool. No nausea or vomiting. Your appetite is normal and no increase in activity at work or home. You are not deliberately trying to lose weight. No problems with your swallowing, no heartburn/reflux, no indigestion. No jaundice or pale stools. No problems passing water. You have had pain in your left knee from arthritis for years, and you used to play a lot of rugby. No swelling, redness, hot joints, no other joints affected.

No mouth ulcers or ulcers anywhere else on your body (genital or oral). No rash elsewhere. You have felt a little lethargic but no temperature and have not had any blood tests from your GP.

## Past medical history:
- Nil of note
- No diabetes, hypertension, raised cholesterol

## Drug history:
- Nil of note

**Social history:**
• Non-smoker and drinks 1–2 pints of standard-strength beer per week

**Other issues including family history:**
• Nil of note

**Your questions for the candidate:**
• *Why isn't it healing with the antibiotics?*
• *Have I got skin cancer?*

---

## Candidate

### History/key questions

#### Dermatology history
Site

Onset of rash and the ulceration – when did the rash start? Chronic with acute exacerbations versus acute onset. When did the ulceration appear?

Description of lesions (small versus large plaques, scaly, pink, any pain, blistering, vesicles, pustules, discharge)

How has it changed since onset?

Distribution of the rash – where is the rash (arms, legs, trunk, soles, palms, face, scalp)?

How does the rash feel (symptoms) – pain, itch, bleeding?

Exacerbants – drugs, alcohol, NSAIDs

Joint symptoms – pain, swelling, erythema, deformity; ask about loss of function

Eye, mouth, nail symptoms or signs

Ever had it before?

Any injury to the site remembered by patient (Koebner's) as this can precede the onset of pyoderma gangrenosum

Initially pyoderma gangrenosum can present as single or multiple erythematous nodules/papules/pustules. Found mainly on legs, but can occur in any area

#### Consider underlying causes
Inflammatory bowel disease (IBD) – ask about diarrhoea, abdominal pain, weight loss, rectal bleeding, mouth ulcers

Haematological disorders or malignancies – IgA monoclonal gammopathy, polycythaemia rubra vera, myeloproliferative disorders, leukaemia, lymphoma

Rheumatological conditions – rheumatoid arthritis, ankylosing spondylitis, seronegative arthritis, psoriatic arthropathy

Also reported in association with:
 SLE
 Liver disease – viral hepatitis, autoimmune hepatitis
 Endocrine – thyrotoxicosis / thyroid disease
 Sarcoid
Anyone else in the family been unwell?

#### Drug history
What treatments has the patient tried – topical, oral (including steroids, antibiotics) and avoidance of precipitants, and how did the patient get on with them? Did they help, and how?

Ask about use of herbal and alternative remedies too

Ask about oral contraceptive pill (OCP) use in women – erythema nodosum

Ask about allergies, including any reactions to chemicals, latex, etc.

#### Past medical history
Any previous episodes of skin complaints

Any evidence of atopic conditions, e.g. hayfever, asthma, eczema/dermatitis

How does patient's skin react to sunlight/use of sunblock?

#### Social history
Alcohol history – units per week

Smoking history in pack-years

Any family history of atopic conditions as above, or skin neoplasia

Currrent occupation

### Address patient's questions and concerns
• *Have you had any thoughts about what is going on?*
• *Is there anything in particular you're concerned about?*
• *Do you have anything you would like to ask?*

## Key areas for examination

Use the guide to skin examination (Section G, Examination *routine* 16).

A list of what to look for (in examination order; describe findings on examination)

Description of rash: usually lower leg, tender erythematous or haemorrhagic nodule. Enlarges quickly, ulcerates rapidly with an irregular bluish, raised edge which overhangs, and an erythematous margin

Surrounding skin is erythematous and indurated

Single or multiple lesions

Overall inspection to look for signs of weight loss, anaemia

Perform a visual survey of the patient, from scalp to sole, remembering that most dermatological lesions have a predilection for certain areas. It is as well to remember some of the regional associations as you survey the patient:

Skin: scalp, face, mouth, neck, trunk, axillae, elbows, hands, nails, legs, feet +/− genitalia

Legs: look at both legs, exposing both completely, describe the ulcerated rash (and make the diagnosis)

Check peripheral pulses, capillary refill, check for oedema: tenderness, temperature, swelling

Leg ulcers (diabetic, venous, ischaemic, pyoderma gangrenosum), necrobiosis lipoidica diabeticorum, pretibial myxoedema, erythema nodosum, Henoch–Schönlein purpura, tendon xanthomata in Achilles tendon, erythema ab igne, pemphigoid (legs and arms), lipoatrophy

Hands: look for koilonychia, evidence of psoriatic arthropathy, nail signs (pitting; onycholysis) and psoriatic plaques

Lymphadenopathy – myeloproliferative disorders

Abdominal examination: is there a palpable abdominal mass (e.g. colonic neoplasia, right iliac fossa mass in Crohn's, hepatosplenomegaly in myeloproliferative disorders)?

Say that you would complete your examination with a rectal examination

Also consider:

Thyroid status, look for goitre, thyroid eye disease, thyroid acropachy, pretibial myxoedema

RA arthropathy, nodules, scleritis/episcleritis

Signs of ankylosing spondylitis (loss of lumbar lordosis)

Signs of liver disease – finger clubbing, spider naevi, jaundice, scratch marks, ascites, etc.

## Differential diagnosis

Pyoderma gangrenosum:

- Need to consider the differential diagnosis of the underlying condition, and be able to decide on the likely cause(s) for the pyoderma
- Need to exclude colonic carcinoma given altered bowel habit and weight loss in a 55-year-old man. Differential also includes IBD (Crohn's and ulcerative colitis)

## Discussion with patient

Explain diagnosis

Explain plan, including investigations and management

Address patient's concerns/answer their questions

You have an ulcer on your leg rather than an infection of the skin. This is why the antibiotics have not helped. It doesn't look like a skin cancer. We will refer you to the dermatology doctors to ask for their help, they may need to take a biopsy and will advise on treatment. This type of ulcer can be linked to certain bowel conditions, and as you have mentioned some weight loss and change in bowel habit we will arrange for the gastroenterologist to see you and arrange further outpatient tests for you.

## Management

Investigations – FBC, ESR, immunoglobulins, protein electrophoresis, LFT, rheumatoid factor, tissue transglutaminase (for completeness given altered bowel habit rather than rash), thyroid function tests, repeat swab

Treat any underlying condition

Refer to dermatology for consideration of biopsy, advice regarding ongoing management including need for immunosuppression

Urgent referral to gastroenterology – say that you'd check if they could see him whilst he's there on the MAU to review change in bowels and weight loss (indication for urgent outpatient colonoscopy)

## Addressing concerns/answering questions

- *Why isn't it healing with the antibiotics?* This is an ulcer on your leg rather than an infection, and doesn't respond to treatment with antibiotics. The inflammation in the skin will need to be settled down in order for the ulcer to heal. We will ask the dermatology team to see you and plan further tests and treatment of the ulcer.
- *Have I got skin cancer?* Your leg ulcer looks like an inflammatory condition called pyoderma gangrenosum rather than a skin cancer. The skin doctors may

well arrange for a biopsy to be taken from the ulcer which will aim to confirm the diagnosis.

## Discussion with examiners

The examiners may ask you to clarify details of the above diagnosis and ask questions about your planned investigations and management.

Investigations and management:
Identify and treat underlying condition
Treatment of pyoderma – topical versus systemic:
Steroids topically (or tacrolimus)
Systemic therapy includes high-dose steroids, cyclosporin, azathioprine and infliximab (anti-TNF-$\alpha$)

A possible question includes:
- *What other conditions can pyoderma gangrenosum be associated with?* Main underlying conditions are inflammatory bowel disease, haematological disorders or malignancies (IgA monoclonal gammopathy, polycythaemia rubra vera, myeloproliferative disorders, leukaemia, lymphoma) and rheumatological conditions (RA, ankylosing spondylitis, seronegative arthritis, psoriatic arthropathy). Other reported asso-

ciations include: SLE, liver disease – viral hepatitis, autoimmune hepatitis; thyroid disease and sarcoid.

See also Section I, Station 5, Skin, Case 50.

---

**Examiners' information and requirements**

The candidate should:

1. Identify key features from the history: non-healing ulcerated rash on leg, weight loss, altered bowel habit

2. Identify key examination findings: identify rash as pyoderma gangrenosum; deep ulcer with a violaceous border that overhangs the ulcer bed; recognize the need to look for an underlying cause

3. Outline a sensible management plan: dermatology referral for management of ulcer on leg; history of altered bowel habit and weight loss prompting urgent gastroenterology referral

4. Give a clear explanation to the patient of your diagnosis and plan, address his concerns and answer his questions

---

# Scenario 2 | Generalized rash: psoriasis

## Candidate's information

**Your role:** you are the SHO in the dermatology clinic. The patient has been referred with a generalized rash, not responding to emollients. It has been causing her some distress and this has prompted the referral to the clinic.

**Your task:** to assess the patient's problems and address any questions or concerns she raises.

## Patient's information

**You are:** Jenny Aslett, a 35-year-old woman.

**Your problem:** you had an itchy rash that came on suddenly with many small flat areas of scaly redness across your body including tummy and chest. You have always had some scalp itching and flaking, but recently it is a little worse. You had a cough, with some green mucus, a few weeks before this started. No history of asthma, but your GP gave you some antibiotics and your chest felt better after a few days. The rash has persisted despite the use of aqueous cream, and remains across your trunk and chest.

  You have had an ache in your right elbow since a sporting injury, but it's been worse recently. You take ibuprofen for this but this made the rash worse for a few days. No rash on your genitals. No joint swelling.

### Past medical history:
• Nil of note

### Drug history:
• Your rash is worse after alcohol, or ibuprofen. You are not on an OCP
• Used aqueous cream which lifts the scale but doesn't help the redness or the itch
• Not tried any tablets

### Social history:
• Nil of note
• Non-smoker
• Drinks 2–3 glasses of wine per week
• If asked about how this has affected you, you've felt low since the rash appeared and worried what people think of you when they see it. You've not been able to go swimming which is your usual hobby
• No current partner

### Other issues including family history:
• Grandfather had a red rash on his elbows but you don't know what it was

**Your questions for the candidate:**

- *Can't I just take tablets for this? I saw an internet site suggesting steroid tablets would help.*
- *Why does alcohol make the rash worse?*

---

## Candidate

### History/key questions

Site

Onset – when did the rash start? Chronic with acute exacerbations versus acute onset

Description of lesions (small versus large plaques, scaly, pink, blistering, vesicles, pustules, discharge)

How has it changed since onset?

Distribution of the rash – where is the rash (arms, legs, trunk, soles, palms, face, scalp)?

How does the rash feel (symptoms) – pain, itch?

Is there any bleeding?

Exacerbants – drugs, alcohol, NSAIDs

Joint symptoms – pain, swelling, erythema, deformity; ask about loss of function

Eye, mouth, nail symptoms or signs

Ever had it before?

Anyone else in the family been unwell, e.g. varicella/chickenpox?

### Drug history

What treatments has the patient tried – topical, oral, avoiding precipitants, and how did the patient get on with them? Did they help, and how?

Ask about herbal and complementary remedies too

Ask about OCP use in women – (erythema nodosum)

Ask about allergies, including any reactions to chemicals, latex, etc.

### Past medical history

Any previous episodes of skin complaints

Any evidence of atopic conditions, e.g. hayfever, asthma, eczema

How does patient's skin react to sunlight/use of sunblock?

### Social history

Alcohol history – units per week

Smoking history in pack-years

Any family history of atopic conditions as above, psoriasis or skin neoplasia

Current and previous occupations

## Address patient's questions and concerns

- *Have you had any thoughts about what is going on?*
- *Is there anything in particular you're concerned about?*
- *Do you have anything you would like to ask?*

## Key areas for examination

Use the guide to skin examination (Section G, Examination *routine* 16)

Consider the distribution of the lesions (e.g. psoriasis on extensor areas). Then, after the visual survey of the patient (which should take a few seconds), examine the lesions, looking in particular for the characteristic features.

If you have made a diagnosis, consider whether you need to look for any **associated lesions**.

This patient has psoriasis – look for:

Scalp: psoriasis (look especially at the hairline for redness, scaling, etc.)

Elbows: psoriasis (extensor)

Hands: psoriatic arthropathy – mainly distal joints

Nails: psoriasis (pitting, onycholysis)

Feet: pustular psoriasis

Body: guttate psoriasis

Koebner's phenomenon (scars, trauma)

Describe scaling in psoriasis

Eye signs – redness/tearing due to blepharitis or conjunctivitis, corneal dryness, corneal disease relatively rare

Chest examination – ensure chest now clear (symptoms of lower respiratory tract infection resolved a few weeks before)

With the above information obtained at examination, you should be able to characterize the type of psoriasis.

- *Chronic plaque psoriasis* is the most common, affecting extensor surfaces, scalp, lumbosacral, posterior auricular areas. Inflamed raised areas (plaques) on the scalp, knees, elbows, trunk; silver/white scale covers the plaques and, if removed, the underlying tissue looks red and inflamed
- *Flexural psoriasis*: beefy-red colour but scales are often lost or just at the edge; well-demarcated plaques on genital area, natal cleft, submammary, axillae, posterior auricular and scalp

- *Guttate psoriasis* (as described by the patient above): multiple small papules (salmon pink) on the trunk, can be scaly, and can occur after a lower respiratory tract infection (group A β-haemolytic streptococcus)
- *Pustular psoriasis*: sterile pustules localized to palms or soles, or over body (more serious and may occur due to injudicious use of topical or systemic steroids). Can cause erythema, pustules then scaling. Widespread pustular psoriasis requires admission as dehydration/metabolic complications may occur
- *Erythrodermic psoriasis*: generalized erythema, pain, pruritus, scaling. Covers nearly the entire body surface and can lead to fluid loss, fever, hypothermia, dehydration. If severe, may need inpatient management to control pain and dehydration/metabolic complications
- *Psoriatic arthropathy*: 10–30% of patients with psoriasis. Hands, feet and occasionally the large joints. Stiffness, pain, progressive joint damage. Nail changes include pitting and onycholysis

## Differential diagnosis

You need to be able to recognize the classic rash of psoriasis (guttate psoriasis)

## Discussion with patient

Explain diagnosis
Explain plan, including investigations and management
Address patient's concerns/answer their questions

Psoriasis is an inflammatory rash that can run in families, can be triggered by a chest infection (as in this case) and can flare up after different medications or alcohol.

It is not an infection and can't be passed on to other people.

It is important to acknowledge the effect of the psoriasis on the patient's quality of life.

## Management

Explain the different ways of treating psoriasis, initially with topical medications (emollients and calcipotriol) with scope to increase the therapy as needed. May need light therapy or tar depending on extent of skin involvement.

Would likely need ongoing dermatology follow-up (already in dermatology clinic)
- Mild-to-moderate disease requires topical therapy: topical emollients and calcipotriol. Alternatives include tar, dithranol, combination calcipotriol/

moderate-strength steroid (Dovobet). Avoid potent topical corticosteroids except for palms/soles and use mild-to-moderate topical steroids in flexural disease
- Moderate-to-severe psoriasis (>5–10% of skin surface affected) – oral treatment plus topical. Guttate psoriasis responds well to a course of phototherapy +/– calcipotriol or tar
- Severe disease: under the care of a dermatologist; systemic therapies or phototherapy needed. Systemic therapies include retinoids (acitretin), methotrexate, cyclosporin and anti-TNF-α inhibitors such as infliximab

## Addressing concerns/answering questions

- *Can't I just take tablets for this? I saw an internet site suggesting steroid tablets would help.* Steroid tablets are not helpful in psoriasis as they can make it worse when they are stopped. Best treated according to extent of psoriasis and if possible with topical preparations.
- *Why does alcohol make the rash worse?* Different things can make the rash of psoriasis flare up including alcohol and some drugs, e.g. β-blockers, antimalarials.

## Discussion with examiners

The examiners may ask you to clarify details of the above diagnosis and ask questions about your planned investigations and management.

Other possible questions include:
- *How would you measure the effect of this patient's psoriasis on her quality of life?* There is a validated tool for measuring this – the DLQI (Dermatology Life Quality Index – see Further reading/resources). There is a maximum score of 20 with severe impairment being anything over 10. It is required for the use of biologics along with the PASI (Psoriasis Area and Severity Index [how much psoriasis there is and how thick, red, scaly it is]). You would not be expected to know the details of the DLQI or PASI.
- *Would you ever consider tablet treatment for patients with mild-to-moderate psoriasis?* Yes, if they were fully informed and their quality of life was severely affected.
- *What are the side-effects of methotrexate?* Potential side-effects of methotrexate: major side-effects include hepatotoxicity, myelosuppression (macrocytosis or pancytopenia), pulmonary toxicity (inflammatory and fibrotic lung disease, infections).

Common potential side-effects include gastrointestinal disturbance including nausea, diarrhoea; stomatitis; rash; headache or fatigue, hair loss/alopecia.

- *What would prompt referral to a skin specialist?* Extent of disease/effect on quality of life/erythrodermic flare/unusual presentation or site/genital involvement.
- *Are there any associated diseases?* Independent risk factor for cardiovascular disease, associated psoriatic arthropathy.
- *Any other drugs that you know would make psoriasis worse?* Lithium, β-blockers, antimalarials.

See also Section I, Station 5, Skin, Case 4 and Station 5, Locomotor, Case 2.

---

**Examiners' information and requirements**

The candidate should:

1. Identify key features from the history: acute-onset rash following lower respiratory tract infection, not improved on current therapy, effects on quality of life, exacerbated by NSAIDs and alcohol
2. Identify key examination findings including rash consistent with guttate psoriasis
3. Outline a sensible management plan, including topical therapy for psoriasis, with option for PUVA if sufficient extent or severity
4. Give a clear explanation to the patient of your diagnosis and plan, address her concerns and answer her questions

---

**Further reading/resources**

Dermatology Life Quality Index (DLQI) www.dermatology.org.uk/quality/dlqi/quality-dlqi.html
Psoriasis Area Severity Index (PASI)
PASI with images: www.dermnetnz.org/scaly/pasi.html
Calculator: pasi.corti.li/

# Scenario 3 | Dermatomyositis and falls

## Candidate's information

**Your role:** on-call in the MAU, you are asked to see this 65-year-old man who has presented with a fall and a history of weight loss.

**Your task:** to assess the patient's problems and address any questions or concerns raised by him.

## Patient's information

**You are:** James Brady, a 65-year-old man.

**Your problem:** you've noticed difficulty getting out of chairs and your family is concerned about you as you've had several recent falls. The weakness has crept up on you over the past few months. You have slight general aches in your muscles but they are not tender. You've had chronic joint aches but you're not sure if these are due to the falls or preceded them. Your appetite is unchanged. You remember the falls as you felt your legs give way. You remember hitting the floor and you didn't feel dizzy or lose consciousness.

You have a red rash on your hands – it has been there for ages and it's not itchy. You've noticed changes in your voice and swallowing; you were previously able to eat and drink anything. Now you need to wash down solids with water. You have lost 3–4 kg over the past 6 months. No heartburn, indigestion or vomiting. Bowel habit is unchanged. No abdominal pain.

You have a chronic smoker's cough with white sputum daily, unchanged for the past 20 or more years. No chest pain, coughing up of blood, wheeze or shortness of breath.

## Past medical history and drug history:
- Not been to hospital before
- Not on any medications

## Social history:
- Smoker: 40/day for 40+ years. Rarely takes alcohol – couple of glasses of wine on special occasions, e.g. Christmas
- Lives with wife and has two adult children who live nearby
- Able to climb the stairs but with difficulty recently. Family help with shopping. Wife independent – looks after everything at home

## Other issues including family history:
- Nil of note

## Your questions for the candidate:
- *Why is the food getting stuck?*
- *What can I do to get back on my feet?*

# Candidate

## History/key questions

Weakness +/− pain/tenderness in muscles – when did it start, how has it changed over time, any relieving/exacerbating factors? Which limbs are affected? Symmetrical or asymmetrical?

Any myalgia, tenderness of muscles? Distribution of muscle weakness in dermatomyositis is proximal and symmetrical, with onset over months. Can have tenderness and myalgia although not as prominent as polymyalgia rheumatica, fibromyalgia or myositis due to viruses

Rash:
  Site
  Onset – when did the rash start? Chronic with acute exacerbations versus acute onset
  Description of lesions
  How has it changed since onset?
  Distribution of the rash – where is the rash (arms, legs, trunk, soles, palms, face, scalp, mouth)?
  How does the rash feel (symptoms) – pain, itch, bleeding?
  Exacerbants

Joint symptoms – pain, swelling, erythema, deformity; ask about loss of function

Eye, mouth, nail symptoms or signs

Ever had it before?

Anyone else in the family been unwell?

Respiratory symptoms (associated with interstitial lung disease) – ask about respiratory symptoms including breathlessness, cough, wheeze, sputum, chest pain, haemoptysis, weight loss

GI symptoms – ask specifically about dysphagia, weight loss, appetite and also causes of dysphagia (dermatomyositis can be associated with oesophageal neoplasia and oesophageal dysmotility) including reflux symptoms. Dysphagia – to what sort of foods (what consistency, e.g. hard, soft) or fluids, sudden or gradual onset, how has it changed over past few months?

Ask about prostatic symptoms – hesitancy, frequency, poor stream (dermatomyositis associated with GI/oesophageal, lung, ovarian, prostatic, breast cancers)

Ask if any arthritis/arthropathy, and in which joints

### Drug history

What treatments has the patient tried – topical, oral (including steroids, antibiotics), avoiding precipitants, and how did the patient get on with them? Did they help, and how?

Ask about use of herbal and alternative remedies

Ask about OCP use in younger women

Ask about allergies, including any reactions to chemicals, latex, etc.

### Past medical history

Any previous episodes of skin complaints

Any evidence of atopic conditions, e.g. hayfever, asthma, eczema/dermatitis

How does patient's skin react to sunlight/use of sunblock?

### Social history

Alcohol history – units per week

Smoking history in pack-years

Check social set-up – who does he live with at home? What support does he have?

Current and previous occupation

## Address patient's questions and concerns

- *Have you had any thoughts about what is going on?*
- *Is there anything in particular you're concerned about?*
- *Do you have anything you would like to ask?*

## Key areas for examination

A list of what to look for (in examination order; describe findings on examination)

Overall: will need to have adequately exposed the patient to see the rash and make the diagnosis early, and guide questioning to look for the underlying cause

Skin: look for cutaneous manifestations of dermatomyositis

Hands: Gottron's papules (erythematous, violaceous raised papules and plaques over bony prominences, e.g. extensor surfaces of phalanges, elbows, feet and knees). Nailfold erythema (due to enlarged capillaries) and periungual telangiectasia. 'Mechanic's hands' – roughened cracked skin on palms/sides of hands

Face: lilac 'heliotrope' rash on face around eyelids, cheeks and other sun-exposed regions (including metacarpophalangeal [MCP] joints and trunk)

Body: telangiectasia, hyperpigmentation in sun-exposed areas (the V-sign rash is discrete and confluent macular erythema in a V shape in the sun-exposed areas of the chest and neck; the shawl sign is confluent macular erythema in the distribution of a shawl (the upper back, posterior neck and shoulders)

Rest of body: Raynaud's phenomenon, alopecia, cutaneous vasculitis, calcinosis, buccal – white plaques

Check temperature (fever can occur in 20%)

Other complications include lung fibrosis/interstitial lung disease, arthralgia, myocarditis

Weakness, possibly tenderness, of proximal muscles on examination; ask patient to stand from the chair without using his arms (test for proximal muscle weakness)

Say you would like to examine the patient completely, including a full neurological exam (there is unlikely to be enough time), as part of the investigations into neoplasia; also need to examine joints and lungs (arthritis and interstitial lung disease)

This patient has a characteristic rash of dermatomyositis on his hands and is unable to get up from the chair without using his arms, e.g. a sign of proximal myopathy

## Differential diagnosis

Combination of cutaneous features/proximal muscle weakness – dermatomyositis

Symptoms of weight loss and dysphagia raise the possibility of oesophageal malignancy (associated with dermatomyositis) – needs urgent investigation

Differential diagnosis of dermatomyositis and polymyositis:
  Consider the other causes for proximal muscle weakness with or without elevated muscle enzymes
  Amyotrophic lateral sclerosis (motor neurone disease)
  Myasthenia gravis
  Muscular dystrophies
  Inclusion body myopathy, vasculitis, overlap syndromes (lupus, RA, scleroderma)
  Endocrine – hypothyroidism, Cushing's
  Electrolytes – low K, Mg, Ca, Na
  Infections – viral (including HIV), fungal, bacterial or parasites
  Rhabdomyolysis
  Drug-induced myopathy

## Discussion with patient

Explain diagnosis
Explain plan, including investigations and management
Address patient's concerns/answer their questions

You have a condition affecting the muscles as well as the skin leading to your weakness and the falls. We need to look into why you've developed this, and I would recommend we carry out some tests. We need to arrange an endoscopy camera test to look into your swallowing problems as an urgent out-patient. We'll also send off some blood tests. We'll need the rheumatology specialists to see you here, and the physiotherapists to see you on the unit here to check you're safe to go home. The rheumatologists may want some other tests before starting medications such as steroids, and would arrange an appointment to see you in clinic.

## Investigations

CK, ALT: CK elevated (muscle enzymes) unless muscle not affected/involved

EMG: characteristic findings

Skin biopsy: not diagnostic but may be supportive

Muscle biopsy: from affected muscle, e.g. quadriceps (shows necrosis of muscle fibres, degeneration and regeneration, and inflammatory cellular infiltrate)

Need to urgently investigate causes of weight loss and dysphagia, initially with upper GI endoscopy; important to investigate for associated malignancy but dermatomyositis is also associated with gut dysmotility. If oesophagogastroduodenoscopy (OGD) normal, barium swallow may demonstrate oesophageal dysmotility

Other investigations may also be required, particularly given the significant smoking history (CXR +/– CT chest)

## Management

Explanation and education of patient

### Skin disease

Avoid sunlight and use sunscreen

Dermatology – skin biopsy

Oral steroids, hydroxychloroquine, methotrexate or mycophenolate mofetil

### Muscle disease

Bedrest if severe muscle inflammation

Referral to rheumatology

Physiotherapy

High-dose steroids (NB: bone protection)

Immunosuppressants used early for steroid sparing in both skin and muscle disease (methotrexate and mycophenolate mofetil; azathioprine for muscle disease)

Immunoglobulins

## Addressing concerns/answering questions

- *Why is the food getting stuck?* Swallowing problems are due to a range of causes, and we need to arrange some tests to find out what's causing your difficulties. This rash can be associated with problems with the muscles in the gullet pumping food down. We need to arrange an endoscopy test to look down the gullet and rule out narrowings, etc.
- *What can I do to get back on my feet?* We need to find the cause for the weakness and treat it, but will probably also need to give you some steroid tablets to reduce the inflammation in the muscles which is making you weak.

## Discussion with examiners

The examiners may ask you to clarify details of the above diagnosis and ask questions about your planned investigations and management.

Other possible questions include:

- *What is dermatomyositis/describe the pathogenesis?* Dermatomyositis is an idiopathic inflammatory myopathy with characteristic skin signs. It is a systemic disorder that most frequently affects the skin and muscles but may also affect the joints, the lungs (interstitial lung disease), the oesophagus (dysphagia), and less frequently the heart (myocarditis). Dermatomyositis can be associated with malignancy and this needs to be considered in the over 40s. Pathogenesis: precise mechanisms for the pathogenesis of dermatomyositis are currently unknown.
- *What investigations would you carry out to investigate the dysphagia and weight loss?* OGD followed by contrast swallow (exclude neoplasia first/mechanical obstruction, then look for dysmotility).
- *How would you treat it?* As above.
- *What are the side-effects of steroid therapy and how would you reduce the risk?* Risk of steroid side-effects is dose-dependent and related to duration of therapy. Need, therefore, to prescribe the lowest effective dose for the minimum required period to minimize the overall dose. Consider the risk factors for some of the more common side-effects (e.g. osteoporosis, diabetes, hypertension), the effect of other side-effects on lifestyle / quality of life (e.g. weight gain, cataracts) and don't forget the central side-effects of insomnia, restlessness, altered mood and increased appetite.

  *Bone health*: lifestyle measures to optimize bone health include an active lifestyle / weight bearing exercise, not smoking or taking excessive alcohol, ensuring adequate calcium intake in the diet +/− calcium / vitamin D supplementation; NHS Clinical Knowledge summary advises to offer bisphosphonates to prevent osteoporosis in people who have been taking oral corticosteroids for more than 3 months, or who are likely to do so, and who are: 65 years of age or more; less than 65 years of age *with* a previous fragility fracture; or less than 65 years of age *without* a previous fragility fracture *and* have a T-score of −1.5 or less. Need to organize a dual energy X-ray absorptiometry (DEXA) scan for people less than 65 years of age with no previous fragility fracture who have been taking oral corticosteroids for 3 months or more, or who are due to start a course that is likely to last for 3 months or more. Consider starting treatment if there is a long wait for DEXA scanning. If drug treatment is not indicated because the T-score is between 0 and −1.5, repeat the DEXA scan in 1 to 3 years if corticosteroid use continues.

  *Diabetes*: if patient is known to have diabetes, then follow management plan closely including monitoring blood glucose levels. Drug therapy (insulin and/or oral hypoglycaemic drugs may need to be increased, or insulin started).

  If patient is not known to have diabetes, advise to check for new onset of diabetes 1 month after initiation of oral corticosteroids, then every 3 months thereafter. If possible, dipstick test urine for glucose at each clinic visit.

  *Other risks include*: an increased risk of infection particularly on higher dose steroids; cataract or glaucoma development; peptic ulceration, particularly in patients on aspirin or NSAIDs – check for dyspepsia and reflux symptoms as patients may need a PPI coprescribed; proximal muscle weakness; thinning of the skin; facial changes (moon face); striae; delayed wound healing. Rarer side-effects also include aseptic / avascular necrosis of the hip.

  If patient on steroids for over three weeks, supply a steroid card (includes information on preparation, dose and duration, and contact details of prescriber). Prescribe the dose in the morning to reduce effects on sleeping.

  With patients on steroids for over three weeks you need to consider the risk of adrenal insufficiency, so withdrawal has to be gradual and clearly prescribed and explained to patients. Patients on long-term steroids, or who have been on steroids in the previous year, need advice on how to adjust their steroid dose if unwell/infection, undergoing surgery, extensive dentistry, etc. Addisons Disease Self Help Group's 'Owners Manual' is a useful practical guide for patients regarding this – see the section on 'crisis management'.

See also Section I, Station 5, Skin, Case 6.

---

**Examiners' information and requirements**

The candidate should:

1. Identify key features from history: dysphagia and weight loss. Rash, difficulty getting out of chair, reduced mobility and several falls without dizziness or syncope (mechanical falls)

2. Identify key examination findings including characteristic rash of dermatomyositis, proximal muscle weakness

3. Outline a sensible management plan, including referral for investigations into dysphagia; input from rheumatology and dermatology opinion

4. Give a clear explanation to the patient of your diagnosis and plan, address his concerns and answer his questions

---

**Further reading/resources**

Callen JP. Dermatomyositis. Lancet 2000;355(9197): 53–7. www.emedicine.medscape.com/article/1064945-overview

Addisons Disease Self Help Group – Owners Manual: www.addisons.org.uk/info/manual/page1.html

NHS Clinical Knowledge Summary on 'What should I consider when initiating oral corticosteroids': www.cks.nhs.uk/corticosteroids_oral/management/scenario_corticosteroids_oral/view_full_scenario_no_prescriptions

# Scenario 4 | Systemic sclerosis and Raynaud's syndrome

## Candidate's information

**Your role:** you are a doctor (ST3) in the rheumatology clinic. Mrs Jacob's GP has referred her to you because of chronic ulcers on her fingertips which aren't healing.

**Your task:** to assess the patient's problems and address any questions or concerns raised by her.

## Patient's information

**You are:** Andrea Jacobs, a 55-year-old lady who has just moved into the area to be closer to your grandchildren.

**Your problem:** your main concern is your hands. They have been changing colour in the cold for a few years but for the past 5–6 weeks you have noticed increased pain in your hands. They go white, then blue and then red again, and are painful. The tips of your fingers have been painful, and a small cut on your finger from a cat scratch took 3 weeks to settle even with antibiotics from the GP. There are now little ulcers on your fingers and you can't remember doing anything to cause them.

You've noticed difficulty swallowing solid foods for the past few years. It gradually crept up on you. Your GP referred you to your local hospital 6 months ago (before you moved here) and an endoscopy test (camera test down the gullet and into the stomach) was completely normal. You had a barium swallow X-ray test and the doctors told you that it was probably just the food pipe not pumping as well as it used to, and they put you on some antiacid medicines. These have helped your swallowing a bit but you still have to avoid larger pieces of meat and dry bread. Your weight is stable. You're not worried about the swallowing as it only causes problems once in a while now that you have changed your diet a bit, and you've had this checked out.

Your BP is controlled on the tablets your doctor has prescribed.

### Past medical history and drug history:
- Hypertension – on ACEI (ramipril 5 mg once per day)
- Raised cholesterol – on atorvastatin 40 mg od
- No known diabetes mellitus or other medical conditions. Not previously diagnosed with Raynaud's or systemic sclerosis

### Social history:
- Ex-smoker: 25/day for 40 years. Stopped 3 months ago, when your GP suggested that the problems in your hands could be related to narrowing of the arteries. You don't think it's helped much though

### Other issues including family history:
- No family history of hand problems

**Your questions for the candidate:**
- *What can you do to make the ulcers heal up?*
- *Why can't I swallow solid foods? What's wrong if my endoscopy was normal?*

---

## Candidate

### History/key questions

Ask about the hand symptoms (patient's primary concern). What precipitates (cold) and eases (heat) the symptoms, how frequent and how severe are the changes?

Ask about the different stages of Raynaud's phenomenon – the exaggerated physiological response to cold leading to spasm and cold white 'dead' ischaemic hands: with rewarming the colour changes to blue (stasis) and then red hands (painful reactive/rebound hyperaemia)

Any sensory changes (paraesthesiae, numbness, stiffness, pain) associated with above stages?

How long has she had it (helps differentiate between Raynaud's syndrome and Raynaud's disease, onset >40 and <40 respectively)?

Any pre-existing conditions known – SLE, rheumatoid arthritis

Having made the diagnosis of systemic sclerosis/scleroderma on inspection early in the interview, you may have time to ask about other associated symptoms

Gastrointestinal symptoms: ask about dysphagia – if present, for how long, has it changed (improved or worsened), does anything improve the swallowing, e.g. PPI use, washing food down with fluid? Are certain foods harder to swallow? Any history of food actually sticking, any vomiting or regurgitation? Ask about reflux symptoms (heartburn, water brash). What investigations carried out so far? Ask specifically about endoscopies and contrast / barium studies

Any alarm symptoms including weight loss, haematemesis

Other problems including diarrhoea, bloating (small bowel malabsorption, dysmotility)

Ask about respiratory symptoms such as SOB and cough, thinking about interstitial lung disease, but remember pulmonary hypertension (or both) may be an explanation for these symptoms

Renal function can be impaired so ask about hypertension

### Drug history

Ask about medicines associated with secondary Raynaud's phenomenon, e.g. β-blockers, ergotamine, sumatriptan, some chemotherapy agents, cocaine, decongestants (long list)

Any allergies to medications?

### Past medical history

Ask if known to have circulation problems in hands or elsewhere, and whether known to have Raynaud's?

### Social history

Occupational history – did patient use vibrating machinery/tools (pneumatic drills, polishing tools)? Do her hand symptoms interfere with any current employment, hobbies or home life?

Smoking history (important vascular risk factor)

Alcohol history

### Address patient's questions and concerns
- *Have you had any thoughts about what is going on?*
- *Is there anything in particular you're concerned about?*
- *Do you have anything you would like to ask?*

## Key areas for examination

A list of what to look for (in examination order; describe findings on examination)

Overall inspection

Face:

Tight skin round face, reduced mouth opening (microstomia), telangiectasia, pinched nose (beaking)

Butterfly rash (SLE)

Sympathectomy scars

Hands:

Tightening of skin with smooth shiny skin (sclerodactyly) with flexion deformity of fingers, atrophy of finger tips; telangiectasia

Cold, cyanosed (or red) fingers: dilated capillaries in nailfolds; digital ulceration or infarction/gangrenous finger tips

Calcinosis: firm, whitish dermal papules, nodules, plaques or subcutaneous nodules

There may be tendon friction rubs as well as an arthritis in the hands

Capillary refill

Radial pulses

Sensation in hands

Assess hand function which can be affected by changes of sclerodactyly in the fingers, but an arthritis and tenosynovitis can occur. The early phase of sclerodactyly has an inflammatory stage with digital swelling, later becoming more chronic with the typical tight, tethered skin. Skin changes more proximal than the wrist/forearm suggest the more generalized form of disease. These skin changes may be present on the chest wall or back with areas of hypo- or hyperpigmentation

Say that you would also like to examine:

Upper limb pulses and L+R arm BP – cervical rib is a differential diagnosis; important to check BP in systemic sclerosis as this is associated with malignant hypertension. Ex-smoker so vascular disease could be contributing

Respiratory system for signs of interstitial lung disease

Cardiovascular system for signs of pulmonary hypertension

In this patient there is microstomia, telangiectasia, sclerodactyly, nailfold capillary dilatation, atrophy of finger tips and digital ulceration; clinical signs of CREST syndrome

## Differential diagnosis

Raynaud's phenomenon secondary to systemic sclerosis leading to digital ulceration/impaired tissue healing

Probable CREST syndrome given Raynaud's, oesophageal dysmotility

The presence of more proximal skin changes suggests that this is the more diffuse cutaneous type of systemic sclerosis and therefore needs monitoring more closely for the more severe internal organ features (though these can all still occur in CREST variant)

## Discussion with patient

Explain diagnosis

Explain plan, including investigations and management (conservative, pharmaceutical and interventional)

Address patient's concerns/answer their questions

You have changes to the blood vessels in the hands due to Raynaud's syndrome and this is in turn caused by a condition called systemic sclerosis. This has affected your swallowing as well. The changes to the blood vessels in the hands has caused the ulcers on your finger tips to develop, and not heal.

## Investigations

Bloods including:

FBC, ESR

U&E (investigate for scleroderma renal crisis)

ANA and anticentromere and antitopoisomerase (Scl-70) antibodies, immunoglobulins and protein electrophoresis

CXR, pulmonary function tests and CT chest may be needed

2D echo to look for evidence of pulmonary hypertension

Urinalysis

Capillaroscopy for dilated nailfold capillaries, capillary dropout and 'bushy' capillaries

Already had an upper GI endoscopy which was normal – clinical history would fit with dysphagia secondary to systemic sclerosis/CREST. If symptoms are unchanged since last investigations (OGD and contrast swallow) then you don't need to repeat these

Need complete drug history from the patient's GP to exclude any drugs exacerbating or causing the symptoms

## Management

Keep hands warm

Treatment of Raynaud's due to systemic sclerosis – vasodilators (such as calcium channel blockers), ACEI, prostacyclin analogues (as infusion and indicated when digital ulceration has occurred), bosentan for pulmonary hypertension

Digital sympathectomy

## Addressing concerns/answering questions

- *What can you do to make the ulcers heal up?* You need to keep your hands warm, and there are several medications we can use to improve the blood flow, and aim to heal the ulcers.
- *Why can't I swallow solid foods? What's wrong if my endoscopy was normal?* The investigations you had done at the previous hospital sound like they showed dysmotility, impaired pumping of the muscles in the food pipe. This is one of the features of systemic sclerosis. It is reassuring that you had a normal endoscopy, and we don't need to repeat this. You need to avoid hard or dry foods, and wash food down with liquid to improve your symptoms.

# Discussion with examiners

The examiners may ask you to clarify details of the above diagnosis and ask questions about your planned investigations and management.

Other possible questions include:

- *What is the difference between Raynaud's disease and Raynaud's syndrome?* Raynaud's disease is primary Raynaud's phenomenon, where the symptoms occur without any associated condition. Raynaud's syndrome (secondary Raynaud's phenomenon) is where it occurs in presence of a related condition, e.g. systemic sclerosis or SLE.
- *What are the different classifications of scleroderma?* Localized (morphoea); systemic – limited (CREST) or diffuse; chemical-induced (e.g. silica, organic chemicals); overlap with other connective tissue disease (e.g. myositis, RA).
- *What other organs can be involved?* GI, heart, lung, kidney.
- *What makes up the CREST syndrome?* Calcinosis, Raynaud's, oesophageal dysmotility, sclerodactyly, telangiectasia.
- *What is scleroderma renal crisis and how would you manage it?* Development of malignant hypertension, managed by prompt commencement of ACEI when evidence of early hypertension, renal impairment or proteinuria.
- *What would be a differential diagnosis if signs were unilateral and what findings would you look for?* Cervical rib; supraclavicular rib causing ipsilateral reduced radial pulse (more so during attack) and neurological signs including wasting of small muscles of hand, and C8/T1 sensory impairment. See Section I, Station 5, Skin, Case 22.

See also Section I, Station 5, Skin, Cases 1 and 22, and Station 5, Locomotor, Case 3.

## Examiners' information and requirements

The candidate should:

1. Identify key features from the history including the classic features of Raynaud's, the progression of symptoms over time and the severity of symptoms. Include management strategies invoked by the patient. Features suggestive of internal organ involvement must be asked for. Need to elicit the history of dysphagia and the investigations already carried out elsewhere
2. Identify key examination findings including sclerodactyly, digital ulcers, nailfold capillary dilation, functional hand problems and identify CREST syndrome
3. Outline a sensible management plan including conservative approaches, vasodilators and possible need for immunosuppression with more aggressive skin disease or lung involvement. Pulmonary hypertension may need management with other vasoactive substances, such as prostaglandin analogues (prostacyclin), endothelin receptor antagonists (bosentan) or phosphodiesterase inhibitors (sildenafil)
4. Give a clear explanation to the patient of your diagnosis and plan, address her concerns and answer her questions

# Scenario 5 | Rheumatoid arthritis and effects on activities of daily living (ADL)

## Candidate's information

**Your role:** you are an ST2 in a care of the elderly clinic. You have been asked to see this 65-year-old lady who has 'long-standing rheumatoid arthritis' and is struggling at home.

**Your task:** to assess the patient's problems and address any questions or concerns raised by her.

## Patient's information

**You are:** Joyce Walker, a 65-year-old woman.

**Your problem:** you've had rheumatoid arthritis (RA) for the past 40 years. Although your hands haven't been red or swollen for some years, they are painful and you're finding it increasingly difficult to do things round the house. You had a knee replacement about 5 years ago which helped a great deal. You've not noticed any new problems in the other parts of your body – your hands are your main concern. You fell about 6 months ago after tripping over, and lost some of your confidence in going up and down the stairs.

You've lost about 6 pounds in weight as your appetite is less than it was before. There is no breathlessness, and you are able to walk to the shops and round them using two sticks, and your daughter has accompanied you since your fall.

You're having difficulties with putting on clothes (doing up your bra is particularly difficult and you've had slip-on shoes for years), problems gripping cutlery, getting in and out of the bath, and getting up and down the stairs since the fall.

### Past medical history and drug history:
- Your GP mentioned occupational therapy when you saw him last month but you haven't heard any more about it. Perhaps he knew that the doctor here in clinic could arrange it

### Social history:
- You live alone. Family live a few hours away (daughter with small children)
- Non-smoker. You don't drink alcohol

### Other issues including family history:
- Nil of note

### Your questions for the candidate:
- *Is there any way you can keep me independent at home?*
- *Are there any medicines that would help?*
- *Will my daughter/grandchildren develop RA?*

# Candidate

## History/key questions

Ask about the current symptoms and how they have progressed with time: pain, stiffness, weakness

You need to establish whether the patient has any active disease that is contributing to her current symptoms, as the approach to management differs if there is active synovitis. The presence and duration of morning stiffness would support active disease

Ask about the patient's ability to carry out ADL

Ask about the effects this is having on the patient's life

Is anyone helping her with any of the ADL (shopping, cleaning, dressing, washing [personal care], able to use cutlery, cooking for herself)?

### Drug history

Current medicines. Ask about analgesia used (NSAIDs, simple, opiates, atypical)

Any DMARDs now or in the past? Did these help and were there any side-effects?

Use of steroids (intra-articular, intramuscular, oral)

Assess need for gastroprotection (PPI) and bone protection (calcium / vitamin D, or bisphosphonates)

Ever been on biological therapy?

### Past medical history

How long has she had RA?

Any joint surgery?

### Social history

Any assessment by occupational therapy (OT) recently? If so, what were the recommendations/any aids installed?

Does she have adapted cutlery or any other aids?

Physio input – joint protection exercises in early disease, exercises for maintaining range of movement and muscle strength

## Address patient's questions and concerns

• *Have you had any thoughts about what is going on?*
• *Is there anything in particular you're concerned about?*
• *Do you have anything you would like to ask?*

## Key areas for examination

A list of what to look for (in examination order; describe findings on examination)

Need to identify features of RA and decide if there is active inflammation or not

Check for pain before starting; get patient comfortable quickly using a pillow to rest the hands/elbows on

Overall inspection

Arms/elbow surfaces: look for rheumatoid nodules, patches of psoriasis on elbows, scars from previous operations

Hairline: scalp psoriasis

Nails: nailfold infarcts, clubbing, onycholysis, pitting (psoriasis)

Hand deformity:

 Ulnar deviation at MCP joints

 Z deformity of thumb (flexion of the MCP joint of thumb and hyperextension of the interphalangeal joint)

 Swan neck deformity (PIP hyperextension and flexion at DIP and MCP joints)

 Boutonnière's deformity (hyperextension at MCP and DIP and flexion at PIP – due to rupture of extensor tendon slip)

 Muscle wasting, due to nerve entrapment, or deformity and disuse (thenar eminence due to median, hypothenar due to ulnar nerve lesions/entrapment; generalized wasting of small muscles of hand)

Palpation: gently palpate each joint individually, checking temperature compared to forearm (normal control) and testing for synovitis (gently palpate joint line); look for effusions, swelling, erythema and pain on movement (active or passive) which all point towards active inflammation. Do this in a systematic way and don't forget the wrists

Active movements: test pincer (make an 'O' and don't let me open it), grip fingers, spread fingers like a fan, make a fist, and don't let me bend your wrist (extension and flexion)

Upper limb movements: it is important to check other upper limb joints as hand function can be significantly impaired in the presence of elbow and shoulder disease

Test function: ask the patient to write a sentence, pick up a coin from the table, undo buttons, and put both hands up to (brush) hair (or behind head); reach behind back as if to undo bra. Holding cutlery, jars, cups

Say that you would like to look for other features of RA; consider neck and lower limb joint examination, features of vasculitis (nailfold infarcts, scleritis, leg ulceration – may be multifactorial – pericarditis, neuropathy, urinalysis), sicca syndrome (dry eyes and xerostomia), lung involvement (pleural effusion, interstitial lung disease), myelopathy from cervical spine disease

## Differential diagnosis

The diagnosis should be fairly straightforward in this case:

Rheumatoid arthritis

Marked deformity causing difficulties with ADL

In others, you may need to consider psoriatic arthritis, polyarticular gout and SLE, all of which can have a symmetrical polyarthritis, but other clinical features normally suggest these diseases

## Discussion with patient

Explain diagnosis

Explain plan, including investigations and management

Address patient's concerns/answer their questions

The difficulties you are having with washing, dressing, cooking, etc., are due to the chronic damage to your joints from the rheumatoid arthritis rather than inflammation in the joints which could be treated with medicines. We need to ask the occupational therapist in the rheumatology department to assess you and provide advice and equipment to improve your ability to carry out your activities of daily living at home. We will also ask the physiotherapist to see you, and arrange for you to see the rheumatology clinical nurse specialist who can also support you.

## Investigations

Basic blood tests (FBC looking for anaemia – chronic disease, blood loss, myelosuppression, low WBC from DMARD myelosuppression or Felty's syndrome [very rare these days]), ESR, CRP (active inflammation), U&E, LFT

Urinalysis (proteinuria/haematuria): consider renal vasculitis, amyloid, urine infection

X-ray hands and feet (reduced joint space, erosions, periarticular osteoporosis)

Flexion/extension view of cervical spine

CXR for interstitial lung disease/pleural effusion

MRI of cervical spine if myelopathy suspected

Nerve conduction studies if possible carpal tunnel syndrome

## Management

Patient information, education and support

Referral to rheumatology OT; introduce to the rheumatology clinical nurse specialist (CNS) in clinic

Patient information (hospital leaflets and Arthritis Reseach Council [ARC])

Occupational therapy: provide splints, adjusted cutlery with larger handles, grips for opening jars, picking things off floors. Link to community teams for household improvements, e.g. bath seats, rails in house, etc.

Physiotherapy: strengthen remaining muscles, and try to preserve joint function (reduce loss of range of movement/mobility in joints)

Analgesia

Bone protection if on steroids / DEXA if any prior fractures

In the absence of disease activity, DMARDs are not indicated. In early active disease, the approach is for early suppression of inflammation with short courses of steroids (intra-articular, IM, oral) and introduction of DMARDs (methotrexate, sulphasalazine, hydroxychloroquine or leflunomide) either as mono- or combination therapy. In the UK, patients who fail on two DMARDs and have persistent disease activity may be eligible for biological therapy (anti-TNF, anti-B cell [rituximab] or anti-IL-6 [tocilizumab] in that order).

## Addressing concerns/answering questions

- *Is there any way you can keep me independent at home?* The occupational therapists can provide aids to help with washing, dressing, eating, carrying, etc., and can help with exercises to improve your hand dexterity to help you remain independent at home. Physiotherapy can help to improve your muscle strength and help to reduce your risk of falling. We can help you get a pendant alarm to call for help if you fall again and can't get up.
- *Are there any medicines that would help?* No, as there are no signs of active inflammation at the moment. There's signs of chronic joint damage due to the long-term RA – medications will not help this damage.
- *Will my daughter/grandchildren develop RA?* Although there are genes which can increase someone's susceptibility to / risk of developing RA, this is only part of the picture. As with many conditions, it is a combination of the genes you're born with and things you come in contact with in the environment that lead to you developing particular conditions. It is difficult to predict an individual's risk of developing RA.

## Discussion with examiners

The examiners may ask you to clarify details of the above diagnosis and ask questions about your planned investigations and management.

A possible question includes:

- *How could you assess and reduce the risk of her sustaining a fracture?* It is important for her to remain active

– encourage her to try to do weight-bearing exercise to improve her bone strength. Assess her risk of fracture with a FRAX score (see links below) and, if indicated, a bone density scan. Depending on the FRAX score, options vary from lifestyle advice, DEXA scanning or treatment. FRAX score requires age, sex, height, weight, smoking status Y/N, previous fracture Y/N, parental hip fracture Y/N, corticosteroid use (current) Y/N, rheumatoid arthritis Y/N, secondary osteoporosis Y/N, alcohol 3 or more units per day Y/N, femoral neck bone mineral density (g/cm³). One can submit the rest of the above data without a DEXA result to obtain a 10-year probability of major osteoporotic fracture or hip fracture, and the site provides guidance on the required next step including whether a bone density scan is required.

See also Section I, Station 5, Locomotor, Case 1.

## Resources

FRAX available at University of Sheffield's dedicated site: www.shef.ac.uk/FRAX/

UK-specific FRAX site: www.shef.ac.uk/FRAX/tool.aspx?country=1

---

### Examiners' information and requirements

The candidate should:

1. Identify key features from the history: identify that the patient is known to have RA, and function is impaired leading to difficulties with ADL. Any symptoms consistent with active disease; any physio or OT input?

2. Identify key examination findings including evidence of RA; need to look for signs of synovitis/active disease but also for other extra-articular manifestations of RA; assess upper limb and hand function

3. Outline a sensible management plan, as detailed above. To include OT and physio, including aids for ADL

4. Give a clear explanation to the patient of your diagnosis and plan, address her concerns and answer her questions

# Scenario 6 | Psoriatic arthropathy

## Candidate's information

**Your role:** you are an ST2 in the rheumatology clinic. A 35-year-old artist presents with a 6-month history of pain and swelling in his fingers, and he is concerned as his painting hand is now affected.

**Your task:** to assess the patient's problems and address any questions or concerns raised by him.

## Patient's information

**You are:** Christopher Brandon, a 35-year-old graphic designer.

**Your problem:** you have pain and swelling in your right thumb. You first noticed problems in your ring finger on the right hand about 3 years ago, when it became swollen and the finger had restricted bending /straightening (flexion/extension). This settled over a few months and you didn't see anyone about it. Then about 6 months ago you first noticed that you had some swelling of the thumb on the same hand, and the main joint of the thumb felt warm/hot. You took some ibuprofen and it settled with this initially but has now been causing problems with your work, and you are worried that it could prevent you working in the future. It's not too bad at the moment as you're quiet at work but is much worse after a long day at the desk drawing. Ibuprofen doesn't seem to help any more and only resting lets it settle. Your thumb feels really stiff in the morning and takes time to get back to normal. You can't afford to lose your job.

### Past medical history and drug history:
- Tonsils removed age 4
- Malaria age 19 years in East Africa
- Scalp and elbow psoriasis – you use topical calcitriol and occasional steroids to control it. Alcohol makes it worse

### Social history:
- Married 4 years ago, trying for a family at present

### Other issues including family history:
- No-one else in the family has any arthritis other than maybe some wear and tear (both parents)

### Your questions for the candidate:
- *Why are my fingers swelling up? Does it leave permanent damage?*
- *Is this rheumatoid arthritis?*
- *Will the medicines interfere with me trying to have children?*

## Candidate

### History/key questions

Which joints have been affected and in which distribution (symmetrical or asymmetrical; large or small joints)?

What do you feel is wrong with them? Ask about pain, swelling, stiffness

When did it start? Did it start suddenly or come on gradually? Are the symptoms continuous or do they come and go?

Does anything make the symptoms better or worse?

Ask about morning stiffness (consistent with inflammatory process) and pain after exertion/activity (OA)

Any past history of joint problems, in childhood and as an adult. If so, same questions as above to characterize the problems

Any other features: back or neck pain (thinking of ankylosing spondylitis), GI symptoms consistent with UC or Crohn's – seronegative arthropathy as extraintestinal manifestation of IBD (weight loss, diarrhoea, abdominal pain, mouth ulcers, perianal abscesses or fistula); ulceration of mouth/genitals – reactive arthritis, Behçet's, SLE

Any rashes (psoriasis, vasculitis)

How is it affecting him in terms of work activities, hobbies, home life?

### Drug history

What drugs have you been using and did they help?

Ask about use of NSAIDs, and ask about any previous use of DMARDs/biologicals

Any topical/systemic treatments for psoriasis

### Past medical history

Past history of any other condition associated with arthropathy, e.g. known to have RA, OA, SLE, IBD (extraintestinal manifestation of IBD), gout/pseudogout

### Social history

Non-smoker, drinks a glass of wine or two per week

### Family history

Psoriasis/arthritis

### Address patient's questions and concerns

- *Have you had any thoughts about what is going on?*
- *Is there anything in particular you're concerned about?*
- *Do you have anything you would like to ask?*

## Key areas for examination

A list of what to look for (in examination order; describe findings on examination)

Look for plaque psoriasis (scalp – hairline, behind ears; extensor aspect of upper limbs/elbows)

Look for rheumatoid nodules, patches of psoriasis on elbows

Hands: in psoriatic arthritis, there may be an asymmetrical arthritis with DIP involvement. Look for dactylitis and any pain from enthesitis

Nails: nailfold infarcts, clubbing, onycholysis, pitting (psoriasis), transverse ridging

Any deformity: features of RA include ulnar deviation at MCP joints, Z deformity of thumb, swan neck deformity and Boutonnière's deformity

Palpation: gently palpate each joint individually, checking temperature compared to forearm (normal control) and testing for synovitis (gently palpate joint space of each joint); look for effusions, warmth, swelling, stiffness, erythema and pain on movement (active or passive) which all point towards active inflammation

Active movements: test pincer (make an 'O' and don't let me open it), grip fingers, spread fingers like a fan, make a fist, and don't let me bend your wrist (extension and flexion)

Upper limb movements: it is important to check other upper limb joints as hand function can be significantly impaired in the presence of elbow and shoulder disease

Test function: ask the patient to write a sentence, pick up a coin from the table, undo buttons, and put both hands up to (brush) hair (or behind head); reach behind back. Holding cutlery, jars, cups

If the history suggests inflammatory back pain, then the spine should be examined as well

## Differential diagnosis

Psoriatic arthropathy but there is a wide differential diagnosis to be considered for an arthropathy affecting the small joints of the hands: RA, seronegative arthropathies such as psoriatic arthropathy, reactive arthritis, OA, gout, pseudogout (ankylosing spondylitis?)

## Discussion with patient

Explain diagnosis

Explain plan, including investigations and management

Address patient's concerns/answer their questions

The swelling of your thumb is due to inflammation of the lining of the joints in the hands, and this is related to your psoriasis. We need to carry out some investigations to find out more before deciding on the best way forward. This will include blood tests and X-rays.

## Investigations
Basic blood tests including FBC, ESR, CRP
X-rays of hands
Check rheumatoid factor

## Management of psoriatic arthropathy
Simple analgesics (paracetamol)
NSAIDs
Corticosteroid injections if single joint
DMARDs – methotrexate, sulphasalazine, leflunomide
Biologicals: criteria for psoriatic arthropathy

## Addressing concerns/answering questions
- *Why are my fingers swelling up? Does it leave permanent damage?* We need to carry out the above investigations to assess how your fingers are currently; on-going active inflammation in your joints can lead to long-term damage so we will need to review the results and discuss management, including a possible need for medications.
- *Is this rheumatoid arthritis?* It would seem to be related to your psoriasis rather than RA.
- *Will the medicines interfere with me trying to have children?* Men taking either leflunomide or methotrexate need to allow a 3-month washout period before trying to conceive. The inflammation in the joint(s) shouldn't affect fertility.

## Discussion with examiners
The examiners may ask you to clarify details of the above diagnosis and ask questions about your planned investigations and management.

Other possible questions include:
- *What are the different types of psoriatic arthropathy?*
  Distal arthritis involving DIP joints
  Asymmetric oligoarthritis, with less than five small and/or large joints (hands and feet initially)
  Symmetric polyarthritis, similar to RA pattern – can be indistinguishable from RA. The most common of the presentations
  Arthritis mutilans, deforming and destructive arthritis leading to 'telescoping' of fingers
  Spondyloarthritis, including sacroiliitis and spondylitis
- *What are the potential side-effects of methotrexate?* Major side-effects include hepatotoxicity, myelosuppression (macrocytosis or pancytopenia), pulmonary toxicity (inflammatory and fibrotic lung disease, infections). Common potential side-effects include gastrointestinal disturbance including nausea, diarrhoea; stomatitis; rash; headache or fatigue; hair loss/alopecia.

See also Section I, Station 5, Locomotor, Case 2.

---

### Examiners' information and requirements
The candidate should:
1. Identify key features from the history: small joint arthropathy in a patient with psoriasis; single joints affected in the past; concerns regarding ability to work, conception/fertility
2. Identify key examination findings, including evidence of psoriasis, nail pitting, etc., an asymmetrical arthritis with DIP involvement consistent with psoriatic arthropathy
3. Outline a sensible management plan, including appropriate blood tests and radiology
4. Give a clear explanation to the patient of your diagnosis and management plan, address his concerns (including issues regarding fertility) and answer his questions

# Scenario 7 | Ankylosing spondylitis: short notes

The case may focus on differentiation of inflammatory from mechanical pain (with or without nerve root symptoms), the association of spinal pain with other features of a seronegative spondyloarthropathy or the impact of the condition on the patient's work. Therefore you may need to elicit a history of spinal early morning stiffness, the progression and severity of symptoms over time and the duration of the current symptoms during the day. Stiffness can be more of a problem than pain. Relieving factors for symptoms often revolve around exercise – ask if the patient has specific exercises that they undertake; how often/how long for and who showed them (physiotherapist, National Ankylosing Spondylitis Society exercise class); do they help? This can lead on to asking about the impact on their work/social life. In early disease patients are better in more active than sedentary employment. With chronic disease, any fixed restrictions in spinal movement can limit physical activity.

Check that the patient does not have any extraspinal disease (arthropathy – lower limb, especially the hip), enthesitis, dactylitis, iritis, psoriasis, inflammatory bowel disease or any family history of any of these.

Examination should check for features that support the diagnosis of ankylosing spondylitis, such as loss of lumbar lordosis, a reduction in the modified Schober index and increased occiput–wall distance. Look for extra-articular features as mentioned above and assess the severity of these problems.

Non-steroidal anti-inflammatory drugs play the main role in treatment (consider gastric, renal and cardiac toxicity), DMARDs are helpful for peripheral joint involvement and anti-TNF agents are useful for spinal inflammation unresponsive to NSAIDs and exercises.

See also Section I, Station 5, Locomotor, Case 6.

# Scenario 8 | Gout: short notes

The diagnosis of gout is often made on the history, with episodes of severe inflammatory joint pain lasting 10–14 days. Swelling and redness are nearly always present and the pain is severe (even light touch from bed clothes gives excruciating pain). Initial episodes nearly always start in the first MTP joint and then spread to involve others.

Normal joint function returns after initial episodes but recurrent attacks can lead to joint damage that gives persistent mechanical symptoms in between attacks. Chronic tophaceous gout can be a combination of inflammatory and mechanical symptoms, where the pattern of joint involvement changes from asymmetrical monoarthritis to a chronic symmetrical polyarthritis.

Don't assume that nodules at the elbow are rheumatoid in nature; look closely for the whitish deposits of uric acid at the elbow and other sites (fingers, ear, heel). Don't forget to ask about risk factors (diet – purine rich, alcohol, drugs – thiazides, family history and renal impairment) and the impact that flare-ups have on work.

Management can be tricky so a clear history of any lifestyle changes and what drugs are used for attacks (options range from NSAIDs versus colchicine versus steroid – oral or intra-articular) and their relative benefits/toxicities is important. Recurrent episodes need uric acid-lowering therapy, for which allopurinol is first line. Uricosurics are very difficult to obtain and thus infrequently used. Check compliance with any medication and whether uric acid levels are monitored. Effective therapy aims to get the uric acid well into the normal range and this can lead to resorption of tophi over a period of years.

See also Section I, Station 5, Locomotor, Case 5.

# Scenario 9 | Steroid toxicity: short notes

Many patients with rheumatic disease may receive steroids and suffer with side-effects. Polymyalgia with or without giant cell arteritis (GCA) is one of the most common rheumatological conditions to be treated with long-term steroids. You may have to elicit the features of steroid toxicity and put these into context of the condition being treated. Ask about other risk factors for some of the more common side-effects (e.g. osteoporosis, diabetes, hypertension), the effect of other side-effects on lifestyle (e.g. weight gain, cataracts) and don't forget the central side-effects of insomnia, restlessness and increased appetite.

Steroid dose for polymyalgia rheumatica (PMR) and GCA should generally be titrated based on symptoms and guided by the inflammatory response (ESR/CRP). PMR symptoms are of pain and stiffness, which improve considerably within 2–5 days of starting steroids, while weakness is more a feature of polymyositis or steroid myopathy. Recurrent relapses or excessive steroid toxicity is an indication for steroid-sparing agents (methotrexate or azathioprine). Remember that the starting dose of steroids for PMR is 15–20 mg a day and for GCA is 60 mg daily. Eighteen months' therapy is needed in most cases and relapses are more frequent when dose reduction is too rapid.

See also Section I, Station 5, Endocrine, Case 6.

# Other reported rheumatology cases

- A person with rheumatoid arthritis (see Section I, Station 5, Locomotor, Case 1) wanting to know side-effects of infliximab infusion
- Middle-aged lady with rheumatoid arthritis (see Section I, Station 5, Locomotor, Case 1) on long-term biological therapy (e.g. adalimumab) presenting with night sweats
- Ankylosing spondylitis (see Section I, Station 5, Locomotor, Case 6) – effects on ADL/work – see notes above
- Ankylosing spondylitis (see Section I, Station 5, Locomotor, Case 6) in an elderly man with chronic diarrhoea and muscle pains
- Mixed connective tissue diseases: history of Raynaud's, Sjögren's and polyarthralgia (see Section I, Station 5, Locomotor, Case 3)
- Shoulder pain/adhesive capsulitis
- Gouty tophi (see Section I, Station 5, Locomotor, Case 5 and notes above)
- OA (see Section I, Station 5, Locomotor, Case 8)
- Acute hot joints are unlikely to be included

# Scenario 10 | Thyroid eye disease

## Candidate's information

**Your role:** you are the SHO in the gastroenterology clinic, and this patient is attending the clinic following an admission and endoscopic retrograde cholangiopancreatography (ERCP) for cholangitis/biliary obstruction due to gallstones.

**Your task:** to assess the patient's problems and address any questions or concerns raised by her.

## Patient's information

**You are:** Denise Kirk, a 55-year-old woman, attending the gastroenterology clinic after an episode of jaundice and fever caused by gallstones. You were told that you would come for a check-up and to see whether you needed to have your gallbladder removed.

**Your problem:** your main concern is that you've noticed gritty eyes over the past 7–8 months, which have been worse more recently. You get slight blurring and perhaps double vision at times, particularly if tired. This is your main concern and something you would like dealt with today. There are no changes in acuity or colour vision, your eyes just feel dry and sore. You have never seen an optician or ophthalmologist previously for this. Your family have mentioned that your eyes look more prominent, sometimes bulging.

You found the ERCP test very uncomfortable – you remember retching a great deal. You don't think you really had enough sedation and you're not keen to repeat it. You've not had any further jaundice or tummy pain. No fever, stools normal, weight stable. If asked, you have an appointment to see the surgeons next week about having an operation to remove your gallbladder to stop the gallstones blocking the tubes again.

### Past medical history and drug history:
- Treated for hyperthyroidism with thyroidectomy about 3 years ago
- Now on levothyroxine 125 µg once per day. The GP last checked thyroid blood tests about 6 months ago. No change in dose for at least the past 18 months
- No drug allergies

### Social history:
- Smoked 30/day for 25 years, now smoking 10/day

### Other issues including family history:
- Nil of note

### Your questions for the candidate:
- *Will I need endoscopy again for the gallstones?*
- *Why are my eyes gritty?*
- *What can be done about the gallstones in the gallbladder?*

# Candidate

## History/key questions

Regarding gallstones:

Any further episodes of abdominal pain, jaundice, pale stools, dark urine, itch (suggestive of biliary obstruction) or fever, pain, jaundice (cholangitis)

Ask if referral for cholecystectomy was discussed during the recent admission. This is carried out to reduce the risk of further episodes of biliary obstruction due to gallstones (although doesn't completely remove risk as they can relatively rarely form even without a gallbladder). Does she have an appointment to see the surgeons in clinic?

Ask about vision/eyes:

Onset – gradual or sudden, and over what duration?

Diplopia

Eye pain/discomfort

Changes in visual acuity/colour vision

Ever seen opticians or ophthalmologists previously for this or other eye problems

Any history of thyroid problems/ever treated for thyroid problems

Medications (levothyroxine, carbimazole, propylthiouracil), radio-iodine or surgery

Need to assess thyroid status: is patient euthyroid or displaying symptoms and/or signs of hypo- or hyperthyroidism?

Hypothyroidism: lethargy, tiredness, weight gain, slow mentation/poor concentration, depression, deep/hoarse voice, constipation, intolerance of cold

Hyperthyroidism: heat intolerance, weight loss, palpitations, diarrhoea, hair loss, irritability

### Drug history

Ask about current medications, doses and frequency; any allergies

Drugs for hypothyroidism – levothyroxine, including dose

Hyperthyroidism – ask about propranolol, carbimazole, propylthiouracil

Ask about drugs which can cause thyroid dysfunction, e.g. amiodarone (hyper- and hypothyroidism), lithium (hypothyroidism)

### Past medical history

Any autoimmune conditions

Ask about past history of thyroidectomy

### Social history

Nil of note

## Address patient's questions and concerns

- *Have you had any thoughts about what is going on?*
- *Is there anything in particular you're concerned about?*
- *Do you have anything you would like to ask?*

## Key areas for examination

A list of what to look for (in examination order; describe findings on examination)

Inspection: any evidence of jaundice?

Assess thyroid status (see Section G, Examination *routine* 19):

Voice – hoarse, deep in hypothyroidism

Signs of tremor/anxiety/weight loss in hyperthyroidism. Thinning of the temporal hair

Sweaty palms, palmar erythema and tachycardia in hyperthyroidism; check whether in AF

Dry skin and bradycardia in hypothyroidism

Thyroid acropachy (1% of Graves'): resembles finger clubbing in hypertrophic pulmonary osteoarthropathy

Eye signs – present in 30% of patients with Graves' disease:

Kocher's sign – fixed staring look

Periorbital oedema

Proptosis/exophthalmos – sclera visible above the lower eyelid when looking straight ahead; also examine from the side

Lid lag and lid retraction (white of sclera visible above the iris when looking forward)

Ophthalmoplegia

Conjunctival oedema/chemosis

Look for keratitis, ulceration of cornea

Pupils – look for relative afferent pupillary defect (RAPD) as compression of the optic nerve can occur with proptosis

Say that you would like to assess visual acuity and colour vision (given time constraints)

Fundoscopy (ask for this to be done, although the examiner will be unlikely to want it in this case given time constraints) – papilloedema, optic atrophy or glaucoma

Assess eye movements (see Section G, Examination *routine* 13): test for diplopia (most often will be on vertical gaze due to inferior rectus muscle involvement) – use the term 'complex ophthalmoplegia' if multiple muscles are involved

Any eye discomfort

Goitre (see Section G, Examination *routine* 18): need to check whether present or not. Examine the neck from behind. Ask the patient to swallow water.

If goitre present, percuss to assess for retrosternal extension and auscultate for bruit

Evidence of previous thyroidectomy – scar

Any proximal myopathy (thyrotoxic): test by asking patient to stand up from seated position without using her hands

Look for pretibial myxoedema (Graves' – see Section I, Station 5, Endocrine, Case 3) (anterolateral lower limbs or thighs) or peripheral oedema/periorbital myxoedema

Slow relaxing ankle reflexes (hypothyroidism): (again, there may not be time to test for this)

Abdomen: any hepatomegaly/tenderness over gallbladder. Scratch marks (itch from jaundice)

Look for signs of associated autoimmune conditions: there may not be time for this so you need to remember to say that you would

In this case the patient has euthyroid Graves' disease with a history of thyroidectomy for hyperthyroidism in the past; signs include exophthalmos with pretibial myxoedema; the pulse is regular and the rate is normal. No signs of hyperthyroidism; thyroidectomy scar present. No jaundice

## Differential diagnosis

Thyroid eye disease: swelling of the orbit's contents due to the retro-orbital inflammation and lymphocyte infiltration. Can be hypo-, hyper- or euthyroid

Gallstones causing biliary obstruction were cleared at a recent ERCP but the patient needs cholecystectomy to reduce the risk of further events. Not jaundiced at present

## Discussion with patient

Explain diagnosis

Explain plan, including investigations and management

Address patient's concerns/answer their questions

Your eye problems would seem to be related to your past history of thyroid disease (overactivity), and you need some blood tests to check on your thyroid. We need to refer you to the endocrinologist and eye specialists who will carry out some investigations to see exactly what is happening with your thyroid and the eyes to cause the double vision, and work out the next step.

For the gallstones, you're due to see the surgeons next week, and they will be able to explain what surgery would involve, and the benefits and risks.

## Investigations and management

Treat any hyperthyroidism; symptom management with propranolol (non-selective β-blocker); carbimazole/propylthiouracil, radioiodine, surgery

Stop smoking as soon as possible (worsens eye disease): perhaps one of the key steps as there is a direct link with eye disease worsening

Urgent involvement of specialists/ophthalmic surgeons if there are concerns about optic nerve compression (reduced vision or papilloedema)

Imaging (CT or MRI) of orbits

Lubrication (topical eyedrops)

Lateral tarsorrhaphy (protects cornea)

High-dose steroids, surgical decompression or radiotherapy may be indicated

Prisms in glasses (can be adjusted as eyes change with treatment)

Cholecystectomy indicated if fit following episode of biliary obstruction and/or cholangitis due to gallstones

## Addressing concerns/answering questions

- *Will I need endoscopy again for the gallstones?* All the stones in the tubes were removed, and you won't need another ERCP unless a stone blocks the tubes again (but there is less risk as during the endoscopy a cut was made to the opening of the bile duct into the bowel, which will allow any stones to pass through).
- *Why are my eyes gritty?* This is due to a condition related to the problems you had in the past with your thyroid gland, and there is swelling in the tissues around and behind the eye causing the lids not to completely close and the eyes to dry up, and this causes the grittiness. We need to explain here that although the thyroid disease *per se* is stable, thyroid eye disease can sometimes follow its own course and be active despite thyroid gland function being normal.
- *What can you do about the gallstones in the gallbladder?* ERCP doesn't treat the gallstones in the gallbladder. Instead an operation (cholecystectomy) is needed to remove the gallbladder (the source of the stones).

## Discussion with examiners

The examiners may ask you to clarify details of the above diagnosis and ask questions about your planned investigations and management.

Other possible questions include:

- *Discussion of Graves' disease.* Features can be seen in hypo-, hyper- and euthyroid patients. Eye disease may precede Graves' by some years and may not improve with treatment of hyperthyroidism. Diffuse goitre, ophthalmopathy, dermopathy (but they don't all have to be present). Eye signs specific to Graves' (not other causes of thyrotoxicosis). Antibodies specific to Graves' – TSH receptor antibody.

- *What else can cause proptosis?* Neoplasia including retro-orbital lymphangioma, lymphoma, meningioma and metastases. Cavernous haemangioma or cavernous sinus thrombosis; orbital varices. Wegener's and other causes of retro-orbital granuloma (sarcoid, histiocytosis X). Orbital cellulitis.
- *What autoimmune conditions are associated with Graves' disease?* See also Section I, Station 5, Skin, Case 8. Pernicious anaemia, Addison's disease, diabetes mellitus, renal tubular acidosis, fibrosing alveolitis, primary biliary cirrhosis, chronic active hepatitis, hypoparathyroidism, premature ovarian failure, atrophic gastritis with iron deficiency anaemia.

See also Section I, Station 5, Endocrine, Case 1.

---

**Examiners' information and requirements**

The candidate should:

1. Identify key features from the history: blurred vision, gritty eyes; no symptoms of hyper- or hypothyroidism; no recent symptoms suggestive of biliary obstruction /cholangitis
2. Identify key examination findings of long-standing thyroid eye disease including proptosis; signs of thyroid status
3. Outline a sensible plan for management of eye disease including referral to specialist endocrinology and ophthalmology clinics; referral for consideration of cholecystectomy (due to see surgeons)
4. Give a clear explanation to the patient of your diagnosis and plan, address her concerns and answer her questions

# Scenario 11 | Acromegaly

## Candidate's information

**Your role:** You are the ST2 in a general medical clinic. A 50-year-old woman is referred to the general medical clinic with intermittent visual blurring and frontal headache. Her only past history is of diet-controlled diabetes mellitus and colonic polyps found at colonoscopy last year.

**Your task:** to assess the patient's problems and address any questions or concerns raised by her.

## Patient's information

**You are:** Jane Grayling, a 50-year-old woman.

**Your problem:** you've noticed problems with your vision over the past 6 months which you think have been giving you headaches. You usually wear glasses to read, and at an appointment 3 months ago, the optician says that these were fine. You've recently had problems driving, particularly parking and being aware of what's around you. You have found it hard to change lanes on the motorway.

If the doctor asks, you've brought some family portraits from the last 20 years as suggested by your GP. You agree that your appearance has changed but who doesn't in their later years?

The headaches can be worse if you've been busy, particularly recently with your work organizing the local Women's Institute, but you've not noticed any other times when they come on. They rarely occur in the morning, and are not worse if you cough. No weight loss or chest problems.

### Past medical history and drug history:
- Your GP diagnosed 'borderline diabetes' 2 years ago, and now you control it with diet only. At the last check it was apparently OK. No known hypertension – haven't had it checked by your GP for a while
- Colonic polyps were found at colonoscopy last year. All benign, and another camera test is scheduled for 5 years hence

### Social history:
- You live alone. You are a retired school dinner lady
- Non-smoker, don't drink alcohol

### Other issues including family history:
- Nil of note

### Your questions for the candidate:
- *What is happening to my vision?*
- *Why have my hands got bigger and what can be done about it?*

## Candidate

### History/key questions

Headache:

Ask about the headache and the associated symptoms

Site, unilateral versus bilateral headache

Character

Onset – gradual, sudden onset

Duration of headache episodes, and when did they start?

Frequency of headaches

Associated features: any auras, nausea, photophobia, hemiparesis?

Exacerbating and relieving factors, e.g. stress/tiredness leading to frontal headaches; variation with time of day

Visual changes:

Onset – sudden versus gradual

Duration – when did they start?

Any exacerbating factors associated with headache?

When does she notice the problems – walking, driving, etc.?

Any diplopia?

Any increase in hand size, shoe size or hat size?

Galactorrhoea, excessive sweating, arthritis

Pins/needles or numbness in fingers

Amenorrhoea, loss of libido

Any other features of acromegaly: sweating, diabetes mellitus, proximal muscle weakness (difficulty getting out of chairs), carpal tunnel syndrome, lethargy, labile mood?

### Drug history

Check current medications, any allergies

### Past medical history

Ask about diabetes or impaired glucose tolerance; hypertension; kidney stones

Hypercalcaemia/hypercalciuria (as part of multiple endocrine neoplasia [MEN] 1)

Colonic polyps/any previous cancers of the bowel

### Social history

Alcohol consumption (units per week) and smoking history

Ask to see any photographs (old ones of the patient) if she has any with her

### Address patient's questions and concerns

* *Have you had any thoughts about what is going on?*
* *Is there anything in particular you're concerned about?*
* *Do you have anything you would like to ask?*

## Key areas for examination

A list of what to look for (in examination order; describe findings on examination)

Need to identify features of acromegaly but also assess vision/visual fields

Inspection:

Acromegaly – 'coarse features' (although avoid using this term)

Prominent supraorbital ridges, large lower jaw. Exaggerated facial wrinkles

Enlarged lips and nose

Increased interdental spaces; prognathism

Macroglossia

Large 'spade-shaped' hands with thickened skin; sweaty

Evidence of carpal tunnel syndrome – look for carpal tunnel release scars/Tinel's sign (Vol. 1, Station 3, Central Nervous System, Case 33)

Bilateral hearing aids

Hirsutism, excessive sweating

Husky voice

CNS:

Test visual fields – bitemporal visual field defect (present in this patient)

Fundoscopy (exclude papilloedema)

Other physical signs of acromegaly:

Skin tags

Acanthosis nigricans

Proximal muscle weakness

Look for mild hirsutism in women

## Differential diagnosis

Mainly should focus on causes of acromegaly

Acromegaly due to pituitary tumour causing bitemporal peripheral visual field defect (95% of acromegaly caused by pituitary adenoma)

Headache a feature of pituitary tumour: no evidence clinically of raised intracranial pressure

## Discussion with patient

Explain diagnosis

Explain plan, including investigations and management

Address patient's concerns/answer their questions

It is likely that a small area in your brain behind the nose, where the master hormone-producing gland is located (called the pituitary gland), is producing higher than usual amounts of a particular hormone which has caused your hands and bones to grow. We need to carry out tests to confirm this, and to find the cause. It is usually due to a small growth in the brain (usually benign) that can be treated with medicines and/or surgery.

## Investigations

Review photos of patient (recent and previous)

Check BP

Random growth hormone (GH). Proceed if any doubt about diagnosis to oral glucose tolerance test (OGTT) with glucose and growth hormone levels to confirm the diagnosis at 0, then every 30 min until 150 min. In normal individuals, GH is suppressed to less than 1.0 ng/mL 2 h after the patient takes 75 g oral glucose (patients with acromegaly due to active pituitary tumours are unable to do this); 15–20% of patients with acromegaly have a paradoxical rise in GH concentration

Serum insulin-like growth factor (IGF)-1 (linked to/correlates with GH secretion in the previous 24 h) will be increased in acromegaly

MRI of head/pituitary fossa

Full pituitary testing: evaluation of the adrenal, thyroid and gonadal axes (free T4, TSH, prolactin, oestradiol [females], testosterone [males], LH, FSH, morning cortisol)

ECHO, ECG

Formal visual fields and acuity assessment

## Management

In view of the visual symptoms, investigation and treatment (surgery) are needed urgently as sight is under threat if tumour is impinging on optic chiasm

The goal of treatment is reduction of symptoms from the local effects of the tumour, increased GH/IGF-I production, or both

Surgery: trans-sphenoidal hypophysectomy. Usual first-line therapy. Remission rates of 80–85% (microadenomas) and 50–65% (macroadenomas)

Medical management: inhibition of GH release using somatostatin analogues (octreotide) or dopamine analogues; these are also sometimes used post-operatively to induce remission if surgery hasn't achieved this

Radiotherapy for refractory disease or if unfit/unsuitable for operation, but slow acting

Criteria for cure of acromegaly: normal IGF-1 and post-OGTT GH levels <1 μg/L and or mean GH levels over 2 h <1 μg/L

In view of visual field abnormality, advise that driving must stop unless ability to meet recommended national guidelines for visual field abnormalities is confirmed (DVLA guidelines). Visual fields will need to be formally assessed

## Addressing concerns/answering questions

- *What is happening to my vision?* The small area in the brain that is making the extra hormone can press on the nerves for vision, affecting your sight.
- *Why have my hands got bigger and what can be done?* We need to find out the cause and treat it, with medications and/or surgery. Unfortunately, the growth of your hands/feet isn't going to change/return to normal as these have developed over some time, even years.

## Discussion with examiners

The examiners may ask you to clarify details of the above diagnosis and ask questions about your planned investigations and management.

Other possible questions include:

- *What are the risks of trans-sphenoidal hypophysectomy?* Cerebrospinal fluid leak, cerebral salt wasting causing transient hyponatraemia, stroke, hypopituitarism.
- *What would you do if there was no mass seen in the pituitary fossa?* Review the films with a neuroradiologist, then arrange investigations to look for ectopic GH or GH-releasing hormone, e.g. pancreatic, adrenal, lung or ovarian neoplasia.
- *What problems are associated with acromegaly?* Colon cancer risk (10% and need for colonoscopic surveillance), diabetes mellitus, cardiomyopathy, hypertension, hyperthyroidism.

See also Section I, Station 5, Endocrine, Case 2.

---

### Examiners' information and requirements

The candidate should:

1. Identify key features from the history: visual disturbance, headache, impaired glucose tolerance, change in appearance
2. Identify key examination findings: clinical signs of acromegaly including bitemporal visual field defect but no signs of raised intracranial pressure
3. Include acromegaly as main differential diagnosis, and outline a sensible management plan including OGTT / GH measurements, urgent imaging (MRI brain/pituitary fossa), and appropriate onward referral to the endocrinologist
4. Give a clear explanation to the patient of your diagnosis and plan, address her concerns and answer her questions

---

# Scenario 12 | Diabetes mellitus and Charcot joint

## Candidate's information

**Your role:** you are a doctor in the diabetes clinic. A patient has been referred by his GP with poor diabetes control despite oral medications.

**Your task:** to assess the patient's problems and address any questions or concerns raised by him.

## Patient's information

**You are:** Andrew Newton, a 66-year-old man.

**Your problem:** your main concern is your swollen ankle rather than your diabetes, and the difficulty your ankle is causing you when you try to get round the house. You can't remember falling, or any other trauma to the ankle, but it did get swollen and hot a few months ago; the warmth settled down but it has remained swollen since. It's not painful but it feels heavy and affects your balance when you bear weight on that side.

You find yourself stumbling at home, and you don't notice if you get small stones in your shoes. This has caused problems at times and you used to see the chiropodist about some of the corns and ulcers on your feet but haven't been for 12 or more months as these healed up.

You know that your GP has referred you to the hospital to get your diabetes under control, but you think that your ankle is your main problem that needs to be sorted out.

### Past medical history and drug history:
- Diabetes mellitus
- Your usual blood sugar levels are mostly between 10 and 14. Any lower than 6 and you feel 'hypo', meaning you feel unwell and need to eat
- On metformin 500 mg bd and gliclazide 40 mg bd. You have not been taking either for several months because of the 'hypo' episodes you frequently had when taking both regularly

### Social history:
- You live alone in a terraced house. The bedroom and bathroom are upstairs. You have a single rail up the stairs to the first floor but no rails or aids in your bathroom
- Your son helps with shopping twice per week, and you call Ring and Ride to get to the day centre 3 days per week. This has been harder as your ankle has got worse, and now you're struggling with a stick. You wonder whether one of those trolleys would help
- Non-smoker

### Other issues including family history:
- Nil of note

**Your questions for the candidate:**
- *Why has the diabetes damaged my joints?*
- *Will I need an operation?*

## Candidate

### History/key questions

#### Diabetes history

How long has he had diabetes and how has his diabetes control been (does he know about his latest HbA1c – blood test measure of overall diabetes control)?

What medications and for how long. Ask about oral hypoglycaemic medications, insulin

Does he monitor his blood sugars and, if so, what is the usual range for blood sugar readings?

What is his target blood sugar (range)?

Date of last eye screening, kidney screening, BP check

Any changes in his weight over the past 6 months

Usual footcare arrangements – does he see a chiropodist?

History of any ankle or lower limb injuries (sprains, 'going over on the ankle', fractures in ankle)

Ever had ulcers on the feet or toes

Any history consistent with intermittent claudication, rest pain, etc. Any other vascular risk factors (smoking, cholesterol, obesity, hypertension) – check what medicines he's on

Ask about symptoms of neuropathy – numbness, burning, pain, paraesthesiae

Changes in walking/unsteadiness, falls

Ask relevant questions about other causes of neuropathy – vitamin B12/folate/alcohol, paraneoplastic, hypothyroidism, autoimmune, etc.

#### Social history

Who lives at home with him? Does he get any assistance from anyone?

Activities of daily living, and the effect of his ankle problem on this

Smoking history (pack-years)

Alcohol history

### Address patient's questions and concerns
- *Have you had any thoughts about what is going on?*
- *Is there anything in particular you're concerned about?*
- *Do you have anything you would like to ask?*

## Key areas for examination

A list of what to look for (in examination order; describe findings on examination)

Examine the affected joint

Charcot joints are painless, deformed and swollen, with an abnormal range of movement; joint instability (hypermobility of the joint) and crepitus will probably be marked, but you should not test for it! See Section I, Station 5, Locomotor, Case 4.

Look for ulcers and callus on the feet

Assess vascular supply to the feet (pulses in the popliteal, dorsalis pedis and posterior tibial arteries) and assess capillary refill

Peripheral nervous system: diabetic neuropathy diagnosed using history and examination of the feet/lower limbs; on examination, there may be loss of vibration and proprioception, loss of pain/fine touch/temperature; also loss/reduction in Achilles tendon reflex

Say that you would like to carry out a full neurological examination of lower limbs

Look for muscle wasting across the affected joint (compare with other side), e.g. distal lower limb

Dry, hairless skin

Tone, power and reflexes

Test sensation: look for loss of light touch, pinprick, proprioception/joint position and vibration (use a 128 Hz tuning fork) – posterior column signs

Check active and passive ranges of movement (probably restricted)

Say that you would like to complete your examination by examining the upper limb for neurology, and by assessing the patient's gait (you would be looking for ataxia, high-stepping gait [loss of proprioception in the ankle], positive Romberg's sign)

You need to look for signs of the other causes of Charcot joint – syringomyelia, tabes dorsalis/neurosyphilis (ulcers on the feet, Argyll-Robertson pupils), paraplegia, leprosy, myelomeningocoele, hereditary sensory neuropathies, congenital insensitivity to pain

## Differential diagnosis

The picture is consistent with longstanding, poor diabetes control due to poor compliance (not taking medications, not attending appointments, not sticking to diet and exercise advice) or insufficient treatment; as a result now complicated by Charcot joint/diabetes neuropathy – sensory only (glove and stocking distribution)

## Discussion with patient

Explain diagnosis

Explain plan, including investigations and management

Address patient's concerns/answer their questions

The nerves in your legs have been affected by your diabetes. Your ankle has been damaged by this as well, as you haven't been able to feel when it's been injured, and this looks to have led to chronic joint damage. We will need to do blood tests to exclude other causes of the nerve problems, and involve a group of professionals to help you with your diabetes and your ankle problems. This will include the diabetes team, podiatrists, orthotists and orthopaedic surgeons. We will need to check you're up to date with your eye and kidney checks too. It is really important that you control your blood sugars as strictly as possible to reduce the risk of further damage to your body from the diabetes.

## Investigations

Blood tests including FBC, ESR, CRP, LFT, glucose, thyroid function test, vitamin B12 and folate, ANA, autoimmune screen

Protein electrophoresis

Urinalysis and albumin:creatinine ratio

Bence Jones protein (urine)

VDRL/TPHA – syphilis serology

HbA1c

## Management of diabetic neuropathy

Tight control of diabetes (blood sugar levels), footcare to reduce risk of complications, analgesia for any neuropathic pain

Footcare – avoid injuries, podiatry (care with nail cutting)

Wash/dry feet, decent socks and well-fitting shoes (risk of blisters with reduced sensation). Footwear is often to be obtained from surgical supplies/orthotist

Analgesia with tricyclic antidepressants, duloxetine, gabapentin, etc.

## Management of Charcot joint (multidisciplinary team approach)

Diabetes specialist support

Diabetes foot clinic review

Full diabetes check-up including BP, eyes, feet, kidneys (U&E, urinalysis, albumin:creatinine ratio)

Initially patient may need a cast (to immobilize) as well as reduction in weight-bearing for prolonged periods, e.g. 3–6 months in a cast (off-loading)

Mainly non-operative approach to management

Long-term protection of foot and ankle/lower limb – professional footcare regularly, patient education, custom footware/brace to protect lower limb

## Addressing concerns/answering questions

- *Why has the diabetes damaged my joints?* The diabetes has affected the nerves in your legs so that they are less sensitive. You haven't, therefore, noticed when you suffered an injury to your ankle, and the damage to your ankle has continued up until now without you realizing. Your ankle joint is now badly damaged and we need a team of specialists to help you with this.
- *Will I need an operation?* The damage to the ankle joint is usually treated initially with a cast or boot to protect the foot and ankle, followed by custom-made shoes, rather than an operation. It is important to protect the feet as you will be at risk of developing foot ulcers due to the loss of feeling in the feet and the ankle joint. Sometimes operations are needed if the instability of your ankle puts you at too high a risk of ulceration or the footwear is ineffective – the diabetes team works in conjunction with orthotists, physiotherapists and orthopaedic surgeons. Surgery does, however, carry a significant risk of infection and other problems due to the damage to the bone and the soft tissue around the joint in conjunction with your diabetes.

## Discussion with examiners

The examiners may ask you to clarify details of the above diagnosis and ask questions about your planned investigations and management.

Other possible questions include:

- *What are the causes of Charcot joints?* Diabetes, alcohol, cerebral palsy, leprosy, tabes dorsalis, syringomyelia, syphilis.
- *What is the prognosis?* The prognosis depends mainly upon early recognition of the problem and effective management which includes patient education, diabetes control and MDT foot clinics. Treatment is essentially medical (bisphosphonates may be of value, particularly in the acute phase) but surgery may also be required.
- *What are the other aspects of diabetes care?* Eyes, kidneys, BP, and especially reduction of cardiovascu-

lar risk, type 2 diabetes being more than anything, a condition associated with premature cardiovascular death.

See also Section I, Station 5, Locomotor, Case 4.

**Examiners' information and requirements**

The candidate should:

1. Identify key features from the history: poorly controlled diabetes, progressive problems with ankle, symptoms of neuropathy
2. Identify key examination findings including evidence of sensory neuropathy with Charcot joint
3. Make diagnosis of Charcot joint, diabetes mellitus and poor concordance
4. Outline a sensible management plan, including MDT foot clinic approach with involvement of diabetes clinical nurse specialists, consultants, podiatrist and orthotists
5. Give a clear explanation to the patient of your diagnosis and plan, address his concerns and answer his questions

# Scenario 13 | Diabetes mellitus: foot ulcer and diabetes control

## Candidate's information

**Your role:** you are an SHO in the diabetes clinic. You have been asked to see a patient by the clinical nurse specialist who is concerned about the patient's foot ulcer which hasn't improved as much as he had hoped with treatment in the community. A GP letter reports HbA1c 9.5 a month ago.

**Your task:** to assess the patient's problems and address any questions or concerns raised by him.

## Patient's information

**You are:** Simon Pinter, a 40-year-old man.

**Your problem:** you've had difficulty with an ulcer under your right big toe for the past 6 months or so. You didn't notice it appearing until your chiropodist commented on it whilst doing your corns. Your GP initially thought you might have narrowing of the arteries in your leg, particularly with your smoking.

You had a recent course of flucloxacillin to treat some infection round the ulcer, and the district nurses came round several times per week to change the dressing. There was a strong smell coming from the ulcer so you went back to your GP who referred you in to clinic. The antibiotics only helped a little with the ulcer.

You get no pain in the legs on walking but you've been having some burning pains in your feet at night.

Your understanding of diabetes mellitus is that as long as your blood glucose is <15, that's fine. You feel a little odd if your blood glucose <6, as if having a 'hypo' and you need to eat.

### Past medical history and drug history:
- Diabetes for past 10 years (diagnosed at GP health check). Usual blood sugar levels 9–13
- Metformin 1 g twice per day – stopped taking it about 4 months ago as you felt well
- Aspirin 75 mg once per day
- Perindopril 2 mg once per day
- Simvastatin 40 mg nocte
- No known drug allergies

### Social history:
- You smoke 5–10/day (previously 20/day for 30 years)
- You don't drink alcohol

### Other issues including family history:
- Nil of note

**Your questions for the candidate:**
- *What can you do to get rid of the ulcer?*
- *Will I go blind (one of my friends with diabetes was recently registered blind)?*
- *Will I need an amputation?*

---

## Candidate

### History/key questions

Diabetes history: how long has he had diabetes and how has his diabetic control been? Is he overweight? Most patients with type 2 diabetes are (diabesity)

Check which diabetes medication he's on, and what he's taking. What has he tried before, any side-effects?

Diabetic control: including patient's understanding of diabetes, target blood glucose range and usual blood glucose range

Has he ever monitored his blood sugars, and if so, what is the usual range for blood sugar readings?

Ask about diet and lifestyle

Date of last eye screening, kidney screening, BP check

Any changes in his weight over the past 6 months

Usual footcare arrangements – does he see a chiropodist?

Ever had ulcers before on the feet or toes, and where? Shoe rub versus weight-bearing areas? Any trauma including surgery/chiropody

Any history consistent with intermittent claudication, rest pain, etc.

Any history of neuropathy/neuropathic pain: ask about symptoms of neuropathy – numbness, burning, pain, paraesthesiae

Any other vascular risk factors (smoking – current, ex, number of pack-years – cholesterol, obesity, hypertension, previous stroke or ischaemic heart disease/MI) – need to check exactly what medicines he's on

Ever had an angiogram or angioplasty of his lower limbs

Ask for recent results – blood sugar monitoring, recent HbA1c, temp. 37.3°C, BP 135/85

### Drug history

Ask for a full drug history, including allergies

Check medicines and allergies. Is he on aspirin, clopidogrel or warfarin?

### Social history

Smoking history (pack-years)

Alcohol history (units per week)

Who lives at home with him? Does he get any assistance from anyone? Activities of daily living and the effect of his foot ulcers on mobility, etc.

## Address patient's questions and concerns
- *Have you had any thoughts about what is going on?*
- *Is there anything in particular you're concerned about?*
- *Do you have anything you would like to ask?*

## Key areas for examination

A list of what to look for (in examination order; describe findings on examination)

Describe ulcers on feet: location (areas of rub, metatarsal heads in diabetes [weight bearing] versus arterial ulcers)

Look carefully for signs of cellulitis/evidence of infection (any aroma of anaerobic infection)

Look also for tinea pedis in toe interspaces – can let in infection

Vascular examination of foot: peripheral pulses, capillary refill, hair loss

Say that you would check pulses with Doppler/Ankle Brachial Pressure Index

Peripheral nervous system: diabetic neuropathy diagnosed from the history and examination of the feet/lower limbs; on examination, there may be loss of vibration sense and proprioception, loss of pain/fine touch/temperature; also loss/reduction in Achilles tendon reflex

Say that you would like to carry out a full neurological examination of lower limbs

Testing sensation: look for loss of light touch, pinprick, proprioception/joint position and vibration (128 Hz tuning fork) – posterior column signs

Ask for a 10 g monofilament to assess fine touch (current gold standard). The patient who cannot feel the 10 g monofilament is at risk of neuropathic foot ulceration

In this patient, capillary refill is <5 s, palpable peripheral pulses but reduced fine touch. No cellulitis. Ulcers over rub area of foot, medial aspect of right great toe

## Differential diagnoses

Diabetic neuropathic ulcer with no evidence of small vessel/large vessel disease

Poor diabetic control

## Discussion with patient

Explain diagnosis

Explain plan, including investigations and management

Address patient's concerns/answer their questions

## Management

Tight control of diabetes (blood sugar levels), footcare to reduce risk of complications, analgesia for any neuropathic pain

Diabetic control: increase treatment to improve control: diet, exercise, metformin, sulphonylureas, pioglitazone, gliptins, SGLT2 inhibitors, GLP1 receptor agonists and insulin are among the treatments available. GLP1 receptor agonists (exenatide, liraglutide, lixisenatide) are a particularly good choice for the obese patient. Tight diabetic control will help healing of any ulcer and protect from other complications

Footcare: avoid injuries, podiatry (care with nail cutting). Wash/dry feet, decent socks and shoes (risk of blisters with reduced sensation)

Analgesia with tricyclic antidepressants, duloxetine, gabapentin

Close monitoring by diabetes CNS (± community input) including education about diabetes/diet, etc.

Vascular input: Doppler at bedside, joint clinic, angiography (MRI versus standard) ± angioplasty

Smoking cessation referral and advise the patient to stop (explain benefits)

Statins and use of protective footwear in close liaison with chiropody

## Addressing concerns/answering questions

- *What can you do to get rid of the ulcer?* Should be covered by the above explanation but overall management is to improve control of diabetes (blood sugar levels) as much as possible, footcare to reduce the risk of complications including further damage, painkillers for any nerve pain and regular check-ups to make sure that everything is healing.
- *Will I go blind (one of my friends with diabetes was recently registered blind)?* The chances of diabetes-related complications in the eyes, similar to that in the feet, will depend on tightening and improving overall diabetic control. Insulin will obviously help achieve this. The care of diabetes involves regular eye checks and treatment of any of the problems associated with diabetes; it is important to control the diabetes, BP, etc., as well as possible to reduce the risk of complications such as visual problems. This includes stopping smoking as it causes narrowing of the blood vessels and worsens the eye problems.

- *Will I need an amputation?* The ulcers seem to be due to the loss of feeling in the soles of the feet, rather than blood vessel problems. We aim to get the foot better with medical treatment, improvement of diabetic control, along with better shoes and socks, regular chiropody, etc., so that we can avoid long-term problems with the feet needing operations.

## Discussion with examiners

The examiners may ask you to clarify details of the above diagnosis and ask questions about your planned investigations and management.

Other possible questions include:

- *What would make you switch the patient to insulin?* See above. Insulin if other treatments insufficient. Insulin tends to increase weight, which is not good in overweight patients, hence, GLP1 receptor agonists are increasingly preferred. This patient needs tighter and improved diabetic control as the chances of diabetes-related complications in end organs such as feet, eyes and kidneys will depend on this.
- *Why does diabetes increase vascular risk?* By increasing or hastening the atherosclerotic process through a complex interplay of endothelial dysfunction, inflammation and augmenting a prothrombotic state.

See also Section I, Station 5, Locomotor, Case 4.

---

### Examiners' information and requirements

The candidate should:

1. Identify key features from the history: diabetes/poor control, vascular risk factors
2. Identify key examination findings of diabetic foot ulcers, distal peripheral neuropathy including reduced fine touch, normal peripheral pulses
3. Outline a sensible management plan, including involving the diabetes multidisciplinary team and vascular team
4. Give a clear explanation to the patient of your diagnosis and plan, address his concerns and answer his questions

---

## Reported variants on this case

- Osteoarthritis of hip and poor diabetic control (see Section I, Station 5, Locomotor, Case 8)
- Diabetic control and diabetic retinopathy (see Section I, Station 5, Eyes, Case 1)

# Scenario 14 | **Goitre and weight loss**

## Candidate's information

**Your role:** you are the ST2 in the gastroenterology clinic. This 35-year-old lady has been referred by her GP with diarrhoea and weight loss. Blood tests at her GP were normal including FBC, CRP and renal function.

**Your task:** to assess the patient's problems and address any questions or concerns raised by her.

## Patient's information

**You are:** Eloise Wickham, a 35-year-old woman.

**Your problem:** your main concern is the lump in your neck. Your partner first noticed a fullness or swelling in the centre of the front of your neck about 8 weeks ago. You don't think it's got any bigger but you're self-conscious about it now, and wear scarves when going out. You mentioned it to your GP but she was more interested in hearing about your bowel habit, and arranged today's appointment in the bowel clinic.

You've noticed some weight loss despite eating a little more than usual – 5 kg over the past 3–4 months.

You've noticed a change in your bowel habit – now stools are softer and more frequent. You get increasingly anxious about where the nearest toilet is, particularly when you're out shopping or socialising. Eveything seems to have crept up on you over the past 8 weeks.

You have also noticed some changes in your eyes – a gritty feeling, and you haven't been able to wear your contact lenses (drying out too fast). No double vision and you can read/see in the distance clearly (unchanged).

Your work colleagues have commented that you are a little cranky at work, short-tempered and impatient. You just can't help yourself, and you had noticed it but put it all down to the shortcomings of your staff.

**Past medical history and drug history:**
• No previous serious illnesses. Never been in hospital
• On oral contraceptive pill. No other medications. No drug allergies

**Social history:**
• Non-smoker. You drink a glass of wine at weekends, sometimes two
• You live with your partner, who works in construction
• You work as a manager in the civil service

**Other issues including family history:**
• Not sure if your mother had an operation on her neck as a young woman, as there was a faint scar there but she never talked about her health

**Your questions for the candidate:**
- *Is it cancer?*
- *Will I need an operation?*
- *Why am I losing weight?*

## Candidate

### History/key questions

Ask about neck lump: when first noticed, any change in size, and over how long? Tender?

    Any change in swallowing, voice, breathing (due to retrosternal extension of thyroid)?

    Any history of a preceding URTI (to rule out thyroiditis)?

Ask about thyroid status:

    Hyperthyroidism – weight loss, heat intolerance, diarrhoea/increased stool frequency, insomnia, irritability, anxiety, depression, increased appetite, palpitations, oligomenorrhoea, hair loss

    Hypothyroidism – weight gain, slowed mentation, depression, constipation, intolerance to cold, myalgia; any history of carpal tunnel syndrome, menorrhagia

Ask about any visual changes:

    Diplopia

    Eye pain/discomfort/dryness or grittiness

    Changes in visual acuity/colour vision

    Onset – gradual or sudden, and over what duration?

    Ever seen an optician or ophthalmologist previously for this or other eye problems

Any history of thyroid problems/ever treated for thyroid problems

Medications (levothyroxine, carbimazole, propylthiouracil), radio-iodine or surgery

### Drug history

Ask about drugs which can cause thyroid dysfunction, e.g. amiodarone (hyper- and hypothyroidism); lithium (hypothyroidism)

Check current medications; any allergies

### Past medical history

Any history of thyroid problems, either under- or overactive? Ever been given medications for this?

Recent pregnancy?

Any previous neck operations or irradiation (associated with hypothyroidism)

### Social history

Anyone in family had thyroid problems or goitre, or operations to remove their thyroid

### Address patient's questions and concerns

- *Have you had any thoughts about what is going on?*
- *Is there anything in particular you're concerned about?*
- *Do you have anything you would like to ask?*

### Key areas for examination

A list of what to look for (in examination order; describe findings on examination)

Overall aim of the examination is to determine the cause of the neck lump

Need to be able to recognize the lump as a goitre and assess thyroid status

In this case it is a firm, diffusely enlarged thyroid with no bruit, retrosternal extension or lymphadenopathy; slight tremor, signs of Graves' disease – pretibial myxoedema, eye signs, thyroid acropachy

Overall inspection: often thin, anxious/restless in hyperthyroidism with tremor and thinning of the temporal hair; overweight in hypothyroidism

Voice: hoarse, deep in hypothyroidism

Hands: look for thyroid acropachy, onycholysis, fine tremor, sweaty palms, palmar erythema in hyperthyroidism

Assess pulse (tachycardia in hyperthyroidism – check whether in AF; bradycardia and dry skin in hypothyroidism)

Thyroid:

    Observe patient from the front and side, then when swallowing water

    Look for scars on inspection suggesting previous thyroid surgery

    Check with patient whether neck lump is painful or tender

    Examine from behind: relax neck muscles to be able to palpate thyroid

    Assess goitre location, size and shape (smooth or nodular: single or multiple nodules), whether moves with swallowing

    Any tenderness over thyroid on palpation

    Percuss for retrosternal extension if inferior margin of thyroid gland is not palpable

    Listen over both lobes of the thyroid for bruits

    Examine for lymphadenopathy in head and neck – hard, fixed (neoplasia), tender and mobile (reactive lymph nodes) or rubbery (lymphoma)

Face:

Look for signs of thyroid eye disease: present in 30% of patients with Graves' disease; periorbital oedema (from myxoedema [hypothyroidism] or Graves'), proptosis/exophthalmos, lid lag and lid retraction, ophthalmoplegia, conjunctival oedema/chemosis

Look for keratitis, ulceration of cornea

Visual acuity:

Pupils – relative afferent pupillary defect (RAPD) (in case of optic nerve compression due to proptosis)

Any papilloedema – fundoscopy (unlikely to be asked to perform but say that you would do it)

Assess for diplopia (particularly on upward vertical gaze due to inferior rectus muscle involvement)

Pretibial myxoedema (Graves') – typical ulceration/ pigmentation/atrophic/scarred area over shin

Proximal myopathy (check standing from chair without use of arms) in hyperthyroidism

## Differential diagnosis

Decide if it is the thyroid that is enlarged; if so, is it smooth or nodular (single versus multiple)?

Assess thyroid status: key signs of thyroid overactivity are tachycardia or AF, lid lag, thyroid bruit

In this case: firm, diffusely enlarged thyroid with evidence of Graves' disease, and symptoms and signs of hyperthyroidism

Causes of firm diffusely enlarged goitre:

Smooth, euthyroid – endemic (iodine deficiency), physiological (puberty), thyroiditis (e.g. viral, post-partum thyroiditis), goitrogens (kelp, seaweed, drugs like amiodarone), Hashimoto's thyroiditis

Smooth, hyperthyroid/toxic – Graves' disease (painless smooth/diffuse goitre in 90%+)

(See also Section I, Station 5, Endocrine, Case 4)

## Discussion with patient

Explain possible diagnosis

Explain plan, including investigations and management

Address patient's concerns/answer their questions

The lump you can feel in your neck is the thyroid gland, and you are showing signs of it being overactive. This has also caused some changes in your eyes, making them feel gritty.

We need to carry out some blood tests and an ultrasound of the thyroid, then refer you to the hormone specialists for further investigation and treatment.

## Investigations

Blood tests including TSH, FT4, FT3 and TPO antibody (TSH receptor antibodies more sensitive but more expensive) and full screen for weight loss/diarrhoea (FBC, U&E, CRP, TTG) if there is doubt over the diagnosis of hyperthyroidism

Most cases will have unrecordable TSH with elevated free T4 and free T3

## Management

Referral to endocrinologist for definitive management

Ultrasound of thyroid – imaging probably not required if clinically and biochemically consistent with Graves'/diffuse goitre/hyperthyroidism

Treatment for hyperthyroidism: based on levels of T3 and T4, as well as symptoms/signs, and underlying cause of hyperthyroidism:

*Symptom management* – manage marked adrenergic symptoms (such as tachycardia/tremor) with propranolol (non-selective β-blocker) if no contraindications. Stop smoking if a smoker as there is a direct link with Graves' ophthalmopathy worsening in smokers. Also candidates should note that thyroid eye disease has no correlation with thyroid gland activity – treating one may not necessarily lead to the other improving and vice versa

*Thionamides* – either carbimazole or propylthiouracil (PTU) (NB: 5% risk of agranulocytosis with carbimazole and only 50% remission in Graves' disease with thionamides). PTU is the preferred choice in pregnancy and if breastfeeding. UK guidelines: in recurrent clinical or biochemical disease, thionamides should be administered (typically for 2–3 months) until the serum FT4 is normal or near normal prior to [131]iodine therapy. All patients proceeding to surgery should also be rendered euthyroid (normal FT4 and FT3) with thionamides. Monitor TFT every 1–3 months until stable

*Radio-iodine* – most patients with recurrent hyperthyroidism require definitive treatment with [131]I. Administered orally, [131]I is then concentrated in the thyroid. It releases β emissions which cause local tissue damage and a reduction in thyroid function over 6–18 weeks. Pregnancy and breastfeeding are contraindications to radio-iodine. Can worsen the ophthalmopathy of Graves' disease compared to drug therapy or surgery (use steroid cover). Restrictions apply for a few weeks (3 weeks roughly, check local guidelines) after the dose is administered, including contact with partner, household members, pregnant women and children, depending on the dose administered. Conception/pregnancy should be avoided for 6 months after the dose, to ensure that the radioactivity is fully cleared, hyperthyroidism is treated successfully and any resultant hypothyroidism controlled

*Surgery* – rarely required for Graves'. Indications include large goitre (particularly if causing dysphagia or airways obstruction), for relapse of hyperthyroidism after treatment, in some cases of exophthalmos, and if radio-iodine is contraindicated or declined by patient (e.g. in pregnant women intolerant of antithyroid medicines, and poorly tolerating hyperthyroidism)

## Addressing concerns/answering questions

- *Is it cancer?* Very unlikely as there are no signs of any worrying isolated lumps on examination – the swelling is due to the whole thyroid enlarging (swelling of the thyroid due to inflammation and lymphocyte infiltration).
- *Will I need an operation?* No, probably not. First treatment is with medicines to reduce the amount of thyroid hormone being produced, and reduce the size of the thyroid.
- *Why am I losing weight?* The overactive thyroid gland is making more of your thyroid hormone which increases your metabolism and burns off more calories.

## Discussion with examiners

The examiners may ask you to clarify details of the above diagnosis and ask questions about your planned investigations and management.

Other possible questions include:
- *What are the other options if oral antithyroid drugs (ATD) fail?* This would lead to a discussion on radio-iodine and surgery.
- *What are the side-effects of carbimazole/propylthiouracil?* Carbimazole side-effects include: bone marrow suppression (agranulocytosis; usually presents as sore throat. Most patients on carbimazole with a sore throat do not have agranulocytosis. Thus, do not stop carbimazole until neutropenia is confirmed by urgent WBC measurement), jaundice, nausea, taste disturbance, headache, fever, malaise, arthralgia, pruritis. Propylthiouracil as for carbimazole but also includes nephritis, SLE-like syndromes, hepatic disorders, hypoprothrombinaemia.
- *Why is this presentation not one of thyroiditis?* It is not viral thyroiditis as there is no history of viral prodrome, neck pain or raised ESR (TFT can be thyrotoxic). In reality, treatment of viral thyroiditis is with beta-blockers if clinically thyrotoxic during the

hyperthyroid phase with simple treatments for the flu-like symptoms and aches and pains whilst they last – the patient may then go into a hypothyroid phase which can last months and may require thyroxine. Clue for thyroiditis is a history of a viral illness at the start and negative thyroid antibodies (e.g. TPO antibodies). Important to get this from the history in order to recognize the possibility of the diagnosis and also be clear that a patient with thyroiditis does not need life-long thyroxine – this can be tailed off in due course.

- *If a discrete solitary lump was found on ultrasound of the thyroid in an otherwise asymptomatic 70-year-old woman, what would you do?* [123]I scintigraphy, fine needle aspiration cytology (FNAC), TFT.
- *What are the possible clinical presentations of a substernal/retrosternal goitre?* Breathlessness/wheeze (tracheal narrowing <8 mm). Cough or choking sensation. Dysphagia less common (oesophagus posterior). Hoarse voice/change in voice due to recurrent laryngeal nerve palsy (vocal cord palsy). Horner's syndrome due to compression of cervical sympathetic chain. Superior vena cava (SVC) syndrome/subclavian steal.

See also Section I, Station 5, Endocrine, Case 4.

---

### Examiners' information and requirements

The candidate should:
1. Identify key features from the history: symptoms of hyperthyroidism, goitre/neck swelling
2. Identify key examination findings including recognizing goitre as the cause of the neck mass, evidence of Graves' disease, and determine thyroid status (hyperthyroid)
3. Outline a sensible management plan, including blood tests to confirm hyperthyroidism, referral to endocrinology, and be able to explain the likely management plan to the patient
4. Explain and reassure the patient clearly that investigations need to be done but most likely the symptoms stem from a possible thyroid disorder which can be treated successfully, with medications; address her concerns and answer her questions

**Further reading/resources**

UK guidelines for the use of thyroid function tests: www.rlbuht.nhs.uk/jps/tft_guideline_summary.pdf

**Reported variants on this case**

- Solitary thyroid nodule (see Section I, Station 5, Endocrine, Case 4) – examination findings, likely differential diagnosis, how to investigate single thyroid nodule
- Euthyroid goitre (see Section I, Station 5, Endocrine, Case 4)

# Other reported endocrinology cases

- Headache in a patient with acromegaly (see Section I, Station 5, Endocrine, Case 2)
- Phaeochromocytoma
- Prolactinoma
- Diabetic control
- Diabetic retinopathy (see Section I, Station 5, Eyes, Case 1)
- Osteoarthritis hip in a patient with poor diabetic control (see Section I, Station 5, Locomotor, Case 8)
- Palpitations – thyroid overactivity (see Section I, Station 5, Endocrine, Case 3)

# Scenario 15 | Retinitis pigmentosa

## Candidate's information

**Your role:** you are the SHO in the acute medicine clinic. A 26-year-old man presents with a 6-month history of visual deterioration.

**Your task:** to assess the patient's problems and address any questions or concerns raised by him.

## Patient's information

**You are:** Phillip Hornby, a 26-year-old male HGV driver.

**Your problem:** you have a 6-month history of gradually increasing difficulty with the vision of both eyes, particularly when out walking the dog at dusk or when in a dimly lit room, and you have been bumping into objects you haven't noticed around you. No headache, redness of your eyes, diplopia or photophobia. You went to your optician 1 year ago and no glasses were required (you felt distance vision was a little blurry at times). You have no weakness in your arms or legs. No change in sensation. No increased thirst, nocturia or polyuria. Distance and reading vision are equally affected with difficulty reading and seeing road signs. You had an episode where you clipped a wing mirror on your truck and this made you seek medical attention as it scared you. No flashes of light in your vision. No changes in your hearing.

### Past medical history:
- No history of diabetes
- No past history of note, no ocular history of note (no cataracts). Normal vision up to this point

### Drug history:
- Regular cocaine use, once every 1–2 weeks. Never injected drugs

### Social history:
- Two children, ages 3 and 5 (boys)
- Non-smoker, occasional alcohol (less than 4 pints per week)
- Milk tanker driver – no exposure to noxious materials now or in the past. Holds HGV licence

### Other issues including family history:
- Two uncles are registered blind and grandfather may also have been blind but he died when you were a little boy

### Your questions for the candidate:
- *Am I going to go blind?*
- *Can I still drive my truck?*
- *What about my kids – will they go blind?*
- *What treatment is there for this?*

# Candidate

## History/key questions

Visual loss: unilateral versus bilateral, near vision versus distance

Gradual versus sudden

Painful versus painless

Pain: in eyes/headache: uveitis can cause headache; subacute angle closure glaucoma can cause pain in eyes and headache, and can also have problems at dusk but get halos round lights, nausea, flashing lights. Can get flashes of light in retinitis pigmentosa (RP)

Reduced night vision (nyctalopia)

Tunnel vision (bumping into objects): RP, advanced glaucoma only, panretinal photocoagulation (PRP) for diabetic retinopathy but tunnel vision only if extensive PRP in peripheries

Distortion of vision, e.g. crooked window frames or words look abnormally small or big in newspaper (macular pathology, e.g. macular degeneration, diabetic macular oedema)

### Drug history

Tobacco/alcohol/methyl alcohol/TB medications/sulphonamides (affect visual acuity)

Recreational drug use including cocaine

### Past medical history

Nutritional deficiencies (vegans/exclusion diets)

### Social history

Smoking, alcohol history

## Address patient's questions and concerns

- *Have you had any thoughts about what is going on?*
- *Is there anything in particular you're concerned about?*
- *Do you have anything you would like to ask?*

## Key areas for examination

A list of what to look for (in examination order; describe findings on examination)

Look for signs of conditions associated with retinitis pigmentosa (see below), e.g. polydactyly in Bardet–Biedl syndrome, hearing aids (associated Usher's, Refsum's, Alport's syndrome) – in this case normal inspection

Visual fields (confrontational)

Colour vision/Ishihara plates

Acuity: finger counting, hand movements, perception of light, Snellen chart (if unable to read, orientation of Es chart, Illiterate Es). In this case acuity is 6/36 both eyes and 6/10 is required for driving

Fundoscopy including red reflex

Ophthalmic signs on fundoscopy of RP

'Bone spicule' pigmentation

'Waxy pallor' of the optic disc

Arteriolar attenuation (fundal vessels appear thin)

Cataract

Can also be associated with cystoid macular oedema (CMO) – can't see on fundoscopy (would need slit lamp)

Pupils: normal size

Pupillary reflexes (direct and consensual): normal

RAPD: not usually, depends on how asymmetrical disease is (not in bilateral and symmetrical RP)

Test II, III, IV, VI nerves

Complete cranial nerve examination: you need to say that you would ideally like to carry out a full neurological examination (to look for signs of syndromes associated with retinitis pigmentosa) – there won't be time for this

## Differential diagnosis

Causes of progressive visual loss: combination of nyctalopia, 'tunnel' vision, reduced vision and family history points strongly towards an inherited retinal dystrophy, most likely retinitis pigmentosa. Clinical findings confirm this

## Discussion with patient

Explain diagnosis

Explain plan, including investigations and management

Address patient's concerns/answer their questions

You have a condition called retinitis pigmentosa which is causing progressive visual loss. This is often an inherited condition and it sounds like your two uncles and your grandfather may also have had it.

Unfortunately there is no curative treatment at the moment, but we can help support you with strategies to optimise the vision you have; research into future treatments is ongoing.

(Use your communication skills, show empathy, treat as 'breaking bad news')

## Investigations

Referral to ophthalmology:

Formal colour vision testing (100 hue test)

Formal visual fields (Humphrey/Goldmann)

Retinal photos to monitor progress

May need fundus fluorescein angiogram

Electrodiagnostic testing – (flash and pattern) electroretinogram and electro-oculogram

## Management

Treatment is supportive

Low-vision clinic for optician refraction and low-vision aids (magnifiers, CCTV readers [desktop video magnifiers], etc.), large-print books

Sight-impaired registration (Certificate of Visual Impairment [CVI])

Sight-impaired registration – 'partially sighted'

Severe sight-impaired registration – 'blind'

Cannot drive HGV or private car, and will need to inform DVLA – will therefore need support with employment

Social services input

Retinitis pigmentosa societies, e.g. www.rpfighting-blindness.org.uk, RNIB or local support groups

Family counselling – possibility of geneticist input

Some evidence that vitamin A may slow progression

Acetazolamide if cystoid macular oedema

Cataract surgery

## Addressing concerns/answering questions

• *Am I going to go blind?* Unfortunately, this is a progressive condition which leads to gradual worsening of vision, mainly in the peripheries. There is no treatment at the moment, although there are some proposed treatments to try and delay it. There may come a time when you will want to be registered as sight impaired, and we can put you in touch with the local support groups. There is a lot of research going on in this area with stem cell treatments and implants, but nothing that's likely to be helpful in the near future.

• *Can I still drive my truck?* Unfortunately, your vision is below what's required from a legal point of view for both your car and HGV licences and you should stop driving now as it is no longer safe to continue. You will need to inform the DVLA about this. As you drive an HGV, the DVLA may want to arrange tests of their own. Your insurance would not be valid if you had an accident. DVLA and GMC have issued guidance about notification to DVLA, and what to do if patients continue to drive despite your advice to stop.

• *What about my kids – will they go blind?* The condition can be inherited and it is possible that this will affect your children. You know that you have a family history but it's difficult to predict. If you want to know, we can refer you to the clinical geneticists. (Alternative scenario – planning family for a patient who doesn't yet have children – refer to the clinical geneticists.)

• *What treatment is there for this?* As above – and see the Management section.

## Discussion with examiners

The examiners may ask you to clarify details of the above diagnosis and ask questions about your planned investigations and management.

A possible question includes:

• *What syndromes can be associated with retinitis pigmentosa?* Abetalipoproteinaemia (learning difficulties, peripheral neuropathy, ataxia, Alport's disease), Usher's syndrome (RP combined with deafness), Laurence–Moon syndrome, Bardet–Biedl syndrome, Kearns–Sayre syndrome (mitochondrial DNA disorder – ophthalmoplegia, ataxia, dysphagia and cardiac conduction defects), mucopolysaccharidosis I–III, Refsum's disease.

See also Section I, Station 5, Eyes, Case 2.

---

**Examiners' information and requirements**

The candidate should:

1. Identify key features from the history: progressive visual loss; combination of nyctalopia, 'tunnel' vision, reduced vision and family history of visual loss

2. Identify key examination findings including findings consistent with retinitis pigmentosa

3. Outline a sensible management plan, including referral to ophthalmology, investigations listed above, and need to focus on patient's needs/effect on his life

4. Give a clear explanation to the patient of your diagnosis and plan, address his concerns and answer his questions

---

# Scenario 16 | **Optic atrophy**

## Candidate's information

**Your role:** you are an SHO in the MAU. You have been asked to see this 55-year-old woman who presented with reduced colour vision and has noticed a slight reduction in her visual acuity. Otherwise well at present.

**Your task:** to assess the patient's problems and address any questions or concerns raised by her.

## Patient's information

**You are:** Wendy Davies, a 40-year-old woman.

**Your problem:** there have been changes to your vision with reduced colour vision – you noticed difficulties when driving and stopping at the traffic lights. Slight reduction in your eyesight, not improved by a visit to the optician. No double vision.

You were treated for pulmonary tuberculosis (TB) 18 months ago with Rifater, and completed the full course of treatment. You have been generally well since coming off treatment but you've noticed this change in your vision since being on the drugs. You've been having difficulty differentiating colours (traffic lights, particularly the red light), difficulty choosing clothes and paint colours.

The rest of your family were screened using X-rays and received tablets to ensure they didn't get TB.

### Past medical history:
- Never had any previous problems with vision and never had weakness, numbness or pins and needles in arms/legs
- No history of diabetes mellitus, raised cholesterol, hypertension, known cardiovascular disease, e.g. IHD, MI, stroke, peripheral vascular disease
- Never had sarcoid, syphilis, HIV, etc.
- Never been diagnosed with glaucoma
- Never had infections in or around eye(s) or any trauma/foreign body in eye(s)

### Drug history:
- Vitamin B12 injections for 7 years. Had been anaemic at the time due to low B12 and has been fine since

### Social history:
- Non-smoker, no alcohol

### Other issues including family history:
- Nil of note

**Your questions for the candidate:**
- *Why has my vision changed?*
- *Will it get better?*
- *Is it related to my vitamin B12 deficiency?*

## Candidate

### History/key questions

Causes for these symptoms include: the causes of optic atrophy (OA) (presents with reduced visual acuity and/or red-green colour blindness) – see list in 'Past medical history' below: questions need to reflect these

Ask about previous episodes of visual loss or disturbance

Blurring, diplopia, limb weakness or paraesthesiae suggestive of multiple sclerosis (MS)

Any risk factors for ischaemic /circulatory causes, e.g. diabetes, raised cholesterol, hypertension, known cardiovascular disease, e.g. IHD, MI, stroke, peripheral vascular disease

Ever been diagnosed with glaucoma?

Any infection in or around eye?

Any trauma/foreign body in eye?

Headache, change in memory or personality, issues with reading, understanding or speech (cerebral lesion, cerebrovascular disease)

Check for headache and temporal arteritis symptoms – although usually older age group

### Drug history

With the history of TB, you need to know which medicines were used, e.g. isoniazid and ethambutol

Ever taken any other drugs associated with optic atrophy – sulphonamides?

### Past medical history

Ask directly for any history of conditions associated with optic atrophy

Following optic neuritis: demyelination/MS

Compressive: papilloedema, cerebral tumour, bony growth, thyroid eye disease, chiasmal pathology, e.g. pituitary tumours, optic sheath meningioma

Glaucoma (increased intraocular pressure)

Vascular: ischaemic optic neuropathy (can be secondary to vasculitis), diabetes

Congenital: DIDMOAD, Friedreich's ataxia, Leber's hereditary optic atrophy

Infections such as TB, Lyme disease, fungal, viral including HIV, viral encephalitis, etc.

Inflammatory causes: sarcoid, TB, SLE, Behçet's, syphilis, meningitis, orbital cellulitis

Drugs, toxins, nutrition: medications, e.g. ethambutol, methanol, vitamin deficiency

Neoplasia: cerebral tumour, lymphoma, leukaemia, glioma

Trauma and radiation can both cause optic neuropathy

### Social history

Alcohol history – current alcohol intake in units per week, ever drunk larger amounts in the past

Ever ingested methanol/methyl alcohol?

Smoking history in pack-years

### Other issues including family history

Any family history of colour blindness or loss of vision in later life

Employment – contact with hydrocarbons, sulphur, lead

### Address patient's questions and concerns
- *Have you had any thoughts about what is going on?*
- *Is there anything in particular you're concerned about?*
- *Do you have anything you would like to ask?*

## Key areas for examination

A list of what to look for (in examination order; describe findings on examination)

This patient looks normal and well

Say that you would check the patient's blood pressure

Neurological:

Pupils: direct and consensual pupillary reflexes. Look for RAPD (normal in this case)

Fundoscopy: red reflex, discs and vessels. She has bilaterally pale discs with distinct margins (optic nerve fibre layer is thinned or lost, appearances probably represent the loss/absence of small vessels in the disc head)

Visual fields: bitemporal (superior) field defects for chiasmal lesions

Look for blind spot with red hat pin – may have enlarged blind spot

Visual acuity – Snellen chart

Test for red-green defect with Ishihara plates

Cranial nerves – particularly III, IV, VI, VII. Say that you would like to carry out complete examination (formal visual fields assessment)

Signs of optic atrophy:

Pupils – may be normal if symmetrical OA, otherwise RAPD present

Visual fields – depends on the cause

Visual acuity – may be normal

Fundoscopy – pale disc(s) with distinct margins

Look for temporal artery tenderness

Say that you would like to carry out a complete neurological examination (look for any cranial nerve or peripheral nervous system neurological signs, as well as cardiological examination including carotid bruits, e.g:

Diplopia/nystagmus, internuclear ophthalmoplegia in a patient with demyelination (previous optic neuritis leading to OA in patient with MS)

Older patient with compressive cause, e.g. history of breast cancer. May present with VI nerve palsy and optic atrophy

Cavernous sinus pathology – combination of lesions (III, IV, V and VI)

Optic atrophy and bitemporal hemianopia from a pituitary tumour (non-functioning)

Say that you would complete your examination with a breast examination

## Differential diagnosis

OA with no other localizing signs/focal neurology

History of TB, and isoniazid/ethambutol associated with OA

OA unlikely to be related to B12 deficiency as has been receiving regular B12 replacement

## Discussion with patient

Explain diagnosis

Explain plan, including investigations and management

Address concerns/answer their questions

You have optic atrophy, which could be due to your previous TB/TB treatment but various other causes also need to be considered. It is unlikely to be due to the vitamin B12 deficiency as you have been on regular replacement before, during and after the TB treatment. We need to carry out some investigations to find the underlying cause for the changes to your vision, and this will include blood tests and scans.

## Investigations

Formal assessment of visual fields (Goldmann rather than Humphrey)

MRI scan of brain and orbits with contrast

CT scan of the brain and orbits with contrast (in addition to space-occupying lesion [SOL], look for bony growth/disease, sinusitis, fibrous dysplasia)

Fasting blood glucose level (look for diabetes)

Blood pressure, cardiovascular examination including carotids; carotid Doppler ultrasound study

Vitamin B12, antinuclear antibody levels, serum ACE/CXR for sarcoid, homocysteine levels, antiphospholipid antibodies

Syphilis serology (VDRL and *Treponema pallidum* haemagglutination [TPHA] tests)

TORCH panel: ELISA for toxoplasmosis, rubella, cytomegalovirus, herpes simplex virus

Electrodiagnostic tests such as visual evoked potential (confirm diagnosis, and to monitor during follow-up/for progressive changes)

## Management

Review with the above investigations: although history may point towards TB medication such as isoniazid/ethambutol as cause of OA, it is important to exclude other causes of optic atrophy in which treatment may reduce risk of progression (treatment with steroids has been shown to help vasculitic/arteritic anterior ischaemic optic neuropathy)

Best treatment for all causes is to adequately treat the underlying condition before the OA has developed, as no treatment for OA exists

## Addressing concerns/answering questions

- *Why has my vision changed?* Changes to the nerve coming into the back of the eye have affected your colour vision, and vision overall. There are no other signs on examination but we will need to carry out tests to look for reasons why this has happened. It may all be related to your previous treatment for TB, as this can happen with some of the medicines.
- *Will it get better?* Difficult to say at this stage whilst investigations are ongoing.
- *Is it related to my vitamin B12 deficiency?* Your vitamin B12 levels sound like they would have been normal since you've been on replacement injections, so it is unlikely to be related.

## Discussion with examiners

The examiners may ask you to clarify details of the above diagnosis and ask questions about your planned investigations and management.

Other possible questions include:

- *What's the pathophysiology?* Loss of axons, shrinkage of myelin. This leads to gliosis and widening of the optic cup.
- *What are the alternative causes for this appearance of the optic disc?* Optic nerve hypoplasia (born with small aberrant optic nerve), myelinated nerve fibres (bright white nerves in area around optic disc), myopic or scleral crescent, or tilted disc (nerve comes into eye at an angle).
- *What is the differential diagnosis of optic atrophy?* See list in past medical history section above.

See also Section I, Station 5, Eyes, Case 3.

---

### Examiners' information and requirements

The candidate should:

1. Identify key features from the history: acquired colour vision and visual acuity defect following TB treatment; no other risk factors identified
2. Identify key examination findings including fundoscopic signs of optic atrophy, without papilloedema
3. Outline a sensible management plan, including investigations to look for the cause of the optic atrophy
4. Give a clear explanation to the patient of your diagnosis and plan, address her concerns and answer her questions

---

## Further reading/resources

Optic atrophy: www.eyewiki.aao.org/Optic_Atrophy (American Academy of Ophthalmology): includes fundoscopic pictures of optic atrophy

NICE TB guidance: www.nice.org.uk/CG033

# Scenario 17 | Visual blurring in a patient with diabetes mellitus

## Candidate's information

**Your role:** you are the SHO in the diabetes clinic. You have been asked to assess this 45-year-old man who has reported blurring of his vision. No diplopia has been reported. He has type 1 diabetes and is under follow-up in this clinic.

**Your task:** to assess the patient's problems and address any questions or concerns raised by him.

## Patient's information

**You are:** Robert Salter, a 45-year-old man.

**Your problem:** you've been getting blurring of your vision over the past few months on and off, and it has been getting in the way of reading and watching TV. You haven't noticed any double vision or episodes of transient complete visual loss. You have no weakness of arms or legs, or headache. You usually wear glasses but these had not been changed for about 5 years without any problems, but you've recently been back and forth to the optician and had several changes to the prescription over the past four to six months.

At times you have felt unwell and tired and can be quite thirsty.

## Past medical history:

- Diabetes mellitus since age 17. You have been on insulin since, and you attend for your regular eye check-ups, including photos. You had laser treatment of your retinas a few years ago but you're no longer under the eye clinic. Last photos a few months ago – haven't heard back with any problems
- You have hypertension but you had a cough with one of your medicines, so you stopped this a while ago, and you missed your last practice nurse appointment regarding your BP monitoring over 2 months ago
- No previous kidney problems, and your feet are checked annually by the practice nurse (no problems)
- Usual range for blood sugars – in the past 4–6 months it has been running at 8–12, and you think that maybe the blurring is worse when your blood sugar goes over 15
- You don't know what the last few blood test results were for your diabetic control

## Drug history:

- Glargine once a day and novorapid three times per day
- If asked, express the view that you don't worry too much about controlling the blood sugars because you usually feel OK, and your eyes are being looked after by yearly photos and the previous laser treatment you had

**Social history:**
- Non-smoker, no alcohol

**Other issues including family history:**
- Mother had diabetes and died age 55 from a stroke

**Your questions for the candidate:**
- *Why do I need to take all these tablets?*
- *I thought the laser treatment would stop any problems with my eyes – why are they blurry?*
- *Have I done myself permanent harm by not taking my BP medications?*

---

## Candidate

### History/key questions

Ask the patient to describe the visual disturbance (blurring in his case), precipitants and relieving factors, any other associated factors

Ask specifically about diplopia (horizontal versus vertical), episodes of loss of vision (amaurosis fugax), any associated changes in speech or limb weakness?

One eye or both?

Any triggers?

Does he know what his blood glucose is when it happens?

Any symptoms consistent with cataract, e.g. halos or glare in vision when driving at night with oncoming headlights

Maculopathy (would lose or get disturbance in central vision)

Neovascularization and vitreous haemorrhage: get black blobs and floaters in vision

Diabetes history: how long has he had diabetes and how has his diabetes control been (does he know about his latest HbA1c – blood test measure of overall diabetes control)? What medications has he been on and for how long? Ask about insulin (injections versus pump) and any oral hypoglycaemic medications

Ask about all other medications (including aspirin, statin, hypertension medications), over-the-counter medications and herbal/alternative medications; assess concordance, i.e. is he actually taking the medicines (non-confrontational, empathetic approach) and if not, why not (patient understanding, side-effects)?

Does he monitor his blood sugars, and if so, what is the usual range for blood sugar readings?

What is his target blood sugar (range)?

Does he get severe hypoglycaemia?

Any changes in his weight over the past 6 months?

Date of last eye screening, kidney screening, BP check

Any kidney problems?

Usual footcare arrangements: does he see a chiropodist?

Ever had ulcers on the feet or toes?

Any history consistent with intermittent claudication, rest pain, etc.?

Think about other vascular risk factors (smoking, cholesterol, obesity, hypertension)

Does he have a diabetes specialist nurse in the community and has he seen a dietitian?

Ask about symptoms of neuropathy: numbness, burning, pain, paraesthesiae

Changes in walking/unsteadiness, falls

*Social history*

Smoking history (pack-years)

ICE (ideas, concerns, expectations): elicit patient's understanding of diabetic control, emphasize the importance of diabetic control and BP treatment in terms of reducing risk of complications from diabetes, and overall cardiovascular risk

### Address patient's questions and concerns
- *Have you had any thoughts about what is going on?*
- *What do you think causes your blurred vision?*
- *Is there anything in particular you're concerned about?*
- *Do you have anything you would like to ask?*

### Key areas for examination

A list of what to look for (in examination order; describe findings on examination)

Overall inspection

Ask to check BP: examiners tell you that it is 180/110 left arm, 175/105 right arm

Cranial nerves

Eyes:

Visual acuity (with and without glasses) – normal in this patient with glasses on

Pupil size, pupillary reflexes (direct and consensual)

Red reflex

Fundoscopy – can see laser burns in the peripheries (not macula) from photocoagulation in this patient. There may be changes of diabetic retinopathy or hypertensive retinopathy. May however be normal other than the laser photocoagulation

Check blood glucose: examiners say that it is 6 at present

Eye movements: ensure no diplopia/III, IV or VI palsy/nystagmus

Ask to see blood sugar diary to assess control (if patient has been completing one)

Ask to see an ECG (LVH, check for AF)

## Differential diagnosis

Visual blurring due to hyperglycaemia

Uncontrolled hypertension due to non-concordance with GP's management plan for patient's BP

## Discussion with patient

Explain diagnosis

Explain plan, including investigations and management

Address concerns/answer their questions

Your blurring of vision is due to your blood sugar levels being higher than aimed for/advised. You have high BP too, and this is due to not being on the medicines that your GP prescribed. Both diabetic control and BP control are important as they reduce the risk of the complications of diabetes (stroke, heart attack, kidney failure, eye problems, narrowing of arteries in legs, etc.).

## Investigations

Urinalysis and albumin:creatinine ratio

Check HbA1c result as done recently

## Management

Diabetes control: set clear target and monitor blood glucose; will need education through practice nurse ± community diabetes team. Check patient has a blood glucose monitor and sufficient test strips

BP control: angiotensin II antagonist and regular monitoring by practice nurse

Regular exercise

Explain that episodes of blurring of vision should settle with improved control of diabetes; provide patient with clear blood glucose targets

Provision of educational materials

Link in with diabetes team 'Think Glucose'

Insulin passport: ensures patient has a record of what he's taking, doses, etc.

## Addressing concerns/answering questions

- *Why do I need to take all these tablets?* Diabetes is associated with high blood pressure and high cholesterol, and it is important to control these as well as the blood sugar to keep you healthy long-term, and reduce the risk of strokes and heart attacks.
- *I thought the laser treatment would stop any problems with my eyes – why are they blurring?* Blurring is due to the high blood sugar levels affecting the lens in the eye and the insides of the eye (hyperosmolar state affects the lens and vitreous humour, causing swelling through osmosis and swelling of the lens). This explains the fluctuating spectacle prescription. The laser treatment he had was to prevent further development of blood vessels in the retina, the back of the eye, to prevent bleeding into the eye and loss of vision.
- *Have I done myself permanent harm by not taking my BP medications?* We will need to check that your kidneys haven't been affected by checking blood tests and urine. You've already had some damage to the back of the eyes requiring laser treatment, so it is really important to take the medicines, and see the practice nurse for regular BP checks.

## Discussion with examiners

The examiners may ask you to clarify details of the above diagnosis and ask questions about your planned investigations and management.

Other possible questions include:

- *What are the possible causes of visual loss in a patient with diabetes?* Diabetes maculopathy, vitreous haemorrhage, branch or central retinal artery occlusion, branch or central retinal vein occlusion, hemianopia/stroke, rubeosis and secondary/subsequent neovascular glaucoma, cataracts, anterior ischaemic optic neuropathy, ocular ischaemic syndrome.
- *What are the stages of diabetes retinopathy and management?*

Background: monitor (back to screening service). May remain under ophthalmological follow-up if poorly-controlled diabetes/concerns about progression.

Preproliferative: optimize medical management of diabetes and keep under regular ophthalmological follow-up.

Proliferative: Panretinal photocoagulation (PRP).

Maculopathy: clinically significant – either focal or grid macular laser; intravitreal steroids (maculopathy resistant to laser, maculopathy involving fovea so can't laser) or anti-vascular endothelial growth factor (VEGF) agents.

Rubeosis: without neovascular glaucoma – PRP and close monitoring; with neovascular glaucoma – requires control of intraocular pressures, PRP if possible (pupils can't dilate often), cyclodiode laser.

See also Section I, Station 5, Eyes, Case 1.

## Further reading/resources

Think Glucose: www.institute.nhs.uk/quality_and_value/ think_glucose/welcome_to_the_website_for_ thinkglucose.html

www.medweb.bham.ac.uk/easdec/index.html

---

**Examiners' information and requirements**

The candidate should:

1. Identify key features from the history: poorly-controlled diabetes and hypertension, poor concordance in part due to poor understanding. Visual changes are those of blurring alone, associated with increased blood glucose

2. Identify key examination findings including retinal photocoagulation scars on fundoscopy, but otherwise normal examination

3. Outline a sensible management plan, including clear explanations to patient, identification of the need for patient education, switch to angiotensin II antagonist

4. Give a clear explanation to the patient of your diagnosis and plan, address his concerns and answer his questions

# Other possible eye cases

- Scleritis
- Marfan's lens dislocation (see Section I, Station 5, Locomotor, Case 9)

# Scenario 18 | Iron deficiency anaemia

## Candidate's information

**Your role:** You are an ST3 in gastroenterology and you have been asked to see a 27-year-old man referred by his GP to the gastroenterology clinic with iron deficiency anaemia. Hb 10.9, MCV 73, ferritin 18 (low).

**Your task:** to assess the patient's problems and address any questions or concerns raised by him.

## Patient's information

**You are:** Colin Vickers, a 27-year-old engineer.

**Your problem:** you went to your GP as you have been feeling more tired than usual over the past 3 months. Your GP carried out some routine blood tests and found that you are anaemic with low iron levels. He then referred you to clinic.

You were diagnosed with irritable bowel syndrome by your GP about 5 years ago as you had noticed looser stools and marked bloating after eating bread, pasta and biscuits. The GP mentioned food intolerances and you now avoid these foods. You had not been to the GP since until the past few months when you started feeling very tired. No weight loss. No rashes.

You have had mouth ulcers for about 3–4 years on the inside of your lips and on your tongue. These can be very irritating but they just settle on their own.

Your bowels are usually regular unless you eat something that sets you off, e.g. bread. No rectal bleeding. You get occasional bloating. If asked, you've been eating bread at least daily on the advice of your GP over the past six weeks in the run-up to this appointment – your bowels have been troublesome, and the bloating uncomfortable.

### Past medical history and drug history:
- On no current medications. No drug allergies
- Never been in hospital

### Social history:
- You work in manufacturing of jet engines
- Non-smoker, rare alcohol – only a couple of glasses of wine at Christmas and one or two beers at the football (once a month)

### Other issues including family history:
- Son aged 2 years (recently diagnosed as having coeliac disease as 'failed to thrive'/ didn't put on weight as quickly as should have done)
- No-one else in your family is known to have coeliac disease
- No-one has had colorectal cancer or inflammatory bowel disease that you know of

**Your questions for the candidate:**
- *Why am I anaemic?*
- *Why would I need an endoscopy? Why can't you just give me some iron?*
- *Do I have coeliac disease like my son?*

If coeliac disease is suggested by the doctor, alternative questions include:
- *Is it curable?*
- *Can't you just give me medicine?*
- *If I have coeliac disease, can I still have a beer at the football?*
- *Doesn't coeliac disease cause cancer? (I've been reading about this on the internet since my son was diagnosed.)*

---

## Candidate

### History/key questions

Upper and lower GI symptoms: dyspepsia, reflux symptoms, dysphagia; ask about bowel habit and any changes (diarrhoea, steatorrhoea), rectal bleeding

Symptoms of anaemia: tiredness, lethargy, shortness of breath, dizziness

Bloating, lethargy and any dietary triggers, e.g. symptoms after wheat (both coeliac disease and gluten intolerance can cause this)

Evidence of blood loss (haematemesis, melaena, haematuria, epistaxis, recent operations)

Arthralgia, gritty eyes (extraintestinal manifestations of IBD)

Mouth ulcers (IBD, coeliac)

Rash: erythema nodosum, dermatitis herpetiformis (itchy rash)

Dietary history: does he eat meat, how often, and which (red meat, chicken, fish versus vegetarian)?

Ever donated blood? If so, how many times? Ever been declined due to anaemia?

### Drug history
Use of aspirin or NSAIDs; oral steroid use

### Past medical history
Check that there's no past history of anaemia

### Social history
Alcohol intake (units per week) and smoking history (pack-years)

### Other issues including family history
Does anyone in the family have coeliac disease, inflammatory bowel disease, GI cancers (gastro-oesophageal, colonic)? – ask about his parents, siblings, and his children's health

### Address patient's questions and concerns
- *Have you had any thoughts about what is going on?*
- *Is there anything in particular you're concerned about?*
- *Do you have anything you would like to ask?*

### Key areas for examination
A list of what to look for (in examination order; describe findings on examination)

Evidence of anaemia (pale conjunctivae), jaundice, lymphadenopathy

Rash: dermatitis herpetiformis (coeliac), erythema nodusum (IBD), pyoderma gangrenosum (IBD)

Angular cheilitis, mouth ulcers, glossitis

Telangiectasia on lips/body

Look for signs of portal hypertension

Abdominal examination: exclude hepatomegaly/splenomegaly; masses, e.g. ileocaecal Crohn's

Say that you would like to carry out a digital rectal examination

### Differential diagnosis
Coeliac disease: reports symptoms consistent with gluten enteropathy (coeliac disease) with diarrhoea, bloating, mouth ulcers; has been found to have iron deficiency anaemia and has a family history of coeliac disease (his son): GP hasn't carried out a TTG/coeliac serology, probably as he needed to be on a diet containing gluten for six weeks before the test.

Other causes of anaemia for this age group include:
   Peptic ulceration, oesophagitis (but no reported dyspepsia and denies NSAID use)
   IBD given history of diarrhoea
   Angiodysplasia, previous blood donation (no history) and rarer causes

**Key facts/areas to consider** (including information available in scenario summary before station starts):

iron deficiency in men and postmenopausal women requires investigation

## Discussion with patient

Explain diagnosis

Explain plan, including investigations and management

Address patient's concerns/answer their questions

The diarrhoea and bloating you've been having, along with the anaemia that your GP diagnosed, all points towards coeliac disease given that your son has this. Your symptoms and the anaemia need investigation to identify the cause and then treat it. We need to perform some blood tests to look for levels of vitamins in the blood and to test for coeliac disease, particularly as your son has it, and it can be inherited. Although there are a variety of causes for anaemia, your symptoms and family history point towards coeliac disease. Explain investigations and management as below.

## Investigations

Plan would be for blood tests to check haematinics (look for coexistent vitamin B12 and folate deficiency), TTG (IgA antibody), immunoglobulins (IgA deficiency in 0.5% of overall population but up to 10% of coeliacs), routine bloods such as U&E, LFT, CRP, ESR and vitamin D.

Endoscopy of upper GI tract (gullet, stomach and small bowel, with small bowel biopsies to confirm/exclude coeliac): the gold standard for diagnosis is upper GI endoscopy and duodenal biopsies ×4 whilst on a gluten-containing diet – one meal per day containing gluten for 6 weeks prior to endoscopy. If he has been very symptomatic after eating wheat/gluten, he may be/have already been on a relatively gluten-free diet, risking false-negative serology and/or duodenal biopsy (TTG being 95% sensitive and 95% specific for detection of coeliac disease; duodenal mucosa should return to normal after about 6 months of an absolutely gluten-free diet). Fortunately his GP has advised him to take daily wheat/gluten in the lead up to the appointment, and he should be advised to continue this until the endoscopy.

Even if negative coeliac serology with normal IgA, explain that he would still need upper GI endoscopy/biopsies to exclude coeliac disease given high clinical probability (symptoms after eating wheat, iron deficiency anaemia, son with coeliac disease).

If no evidence of coeliac disease, he will require further GI investigations, e.g. colonoscopy.

Explain OGD procedure: throat spray or sedation (not general anaesthesia); benefits include the confir-

mation or exclusion of coeliac disease before committing him to a lifelong gluten-free diet; and risks of the procedure include bloating and belching during the procedure, sore throat afterwards, drug reaction, incomplete procedure, bleeding and very rarely perforation requiring an operation.

## Management

If coeliac disease confirmed, he will need:

Referral to dietitians for advice on complete/absolute and lifelong removal of gluten from diet (wheat, rye, oats, barley)

Replacement of vitamin deficiencies

DEXA scan to assess bone density at baseline (look for osteopenia/osteoporosis)

A fixed supply of 'units' per month of gluten-free food is available on GP prescription from the NHS to patients formally diagnosed with coeliac disease and/or dermatitis herpetiformis

Patient associations such as Coeliac UK provide information on gluten-free foods in the UK, patient support groups, information via newsletters and the web

## Addressing concerns/answering questions

- *Why am I anaemic?* Your GP has found that you have low iron levels, and this is why you have become anaemic. We do need to find out why your iron levels have become low, and treat the underlying condition as needed. We need to find out whether you have coeliac disease as this leads to reduced absorption of iron, leading to low iron levels and anaemia.
- *Why do I need an endoscopy? Why can't you just give me iron?* We need to find out the cause and treat this, rather than just treating the symptoms (the anaemia).
- *Do I have coeliac disease like my son?* You may well do, given your symptoms and the anaemia, and we need to send blood tests and arrange an endoscopy to find out.
- *Is it curable?* Coeliac disease is managed by removing wheat from the diet long term, rather than 'curing'. The small bowel returns to normal over the next 6 months or so and returns to absorbing nutrients normally again. It is essential to avoid all gluten, as the bowel only stays settled if there is no gluten in the diet. Small amounts of gluten may not cause you trouble with your bowels, but will make the lining of the bowel change back and the absorption of nutrients will reduce.
- *Can't you just give me medicine?* The best 'treatment' available currently is dietary through the removal of

wheat to allow the lining of the bowel to return to normal; medicines are only used in a very small minority of patients who remain unwell despite being strictly on the diet.

- *Can I still have a beer at the football?* Unfortunately not. There are a few breweries producing gluten-free beer but it is expensive and not sold at the football!
- *Doesn't coeliac disease cause cancer?* Cancer is fortunately a rare complication of coeliac disease and usually arises in people whose bowel fails to respond to the complete removal of wheat from the diet.

## Discussion with examiners

The examiners may ask you to clarify details of the above diagnosis and ask questions about your planned investigations and management.

Other possible questions include:
- *What is the possible differential diagnosis?* There is a high clinical suspicion of coeliac disease given the iron deficiency anaemia and symptoms of IBS which could be due to coeliac disease (rather than IBS), and the family history.
- *If you confirm coeliac disease on duodenal biopsies, does the patient need further investigations into his iron deficiency anaemia (e.g. a colonoscopy)?* Hold off colonoscopy as a first-line investigation as the clinical picture points strongly towards coeliac disease as the main differential, and he has no colonic or abdominal symptoms to suggest IBD (low clinical suspicion of IBD). At his young age colonic malignancy would be very rare indeed (important to check whether any family history of colon cancer which could increase his risk); upper GI pathology such as peptic ulceration should be excluded at OGD. Review the need for colonoscopy if the biopsies were normal, excluding coeliac disease.
- *If his TTG was negative, how would you investigate?* In view of his GI symptoms (reports symptoms after ingesting wheat), iron deficiency anaemia and positive family history, upper GI endoscopy and duodenal biopsies would be indicated to exclude coeliac disease, even if TTG was negative (and IgA deficiency excluded) as he may be one of the very few who have coeliac disease but are TTG negative. If there is no evidence of coeliac disease (NB: on a gluten-containing diet) then we will need to consider lower GI endoscopy (colonoscopy) ± capsule endoscopy. Other causes of villous atrophy (with a negative TTG)

include giardiasis, bacterial overgrowth, use of NSAIDs, tropical sprue, Whipple's disease, lymphoma, hypogammaglobulinaemia. Genetics of coeliac disease: 95% HLA DQ2 (genotyping not widely available).

- *What are some other associations with coeliac disease?* Dermatitis herpetiformis (70% have coeliac disease), diabetes (3–7% have coeliac disease), thyroid/adrenal disease (7%), IBS (5%), SLE, psychiatric disease, temporal lobe epilepsy, psoriasis, elevated liver function tests.
- *What are the complications?* Osteoporosis, splenic atrophy, GI lymphoma (enteropathy associated T-cell lymphoma), ulcerative jejunitis, oesophageal cancer (squamous cell), small bowel adenocarcinoma.

---

### Examiners' information and requirements

The candidate should:

1. Identify key features from the history: features of coeliac disease (these include iron deficiency anaemia in a young man reporting lethargy, bloating and mouth ulcers, with a family history of coeliac disease)
2. Identify key examination findings including any signs of anaemia; examination may well be entirely normal (e.g. when the patient is an actor)
3. Outline a sensible management plan, blood tests including TTG/coeliac serology and referral for endoscopy/biopsy (would carry out OGD + biopsies even if TTG was negative, given strength of clinical suspicion)
4. Give a clear explanation to the patient of your diagnosis and plan, address his concerns and answer his questions

---

### Further reading/resources

www.coeliac.org.uk – see the health professional resources on prescribing

NICE guidance on coeliac disease (2009): www.nice. org.uk

British Society of Gastroenterology (2011): iron deficiency anaemia guidelines: www.bsg.org.uk/clinical-guidelines/general/guidelines-by-date.html

# Scenario 19 | Haematemesis

## Candidate's information

**Your role:** you are an ST2, covering the acute medical unit on-call. A 27-year-old female presents via the emergency department with a single episode of vomiting fresh red blood. The observations recorded on arrival were pulse 70, BP 115/75, Hb 14.5, MCV 83 on bloods in the emergency department, and she has been referred to you for further assessment including endoscopy.

**Your task:** to assess the patient's problems and address any questions or concerns raised by her.

## Patient's information

**You are:** Sue Barnet, a 27-year-old woman.

**Your problem:** you went out last night and bought a take-away and drank four pints of lager. You felt unwell about an hour after having the lager and eating the fried chicken from somewhere on the High Street, and you started vomiting shortly afterwards. You vomited three times, then saw streaks of fresh red blood in the vomit on the fourth time, and several eggcupfuls of blood in the last (fifth) vomit. You haven't vomited for about 7 h and feel much better. You had breakfast this morning without any problems. Your bowels have been opening normally with no change in colour or consistency. Your weight has been stable and you've not had any reflux/ indigestion or abdominal pain after eating, or swallowing problems. Your partner has been fine throughout.

### Past medical history and drug history:
- You are usually well and take no regular medications
- You don't take aspirin, NSAIDs or steroids
- You've never had any operations and no significant medical history
- You can't remember when you last saw your GP or why

### Social history:
- Unemployed
- Non-smoker
- Alcohol: Drinks 1–2 pints of 4% lager per night during the week, and up to 6 pints of lager on a Friday and Saturday night out – up to 50 units/week

### Other issues including family history:
- You are concerned about the blood you vomited up, and you wonder whether you're still bleeding
- Your uncle had stomach cancer about 10 years ago, age 60; the cancer was diagnosed 'late' by his GP. He subsequently died. He had alcohol problems for years before he died

## Your questions for the candidate:

- *Where's the blood coming from?*
- *Do I need to stay in hospital?*
- *What's the chance of it being stomach cancer like my uncle (diagnosed age 60)?*
- *Can I still drink alcohol?*

## Candidate

### History/key questions

Check sequence of events carefully (vomiting repeatedly leading to minor haematemesis [streaks only then small amounts] points towards Mallory–Weiss tear – now settled, with no vomiting since)

Type of haematemesis ('coffee grounds' – black digested blood versus fresh red blood; quantity/how often)

Any melaena (black, tarry stool), dark red blood PR suggesting brisk upper GI bleeding or fresh blood in lower GI bleeding

Any other factors suggesting peptic ulceration: NSAID, aspirin or steroid use; symptoms of dyspepsia, reflux; need to ask about alarm symptoms including weight loss, dysphagia. Any past history of ulcers?

Any suggestion of varices as a possible cause: any known liver disease, previous endoscopies and the results of these if known, any history of varices/portal hypertension or GI bleed in the past; clinical signs of portal hypertension on examination

### Drug history

Usual medications, over-the-counter medicines, particularly use of NSAID/aspirin, steroids

Need to watch for propranolol/β-blockers particularly in cirrhotics who take them for varices prophylaxis: patients on β-blockers will have an 'inappropriately' low pulse rate despite blood loss as rate-limited by the medications

### Past medical history

Any past history of peptic ulceration; any operations for ulcers?

### Social history

Alcohol intake (units per week)

Smoking history (pack-years)

### Address patient's questions and concerns

- *Have you had any thoughts about what is going on?*
- *Is there anything in particular you're concerned about?*
- *Do you have anything you would like to ask?*

## Key areas for examination

A list of what to look for (in examination order; describe findings on examination)

ABCDE approach

Cardiovascular (pulse, BP, capillary refill, temperature of peripheries, GCS/consciousness level) – any evidence of shock?

Any signs of anaemia

Signs of portal hypertension (spider naevi, ascites) or decompensated cirrhosis (hepatic flap, jaundice, ascites)

Abdominal examination: look for masses, tenderness (non-specific over epigastrium)

Say that you would complete your examination with digital rectal examination (to exclude melaena)

Ask to see observations chart including pulse, BP, urine output, respiratory rate, drug chart

Examination is normal in this patient

## Differential diagnosis

A Mallory–Weiss tear is the most likely diagnosis given the history of repeated vomiting (without blood in the vomit) followed by haematemesis. MW tears can still cause significant GI bleeding (active bleeding from visible vessels leading to haemodynamic compromise) but usually settle with conservative management, as in this case. This patient has been stable, no signs of shock

Peptic ulceration: less likely in the absence of dyspepsia symptoms; history fits with MW tear

Varices unlikely in the absence of chronic liver disease

## Discussion with patient

Explain diagnosis

Explain plan, including investigations and management

Address patient's concerns/answer their questions

The likely cause of your symptoms is a minor tear in the lining of your oesophagus/gullet due to the repeated vomiting (a benign cause of vomiting blood). We will request urgent blood tests and if these are normal, and you're able to eat and drink OK without further vomiting, then you can go home with a plan to carry out an urgent outpatient endoscopy which will complete the full check-up. You don't need to stay in hospital for this endoscopy. The endoscopy may well be completely normal as the minor tear heals up quickly (explain the ambulatory care of low-risk GI bleeds). Gastric cancer is very unlikely given your young age, and your presentation with a classic history of a tear in the lining of the gullet. The endoscopy will give you a check-up and exclude ulcers, as well as reassure you that you don't have gastric cancer. We would advise you to return to hospital if you have any further episodes of vomiting blood.

I would advise reducing your alcohol intake, as the vomiting and then bringing up blood is likely to be related to the alcohol (causing the vomiting in the first place), and to avoid long-term problems from alcohol. See the brief advice section below.

## Investigations

History suggestive of MW tear; cardiovascularly stable with no melaena

Basic investigations required: FBC, INR, U&E, LFT, group and save

Use of Blatchford and Rockall scores to triage/assess risk of mortality (Rockall) or need for endoscopic intervention (Blatchford): see Tables H19.1–19.3

This patient has low-risk bleeding (SIGN guidelines): Rockall 0 and Blatchford 0

### Rockall score

Predictive of the risk of mortality in patients with an upper GI bleed. Add endoscopy findings to the pre-endoscopy score to obtain the post-endoscopy score and this can be used to estimate the risk of rebleeding.

Table H19.1 Pre-endoscopy Rockall score

| Age (years) | | Evidence of shock | | Comorbidity | |
|---|---|---|---|---|---|
| <60 | 0 | None | 0 | None | 0 |
| 60–79 | 1 | Pulse >100 Systolic BP >100 | 1 | CCF, IHD or any other major comorbidity | 2 |
| 80+ | 2 | Systolic BP <100 | 2 | Renal/liver failure, disseminated malignancy | 3 |

Table H19.2 Post-endoscopy Rockall score: add to pre-endoscopy total to make total score

| Endoscopic stigmata | | Diagnosis | |
|---|---|---|---|
| None or dark spot seen | 0 | Mallory–Weiss tear; no lesion seen and no stigmata of recent haemorrhage | 0 |
| | | All other diagnoses | 1 |
| Blood in upper GI tract, adherent clot, visible or spurting vessel | 2 | Malignancy of upper GI tract | 2 |

A pre-endoscopy score of 0 identifies patients with a very low risk of death (0.2%) and rebleeding (0.2%) and who may be suitable for early discharge or non-admission (SIGN guidelines – see references).

### Blatchford score

This score predicts the need for intervention. You wouldn't be expected to remember the details but perhaps the basic components required (sex, Hb, urea, presence of shock, melaena, syncope, hepatic/cardiac disease). Fortunately, there are many online calculators available.

Table H19.3 The Blatchford score

| Admission risk marker | Score component value |
|---|---|
| **Blood urea** | |
| <6.5 | 0 |
| ≥6.5 <8 | 2 |
| ≥8 <10 | 3 |
| ≥10 <25 | 4 |
| ≥25 | 6 |
| **Haemoglobin (men)** | |
| >13 | 0 |
| ≥12 <13 | 1 |
| ≥10 <12 | 3 |
| <10 | 6 |
| **Haemoglobin (women)** | |
| >12 | 0 |
| ≥10 <12 | 1 |
| <10 | 6 |
| **Systolic blood pressure (mmHg)** | |
| >110 | 0 |
| 100–109 | 1 |
| 90–99 | 2 |
| <90 | 3 |

(Continued)

**Table H19.3** (*Continued*)

| Other markers: (add if present) | |
| --- | --- |
| Pulse ≥100 | 1 |
| Presentation with melaena | 1 |
| Presentation with syncope | 2 |
| Hepatic disease | 2 |
| Cardiac disease | 2 |

A patient scoring 0 with Blatchford has a minimal risk of needing an intervention such as transfusion, endoscopy or surgery. These patients can be considered for an early discharge and outpatient management on ambulatory care pathways for low-risk GI bleeds. A score >0 has a higher risk of needing medical intervention (transfusion, endoscopy) or surgery. Patients scoring >6 have a greater than 50% risk of requiring an intervention.

## Management

Outpatient OGD (urgent) as part of ambulatory care pathway for GI bleeding, e.g. if Blatchford score = 0

Copy of discharge letter for patient and GP: advise to reattend if further haematemesis (would then need to consider inpatient OGD)

Can give proton pump inhibitor, e.g. for 1 month, to assist healing

Brief advice regarding alcohol (potentially harmful drinking levels). National limits for women advise 14 units per week (maximum of 2–3 units per night with several alcohol-free days per week). She is currently drinking over three times the recommended limits, and it will have been one of the causes for the vomiting and then the bleeding

Brief advice regarding alcohol should be based on the FRAMES approach:

   Feedback – patient's risk of having alcohol problems, units, risk levels, knowing position on scale, potential harm caused by her level of drinking; Reasons for changing the behaviour (benefits of reduction) including health and well-being benefits; barriers to change

   Responsibility – change is her responsibility

   Advice – provision of clear advice when requested

   Menu – what are the options for change? Outline practical strategies to help reduce alcohol consumption ('menu'): alcohol-free days, plan alternative activities, workout not drink, other interests, no pub after work, eat then drink, quench thirst with soft drinks. This leads to a set of goals

   Empathy – an approach that is warm, reflective and understanding; non-judgemental

   Self-efficacy – optimism about the behaviour change

Offer referral to local alcohol services for confidential advice/guidance/support (see local protocols) – based on drinking 12 units per night two nights per week, and presenting to hospital with alcohol-related vomiting and haematemesis

## Addressing concerns/answering questions

- *Where's the blood coming from?* Likely to be a minor tear of the gullet/foodpipe; no signs of any significant bleeding.
- *Do I need to stay in hospital?* No – all your observations have been normal and you can quite reasonably be discharged home with a plan for outpatient endoscopy to check that all has healed up.
- *Can I still drink alcohol?* Yes, but advice re alcohol as above: less than 14 units per week/several alcohol-free days, etc. See section on brief advice above.
- *What's the chance of it being stomach cancer like my uncle?* It is very unlikely given your young age and lack of previous symptoms; unlikely to be at increased risk as uncle was 60 years of age. The endoscopy will provide a full check-up of the stomach.

## Discussion with examiners

The examiners may ask you to clarify details of the above diagnosis and ask questions about your planned investigations and management.

Other possible questions include:

- *Does she really need an endoscopy?* Ambulatory care pathways for low risk upper GI bleeding will include an outpatient upper GI endoscopy (next 1–2 weeks).
- *What are the recommended alcohol units per week for a man?* 21 units per week, maximum of 3–4 units per day with several alcohol-free days per week.
- *What are the potential health consequences of her alcohol consumption?* Wide range of potential health consequences including liver disease, effects on fertility, hypertension, risk of breast cancer.

## Examiners' information and requirements

The candidate should:

1. Identify key features from the history: history consistent with a Mallory–Weiss tear (vomiting → flecks of blood → small amounts of blood); alcohol history including units of alcohol per week; low-risk GI bleed (Rockall 0, Blatchford 0). Discuss low-risk parameters: need to be aware of Blatchford/Rockall; safe to discharge
2. Identify key examination findings: normal examination likely; cardiovascularly stable
3. Outline a sensible management plan, including ambulatory GI bleed pathway/ urgent outpatient OGD
4. Give a clear explanation to the patient of your diagnosis (GI bleed, alcohol use above recommended limits) and management plan (outpatient endoscopy). Provide brief advice regarding alcohol, address her concerns and answer her questions

## Further reading/resources

Brief advice on alcohol: www.sips.iop.kcl.ac.uk/ba.php
e-learning package on how to screen for alcohol use and provide brief advice: www.alcohollearningcentre. org.uk
SIGN guidelines on GI bleeding: www.sign.com
Calculators for Rockall and Blatchford scores: www. gastrotraining.com
NICE guidance on acute upper GI bleeding: www. guidance.nice.org.uk/CG141

# Scenario 20 | Elevated liver function tests: non-alcoholic fatty liver disease (NAFLD)

## Candidate's information

**Your role:** you are an ST2 in the diabetes clinic and a patient has come to see you. His GP has forwarded to you some recent blood results which show an elevated ALT of 92 (usual <41), γ-GT 102 (usual <50). The GP reports that the patient has diabetes with good control, with slightly raised cholesterol and a BMI of 32, and the GP is asking for your help in investigating why the liver tests are elevated. The patient's recent HbA1c was only very slightly above normal. ALT was 60 2 years ago with otherwise normal LFT. Ferritin 500.

**Your task:** to assess the patient's problems and address any questions or concerns raised by him.

## Patient's information

**You are:** Jeremy Somers, a 65-year-old man.

**Your problem:** you went to your GP to have some routine blood tests taken for monitoring as you're on a 'statin' tablet for your cholesterol. He had mentioned to you that you had slightly raised liver tests last year but said that it was probably due to your diabetes. A new 'locum' GP was there because your usual GP was on holiday, and he called you back in and told you that your liver was not working as well as it should, and you may need a biopsy of your liver. He explained that the diabetes specialists were due to see you and they could decide. You've put on about a stone in the past year, despite trying to lose weight.

## Past medical history and drug history:
- Diabetes for 10 years. On treatment for raised cholesterol and on treatment for blood pressure
- No previous operations, blood transfusions, piercings, tattoos
- Never injected medicines or drugs
- No recent foreign travel (last time Spain about 5 years ago) and never been unwell whilst away
- Never been jaundiced, and no-one in your family has ever been jaundiced
- Metformin 1g bd, gliclazide 80mg bd, atorvastatin 40mg od (nocte), ramipril 2.5 od
- No allergies to medicines, and not taking any herbal/alternative medicines

## Social history:
- Alcohol: you have 3 pints of lager (4%) every Saturday night, and avoid drinking during the week

- Never had a problem with drink, and you don't think that you drink excessively. You have never been told what the right amount is to drink per day or per week. It's never caused you any health problems in the past
- You are an office worker

### Other issues including family history:
- Your father had problems with alcohol and developed cirrhosis from which he died aged 65
- No family history of haemochromatosis and no-one in family ever needed venesections

### Your questions for the candidate:
- *Why is my GP worrying about my liver now after 2 years?*
- *Do I need a liver biopsy?*
- *How much alcohol can I drink every day?*

## Candidate

### History/key questions
Full liver history: includes past history of jaundice, liver disease

Any blood transfusions in the past (and where), medical procedures (and where), piercings, tattoos, ever injected drugs?

Alcohol intake: ask patient to describe in pints/bottles per day, and what strength drunk (1 pint of 4% lager is 2.3 units, 1 pint of 5% lager is 2.8 units per pint ) – see www.DrinkAware.co.uk for units calculator. You can then use this information to calculate units per day and total units per week

Patient's understanding of diabetes control/tablets, etc.

### Drug history
Hepatotoxicity caused by medicines: check his prescribed and over-the-counter medications including alternative and herbal medicines, Chinese herbal medicines

### Other issues including family history
Any family history of jaundice, liver disease or chronic viral hepatitis infection (e.g. any partner(s) ever been ill with jaundice, or diagnosed with chronic hepatitis B or C)

Anyone in the family have haemochromatosis

### Address patient's questions and concerns
- *Have you had any thoughts about what is going on?*
- *Is there anything in particular you're concerned about?*
- *Do you have anything you would like to ask?*

## Key areas for examination
A list of what to look for (in examination order; describe findings on examination)

BMI / is he obese or overweight?

Lymphadenopathy (cervical/supraclavicular)

Tattoos, piercings, injection sites (injecting drug use)

Signs of chronic liver disease: protein calorie malnutrition (muscle wasting), leuconychia, clubbing, Dupuytren's, palmar erythema, hepatic flap, jaundice, parotid enlargement, gynaecomastia, spider naevi, hepatomegaly (if fatty/enlarged), ascites, oedema

Any signs of haemochromatosis: skin pigmentation (bronzed/grey), hepatomegaly ± splenomegaly; may have signs of chronic liver disease as above

(This patient will have central obesity but no features of chronic liver disease)

## Differential diagnosis
The most likely cause for the elevated liver blood tests is non-alcoholic fatty liver disease (NAFLD). Predisposing causes for this include obesity, diabetes, raised cholesterol (metabolic syndrome) – leads to fat deposition in the liver

Mention haemochromatosis (raised ferritin in patient with diabetes): needs HFE genotype test to look for genotype consistent with haemochromatosis. Important to note that raised ferritin can also be due to increased alcohol intake or inflammation, e.g. viral hepatitis or other acute phase reaction (e.g. the acute phase of viral hepatitis can lead to an elevated ferritin which then settles over time)

## Discussion with patient

Explain diagnosis
Explain plan, including investigations and management
Address patient's concerns/answer their questions

The elevated liver blood tests found by your GP are probably due to increased amounts of fat in the liver, a condition called fatty liver. This is related to you having diabetes, raised cholesterol and being overweight. We will send off a collection of blood tests to look for other causes of raised liver blood tests such as infections in the liver, or inflammation, and arrange an ultrasound scan to look at the liver. I'll arrange for you to go and see the liver doctors after these tests have been done. The main treatment of fatty liver is through the ongoing treatment of your diabetes and cholesterol, as well as weight loss (reduced intake, increased exercise, aiming for gradual sustainable weight loss, and healthy living). Although the risk of developing cirrhosis or scarring in your liver from having fatty liver is low, it is really a warning shot for the need for healthier eating, more exercise, weight loss etc. to reduce the risk of diabetes-related vascular complications in the long term, e.g. stroke, heart attacks, etc.

## Investigations

To exclude other causes of raised LFT (e.g. viral hepatitis, autoimmune liver disease, haemochromatosis) and assess synthetic function (INR, bilirubin, platelets) to help assess whether there is evidence of cirrhosis (are there signs of cirrhosis on examination?)

Full liver screen: hepatitis B surface antigen, hepatitis C antibody, immunoglobulins, antimitochondrial antibody, anti-smooth muscle antibody, anti-liver kidney microsomal antibody, antinuclear antibody, ferritin, α1-antitrypsin, INR, LFT, FBC, γ-GT, α-fetoprotein; caeruloplasmin if <40 years of age

Ultrasound to exclude focal lesion(s), biliary obstruction. Often echogenic livers noted, consistent with 'fatty change'. Ultrasound has poor sensitivity/specificity for cirrhosis

## Management

Alcohol: as above. Not drinking excessively at present, advise patient to stick to recommended limits in diabetes. Need to bear in mind the increased risk of hypoglycaemia with alcohol, and the 180 calories in each pint of standard strength 4% lager (as weight loss is a core part of the management of fatty liver)

NAFLD: weight loss and management of the metabolic syndrome (diabetes, cholesterol, obesity) are the two key parts of NAFLD management

Suggest referral to gastroenterology to investigate the elevated LFT. They will decide on the likelihood of him having fatty liver/NAFLD, non-alcoholic steatohepatitis or cirrhosis, and whether he needs a liver biopsy based on the results of the full liver screen and imaging. Non-invasive methods for guiding the decision on whether a biopsy is required include scoring systems such as the BARD or Angulo scores, and newer, non-invasive assessments of the degree of liver fibrosis such as 'fibro-scans' are available in some centres; these methods all aim to assess the degree of fibrosis in the liver without the need for a biopsy. Liver biopsies may then be carried out in patients with scores suggestive of fibrosis or cirrhosis, as this can guide further management (you won't be expected to know about the different scoring systems.).

## Addressing concerns/answering questions

- *Why is my GP worrying about my liver now after 2 years?* One of the liver blood tests (ALT) was higher this year compared to the previous time (last year) and your GP wanted a full check-up of the liver, an MOT, to rule out any other causes (unrelated to diabetes/fatty liver) requiring different treatment.
- *Do I need a liver biopsy?* We will send off all the tests, arrange the scan and the liver doctors will see you and decide on further management. They may advise a biopsy if they think that it will provide useful information that blood results don't.
- *How much alcohol can I drink every day?* The standard advice is <21 U/ week for a man (maximum of 3–4 units per day with several alcohol-free days per week) but you need to be aware of the calorie intake associated with alcohol, and the risk of weight gain due to this.

## Discussion with examiners

The examiners may ask you to clarify details of the above diagnosis and ask questions about your planned investigations and management.

A possible question includes:
- *What are the features of the metabolic syndrome?* Various definitions exist. The International Diabetes Federation criteria in 2006 require central obesity (waist circumference) combined with two of:

Hyperlipidaemia:
    elevated triglycerides or on treatment for this
    low HDL or on treatment for elevated HDL
Hypertension or on treatment
Elevated fasting plasma glucose (>5.6 mmol – prefer-
    ably confirm with oral glucose tolerance test) or
    previously diagnosed type 2 diabetes.

**Further reading/resources**
www.drinkaware.co.uk

---

**Examiners' information and requirements**

The candidate should:

1. Identify key features from the history: risk factors for elevated LFT, an accurate number of units of alcohol per week, risk factors for NAFLD including metabolic syndrome (central obesity, hypertension, diabetes, raised cholesterol)

2. Identify key examination findings, including obesity but no signs of cirrhosis/ chronic liver disease

3. Outline a sensible management plan, including further investigations to find the cause of the abnormal LFT, the components of a standard liver screen, and the need for an ultrasound; referral to gastroenterology; fatty liver as the cause, and management through weight loss and control of risk factors

4. Give a clear explanation to the patient of your diagnosis and plan, address his concerns and answer his questions

# Other possible alcohol-related gastroenterology cases

- Raised LFT due to alcohol/no signs of chronic liver disease. Brief advice about alcohol/advise reduction/long-term consequences
- Decompensated cirrhosis (see Vol. 1, Station 1, Abdominal, Case 3) due to alcohol, still drinking 80 units per week. Give advice about alcohol, discuss referral to alcohol services for support, advise life-long abstinence but need to gradually reduce alcohol intake down to zero under the supervision of alcohol services (rather than an abrupt stop which could precipitate alcohol withdrawal), arrange full liver screen including ultrasound of liver, refer to gastroenterology for ongoing management of decompensated cirrhosis

# Scenario 21 | Elevated liver function tests and hepatitis B serology

## Candidate's information

**Your role:** you are the ST2 in the general medical clinic, and a 35-year-old male patient has been referred by his GP. Elevated liver function tests were found on routine testing by the GP, and a liver screen was sent by the GP. Hepatitis B serology included with the GP letter has shown that he is hepatitis B surface antigen positive, core antibody positive, e antigen positive, e antibody negative. Normal liver ultrasound.

**Your task:** to assess the patient's problems and address any questions or concerns raised by him.

## Patient's information

**You are:** Jason Dundas, a 35-year-old man.

**Your problem:** your GP checked your liver blood tests as you were feeling a bit tired, and found that one of your liver function tests was higher than it should be, and then sent off a lot of different blood tests. He called you in to say that you have hepatitis B but didn't say much more. You checked the internet and several of the websites mentioned that hepatitis B causes cirrhosis, cancer and death. It also mentioned that it can be caught sexually.

You had an episode of jaundice (felt unwell, had yellow eyes and dark urine) about a year or more ago, and this settled over a few weeks. You felt a bit tired for a few weeks afterwards but you feel well now. You didn't go and see your GP at the time. You split from your long-term female partner about 18 months ago (she's been well since) and have had unprotected vaginal intercourse with two women since (no sex with men). The first was just after you split up with your long-term partner (over a year ago but before the jaundice), and the last about 3 months ago.

You don't know the first woman as you were on holiday in the UK but your most recent sexual encounter was with a female friend of yours. She doesn't know about the hepatitis B and you're worried that you'll have to tell her. She's married to someone else. You've had protected vaginal intercourse with her (no anal intercourse).

### Past medical history and drug history:
- No other past history of note, and no usual medications
- No herbal or alternative medicines
- Never had any operations, blood transfusions or injected medications or drugs. No tattoos or piercings

### Social history:
- Non-smoker
- Lives alone. No current partner
- Up to 4–5 pints of (4.2%) lager per week

**Other issues including family history:**

- No family members are known to have liver disease or hepatitis

**Your questions for the candidate:**

- *How did I get it?*
- *Can I get rid of it?*
- *Do I have cirrhosis? Will I get cancer?*
- *Should I tell my friend?*

## Candidate

### History/key questions

Liver history:

Ever had any blood transfusions, tattoos or piercings

Ever injected drugs

Herbal or alternative medicines

Ever been jaundiced. If so, when, how long did it last, and any investigations carried out after it happened to find out the cause?

Alcohol intake in units per week

Need to take a full sexual health history:

Symptoms: dysuria, urethral discharge, skin problems, oral and perianal symptoms

Any eye symptoms (e.g. gritty or red eyes) and/or arthropathy consistent with sexually acquired reactive arthritis (previously called Reiter's syndrome)

Bridging questions: tactful ways of linking general health questions to more specific sexual health questions (easier if you have already identified that the patient is concerned about a possible STI)

Last sexual intercourse: which gender; type of sexual intercourse (oral, anal, vaginal); condom use/barrier contraception – used throughout and remained intact?

Relationship with partner – long-term, ?duration

Any casual sexual contacts, traceable versus non-traceable partners' health, any symptoms

Previous partner(s) in last couple of years given timing of jaundice: questions as above for each, including the nationality/country of birth of the sexual partners (part of risk assessment process)

If no partners in last 3 months: when was last sexual intercourse?

All men should be asked if they have had sex with another man in the past

Is current partner aware of his symptoms, had recent sexual health check or known to have any previous STI?

Is partner with him today?

Risk assessment for viral hepatitis/HIV:

Any previous STIs

Ever had any testing in the past (GUM clinic, GP, hospital) for HIV or STI

Any vaccination history for hepatitis B

Ever had sex abroad other than with partner with whom he was travelling

Medical treatment abroad

Ever exchanged money in return for sex (UK or abroad)

Ask about medications and any drug use (injecting drug use, sharing of needles, syringes, drug preparation equipment)

### *Other issues including family history*

Anyone in the family ever had jaundice or liver disease?

Anyone known to have hepatitis B, e.g. parents or siblings (consider vertical transmission of hepatitis B)

Country of origin

Any children? If so, have they been tested for hepatitis B, and if non-immune have they been vaccinated?

### Address patient's questions and concerns

- *Have you had any thoughts about what is going on?*
- *Is there anything in particular you're concerned about?*
- *Do you have anything you would like to ask?*

### Key areas for examination

A list of what to look for (in examination order; describe findings on examination)

Overall inspection

Look for signs of chronic liver disease: palmar erythema, spider naevi, hepatic flap, gynaecomastia

Tattoos, piercings, needle marks (injecting drug use)

Lymphadenopathy

Abdominal examination: hepatomegaly, splenomegaly, ascites

Oedema

On examination this patient has no signs of chronic liver disease; patient feels well. No tattoos, piercings, needle marks

## Differential diagnosis

Chronic hepatitis B; based on the history and the serology

Twelve months or more after an episode of jaundice, he remains hepatitis B surface antigen positive, which suggests that he has had an episode of acute hepatitis B and failed to clear the virus/become immune. He now has chronic hepatitis B (chronic hepatitis B is defined as persistence of HBsAg in the circulation for more than 6 months). The surface antigen is found on the hepatitis B virion and its presence in the blood means that there is virus present

## Discussion with patient

Explain diagnosis

Explain plan, including investigations and management

Address patient's concerns/answer their questions

You have an infection with a virus called hepatitis B, and this appears likely to have caused your jaundice a year ago. It looks like it has become a chronic infection with hepatitis B based on the blood results and the history of an episode of acute jaundice a year or so ago. The body hasn't cleared the virus so we need to arrange some blood tests today to see how much virus is present in the blood, a scan of the liver, and we will refer you to one of the liver specialists.

## Investigations

Will need hepatitis B virus DNA levels to assess the level of viral load. This will help guide the next steps in management

All hepatitis B surface antigen positive patients should be referred to a hepatologist who will decide on the need for antiviral therapy. A liver biopsy may be required for assessment of the degree of inflammation, fibrosis and cirrhosis, as further management would be required in the presence of cirrhosis (screening for varices/HCC). Antiviral therapy in hepatitis B is a specialist field

Check results of GP's full liver screen: needs hepatitis C antibody, immunoglobulins, anti-mitochondrial antibody, anti-smooth muscle antibody, anti-liver kidney microsomal antibody, anti-nuclear antibody, ferritin, α1-antitrypsin, INR, LFT, FBC, γ-GT, α-fetoprotein (and caeruloplasmin if <40 years of age). Ultrasound to exclude focal lesion(s), biliary obstruction

HIV testing (opportunistic) is important: co-infection with HIV alters management (although some of the antivirals used for HIV are also used for HBV infection, it is more complicated)

## Management

Treatment of chronic hepatitis B infection aims to reduce viral replication and therefore the viral load, aiming to delay or prevent the development of fibrosis or subsequent cirrhosis and its complications (portal hypertension/variceal bleeding, HCC and death). Other aims include seroconversion (loss of e antigen and development of e antibodies) and then later loss of the hepatitis B surface antigen

Referral to hepatologist (viral hepatitis expert)

GUM clinic for sexual health check: provide contact details for the GUM clinic

HIV serology and counselling: although this could also be carried out at the GUM clinic, opportunistic testing is important (and encouraged by GU physicians), particularly as coinfection with HBV and HIV is complicated. HIV is now managed as a chronic disease; counselling in this consultation would be appropriate

Household and sexual contacts: check hepatitis B status (vaccination if non-immune, referral to specialist if chronic hepatitis B). Sexual contacts should also attend the GUM clinic

Advise patient to avoid sharing toothbrushes and razors

Recommend only protected intercourse using condoms. Non-immune sexual partners should be vaccinated

## Addressing concerns/answering questions

- *How did I get it?* The most likely cause is through the unprotected intercourse given the timing of the jaundice. Unfortunately, 5% of adults fail to clear the acute infection, resulting in chronic infection.
- *Can I get rid of it?* The specialists will decide on the need for medical treatment for the chronic hepatitis B infection – this aims to keep the levels of the virus as low as possible, reduce the ongoing damage to the liver, and reduce the risks of future complications. (A small proportion of people clear the hepatitis B virus surface antigen [5% of hepatitis B e-antigen negative patients with hepatitis B lose their surface antigen positivity after five years of therapy].)

• *Do I have cirrhosis? Will I get cancer?* There are no signs of cirrhosis on examination but you need to be referred to the liver specialists (gastroenterologists) who can decide regarding further investigations; these will include an ultrasound scan, blood tests and fibroscan (non-invasive method of assessing liver fibrosis) and possibly a liver biopsy. Cirrhosis is scarring of the liver and this can develop due to the virus in the liver. It is important to reduce the risk of cirrhosis developing e.g. with antiviral medicines, and to manage it if it's already developed. One of the potential complications of cirrhosis is the development of cancers of the liver and we monitor patients with six monthly special blood tests and ultrasound scans to pick these up if they occur.
• *Should I tell my friend?* The Health Protection Agency will be contacting you regarding the hepatitis B infection, and contact tracing is one of their key jobs. Your friend needs to know for her own health (and her current partner), as it has serious implications for her (if positive, she would need assessment by a hepatologist, and her sexual partner(s) and household contacts would need testing for hepatitis B, and vaccination if non-immune). Both of you should go to the GUM clinic and have a full sexual health check (confidential).

## Discussion with examiners

The examiners may ask you to clarify details of the above diagnosis and ask questions about your planned investigations and management.

Other possible questions include:
• *What are the liver-related consequences of chronic hepatitis B?* Cirrhosis and its complications (decompensation of cirrhosis with ascites, encephalopathy, portal hypertension including varices / bleeding, renal impairment, protein calorie malnutrition, hepatocellular carcinoma).
• *What other viral infections should be screened for in patients newly diagnosed with hepatitis B?* HIV and hepatitis C need to be screened for as the presence of one or both of these influences the drugs used to treat hepatitis B and HIV coinfection.

See also Vol. 1, Station 1, Abdominal, Case 3.

---

### Examiners' information and requirements

The candidate should:
1. Identify key features from the history: unprotected sexual intercourse followed by an episode of acute jaundice, and now a year or more later diagnosed with chronic hepatitis B
2. Identify key examination findings including no signs of chronic liver disease. Interpret the hepatitis B serology correctly as chronic carrier
3. Outline a sensible management plan including basic investigations (US/full liver screen), HIV serology, and onward referral to hepatologists and GUM physicians
4. Give a clear explanation to the patient of your diagnosis and plan, address his concerns and answer his questions

---

### Further reading/resources

NICE hepatitis B guidelines: www.guidance.nice.org.uk
BASL/EASL guidelines: www.basl.org.uk
British Liver Trust leaflet – A Professional's Guide to Hepatitis B: www.britishlivertrust.org.uk

# Scenario 22 | Crohn's disease/ inflammatory bowel disease

## Candidate's information

**Your role:** you are an ST2 in the MAU. A patient has been referred to the medical team by the emergency department doctors with a history of abdominal pain and weight loss.

**Your task:** to assess the patient's problems and address any questions or concerns raised by him.

## Patient's information

**You are:** Liam Kingston, a 22-year-old man.

**Your problem:** your main concerns are the abdominal pain and weight loss that you have been having. You have had about 3 months of pains in the lower right area of your tummy; these start about 1 h after eating and you feel bloated and full. Your family have told you that they can hear your bowel rumbling across the room. You've had some mouth ulcers and some right elbow pains. Last week, your GP mentioned that you were anaemic after your blood test results came back. You had gone to your GP as you were feeling sick and bloated. You had a more severe episode of pain last night, which came on about an hour after eating. It felt like a cramping, gripping pain in the lower right part of your stomach. Hot water bottles and paracetamol didn't help. You vomited last night for the first time and this did ease the tummy pains for a few hours. The pains have settled now as you haven't eaten for a few hours.

You've not had any fever but you have lost 5 kg of weight over the past 3 months – you're active and you put it down to stress initially but you now think it might be related to the pains.

You've been having diarrhoea up to three times per day with custard-consistency motions. You haven't been opening your bowels at night. No blood in the stools or having to rush to the toilet. Before this all started, you were opening your bowels once per day with formed motions.

You have also been feeling tired and drained for the past few months and have been struggling to keep up with your studies.

### Past medical history and drug history:
- Nothing of note. Tonsils removed age 5
- No regular medications or allergies

### Social history:
- Smoked 20/day for past 3 years
- Alcohol: 3 pints of 5.3% lager on a Friday night

### Other issues including family history:
- Your grandmother had bowel cancer age 75 and died shortly afterwards

---

## Candidate

### History/key questions

Pain: site, onset, character (colicky, squeezing in incomplete obstruction), duration, relieving and exacerbating factors (including opening bowels, vomiting, analgesia, not eating)

Diarrhoea (motions per day and per night, consistency, presence of blood in/on stools)

Urgency

Rectal bleeding

Weight loss: need to quantify (in kilograms)

Appetite

Pain/bloating/vomiting/nausea suggestive of obstruction

Extraintestinal manifestations of IBD: ask about uveitis (gritty eyes), arthralgia, mouth ulcers, rash such as erythema nodosum or pyoderma gangrenosum

#### Social history

Smoker? Quantify in pack-years (cessation important in Crohn's disease)

#### Other issues including family history

Family history of IBD?

### Address patient's questions and concerns

- *Have you had any thoughts about what is going on?*
- *How much is being unwell interfering with your studies?*
- *Is there anything in particular you're concerned about?*
- *Do you have anything you would like to ask?*

## Key areas for examination

A list of what to look for (in examination order; describe findings on examination)

Signs of weight loss/protein calorie malnutrition

Any joint swelling or redness

Erythema nodosum, pyoderma gangrenosum

Mouth ulcers/angular cheilitis/glossitis/pale conjunctivae

Abdominal signs:
  Visible peristalsis (obstruction)
  Tenderness RIF ± palpable mass (?ileocaecal Crohn's)
  High-pitched bowel sounds in obstruction

Say that you would like to carry out a digital rectal examination; may show lateral rectal wall tenderness if pelvic/small bowel mass in RIF; blood on finger

Examination findings: tenderness RIF on deep palpation, no guarding. Bowel sounds normal

## Differential diagnosis

IBD: Crohn's disease given pain, weight loss, change in bowel habit and anaemia in young man

Differential diagnosis includes ulcerative colitis (diarrhoea, pain, weight loss but no rectal bleeding/urgency, and opening only three times per day; Crohn's is main differential diagnosis with pain and weight loss his main symptoms)

Generally, consider coeliac disease in all patients with anaemia, diarrhoea and/or weight loss but here wouldn't give the obstructive symptoms (pain)

Colon cancer/neoplasia unlikely given age

Extraintestinal manifestations of IBD: mouth ulcers, arthralgia

## Discussion with patient

Explain diagnosis

Explain plan, including investigations and management

Address patient's concerns/answer their questions

Symptoms of diarrhoea, weight loss, abdominal pain and anaemia raise the possibility that there is inflammation of the lining of the bowel, a condition called inflammatory bowel disease. We need to carry out a set of tests to find out, and refer you to the gastroenterologists (bowel specialists) who will either see you here in the unit or soon as an outpatient.

### Investigations

Examination: complete by DRE/PR examination

Basic bloods including FBC, ESR/CRP, TTG, LFT, albumin and haematinics (anaemic)

Abdominal X-ray/CXR to rule out obstruction (look for dilated small bowel loops due to ileocaecal Crohn's/stricturing small bowel disease)

As part of investigations into possible IBD, patient is likely to need colonoscopy and small bowel imaging (MR enterography or small bowel follow-through, depending on local availability)

## Management

Inpatient versus outpatient management: find out if the gastroenterologists can see him in the MAU with the results of the above blood tests and plain X-ray, and plan further investigations and follow-up as an outpatient

Important to stress the need to stop smoking completely if diagnosed with Crohn's; offer referral to smoking cessation services. General health benefits outside the gut too

Suggest holding off treatment (steroids, etc.) until diagnosis made (confirmed by endoscopy, histology, radiology)

Gastroenterology multidisciplinary team approach involving physicians, clinical nurse specialists, radiologists, surgeons, pathologists, dietitians

Travel insurance essential: the patient will need to inform his insurance company as he may not be covered if he has been under investigation as an inpatient and doesn't tell them, and then needs to claim (worst case is being admitted to a US hospital when uninsured)

## Addressing concerns/answering questions

- *What's causing it? Anything serious?* We need to find out what is causing you to become unwell and suffer the pain, diarrhoea and weight loss. The most likely cause is inflammation of the bowel, and we need to carry out some tests, and ask the bowel doctors to see you about it.
- *Is it cancer? My gran had colon cancer.* All the symptoms fit with inflammation of the bowel, and bowel cancer in the young is very rare indeed.
- *Can I go on holiday in 2 months to Barbados – it's all booked?* We need to arrange for you to see the gastroenterologists, and probably need to wait and see how you get on over the next few months. It is important to have travel insurance for your holiday and you will need to inform the company of the change in your medical circumstances so that you are covered in Barbados if you become unwell there.
- *Will I still be able to go to university (final year of studies in management) – exams coming up in a couple*

*of months?* We need to carry out the investigations/ refer you to the gastroenterologists and then start treatment once a diagnosis has been made. The aim of treatment will be to get you well so that you are able to attend university and sit your exams as planned.

## Discussion with examiners

The examiners may ask you to clarify details of the above diagnosis and ask questions about your planned investigations and management.

Other possible questions include:

- *What is the typical management of Crohn's disease?* Use of immunosuppression to settle the inflammation in the GI tract and keep the patient well. Early control of inflammation aims to reduce the progression to fibrosis, stenosis/stricturing of bowel and subsequent complications such as perforation, fistulation, abscesses and the need for surgery: immunosuppression includes steroids, thiopurines (azathioprine, 6-mercaptopurine), methotrexate or anti-TNFα, 'biological' drugs such as infliximab and adalimumab.
- *What are the side-effects of steroids?* See Section I, Station 5, Endocrine, Case 6 and Scenario 3, 'Dermatomyositis and falls', What are the side-effects of steroid therapy and how would you reduce the risk?

See also Vol. 1, Station 1, Abdominal, Case 9.

## Further reading/resources

ECCO guidelines: www.ecco-ibd.eu and go to guidelines
BSG guidelines: www.bsg.org.uk/clinical/general/guide lines.html

# Scenario 23 | Dysphagia and weight loss

## Candidate's information

**Your role:** you are an ST2 in elderly care. Mrs Driver has been referred urgently by her GP to the medical outpatient clinic with dysphagia.

**Your task:** to assess the patient's problems and address any questions or concerns raised by her.

## Patient's information

**You are:** Jessica Driver, a 66-year-old retired secretary.

**Your problem:** swallowing problems. You started bringing food back up about 4 weeks ago. Initially this was only hard meat that you hadn't chewed properly but for the past week softer foods feel like they stick in the lower part of your chest. You find that you have to drink liquids to wash down the food; liquids go down OK. About once or twice per day you are bringing up small amounts of recently eaten foods.

You have lost about 7 kg in weight over the past 3 months. You had initially put it down to a change in medications (you started a statin for raised cholesterol about 4 months ago) as you thought that this had made you lose your appetite, but your appetite didn't come back when you stopped the medicine. You know that you are overweight and you were happy to be losing the weight, at least initially. No chest pain or abdominal pain. Slight heartburn after certain spicy foods but this is a long-standing problem, only a little worse recently. Usually eased by Gaviscon.

### Past medical history and drug history:
- No medications. Uses Gaviscon occasionally if heartburn is particularly bad

### Social history:
- Alcohol: 3 or 4 small glasses of wine per week
- Smoked 25/day for past 30 years

### Other issues including family history:
- You are the main carer for your husband who gets confused and isn't very good on his feet. He finds it hard to cope for long at home on his own, and you're particularly worried that he'll fall over and injure himself. You feel that you can't stay at the hospital much longer, and certainly not overnight
- You're worried about the idea of having an endoscopy. Your GP mentioned that you might need one, and one of your friends had one up the bottom and found it uncomfortable

### Your questions for the candidate:
- *What's the problem with my swallowing?*
- *Is it cancer?*

- *Is the endoscopy painful?*
- *Is there any other way to find out what's causing my swallowing problems?*
- *Do I have to stay in hospital?*

---

## Candidate

### History/key questions

Dysphagia: when did it start and what foods is she able to swallow? Sudden or gradual onset? Progressive over time?

Vomiting or regurgitation: what comes up and how long after eating? Regurgitation often immediate, bringing up very recently eaten food

Is she able to swallow her own saliva (the inability to do so, leading to drooling of saliva, are symptoms of complete dysphagia)?

Pain on swallowing (odynophagia)

Ask about bloating/epigastric pain after eating (dyspepsia)

Associated alarm features: weight loss, haematemesis, abdominal mass

Any past history of dysphagia?

Any previous investigations into her dysphagia (this episode or any previous episodes), e.g. upper GI endoscopy, contrast swallow or oesophageal pH and manometry studies?

Any comorbid illnesses, particularly those associated with oesophageal problems/dysphagia, e.g. scleroderma, Parkinson's, diabetes and oropharyngeal candidiasis

Symptoms of reflux (heartburn, water brash, chest pains) which could cause GORD-related stricture or oesophageal dysmotility

Respiratory conditions can also cause dysphagia through extrinsic compression of oesophagus, e.g. lung cancer, so ask about respiratory symptoms (cough, SOB, wheeze, haemoptysis, chest pain)

Other causes include previous ingestion of caustic agents which cause strictures, e.g. bleach, caustic soda

### Drug history

Steroids, steroid inhalers (oesophageal candidiasis)

Any PPI use

### Past medical history

Barrett's oesophagus (potentially premalignant condition predisposing patient to oesophageal cancer)

Asthma or COPD on inhalers, diabetes (all associated with oesophageal candidiasis)

### Social history

Smoking (record in pack-years)

Alcohol history (units per week)

### Address patient's questions and concerns

- *Have you had any thoughts about what is going on?*
- *Is there anything in particular you're concerned about?*
- *Do you have anything you would like to ask?*

## Key areas for examination

A list of what to look for (in examination order; describe findings on examination)

Any signs of weight loss

Oropharyngeal candidiasis

Supraclavicular lymphadenopathy (Virchow's node in gastric cancer)

Signs of weight loss (loose skinfolds) or evidence of protein calorie malnutrition/muscle wasting

Abdominal examination: any masses or hepatomegaly

Ask to do a DRE (consider other causes of weight loss)

Examination for this patient may well be normal (actor)

## Differential diagnosis

Key differential is that of gastro-oesophageal malignancy (e.g. oesophageal cancer leading to symptoms of progressive dysphagia, regurgitation and weight loss)

## Discussion with patient

Explain diagnosis

Explain plan, including investigations and management

Address patient's concerns/answer their question

Use your communication skills to explain the diagnosis and plan to this patient - you will need to find out what she thinks is going on, and ask her if she is the kind of person who likes to know what's going on, for better or for worse.

The causes of your swallowing problems range from acid-related inflammation of the lining of the gullet through to more serious causes including the most serious, cancer of the gullet or food-pipe. I am concerned that something serious is going on because you have been having difficulty swallowing, you've lost weight and your appetite has been poor. I think we need to do some tests to find out what is happening. We will carry out some blood tests and a chest X-ray today, and I will arrange an urgent outpatient endoscopy test to look down the food-pipe (the oesophagus) and into the stomach. (You need to request the test yourself to be carried out as an urgent outpatient [within the next 2 weeks] to minimize delay rather than via a referral to the gastroenterology clinic.)

I will give you the appointment date and time and the information sheet about the endoscopy before you go home today. The endoscopy itself takes 5–10 min, and you have a choice between sedation to make you sleepy and relaxed, and local anaesthetic throat spray which numbs the back of the throat and tastes like bad banana. The benefits of having the endoscopy are that it is the best way to diagnose the cause of swallowing problems, and allows us to take pictures and samples from the lining of the gut, not possible with an X-ray. Risks include pain, drug reaction, bleeding and, very rarely, perforation requiring an operation to fix it. Please read the information sheet when you get home and you'll be able to ask the endoscopist questions before the test when you attend for the procedure, and the results of the test will be discussed with you after the procedure.

## Investigations

Oesophago gastro duodenoscopy (OGD) is the best investigation for dysphagia and needs to be urgent (within the next 2 weeks). Alternative investigations such as barium swallow or CT scanning don't allow direct visualization or biopsies

If she had high dysphagia (e.g. pointing at throat), then the differential diagnosis would include oropharyngeal cancers (ENT and nasal endoscopy of oropharynx likely to be needed as these high cancers can be missed at OGD). If she gave a chronic history of regurgitation without alarm symptoms, this can point towards a pharyngeal pouch (may need a barium swallow first as there is an increased risk of perforation at OGD)

## Management

Discussion with patient – the plan after the endoscopy depends on the diagnosis at endoscopy

Discussion with examiners regarding options if oesophageal cancer diagnosed (key differential)

Options depend on various factors including histological type and stage of cancer, patient's fitness and comorbidities. Possible options range from surgery (if fit for operation and only if staging scans demonstrate that a cancer would be potentially cured by an operation), radiotherapy, chemotherapy or a palliative approach (stenting to ease swallowing/improve intake, symptom control)

Patients with upper GI cancers are managed through their staging and treatment by a multidisciplinary team including clinical nurse specialists who will provide support to patients and their families throughout the process

PPI (in an orodispersible form), liquid supplements aiming to maintain nutrition and weight (otherwise she will lose weight and her physical condition will deteriorate, potentially to the point where she would be unfit to undergo treatment)

Would also need to involve the patient's GP; care for her husband will need to be addressed by her GP, particularly if she is diagnosed with cancer requiring palliative treatment/end-of-life care as she is his main carer

If a benign/peptic stricture is found at OGD: she will need a full-dose PPI long term, to address any modifiable risk factors (e.g. avoid exacerbants such as alcohol; lose weight; stop smoking) and she will need a repeat endoscopy ± dilation in a month (dilation only performed if benign histology)

She will need referral to gastroenterology (and if malignancy confirmed, the upper GI cancer multidisciplinary team) for subsequent management following OGD

Explain the need to exclude serious causes of swallowing problems through these urgent investigations

Pre OGD, suggest soft/mashed/liquids only (no 'solids'); if only able to take liquids then needs oral liquid supplements (Fortijuice, Ensure, etc.) to maintain nutrition

## Addressing concerns/answering questions

- *What's the problem with my swallowing?* See explanation above in discussions with patient.
- *Is it cancer?* See explanation above in discussions with patient.
- *Is the endoscopy painful?* The endoscopy can be uncomfortable, with bloating and belching, but shouldn't be painful; can cause a slight sore throat afterwards.
- *Is there any other way to find out what's causing my swallowing problems?* The alternatives include X-rays (contrast/barium swallow) but although they would show if there's a narrowing, they don't allow us to see

the lining of the gullet directly and take samples. Endoscopy is the best test to find out what's happening and help us develop a plan.

- *Do I have to stay in hospital?* These tests can be done as an outpatient on an urgent basis, but if your swallowing gets worse in the meantime, you need to come back (safety-netting – either to MAU or emergency department) because if your oral fluid intake is limited by dysphagia, you would need IV fluids and the tests would be carried out as an inpatient.

## Discussion with examiners

The examiners may ask you to clarify details of the above diagnosis and ask questions about your planned investigations and management.

Other possible questions include:
- *What are the causes of dysphagia?* Causes range from peptic stricture or oesophagitis (due to acid reflux), gastro-oesophageal cancer, eosinophilic oesophagitis, oesophageal dysmotility (various disorders including diffuse oesophageal spasm, 'nutcracker' oesophagus), oesophageal webs, achalasia, stricturing due to previous caustic injury, Sjögren's, scleroderma, or functional (normal investigations).
- *What other tests can be used to diagnose the cause of her dysphagia?* Contrast swallow (barium swallow) can demonstrate e.g. stricturing, dysmotility and /or gastro-oesophageal reflux; CT scanning can demonstrate thickening of the oesophagus, an oesophageal mass or lymphadenopathy, and is used to look for evidence of local and distant spread of an oesophageal cancer. It is not possible to get biopsies or histology with barium swallow or CT scans. Oesophageal manometry is used to demonstrate dysmotility, often in conjunction with pH studies (GORD is a cause of dysmotility) but is not a first-line investigation into dysphagia.

---

**Examiners' information and requirements**

The candidate should:
1. Identify alarm symptoms of dysphagia to solids, regurgitation and weight loss
2. Include cancer of oesophagus in the list of differential diagnoses. This list also includes benign reflux-related stricture but patient has marked alarm symptoms
3. Outline a clear management plan, including urgent outpatient OGD and plan for follow-up with gastroenterology
4. Give a clear explanation to the patient of your diagnosis and plan, address her concerns and answer her questions

---

# Scenario 24 | Diarrhoea: recent antibiotics

## Candidate's information

**Your role:** you are a medical ST2 covering the medical wards this weekend, and you are asked to see Mrs Carter who is a 70-year-old on the care of the elderly medical ward. She has developed diarrhoea after a course of antibiotics for a urinary tract infection.

**Your task:** to assess the patient's problems and address any questions or concerns raised by her.

## Patient's information

**You are:** Joan Carter, a 70-year-old woman.

**Your problem:** you've been in hospital for about 10 days after you had a water infection which made you go off your legs. You had some antibiotics called cefalexin from your GP at your nursing home but you then got worse with a burning sensation when passing urine, fever and right lower back pain; you came into hospital and were given a different antibiotic (co-amoxiclav) and you feel better.

Over the past 4 days or so, you have been getting back on your feet with the physio (usually you're able to transfer from bed to chair) but over the past 2 days you have started having green, foul-smelling diarrhoea and aching in your lower tummy, and you've lost your appetite. You've been opening your bowels about six times per day with runny/softer than custard consistency stool. Not opening bowels at night. Usually you open your bowels once per day with formed stool, like when you first came into hospital. Prior to coming into hospital, you had been living in a nursing home for one year because of needing help with your diabetes and poor mobility.

## Past medical history:
- Diabetes mellitus; no hospital admissions in past year or two. Never had any steroids, chemotherapy

## Drug history:
- On chart – omeprazole 40 mg od, enoxaparin 40 mg sc od, metformin 500 mg bd, perindopril 2 mg, simvastatin 40 mg od. Lantus insulin
- Co-amoxiclav course finished 5 days ago

## Social history:
- You live in a nursing home – you've not heard of anyone else there with diarrhoea. You moved there a year ago as you need help with your medicines and your diabetes, and you had been struggling at home
- Daughters visit you daily in the hospital with your grandchildren (15 and 16 years old) who are on their school holidays at the moment – they've been well
- Not been abroad for 10 years. You go on holiday in the UK

**Other issues including family history:**
- Nil of note

**Your questions for the candidate:**
- *Will I give it to my grandchildren?*
- *Why do you want to give me antibiotics to treat the bug in the bowel if the antibiotics gave me diarrhoea in the first place?*

## Candidate

### History/key questions

Diarrhoea: how often (day and night), consistency (use real-world comparators similar to the Bristol Stool Chart pictures, e.g. formed/sausage-shaped, blobs, custard consistency, watery/loose, or use the photos on the Bristol Stool Chart if one is present); did she see any blood in stool or on wiping?

Duration of diarrhoea (days, weeks or longer); continuous or intermittent. If intermittent, what happens in between episodes?

Urgency, rectal bleeding?

Any obvious precipitant (eating out, new medications, 'gastroenteritis', antibiotic use, any outbreaks at home or long-term care facility – nursing home, intermediate care, prison, hospital or school)

Medications such as metformin, lansoprazole can cause diarrhoea

Admissions to hospital in past year?

Foreign travel in past year and to where?

Associated symptoms: weight loss, abdominal pain

Ask about arthralgia, mouth ulcers, uveitis (extraintestinal manifestations of IBD)

### Drug history

Ask to see the patient's drug chart

Ask about PPI use (linked to *C. difficile*); long-term antibiotic use for UTI prophylaxis

### Past medical history

Any abdominal surgery?

### Social history

Where does the patient live?

### Address patient's questions and concerns

- *Have you had any thoughts about what is going on?*
- *Is there anything in particular you're concerned about?*
- *Do you have anything you would like to ask?*

## Key areas for examination

A list of what to look for (in examination order; describe findings on examination)

Overall appearance

Fluid balance: JVP

Pulse, BP, capillary refill/peripheral perfusion: the patient looks well, pulse 80, BP 135/75, mild tenderness only

Abdominal examination: examine carefully; look for tenderness including guarding, masses and percussive tenderness (peritonism)

Say that you would like to carry out a DRE

Also ask to assess oral intake (fluids/nutrition) on charts

See stool/temp/pulse/BP charts

## Differential diagnoses

*Clostridium difficile* is the key differential: the given history of antibiotic use (and types), age, nursing home resident, PPI use

Infective: viral (no vomiting reported); exclude salmonella/shigella/campylobacter

Altered bowel habit with diarrhoea, abdominal pain and fever – differential diagnosis includes diverticulitis; IBD can present acutely with similar symptoms; neoplasia always needs to be considered but this is an acute history

Acute presentation whilst in hospital, and after antibiotics, points strongly towards *C. difficile* (main differential)

## Discussion with patient

Explain diagnosis

Explain plan, including investigations and management

Address patient's concerns/answer their questions

You've developed diarrhoea since coming into hospital and we need to find out the cause. We'll send off a stool sample to look for any infection in the bowel, we'll do an X-ray of your stomach, and do some blood tests. The diarrhoea may be related to the antibiotics that we gave to you for your urine infection. These antibiotics can disturb the balance of bugs in the bowel, allowing overgrowth of diarrhoea-causing bacteria. This would be treated with a different antibiotic. We've prescribed some supplement drinks, and please keep eating your meals. We'll move you to a single room. Your family need to wash their hands when they come and visit, to reduce the risk of them catching the same infection.

## Investigations

Need to follow local trust clinical guidelines/flowchart for *C. difficile* management

Blood tests including FBC, U&E, ESR, CRP, albumin

Stool for MCS and *C. difficile*: urgent/need same-day result. Any source will do (take stool from commode pan/pads/bed)

Abdominal X-ray (±CT in severe disease)

Isolation

Decide on whether mild, moderate or severe disease based on clinical criteria (mild-to-moderate: can include <5 stools per day and WCC <15; severe: includes WCC >15 (often >40), CRP >150, dry/hypovolaemia, acute renal impairment including acidosis and raised lactate, temp 38.5+, evidence of severe colitis, severe abdominal pain/diffuse; abdominal X-ray – colitis/toxic megacolon [7 cm])

## Management

Review any antibiotics and discuss with microbiology about whether possible to stop

Empirical antibiotics early for *C. difficile*: choice depends on local protocols based on the severity of probable *C. difficile* to decide between metronidazole or vancomycin for severe disease

Urgent isolation of patient: side ward/gloves/gowns/handwashing

Stool chart (stool type as per Bristol Stool Chart, size/amount, presence of blood)

Nutrition: sip feeds/supplements and nutritional charting

Stop PPI unless necessary (risk/benefit balance depends on past history)

Stop laxatives/antidiarrhoeals

Caution with opiates

## Addressing concerns/answering questions

• *Will I give it to my grandchildren?* Visitors and family need to wash their hands with soap and water when leaving the room; check if anyone is unwell/immunosuppressed. Advise against bringing in small children, pregnant women.

• *Why do you want to give me antibiotics to treat the bug in the bowel if the antibiotics gave me diarrhoea in the first place?* We use the new antibiotics to treat the *C. difficile* bug that is causing the diarrhoea, and allow the balance of bugs in the bowel to recover.

## Discussion with examiners

The examiners may ask you to clarify details of the above diagnosis and ask questions about your planned investigations and management.

Other possible questions include:

• *What are the risk factors for C. difficile-associated diarrhoea?* Antibiotic use, age, hospitalization or long-stay facilities (nursing homes); severe illness and immunosuppression; IBD, NG feeding and PPI.

• *What antibiotics are associated with C. difficile?* Frequently associated antibiotics include fluoroquinolones, clindamycin, penicillins (broad spectrum), co-amoxiclav, cephalosporins (broad spectrum).

• *What is the pathogenesis?* Antibiotic use → disturbed colonic microflora/loss of colonization resistance → *C. difficile* exposure and colonization → toxin A and B production → toxin-mediated marked proinflammatory response → diarrhoea and colitis/intestinal injury.

• *What are the options for therapy?* Local protocols do differ slightly and need to be consulted. If in doubt, consult local microbiologists (who will be involved with ongoing care of patients with *C. difficile* colitis). Mild-to-moderate: criteria can include <5 stools per day and WCC <15. Initially treated with po metronidazole, switching to po vancomycin if no response after 7 days. Criteria/features of severe *C. difficile* colitis include: WCC >15 (often >40), CRP >150, dry/hypovolaemia, acute renal impairment including acidosis and raised lactate, temp 38.5+, evidence of severe colitis, severe abdominal pain/diffuse; abdominal X-ray – colitis/toxic megacolon (7 cm). These patients receive IV metronidazole 500 mg tds and NG/po vancomycin 125–500 mg qds. Further therapies include rectal vancomycin enemas, immunoglobulin therapy and surgery (colectomy for medically refractory disease or complications such as perforation). Endoscopy (limited flexible sigmoidoscopy) only indicated if *C. difficile* negative on stools, and then to look for a pseudomembrane (evidence of possible CDAD) or to exclude other causes of diarrhoea (e.g. coexistent IBD, cancer, diverticulitis). The use of probiotics to prevent *C. difficile*-associated diarrhoea in patients receiving antibiotics is currently being studied in several UK-based randomized controlled trials.

## Further reading/resources

Kelly CP, Clostridium difficile – more difficult than ever. NEJM 2008;359:1932–40

Patient information leaflet on *C. difficile*: www.Uptodate. com

---

## Examiners' information and requirements

The candidate should:

1. Identify key features from the history: diarrhoea following course of antibiotics, also inpatient, resident at nursing home, PPI use
2. Identify key examination findings including diffuse tenderness (mild)
3. Outline a sensible differential diagnosis and management plan; differential diagnoses must include *C. difficile*; be able to plan appropriate treatment of *C. difficile* according to severity
4. Give a clear explanation to the patient of your diagnosis and plan, address her concerns and answer her questions

# Scenario 25 | Weight loss

## Candidate's information

**Your role:** you are an ST2 in the gastroenterology clinic. Mrs Stone (70 years old) has been referred by her GP as an urgent outpatient (2-week wait pathway in the UK) with dyspepsia and weight loss (you are given the 2-week wait referral form containing this information only).

**Your task:** to assess the patient's problems and address any questions or concerns raised by her.

## Patient's information

**You are:** Philippa Stone, a 70-year-old woman.

**Your problem:** you have lost 2 stone in weight over the past 3–4 months. You've noticed that you get an ache in your upper stomach after eating and feel fully easily, but your swallowing is fine. You've never had food get stuck in the gullet. Your GP recently started you on omeprazole which has helped the aching a little, but not taken it away. You have felt sick a few times, and vomited twice last week. Your appetite has been smaller than usual over the past couple of months – you've just not felt particularly hungry, and you attribute your weight loss to this.

**Past medical history and drug history:**
- Hypothyroidism diagnosed 2 years ago. GP says blood tests a month ago for the thyroid were fine, and not the cause of the weight loss and other problems
- Never been admitted to hospital, no operations
- Only medications are levothyroxine 50 µg once per day and omeprazole 20 mg once per day
- No aspirin or NSAID use

**Social history:**
- Never smoked
- Drinks 2–3 small apricot brandies per week

**Other issues including family history:**
- Father had an ulcer – took lots of tablets, but always suffered with his indigestion
- No-one in the family has had stomach, oesophageal or colonic cancer
- Nothing runs in the family
- No known contact with anyone with TB

**Your questions for the candidate:**
- *Don't I just have an ulcer?*
- *Do I have cancer?*
- *Is the endoscopy painful?*

# Candidate

## History/key questions

Dyspepsia (upper abdominal pain after eating), reflux symptoms (retrosternal burning, water brash – bitter taste in mouth). Bloating of upper abdomen

Ask about dysphagia (to solids or liquids), ever had food sticking, ask if food goes down OK

Early satiety, anorexia, weight loss (quantify in kg/stone, and over what period) – intentional versus unintentional

Consider other causes of weight loss:

Colorectal cancer, IBD – change in bowel habit, rectal bleeding, anaemia, abdominal pain

Respiratory – ask about smoking history, respiratory symptoms (breathlessness, cough, sputum, haemoptysis, chest pain, wheeze, stridor, weight loss), occupational history (asbestos exposure, for example)

Thyroid function

Pancreatic cancer – can present with upper abdominal pain; ask about symptoms of obstructive jaundice (painless): jaundice, dark urine, pale stools, itch

### Drug history

Consider causes of dyspepsia including aspirin, NSAID, steroids

Drug allergies

### Past medical history

Previous operations, medical conditions

### Social history

Smoking history (in pack-years)

Alcohol intake in units per week

## Address patient's questions and concerns

- Have you had any thoughts about what is going on?
- Is there anything in particular you're concerned about?
- Do you have anything you would like to ask?

## Key areas for examination

A list of what to look for (in examination order; describe findings on examination)

Stigmata of weight loss: loose skinfolds, ill-fitting clothing

Clubbing/tar stains (non-smoker in this case)

Tremor or tachycardia in thyrotoxicosis

Jaundice, signs of anaemia

Lymphadenopathy (supraclavicular lymphadenopathy in gastric cancer – Troisier's sign or Virchow's node)

Abdominal examination: look for abdominal masses (gastric/liver/pancreas, etc.) as well as succussion splash in gastric outflow obstruction (large fluid-filled stomach caused by, for example, an obstructing tumour or ulcer at the pylorus)

DRE to look for rectal cancer

## Differential diagnosis

Need to exclude gastric/oesophageal malignancy with above symptoms

Differential diagnosis pancreatic cancer (given pain and weight loss) but await LFT and OGD results

**Key facts/areas to consider** (including information available in scenario summary before station starts): combination of dyspepsia and weight loss requires urgent investigation with upper GI endoscopy

## Discussion with patient

Explain diagnosis

Explain plan, including investigations and management

Address patient's concerns/answer their questions

We need to arrange some tests to find out the cause of your stomach pain and weight loss. We will arrange blood tests and a chest X-ray today, and book you for an urgent outpatient endoscopy test to look for causes of the tummy discomfort and weight loss. I'll arrange follow-up in this clinic with the gastroenterology consultant after endoscopy.

## Investigations and management

Basic blood tests including FBC, U&E, LFT, INR, ESR, CRP, TTG, immunoglobulins

Chest X-ray

Urgent upper GI endoscopy with biopsies of ulcers or neoplasia, CLO test (*H. pylori* urease test), duodenal biopsies to exclude coeliac disease (given weight loss)

You need to be able to explain the OGD procedure:

Takes 5–10 min; patients have a choice between sedation to make you sleepy and relaxed (not completely unconscious like a general anaesthetic) or local anaesthetic throat spray to numb the back of the throat

Benefits (diagnose cause of pain and weight loss)

Risks of the procedure (bloating and belching during the procedure, and sometimes a sore throat later on; reaction to the medications, rarely bleeding, and very rarely a perforation requiring operation)

Allay anxiety about procedure through your explanations. Patient will receive an information sheet about the procedure, and the endoscopist will answer any questions or queries on the day

The patient will receive the result of the endoscopy on the day, and then you will arrange further follow-up (will need to consider arranging a CT scan if the OGD is normal)

Follow-up in the gastroenterology clinic

### Addressing concerns/answering questions

- *Don't I just have an ulcer?* Ulcers can cause pain and loss of appetite which can lead to a degree of weight loss, but we need to carry out the endoscopy test to look for all the possible causes and then treat the cause.
- *Do I have cancer?* Explain that we need to give her a full check-up, and diagnose what is causing her symptoms. Explain that causes of ulcer-like pain with weight loss range from benign acid-related ulcers through to the most serious causes, including cancer. The best test to give her a full check-up would be an endoscopy, and we can arrange this for her today as an outpatient.
- *Is the endoscopy painful?* As detailed above, OGDs can be uncomfortable due to bloating and belching, and sometimes a sore throat afterwards, but shouldn't be painful. If she is anxious regarding the procedure, she could opt for sedation rather than throat spray but would need someone to take her home afterwards and stay with her overnight. No driving for 24 h or operating heavy machinery.

## Discussion with examiners

The examiners may ask you to clarify details of the above diagnosis and ask questions about your planned investigations and management.

A possible question includes:

- *If the endoscopy is normal, what next?* Depends on results of above tests. If there is iron deficiency anaemia, will need colonoscopy to exclude colorectal neoplasia. Would need CT abdomen/thorax/pelvis to look for evidence of, for example, pancreatic cancer or lymphoma causing pain and weight loss.

### Further reading/resources

NICE dyspepsia guidelines (quick reference guide): www. nice.org.uk/CG017

# Scenario 26 | Gastrointestinal bleed: significant bleed

## Candidate's information

**Your role:** you are an ST2 in the MAU. You have been asked to see this 65-year-old man who has presented having had a collapse in his garden. A&E report melaena on rectal examination. Pulse 105, BP 90/60 in the ambulance. A&E report that he has improved with fluids.

**Your task:** to assess the patient's problems and address any questions or concerns raised by him.

## Patient's information

**You are:** Bert Field, a 65-year-old recently retired gardener.

**Your problem:** nausea and upper abdominal pain after eating then some vomiting this morning. You have had chronic hip pain for a year, worse this past 3 months, which has started to limit your mobility. Been to see GP who diagnosed wear and tear arthritis of your hip. Due to have X-rays of both hips in a couple of days' time. Your GP prescribed painkillers (diclofenac MR 75 mg bd) which you have been taking regularly for the past 3 weeks. For the last 4 days you've started having pains in the upper part of your stomach after eating, and continuous nausea for the past 2 days. No problems swallowing. Your stools have been black for the past 24 h and runnier than usual.

You went out into the garden today and whilst working in your greenhouse, you suddenly felt very dizzy. You had to lie down and then you vomited up a large amount of black vomit whilst in the potting shed. Fortunately, your partner was nearby and called the ambulance. She reports that you passed out briefly but came round within seconds. The dizziness went completely after you were given a drip in the ambulance. BP 90/60 with pulse of 105 in the ambulance: pulse 90 and BP 105/75 after 1 litre of IV Hartmann's in the ambulance/A&E.

**Past medical history and drug history:**
- Indigestion in the past (on/off for 10 years, but usually much less than today). Settled after some Zantac you bought over the counter
- Never been to hospital for anything

**Social history:**
- Alcohol: 1 glass of wine per night. Bottle lasts two nights shared with partner
- Never smoked
- Lives with partner, only retired earlier this year

**Other issues including family history:**
- Father had terrible trouble with his ulcers – on lots of antacids then had operation for burst ulcer in his 70 s. Nearly died from that

**Your questions for the candidate:**

- *What's happening?*
- *Is it an ulcer – will I need an operation like my father?*
- *What painkillers can I take for my hip?*
- *Is there something wrong with my heart to make me collapse?*

---

## Candidate

### History/key questions

Ask about vomiting and haematemesis; fresh red blood versus coffee ground vomiting

Melaena (black tarry digested blood versus dark red blood of brisk upper GI bleeding)

PR blood (fresh red blood pointing to lower GI source)

Dyspepsia, reflux symptoms

Alarm symptoms raising possibility of malignancy: dysphagia, weight loss, epigastric mass, early satiety

#### Past medical history

Previous ulcers/surgery for ulcers

Any previous upper GI endoscopy

#### Drug history

NSAID/aspirin/steroid use

#### Social history

Alcohol history (units per week), smoking history (pack-years)

### Address patient's questions and concerns

- *Have you had any thoughts about what is going on?*
- *Is there anything in particular you're concerned about?*
- *Do you have anything you would like to ask?*

### Key areas for examination

A list of what to look for (in examination order; describe findings on examination)

'ABCDE' approach

A: Airway/oxygenation

B: Breathing/ventilation

C: Circulation/shock management

D: Disability/neurological

E: Exposure/examination – any signs of chronic liver disease

Abdominal examination: mild epigastric tenderness (non-specific sign)

Ask to see observations chart and the results from any blood tests, if available

Say you would complete the examination with a DRE to look for melaena, rectal blood

Upper part of abdomen is tender, nothing else on examination

### Differential diagnosis

Upper GI bleed with shock and leading to near-syncope

Likely cause is peptic ulceration: gastric or duodenal given dyspepsia following NSAID use

No signs of decompensated liver disease to point towards oesophageal varices

### Discussion with patient

Explain diagnosis

Explain plan, including investigations and management

Address patient's concerns/answer their questions

It looks likely that you are bleeding from your stomach or gullet, possibly from an ulcer as a result of your pain-killing tablets. We need to put a drip into your arm and check your blood tests, and you may need a blood transfusion. We need to carry out an endoscopy test to find the cause of the bleeding and treat it. Explain the OGD and its risks and benefits. Risks include pain, drug reaction (due to sedation), bleeding and rarely a leak of air or bowel contents requiring an operation. Sometimes we can't stop the bleeding during the endoscopy and an operation is needed to stop the bleeding. Rarely the ulcer itself can perforate, or as a result of the endoscopy and the treatment and this can also need an operation.

### Investigations

ABCDE approach

Two large IV cannulae

Fluid resuscitation

Bloods for FBC, U&E, INR, cross-match 6 units

ECG given near-syncope

Erect chest X-ray (exclude perforation)

### Management

Correct any coagulopathy

Stop NSAID

Fluid resuscitation: transfuse aiming for Hb 8–9

Monitored bed: close (hourly at least) observations of pulse, BP, respiratory rate, $SaO_2$, urine output via catheter

Urgent inpatient endoscopy – need to calculate Rockall/ Blatchford scores. (See Scenario 19, where these scores are explained in full)

The Rockall score has been validated in the prediction of mortality from GI bleeding using clinical parameters on presentation (e.g. when the ambulance arrives, not post-resuscitation). This patient has a (pre-endoscopy) Rockall score of 3 (age 65 = 1, systolic <100 = 2)

The Blatchford score is a screening tool designed to determine the patient's likelihood of needing intervention (medical and/or endoscopic); it is more complicated than the Rockall score as it involves lab values such as Hb and urea, but even before the blood results are available the systolic BP of 90 (2 points), melaena (1), syncope (1), pulse >100 (1) give a score of at least 4. Only patients with a low-risk GI bleed, e.g. a Blatchford score of 0, can be considered for outpatient management (ambulatory care of GI bleeds) with an urgent outpatient OGD

You wouldn't be expected to be able to work out the Blatchford score without it in front of you, but you need to know the Rockall score

Discuss with endoscopy department or endoscopist on-call regarding arranging urgent inpatient upper GI endoscopy once he has been resuscitated adequately/stabilized

Liaise with surgical team on-call so that they are aware in case this patient requires laparotomy (if endoscopy fails to control bleeding)

## Addressing concerns/answering questions

- *What's happening?* Covered by explanation of diagnosis and plan as above.
- *Is it an ulcer – will I need an operation like my father?* If the source of the bleeding is inside the stomach/ gullet/first part of the small bowel, we would aim to treat it at the time of endoscopy and it is usually possible to avoid the need for an operation. Sometimes, we can't stop the bleeding at endoscopy or the bleeding starts again over the next 24 h, and then an operation is needed. Rarely an ulcer can cause a leak of air and bowel contents outside the stomach, and this can also need an operation to fix.
- *What painkillers can I take for my hip?* Suggest simple analgesia (paracetamol, codeine), and that you can review this once he's had the endoscopy.

- *Is there something wrong with my heart to make me collapse?* The collapse appears to have been due to low blood pressure because of bleeding from your gut, for example, an ulcer. It doesn't mean that there's anything wrong with your heart. We will, however, check a heart tracing.

## Discussion with examiners

The examiners may ask you to clarify details of the above diagnosis and ask questions about your planned investigations and management.

A possible question includes:
- *What are the Rockall and Blatchford scores used for and what do they tell us about a patient?* Rockall has been validated for a patient's risk of mortality from the GI bleed, and Blatchford has been validated for the need for intervention at the first endoscopy.

---

### Examiners' information and requirements

The candidate should:
1. Identify the significant GI bleed (haematemesis/NSAID use/dyspepsia/ syncopal episode). FBC, U&E results and obs chart may be available on request
2. Demonstrate use of Blatchford and Rockall scores to risk-stratify GI bleeds
3. Perform a focused examination of abdomen/pulse/BP/capillary refill – elicit epigastric tenderness; no cardiovascular compromise at time of examination
4. Consider differential diagnosis (peptic ulceration, erosions, duodenitis – varices less likely given lack of signs of chronic liver disease)
5. Outline a clear management plan, including admission, resuscitation and early endoscopy. Surgery may be required if bleeding is uncontrolled by endoscopy
6. Give a clear explanation to the patient of your diagnosis and plan, address his concerns and answer his questions

---

## Further reading/resources

SIGN guidance on GI bleeding: www.sign.ac.uk

# Other possible gastroenterology cases

### Systemic sclerosis and dysphagia

Patient with unrecognized systemic sclerosis and gradual-onset dysphagia. Need to recognize the signs of systemic sclerosis and that oesophageal dysmotility is a recognized complication. Need to exclude other causes of dysmotility including malignancy, GORD, achalasia, etc.

### Irritable bowel syndrome

Young patient with classic symptoms of chronic alternating bowel habit, pain relieved by defaecation, bloating; no alarm symptoms. Normal FBC, U&E, CRP, ESR from GP on letter. Weight stable. Needs TTG, explanation of 'sensitive bowel' and reassurance.

### Liver transplant 'rejection'

(Likely to use a well patient who would need the correct scars for liver transplant.) Patient admitted feeling generally unwell, history of fever. Reported to have ALT 1000, bilirubin 30, INR 1.7 by emergency department team. Usual medications include immunosuppression, e.g. tacrolimus. Alcohol history is important, as is an assessment of drug concordance (taking the medicines as needed?). Examination: look for signs of jaundice, encephalopathy, chronic liver disease, scar from operation.

Key tasks: full liver screen, same-day US liver with portal and hepatic vein Doppler. Seek advice from specialist centre and local gastroenterology team as soon as possible: contact transplant unit urgently and seek advice on further management, including transfer (if stable) to liver unit, immunosuppressant use, drug levels (tacrolimus).

# Scenario 27 | Anaemia

## Candidate's information

**Your role:** you are the ST2 in the gastroenterology clinic. The letter from the patient's GP says, 'Mrs Bibi has been found to be anaemic. Please see and advise regarding her need for an endoscopy. Blood results: Hb 7.8, MCV 72, ferritin 5 (normal range 25–180), B12 and folate normal. Pulse 72, BP 120/75. No melaena on PR examination'.

**Your task:** to assess the patient's problems and address any questions or concerns raised by her.

## Patient's information

**You are:** Kiran Bibi, a 33-year-old woman.

**Your problem:** a couple of months ago you saw your GP who checked some routine blood tests and found that you were anaemic. He sent you up to the hospital because he wanted you checked out before starting you on iron, and you've been worried ever since your GP mentioned that you may need an endoscopy.

You are well, but your GP did bloods for a 'well woman check' as you have been feeling a little tired recently. You have never been told that you're anaemic before and it's come as a bit of a surprise, but you remember being put on a course of iron when you were pregnant 10 years ago.

You are usually able to walk for at least a few miles without getting SOB, and no dizziness, tiredness or lethargy, but you've found it all a little harder over the past few months, mainly due to being generally tired.

No mouth ulcers. No current medications. Your weight is stable.

Your periods last 5 days, 3 heavy, requiring pads and tampons as you get clots and flooding during those 3 days. Your GP has never really asked about your periods and you forgot to mention them.

No diarrhoea – bowels regular once/day with no abdominal pain. No mouth ulcers. No pain after eating and no heartburn. No vaginal discharge and no pain during/after intercourse. Vegetarian diet.

No-one in your family has had cancer of the colon or stomach/gullet. No family history of coeliac disease.

### Past medical history:
- Thalassaemia trait – you have the card with you
- No allergies

### Other issues including family history:
- You live with your husband and two children
- Your sister is also slightly anaemic, and her doctor has told her it was something she was born with

**Your questions for the candidate:**
- *Why am I anaemic?*
- *What can I do about my periods?*
- *Do I need the endoscopy my doctor told me I might need?*
- *Could I have an ulcer?*

## Candidate

### History/key questions

Symptoms of anaemia (lethargy, tiredness, breathlessness particularly on exertion, reduced exercise tolerance, dizziness)

History of blood loss (menstrual loss in women; PR, PV, urinary loss)

Menstrual history: quantify loss (number of days bleeding per cycle, how many pads/tampons per day, passage of clots/flooding through pads/tampons, any previous treatments)

Risk factors for anaemia

Ever anaemic before? Was a cause found?

History of aspirin or NSAID use, on supplements or vitamin replacement?

History of blood donation (if so, how many units), recent operations

Symptoms associated with GI causes: dyspepsia, reflux symptoms, dysphagia, weight loss, mouth ulcers, diarrhoea, bloating/pain (causes for anaemia include bleeding, malabsorption, IBD; malignancies such as colorectal/gastro-oesophageal cancer in older age groups)

Also need to consider travel history: tropical sprue/hookworm

### Address patient's questions and concerns

- *Have you had any thoughts about what is going on?*
- *Is there anything in particular you're concerned about?*
- *Do you have anything you would like to ask?*

## Key areas for examination

A list of what to look for (in examination order; describe findings on examination)

Signs of anaemia: koilonychia, angular cheilitis, angular stomatitis

Abdominal examination: may be able to feel pelvic mass of fibroids coming out of the pelvis

Express your wish to carry out a digital rectal examination (DRE)

## Differential diagnosis

Menorrhagia likely cause of anaemia

Need to exclude coeliac disease with coeliac serology

Causes of iron deficiency anaemia in premenopausal women is most likely due to menstrual, previous pregnancies and breastfeeding, and dietary

Thalassaemia trait: would give only mild anaemia with reduced MCV

## Discussion with patient

Explain diagnosis

Explain plan, including investigations and management

Address patient's concerns and answer their questions

You have anaemia due to low iron levels and the cause of this looks to be your heavy periods. In females with anaemia before their menopause it is usually menstrual blood loss, previous pregnancies and deliveries, breastfeeding and dietary (low iron intake in the diet). Your thalassaemia trait usually only causes a mild anaemia. We will carry out tests to exclude coeliac disease which can cause anaemia without bowel symptoms.

### Investigations

Aim is to find cause, investigate appropriately and treat

Patient is asymptomatic from the anaemia: looks like anaemia related to menorrhagia (long-standing). No GI symptoms are reported

Basic bloods including haematinics, TTG (the screening test for coeliac disease which has 95% sensitivity and specificity) and immunoglobulins (exclude IgA deficiency, present in 0.5% of general population and up to 10% of coeliacs)

CRP (although no history or clinical signs consistent with, e.g. inflammatory bowel disease)

ESR will increase in any cause of anaemia (increase in ESR of 10 for every 1 g fall in haemoglobin)

## Management

Iron replacement orally – six months to fully replenish stores

Endoscopy not indicated in this case unless positive coeliac serology, and then it would be to confirm the diagnosis prior to lifelong exclusion of gluten from the diet

Needs GP review regarding menorrhagia

## Addressing concerns/answering questions

- *Why am I anaemic?* Based on today's discussion and examination, it looks very likely to be due to your heavy periods.
- *What can I do about my periods?* See your GP regarding management which can vary from going onto non-hormonal or hormonal treatments. The non-hormonal are tranexamic acid and mefenamic acid, and hormonal include the oral contraceptive pill or use of a coil which releases hormone to reduce the blood loss during periods by up to 95%.
- *Do I need the endoscopy my doctor told me I might need?* At the moment, no, as it wouldn't help or add anything to improve your anaemia, so it isn't indicated at this stage. If the coeliac blood tests come back positive, then we would need to carry out a camera test to confirm whether or not you have coeliac disease, but not at the moment. We will write to you and your GP with the results of today's blood tests.
- *Could I have an ulcer?* You don't have any symptoms of ulcers or heartburn, and you've not been on any medicines which put you at risk of ulcers, so it's very unlikely that an ulcer is causing your anaemia.

## Discussion with examiners

The examiners may ask you to clarify details of the above diagnosis and ask questions about your planned investigations and management.

Other possible questions include:

- *If there was no history of menorrhagia, what would you do?* The cause of anaemia in this premenopausal woman with no gastrointestinal symptoms is still likely to be one or more of menstrual blood loss, previous pregnancies / deliveries / breastfeeding and low dietary intake. Coeliac serology will help by excluding coeliac disease as a cause.
- *If patient was 50 and premenopausal would your plan be the same?* Investigation is advised for all males and postmenopausal women with iron deficiency anaemia, but if over 50 and premenopausal, British Society of Gastroenterology guidelines recommend investigation with OGD and duodenal biopsies and colonoscopy (age is the strongest predictor of pathology in iron deficiency anaemia).
- *When would you use intravenous iron?* If patient intolerant of oral iron tablets, try liquid preparations first. Intolerance is related to the amount of elemental iron in the preparation. Use of intravenous iron is indicated if intolerant to oral iron preparations, if there is a clinical requirement for rapid replenishment of iron stores or in IBD when oral preparations may not be tolerated or contraindicated (e.g. due to side-effects).

---

**Examiners' information and requirements**

The candidate should:

1. Identify key features from the history: young woman with iron deficiency anaemia, lack of GI symptoms or risk factors, marked menorrhagia. History of thalassaemia trait
2. Identify key examination findings (likely normal examination)
3. Outline a sensible management plan, including bloods, coeliac serology and then referral back to the GP to manage menorrhagia; full course of iron to replenish stores
4. Give a clear explanation to the patient of your diagnosis and plan, address her concerns and answer her questions

---

# Scenario 28 | Easy bruising/idiopathic thrombocytopenic purpura

## Candidate's information
**Your role:** you are on-call in the MAU. You have been asked to see this 53-year-old woman with a history of easy bruising who was found to have a platelet count of $9 \times 10^9/L$ (150–450 $\times 10^9/L$ usual range) by her GP.

**Your task:** to assess the patient's problems and address any questions or concerns raised by her.

## Patient's information
**You are:** Angela Morris, a 53-year-old bank worker.

**Your problem:** you have been feeling under the weather for the past 2 weeks with your body aching, you've had a bit of a fever, and you've generally felt like you might have flu. You noticed that you were bruising easily over the past week, at the slightest knock or bang.

You saw your GP after you had felt unwell for a week, because you really needed to get back to work. This was earlier in the week and you went back today because you felt so tired and lethargic. Your son suggested it might be due to anaemia after searching the internet. The GP checked your blood count and called you because the platelet level was low.

The GP has been treating you for high blood pressure and it has been normal on treatment. You have been taking a small aspirin tablet daily after you read about it reducing the risk of developing bowel cancer.

You had a period this last week that was much heavier than normal and you couldn't work out why.

You've never been into hospital. No new medications (no heparin, warfarin). No vomiting/blood in vomit, blood in urine or in your stool, and no nosebleeds.

### Past medical history and drug history:
- High blood pressure, diagnosed age 50, controlled on treatment after you lost about a stone in weight last year
- Current medications: ramipril 5 mg once per day, aspirin 75 mg od
- No known drug allergies

### Social history:
- You live with your husband; you have two sons age 23 and 19. All healthy. You have been married for 26 years. If asked, no other sexual partners during this time and no known sexually transmitted infections. Vaginal intercourse only and no discharge or urinary symptoms
- Alcohol: a few glasses of wine per weekend. Never had problems with alcohol in the past, and never drunk more than this

## Other issues including family history:

- Your father had bowel cancer age 72 and you are worried that you could die young from this
- Nothing else runs in the family. No history of TB
- Bowels regular and unchanged. No rectal bleeding

## Your questions for the candidate:

- *Why are my platelets low?*
- *Am I going to get bowel cancer like my dad did?*

---

# Candidate

## History/key questions

Ask about the easy bruising, the presenting complaint

Ask about any exacerbating factors (ask about a history of trauma, and how much trauma caused bruising)

Any signs of blood loss (epistaxis, haematuria, rectal bleeding, haemoptysis, haematemesis or any increased menstrual blood loss?)

Any known bleeding disorder? Ever been diagnosed with hereditary haemorrhagic telangiectasia (HHT) (Osler–Weber–Rendu syndrome)?

Anyone in the family had problems with bleeding from bladder, bowel, lungs, brain or nose?

Ever had low platelets in the past?

Any recent illnesses including flu-like symptoms/viral illness, diarrhoea, rectal bleeding?

Any rash (petechial rash)?

Any history of TB, SLE?

Any recent transfusions?

Regarding the bowel cancer concerns, have any other members of her family had bowel cancer, and if so at what age were they diagnosed? A single first-degree relative developing bowel cancer at age 72 means that she is only at population risk of developing colorectal cancer (she doesn't have an increased risk of developing colorectal cancer and therefore doesn't require surveillance colonoscopies)

### Drug history

Ask about anticoagulant use (warfarin, heparin, any recent admissions to hospital) and antiplatelet use (aspirin, clopidogrel). Heparin can cause low platelets and being on warfarin can give you easy bruising

Any changes to medications, e.g. recent introduction of bendroflumethiazide for hypertension

Ask about herbal and alternative medicine use

## Address patient's questions and concerns

- *Have you had any thoughts about what is going on?*
- *Is there anything in particular you're concerned about?*
- *Do you have anything you would like to ask?*

## Key areas for examination

A list of what to look for (in examination order; describe findings on examination)

Look for petechial rash and ecchymoses. Look at palate for blood blisters

Inspect for bruising

Say that you would check for fundal haemorrhages

Any signs of SLE?

Lymphadenopathy

Look for signs of HHT: telangiectasia (face, lips, tongue [and underneath], buccal and nasal mucosa, palate and on fingers); can also be cyanosed and clubbed

Abdominal examination: any palpable splenomegaly?

## Differential diagnosis

Idiopathic thrombocytopenic purpura (ITP) is the most likely diagnosis with low platelets following a viral illness

Causes of thrombocytopenia:

Destruction/reduced survival of platelets: ITP, viruses, drugs, SLE, thrombotic thrombocytopenic purpura (TTP), disseminated intravascular coagulation (DIC), lymphoma, hypersplenism

Platelet aggregation

Reduced production (bone marrow failure)

## Discussion with patient

Explain diagnosis

Explain plan, including investigations and management

Address patient's concerns/answer their questions

It is likely that you have a condition affecting the level of platelets, called idiopathic thrombocytopenic purpura (ITP). The platelets are cells in the blood which help the blood clot, and low levels of platelets would explain the bruising you have been having. It may well be due to a viral infection. We need to find out why it has happened, as well as giving you some treatment to increase the level of platelets in the blood. I'll refer you to the haematologist, the blood doctors, and they will see you here.

## Investigations

FBC, blood film, PT, APTT, fibrinogen – to look for disseminated intravascular coagulation (DIC)

Recheck the Hb – FBC (rest of FBC: Hb 11.3, MCV 87, WCC 6.5, platelets 10). Eosinophils can be increased

Blood film is important to check platelets and look for other haematological pathology, e.g. lymphoproliferative disorders, leukaemia, etc.

Blood film: red cell fragments – microangiopathic haemolytic anaemias, e.g TTP, HUS

LFTs

Autoimmune serology: ANA positive in 44%

HIV serology: NB need to explain to patient why this is being sent, obtain verbal consent, and plan for the result to be communicated back to the patient (patient is being admitted and haematology will follow-up as inpatient). It is increasingly a standard part of the medical work-up for many conditions, and it is important to check for it as it is a treatable condition once diagnosed, with good long-term outcomes

Viral hepatitis serology

Contact haematology for advice on further management

## Management

Management of acute ITP (symptomatic thrombocytopenia when platelets <10):

Immunosuppressive therapy – prednisolone 1 mg/kg; aim for platelets >30, usually achieves this in a few days

Intravenous immunoglobulin if bleeding

Second-line therapy: splenectomy, azathioprine

## Addressing concerns/answering questions

• *Why are my platelets low?* Your platelets are low because your immune system has reacted to the viral

infection by damaging and destroying your own platelets. Treatment will involve reducing this, and allowing the platelet count to increase. Other blood tests are being sent to check for the cause.

• *Am I going to get bowel cancer like my dad did?* Your father developing bowel cancer at age 72 means that you are at the same risk of developing colorectal cancer as the rest of the population – your father's history doesn't put you at an increased risk of developing colorectal cancer. You don't need any investigations/examinations, e.g. colonoscopy, for this. If you had a first-degree relative under 50, or two first-degree relatives, who had colorectal cancer then under British Society of Gastroenterology guidelines, screening colonoscopy would be indicated +/– clinical genetics input (see www.bsg.org.uk for further details).

## Discussion with examiners

The examiners may ask you to clarify details of the above diagnosis and ask questions about your planned investigations and management.

Other possible questions include:
• *What are the causes of low platelets?*
  – Destruction/reduced survival of platelets: ITP, viruses (EBV, CMV), drugs (heparin, valproate, quinidine and others), SLE, thrombotic thrombocytopenic purpura (TTP), disseminated intravascular coagulation (DIC), lymphoma, hypersplenism, and in pregnant women HELLP (Haemolytic anaemia, Elevated Liver enzymes and Low Platelets).
  – Platelet aggregation.
  – Reduced production (bone marrow failure) – causes include viral infections (mumps, varicella, hepatitis C, rubella, EBV, HIV); irradiation; alcohol; vitamin B12 and folate deficiency.
• *How does TTP present?* Clinical presentation classically reported as five components: microangiopathic haemolytic anaemia (MAHA), thrombocytopenia / purpura, neurological impairment, renal impairment, fever (e.g. young woman with fluctuating neurological signs, fever, renal impairment and microangiopathic haemolytic anaemia).

See also Section I, Station 5, Skin, Case 25.

**Examiners' information and requirements**

The candidate should:

1. Identify key features from the history: low platelet count after viral illness
2. Identify key examination findings including bruising, no active bleeding
3. Outline a sensible management plan as described above, including seeking advice from haematology specialists as appropriate. Assess risk of colorectal cancer in order to answer her query
4. Give a clear explanation to the patient of your diagnosis and plans. Need to address concerns about low platelet count and risk of developing colorectal cancer given father's history

# Scenario 29 | Epistaxis/elevated international normalized ratio (INR)

## Candidate's information

**Your role:** you are on-call in the MAU and you have been asked to see Mr Haynes by the practitioners in the anticoagulant clinic. He was found to have an INR >10 on his routine scheduled appointment, and mentioned to the anticoagulant clinic nurse practitioners that he had been having nosebleeds this week. He is due to go on holiday next week.

**Your task:** to assess the patient's problems and address any questions or concerns raised by him.

## Patient's information

**You are:** Joseph Haynes, a 65-year-old man.

**Your problem:** you have been on warfarin for atrial fibrillation for the past 5 years. Your INR is usually well controlled around your target INR of 2.5, and you have monthly to 6-weekly checks. You thought that you had got the hang of it, but this nose-bleeding has worried you as you hadn't been doing anything different for the past few weeks, and you always follow the instructions the nurses give you in your book. You've brought your yellow book (anticoagulant record) for the doctor to see if he asks for it. Usually you take warfarin 3 mg Monday–Saturday with 4 mg on Sundays. You've never had any operations, no known valve problems, and you've never had a clot on the lungs or in the legs. Your only other medicine is bisoprolol 5 mg once per day. You have no drug allergies. The last INR was 2.9 three weeks ago.

You never usually have nose-bleeds, so you were surprised when they started 3 days ago. You had been down to see your daughter 10 days ago, and had a bit of a chest infection. You saw an out-of-hours GP in Dorset who gave you a course of antibiotics (you can't remember which) for 5 days. You stopped these a few days ago.

The last episode of nosebleeding was about 5 h ago. No active bleeding at present/ you've not seen any blood since. No falls, no head injury and no signs of blood loss from bladder, bowel or lungs.

## Past medical history and drug history:

- Intermittently, you have an irregular rhythm called atrial fibrillation
- Warfarin, bisoprolol 5 mg od
- Recent course of antibiotics

## Social history:

- Member of the Independent Monitoring Board at the local prison
- Retired businessman (exporting machine tools)

- You have a glass of wine at the weekend and you stopped drinking during the week when you started warfarin (on the advice of your GP)
- You have never smoked

**Other issues including family history:**
- No-one in family has had problems with bleeding, including nose-bleeds

**Your questions for the candidate:**
- *Why did I start having nose-bleeds if I never had them before?*
- *Will I need to stop taking warfarin?*

## Candidate

### History/key questions

Ask about warfarin treatment, who follows him up and how stable the INR has been. When was the last INR and what was it? Any difficulties with warfarin in the past?

Ask to see his yellow anticoagulant record book; check whether any recent dose changes

Ask about factors that could cause instability in INR: alcohol excess (recent binges), any changes to existing medications or recent courses of new medications such as antibiotics, allopurinol, simvastatin, amiodarone; many medications cause changes in warfarin metabolism and therefore affect INR (see BNF for full list)

Ask about bleeding: urine (haematuria), GI tract (haematemesis, melaena, fresh rectal bleeding), haemoptysis, menorrhagia, epistaxis, wounds. Any recent head injury/falls/trauma

Ask about precipitants for the epistaxis, e.g. trauma including nose-picking or nose-blowing

Any history of bleeding from these sites in the past? Ever had, for example, peptic ulcer in past?

Recent changes in diet?

Any symptoms of anaemia? These include shortness of breath, lethargy, dizziness, chest pain, reduced exercise tolerance

### Drug history

Medications including doses, frequency: ask about recent changes/additions to medications

### Past medical history

Need to be absolutely clear about the indication for warfarin as this will influence the management of the elevated INR/advice to give the patient (in particular check whether patient has a heart valve replacement [metal/which site – aortic versus mitral])

### Social history

Ask about alcohol (regular use and level of use versus sporadic large intake)

### Address patient's questions and concerns
- *Have you had any thoughts about what is going on?*
- *Is there anything in particular you're concerned about?*
- *Do you have anything you would like to ask?*

## Key areas for examination

A list of what to look for (in examination order; describe findings on examination)

Pulse: may be in sinus rythym or AF

Check BP (patient cardiovascularly stable)

Cardiovascular examination

Basic ENT: look in ears, nose and throat. No signs of epistaxis on examination

Look for signs of hereditary haemorrhagic telangiectasia: red nodules and telangiectasia on lips and face

## Differential diagnosis

Epistaxis as a complication of elevated INR: elevated INR is probably due to recent course of antibiotics as INR had been well-controlled previously

## Discussion with patient

Explain diagnosis

Explain plan, including investigations and management

Address patient's concerns/answer their questions

Your bleeding tendency is increased by the blood being thinner than usual. The INR is high because of the recent course of antibiotics, and we will need to give you some medicines to reduce the INR (although not completely reverse it) and then keep an eye on the levels over the next few weeks. Lots of things can alter the INR even when you've been stable for a while – these include changes in diet, medications like antibiotics, and varying the amount of alcohol you drink.

## Investigations
Formal FBC, INR, U&E. Group and save (cross-match if severe/major bleeding)
ENT opinion if ongoing epistaxis

## Management
If INR confirmed as >10, then manage as per BNF and the advice of local haematologists
As per BNF for this INR: the appropriate step given the recent history of epistaxis is:
>8, minor bleeding – stop warfarin, give phytomenadione (vitamin K1) 1–3 mg by slow IV injection (if complete reversal required – 5 mg by slow IV injection); repeat dose of phytomenadione if INR still too high after 24 h; restart warfarin when INR <5
Other advice for INR >8 includes:
>8, major bleeding – stop warfarin, give phytomenadione (vitamin K1) 5 mg by slow IV injection; give dried prothrombin complex (factors II, VII, IX, X) 25–50 units per kilogram (if dried prothrombin complex is unavailable, fresh frozen plasma 15 mL/kg can be given but is less effective)
>8, no bleeding – stop warfarin, give phytomenadione (vitamin K1) 1–5 mg by mouth using the intravenous preparation orally (unlicensed use)
See BNF for full text including advice for INR <8

## Addressing concerns/answering questions
- *Why did I start having nose-bleeds if I never had them before?* It doesn't take a great deal of trauma to cause nose-bleeds and, if your INR is higher than usual, your blood will take longer to clot.
- *Will I need to stop taking warfarin?* No reason to stop warfarin if you've been stable before and we can find the cause for the increase in the INR. In your case it is likely to be the recent course of antibiotics, which is a common cause. You will need closer monitoring of your INR once we've restarted your warfarin at a lower dose.

## Discussion with examiners
The examiners may ask you to clarify details of the above diagnosis and ask questions about your planned investigations and management.

Other possible questions include:
- *How would you manage an INR over 10 with a metallic aortic valve?* If the patient presents with bleeding and an elevated INR, and is on warfarin for a metallic heart valve replacement, you need to discuss with both the haematology and cardiology teams regarding management of the anticoagulation. You will need to know the severity of the bleeding (e.g. minor versus life-threatening), site of the valve (mitral versus aortic) and whether mechanical / metal (you should hear it on examination or from end of bed) or tissue, and what usual target range is. Mitral position has a higher risk of thromboembolic complications than aortic.
- *What is the usual target value for a patient in AF or for a patient with a metal heart valve?* AF target INR is 2.5 (target rather than a range); target INR for mechanical prosthetic heart valves depends on the type of valve, its position, and other patient factors that contribute to an individual's risk of thrombosis (cardiac rhythm) – see British Committee for Standards in Haematology (BCSH) guidelines.
- *How would you manage life-threatening gastrointestinal bleeding in a patient with a metal aortic valve?* ABCDE approach required. Identify site of bleeding from history and examination (e.g. fresh red haematemesis due to upper GI bleed) as well as the indication for anticoagulation (site, type of valve, any associated AF, history of thromboembolic disease, etc.) and the usual target INR. Will require two large cannulae, resuscitation, blood tests including FBC, INR, cross match, close observations and a multi-specialty approach; will need to discuss with haematology, cardiology and gastroenterology with regard to management of the bleeding, decisions about severity (e.g. minor single coffee-ground vomit compared to shocked/profuse rectal bleeding) and further management of anticoagulation over the next hours, next 24 h and beyond. Bleeding source will need to be controlled at, e.g. endoscopy; discussions with the specialist teams will need to cover management of anticoagulation (e.g. period of anticoagulation [after reversal]) to allow control of bleeding, then anticoagulation with IV heparin if life-threatening bleeding); if stable after minor bleeding may well be appropriate to leave INR unchanged, carry out endoscopy and decide on management of anticoagulation with results of endoscopy. Always seek help from haematology, gastroenterology and cardiology.

**Examiners' information and requirements**

The candidate should:

1. Identify key features from history: recent onset of epistaxis – now settled. On warfarin for AF (no history of valve replacement). Recent course of antibiotics. Last episode about 5 h ago. No active bleeding at present. Cardiovascularly stable

2. Identify key examination findings including AF. Nothing else of note

3. Outline a sensible management plan including appropriate control of anticoagulation; needs to be aware of BNF and haematologists as sources of information

4. Give a clear explanation to the patient of your diagnosis and plan, address his concerns and answer his questions

**Resources**

Guidelines on oral anticoagulation with warfarin edition: www.bcshguidelines.com

British Committee for Standards in Haematology lines: www.bcshguidelines.com

# Scenario 30 | Neutropenic sepsis

## Candidate's information
**Your role:** you are the ST2 in the MAU. You have been asked to see a patient who has been transferred from the acute oncology unit. The oncology clinical nurse specialist referred the patient with a neutrophil count of 0.1 and fever of 38.3°C. Pulse was 120, BP 90/55 in oncology, and he was given some intravenous fluids.

**Your task:** to assess the patient's problems and address any questions or concerns raised by him.

## Patient's information
**You are:** Len Rayburn, a 62-year-old man.

**Your problem:** you had an operation 6 weeks ago for bowel cancer (Duke's C) and recovered well. You started chemotherapy a week ago, with capecitabine and oxaliplatin. You've been having hot and cold attacks with sweats for the past 48 h, and have been generally feeling unwell. You thought you might have the flu, so stuck it out for two nights, but then your wife made you call the specialist nurse in the oncology unit. She had you come in right away, checked your temperature and your blood tests, and referred you here to see the medics.

You've had slightly softer bowel motions for the past couple of days, and going three times instead of once/day, but no cough, SOB or urinary problems (no burning/frequency or going at night). Very poor appetite and intake for the past few days. Felt a bit light-headed walking in today from the car. Feel a bit better after the fluids through the veins.

## Past medical history:
- Bowel cancer diagnosed at colonoscopy (as part of the investigations into a low blood count due to low iron levels) earlier in the year
- Hypertension
- No other operations

## Drug history:
- On ramipril 5 mg od
- No known drug allergies, and have taken penicillins (amoxicillin) without problems (for sore throats in the past)

## Social history:
- Lives with wife, who is well
- Non-smoker
- Drinks a glass of wine on three or four nights per week
- No foreign travel

**Other issues including family history:**
- No-one in family has had any bowel cancer. Rest of family well

**Your questions for the candidate:**
- *Does this mean I can't have chemo again?*
- *Has it permanently damaged my immune system?*
- *Will it happen every time I have the chemo?*
- *Will it delay treatment?*

---

## Candidate

### History/key questions

Which cancer? Which chemotherapy agents? When/ how many days since chemotherapy and which cycle (number)?

Any steroids?

What has been happening since he had chemotherapy a week ago?

Ask about chest symptoms (cough, SOB, sputum, haemoptysis, chest pain, wheeze), urinary symptoms, diarrhoea/rectal bleeding/abdominal pain

Any rash, headache, photophobia, neck stiffness?

Any skin toxicity (palmar plantar syndrome – blistering and soreness) from capecitabine?

Nausea, vomiting?

Anyone else in household unwell?

Ask the patient who his oncologist is, and does he have a card with him with details of his chemotherapy/ advice on what to do if he has a fever?

### Drug history

Which chemotherapy agents?

Check what other medicines he's on for his hypertension

Ask about drug allergies, including antibiotics

How is the chemotherapy administered (peripherally versus a tunnelled line [itself a potential source of sepsis])

### Past medical history

Any comorbid conditions

### Social history

Alcohol and smoking history

Who lives at home with you?

Employment

### Address patient's questions and concerns
- *Have you had any thoughts about what is going on?*
- *Is there anything in particular you're concerned about?*
- *Do you have anything you would like to ask?*

## Key areas for examination

A list of what to look for (in examination order; describe findings on examination)

Inspection

Any tunnelled line in place?

Pulse/BP/peripheral perfusion: BP now 110/80, pulse 75

JVP

Oropharynx: any mouth ulcers/tonsillitis

Check for neck stiffness

Chest examination

Abdominal: given history of diarrhoea

Full skin examination – look for rash, cellulitis, petechiae, swollen/erythematous joints, blistering on hands and/or feet

Avoid rectal examination in neutropenic patients – increases risk of bacterial translocation

Ask to see urinalysis, chest X-ray, blood results

## Differential diagnosis

Neutropenic sepsis as consequence of chemotherapy: assume neutropenic sepsis in any pyrexial patient within three weeks of chemotherapy. Don't delay broad-spectrum antibiotics – give antibiotics after cultures and within 1 hour of presentation. Cause may not be identified. Consider bacterial, viral, fungal causes

Remember standard 'conventional' causes of sepsis in patient immunosuppressed by chemotherapy, e.g. community-acquired pneumonia/UTI

## Discussion with patient

Explain diagnosis

Explain plan, including investigations and management

Address patient's concerns/answer their questions

The results available so far suggest that the chemotherapy you've had has caused a reduction in the white cells in the blood. These are the cells in the blood that attack infection. We need to look for any infections, as well as giving you some strong antibiotics, and the white cell count should gradually increase over the next few days. We may also need to give you a specific medication to increase the neutrophil count.

## Investigations

Isolation/reverse barrier nursing: gloves/gowns

Blood tests: FBC (neutrophil count), U&E, LFT, CRP, ESR, lactate, glucose

Blood cultures: peripheral (and central if central / Hickman line – needs to be carried out by personnel trained to access line safely as needs sterile/aseptic technique, e.g. oncology CNS)

Have blood cultures been taken earlier with routine bloods, and was the first dose of antibiotics administered by the acute oncology unit (NB: golden hour in sepsis)?

Venous gas (pH/lactate): arterial if platelets >50

CXR: exclude pneumonia

Urinalysis/MSSU

Stool culture for MCS and *C. difficile* testing (recent inpatient stay)

May need throat swab

## Management

Empirical antibiotics: follow local neutropenic sepsis protocol (give 4.5 g tds IV tazocin, if not penicillin allergic [NICE 2012 guidance] – often source not identified). Needs first dose of antibiotics as soon as possible after presentation (less than 1 h – the golden hour principle) following cultures of blood, urine

Intravenous fluid resuscitation: aim for systolic BP >100, urine output >0.5 mL/kg/h

Daily bloods

Refer to acute oncology regarding use of granulocyte-colony stimulating factor (G-CSF) to increase neutrophil count

If tunnelled/Hickman line *in situ*, seek advice regarding intravenous antibiotic therapy, and if thought to be the source, need to discuss with microbiology as antibiotic regime may be different. Line infection may result in the line being removed/replaced – this decision would need to be made in conjunction with oncology and microbiology

## Addressing concerns/answering questions

- *Does this mean I can't have chemo again?* See below 'Will it happen every time'.
- *Has it permanently damaged my immune system?* No it hasn't. We expect your neutrophil count to recover on its own within the next few days.
- *Will it happen every time I have chemo?* Oncology will review how you respond to this episode. You may need

prophylactic antibiotics, prophylactic G-CSF or dose reduction for your next cycle of chemotherapy. However, if you get a temperature or symptoms of infection after future cycles of chemotherapy, you should present straight away as it has the potential to get worse rapidly.

- *Will it delay treatment?* It will only delay treatment if neutrophils haven't recovered by the time the next treatment is due.

## Discussion with examiners

The examiners may ask you to clarify details of the above diagnosis and ask questions about your planned investigations and management.

Other possible questions include:
- *What is the role of G-CSF, when to start, and when to stop?* Need to liaise with the acute oncology team. Consider if haemodynamically compromised or very prolonged period of neutropenia.
- *How do you reduce the risk of chemotherapy-induced neutropenic sepsis in future?* Oncology will review how the patient responds to this episode. For future cycles of chemotherapy, may need prophylactic antibiotics, prophylactic G-CSF or dose reduction. Patient factors also important: diet – stay away from products that may have bacterial content (similar diet to pregnancy). Stay away from swimming pools, primary schools. Need to ensure no active sepsis prior to next chemotherapy cycle.

---

**Examiners' information and requirements**

The candidate should:
1. Identify key features from the history: fever and neutropenia in a patient who has recently received chemotherapy for colon cancer
2. Identify key examination findings, including fever. No other signs elicited
3. Outline a sensible management plan, following the local neutropenic sepsis protocol, and contacting oncology and haematology. First dose of antibiotics need to be given within an hour of presenting
4. Give a clear explanation to the patient of your diagnosis and plan, address his concerns and answer his questions

---

### Resources

NICE guidance for neutropenic sepsis: www.guidance.nice.org.uk/CG151

# Other possible haematology cases

### Sickle crisis

Various presentations but pain crisis could easily be used in the exam. Patient may well have normal examination in a pain crisis; no features of sepsis or chest crisis.

Outline basic management. Seek help from haematology; only transfuse on the advice of a haematologist.

Analgesia as indicated on the patient's sickle card (individualized care plan).

For more advice, see: local trust guidelines; British Committee for Standards in Haematology guidelines: www.bcshguidelines.com

# Scenario 31 | Young syncope

## Candidate's information

**Your role:** you are an ST2 in the MAU. You have been asked by the emergency department to see Mr Sawyer, a 25-year-old man, who was brought in by ambulance after he collapsed whilst running.

**Your task:** to assess the patient's problems and address any questions or concerns raised by him.

## Patient's information

**You are:** Julian Sawyer, a 25-year-old man.

**Your problem:** you are an amateur athlete, and you collapsed today during a cross-country running race. You have not been feeling all that well for the past few days, and hadn't taken in as many calories as you usually would in the build-up to the race, and during the race. You had no warning; you remember being in the last few kilometres of the race and doing OK when you suddenly collapsed. No dizziness beforehand.

The paramedics told you that bystanders helped; they apparently saw you fall over and not get up immediately so they went over to help. They said that you appeared to wake up pretty quickly; no incontinence or confusion. No other information available.

You have had some feelings of dizziness and nausea when you haven't eaten properly before a race, but never passed out, and the episode felt different.

You don't drive to work but cycle instead.

This event was sudden, with no warning. You don't remember hitting the ground. You woke up on the ground with race officials standing over you. You were told that you woke up quickly.

No-one who witnessed the event has come with you to hospital – history from bystanders is limited to the information above.

There was no preceding nausea, dizziness, changes to vision (e.g. blurring). No breathlessness or chest pain.

## Past medical history and drug history:
- Fit and well
- No regular medications. Occasional ibuprofen use for aches and pains after races
- Never been in hospital before. Saw GP for ingrowing toenail last year but nothing else in past few years

## Social history:
- Trains hard for triathlons – swims several times per week
- No alcohol or smoking

- You don't drive a car (don't own a car) but occasionally you drive the running team to races in the minibus
- You work as an intellectual property lawyer for the local university

**Other issues including family history:**
- No history of sudden death in family
- Both parents still alive. No siblings

**Your questions for the candidate:**
- *Can I race again this weekend?*
- *Is it because I didn't eat enough?*
- *Can I cycle to work?*
- *Will it happen again?*

# Candidate

## History/key questions

Was loss of consciousness (LOC) complete?

Was LOC transient with rapid onset and short duration?

Did the patient recover spontaneously, completely and without sequelae?

Did the patient lose postural tone?

If all the above are positive then syncope very likely

If negative, exclude other causes of LOC (epilepsy, metabolic disturbances including hypoxia, vertebro-basilar TIA, etc.)

You must answer three key questions:

Is it a syncopal episode or not (i.e. caused by transient global cerebral hypoperfusion)?

Has the aetiological diagnosis been determined?

Are there data suggestive of a high risk of cardiovascular events or death?

Treat as an emergency (within 24 h) anyone with transient LOC who also has any of the following (red flags):

ECG abnormality

Heart failure

Transient LOC on exertion

Family history of sudden cardiac death in a person younger than 40 years and/or an inherited cardiac condition

Aged older than 65 years with no prodromal symptoms

New or unexplained breathlessness

A heart murmur

Collateral history essential:

Bystanders (in person or over the phone)

Paramedics who can verbally pass on information gained from bystanders; need to see their transfer sheet (notes, contain observations [BP, pulse, $SaO_2$, etc.] and some history, but less detailed than narrative handed over in person)

Eyes are usually open during vasovagal syncope and epilepsy but closed in functional 'attacks'

Recovery times of up to 15 min not uncommon in pseudosyncope

Ask how he felt immediately before the collapse: any warning symptoms or signs (prodromal symptoms) such as dizziness, visual changes, nausea (suggests neurally-mediated syncope); aura may suggest seizure; chest pain, palpitations, dizziness, SOB (cardiac/arrhythmia); lack of any prodrome suggests arrhythmia

What was he doing immediately before the collapse? Provides clues as to cause: exercise-induced, need to exclude cardiac causes; postural hypotension (e.g. standing from sitting position); vasovagal (hot rooms, anxiety/upset); seizure activity (known triggers include lack of sleep, drugs including illicit drugs, alcohol, illness, hunger, strobe lights); hypoglycaemic (history of diabetes, fasting). Passing urine (micturition syncope), cough syncope, etc.

Any previous episodes and their precipitants?

What happened during the episode?

Does he remember collapsing/hitting the ground (helps differentiate from fall)?

Did he lose consciousness? Duration of LOC

Any signs consistent with a seizure (patients who have a vasovagal syncope may twitch a little; patients with VT/VF may also appear to 'fit' – this is seen particularly with torsades de pointes tachycardia which is typically paroxysmal. This is short-lived and occurs *after* the loss of consciousness [cf. at same time as LOC in seizure])

Ask how he felt after the collapse. Ask about confusion, incontinence, headache (suggests seizure)

Speed of recovery important: fast in vasovagal compared to more prolonged following a seizure, often with postictal confusion/headache or transient limb weakness (Todd's paresis)

Associated symptoms: any tongue-biting, urinary incontinence or weakness in arms or legs after the event?

### Drug history

Prescribed medications including β-blockers, BP medications, ACE ihibitors, oral hypoglycaemic drugs/ insulin

Over-the-counter medications

Drugs which prolong QT

Illicit drugs including amphetamine, cocaine, ecstasy, any performance-enhancing drugs

### Past medical history

Previous episodes?

Diabetes: autonomic neuropathy

Any IHD, epilepsy

### Social history

Alcohol history

Any family history of sudden death (ask about siblings and rest of family), epilepsy, IHD

Does he drive? Or swim?

### Address patient's questions and concerns

• *Have you had any thoughts about what is going on?*
• *Is there anything in particular you're concerned about?*
• *Do you have anything you would like to ask?*

## Key areas for examination

A list of what to look for (in examination order; describe findings on examination)

Overall inspection

Evidence of urinary incontinence

GCS/Abbreviated Mental Test: exclude confusion

Look for signs of tongue-biting

CVS examination

Pulse, BP: carotid pulse may be jerky in hypertrophic cardiomyopathy (HOCM), slow-rising in true aortic stenosis (AS)

Apex beat: double impulse (forceful atrial systole followed by LV heave) in HOCM

Heart sounds

Murmurs: aortic late ejection systolic murmur (ESM) (left sternal edge) ± thrill; murmur of mitral regurgitation (dynamic obstruction of the LV outflow tract with functional MR, due to HOCM)

Quiet or absent A2 with ESM in aortic area ± thrill with aortic stenosis

Manoeuvres to accentuate the murmurs: HOCM – louder with Valsalva and on standing, softer if patient squats

Ask to see blood glucose reading, blood results, transfer sheet from paramedics including any ECG rhythm strips, resting 12-lead ECG and rhythm strip (for evidence of electrical or structural abnormalities: long QT syndrome, ST/T wave abnormalities in V1–V3 [Brugada syndrome], PR interval, etc.; LVH in AS, widespread T-wave changes in chest leads [HOCM], etc.)

Important to note that examination may well be entirely normal (good case to use an actor for)

This case – normal examination

## Differential diagnosis

Reflex (neurally mediated) syncope: (a) vasovagal (emotional distress, pain, orthostatic stress); (b) situational: cough, micturition, postexercise, etc.; (c) carotid sinus syncope. NB: in this particular case, most likely vasovagal

Orthostatic hypotension (primary or secondary autonomic failure, drug-induced, volume depletion)

Cardiac syncope (bradycardia, tachycardia, structural heart disease [AS, HOCM], pulmonary embolism, aortic dissection, pulmonary hypertension)

Need to exclude HOCM (exercise-induced syncope) with sudden collapse in young athlete

Differential diagnosis includes aortic stenosis due to bifid aortic valve: pulse would be slow-rising, fixed murmur with Valsalva/other manoeuvres, different murmur (AS murmur versus late systolic murmur in HOCM)

In the ED/medical assessment unit, the main objective is to (a) recognize patients with life-threatening conditions and admit them to hospital, (b) recognize those at low risk who can be discharged pending further investigation

Overall, more than 50% of genuine syncope is 'reflex'; only 10–20% is 'cardiac'. In the young, reflex syncope is by far the most frequent, whilst in the elderly multiple causes may be present. In up to 20% of cases, syncope is unexplained. Syncope accounts for approximately 1% of presentations to the ED; 5% present with major injury, with minor injury present in 30%.

## Discussion with patient
Explain diagnosis
Explain plan, including investigations and management
Address patient's concerns/answer their questions

When a fit athlete collapses suddenly during exercise we need to rule out heart problems, which can cause the collapse, using heart tracings and heart scans. Please don't drive, swim or cycle until the investigations are completed and the doctors have reviewed the results. This is in case you have a further collapse, e.g. whilst swimming or driving. These driving rules are laid down by the DVLA, and you may not be insured if you have an accident whilst the tests are ongoing.

## Investigations
Collateral history from passers-by if possible
Bloods including blood glucose at time of incident (ambulance sheet)
L/S BP
12-lead ECG (exclude long QT; LVH; heart block; ischaemic changes in older patients. May be normal in HOCM but more usually shows LVH, Q-waves, conduction defects). Ask to see a copy of his resting ECG
ECHO (exclude structural heart disease/HOCM/aortic stenosis and assess LV function)
ECG monitoring: 24 h tapes will often miss subsequent events as they only pick up those events which happen in that 24 h period. Seven-day event monitoring is more helpful
Exercise test (appropriately supervised by medical team)
Tilt-table testing to evaluate reflex syncope and orthostatic hypotension, if necessary

## Management
Implantable loop recorder if recurrent unexplained syncope

## Addressing concerns/answering questions
- *Can I race again this weekend?* No – I would advise against this whilst we carry out some tests to look at the heart and rule out heart muscle and heart rhythm

conditions that can cause you to collapse. See investigations above.
- *Is it because I didn't eat enough?* Probably not. Exercise can bring on certain types of collapses, and no cause is identified in a proportion.
- *Can I cycle to work?* No, I would advise against this in case you have a further event whilst cycling which could cause an accident and harm to yourself. I would also advise against swimming.
- *Will it happen again?* There is a risk of it happening again but we will be able to explain further/clarify once the investigations have been carried out.

## Discussion with examiners
The examiners may ask you to clarify details of the above diagnosis and ask questions about your planned investigations and management.

Other possible questions include:
- *What features suggest that this is likely to be reflex syncope rather than a seizure?* Quick recovery, no post-event confusion, drowsiness or incontinence. Red Flag of transient LOC on exertion means he requires urgent assessment (e.g. on the medical assessment unit) including investigations listed above.
- *In general, when is tilt-table testing indicated?* The European Cardiology Guidelines for syncope list indications as follows:
  'In the case of an unexplained single syncopal episode in high risk settings (e.g. occurrence of, or potential risk of physical injury or with occupational implications) or recurrent episode in the absence of organic heart disease, or in presence of organic heart disease after cardiac causes of syncope have been excluded'
  '. . . when it is of clinical value to demonstrate susceptibility to reflex syncope in a patient'
  '. . . to demonstrate between reflex and orthostatic hypotension'
  '. . . may be considered for differentiating syncope with jerking movements from epilepsy'
- *What response would you expect to see with a positive tilt test in a patient with reflex syncope?* Following a period of lying flat, the table is moved to an upright position (60–70 degrees). A loss of consciousness or an inability to maintain posture associated with a significant fall in heart rate or BP constitutes a positive test and the patient is returned to the supine position.

**Further reading/resources**

Latest DVLA driving guidance: www.dft.gov.uk/dvla/medical/ataglance.aspx

European Society of Cardiology Guidelines for diagnosis and management of syncope (2009): www.escardio.org/guidelines-surveys/esc-guidelines/GuidelinesDocuments/guidelines-syncope-FT.pdf

European Society of Cardiology Guidelines for diagnosis and management of HCM (2003): www.escardio.org/guidelines-surveys/esc-guidelines/GuidelinesDocuments/guidelines-HCM-FT.pdf

NICE guidance for transient loss of consciousness (TLoC) management in adults: www.guidance.nice.org.uk/CG109

# Scenario 32 | Angina/chest pain

## Candidate's information

**Your role:** you are an ST3 on the MAU and you have been asked to see Mr Bolton, a 65-year-old man who was admitted with chest pain. Currently pain free, BP 150/75, pulse 75.

**Your task:** to assess the patient's problems and address any questions or concerns he raises.

## Patient's information

**You are:** Frederic Bolton, a 65-year-old man.

**Your problem:** you have been having chest pain on exertion for several months; it usually lasts 5 minutes at a time and settles quickly with rest. You weren't concerned but episodes have got more frequent recently, and come on more easily (with less exercise). You haven't been to your GP as you hadn't been worried. This episode today happened at work whilst lifting heavy boxes in the office, so you were sent to hospital by the boss of the taxi firm you work for. The pain lasted 25 min and didn't settle as quickly with rest as it usually does. After 10 min of resting, your manager noticed you looked pale and called an ambulance. The pain had settled by the time the ambulance arrived but they persuaded you to come in for a check-up.

The pain is not altered by breathing in or coughing. No change with posture, only rest helped. You very rarely get indigestion or heartburn, perhaps at Christmas after a couple of big meals in a row and more alcohol than usual.

Risk factors: you smoke 25/day; you don't know about your cholesterol or BP as you have not seen your GP for years.

Exercise tolerance: limited by painful ankle (you fractured your ankle when you fell off a kerb 2 years ago). You are able to walk for a couple of hundred yards at a reasonable pace but not briskly, and you can't run.

### Past medical history and drug history:

- Had chest pains about 5 years ago which your GP diagnosed as angina, and started you on medicines. Well until a few months ago. You stopped taking the medications about 6 months ago as you hadn't had any angina for years. You had been on bisoprolol 5 mg once per day and 75 mg aspirin, as well as a cholesterol tablet
- You are not aware of having diabetes or raised cholesterol
- You don't have any contraindications to aspirin or β-blockers as you tolerated them fine the last time
- No indigestion or history of peptic ulcer disease, no asthma or peripheral vascular disease

### Other issues including family history:

- MI – father at 58, brother at 53

**Social history:**

- Black taxi cab driver. You were thinking about retiring in a few months anyway, so you wouldn't be too bothered if you had to stop being a cabbie a few months early on medical grounds. You do have a car at home though

**Your questions for the candidate:**

- *Have I had a heart attack?*
- *What can I do to prevent having a heart attack in the future?*
- *Can I drive my cab for the last few months before I retire?*

---

## Candidate

### History/key questions

History regarding chest pain:

    Describe pain (open question) then more specific:

        site – central, lateral chest

        onset – sudden, gradual

        character – heavy/crushing/brick-like; stabbing, pleuritic pain worse on coughing or breathing in deeply; burning retrosternal pain

    Any associated breathlessness, nausea, sweating, dizziness, water brash (bitter liquid in mouth), heartburn/indigestion

    Radiation of pain – down arm(s), up to neck, jaw or teeth; through to back

    Exacerbating/relieving factors – exertion, eating, emotion. How much exercise? Heavy lifting; coughing/deep breathing; postural (lying down – GORD/pericarditis)

Any SOB, cough, fever, haemoptysis, weight loss

Current medications. Any allergies to medicines

Past history of chest pain, and what the diagnosis was

Has he ever been diagnosed with angina, MI, raised cholesterol, diabetes, high blood pressure?

Any known respiratory problems such as asthma, COPD

Ever had a collapsed lung/pneumothorax?

Ask about other cardiac risk factors such as smoking (quantify as pack-years: 20/day for 1 year = 1 pack-year); alcohol history per week in units

Any family history of MI, stroke, diabetes

At what age did brothers, sisters, parents have MI (positive family history if first-degree relative(s) MI <55)?

### Address patient's questions and concerns

- *Have you had any thoughts about what is going on?*
- *Is there anything in particular you're concerned about?*
- *Do you have anything you would like to ask?*

## Key areas for examination

A list of what to look for (in examination order; describe findings on examination)

Above history consistent with cardiac cause but need to exclude other common and/or important differentials (GORD, musculoskeletal pain, pneumothorax, pericarditis, etc.)

General inspection: any pain at present at rest, or if takes deep breath or coughs

Look for xanthelasma, tar stains on the fingers, clubbing

Respiratory rate

CVS examination:

    Pulse, BP

    JVP

    Apex beat, parasternal heave, thrills. Any chest wall tenderness?

    Heart sounds, murmurs, pericardial rub, carotid bruits

    Lung bases, signs of peripheral oedema/DVT

Information to ask for:

    BP/observations

    Resting ECGs, blood results including troponin

### Differential diagnosis

Ischaemic heart disease/stable angina; clear cardiac risk factors and consistent history

### Discussion with patient

Explain diagnosis

Explain plan, including investigations and management

Address patient's concerns/answer their questions

Your chest pain sounds like angina due to narrowing of the arteries of the heart. First we need to do some blood tests to make sure that you haven't had a heart attack. If these tests are clear, and you don't get any more pain, we can start you back on the tablets you were on before from your doctor. We will then arrange some tests as an outpatient to look at the arteries in the heart.

We also need to address the driving issue; you shouldn't drive your private car until symptoms are controlled; don't drive the taxi cab until this is sorted – you will need to meet certain criteria before relicensing. You will need to inform the DVLA too.

## Investigations
ECG

Blood tests including troponin (given duration of pain, important to exclude NSTEMI)

CXR

Admit for monitoring

## Management
What does ECG show? Are serial ECGs identical or are there dynamic changes?

Any ongoing chest pain?

Check troponin: if troponin negative *and* there are no dynamic ECG changes, patient may go home with outpatient investigations

Consider as new-onset chest pain and assess likelihood of pain being of cardiac origin:

If <10% reassure and discharge

10–30% consider CT calcium scoring

30–60% non-invasive stress imaging (nuclear or MRI)

>60% refer to cardiology for coronary angiography. ETT now has little role in the investigation of chest pain

Aspirin 75 mg od and β-blocker given history. Previously tolerated them. Consider rate-limiting calcium antagonists (e.g. diltiazem) if asthmatic, etc.

If troponin positive and/or there are dynamic ECG changes – referral to cardiology, aspirin 300 mg, clopidogrel (or similar), low molecular weight heparin + angiography with a view to revascularization

Risk factor management:

Manage hypertension, high cholesterol (regular statin), exclude diabetes (consider OGTT). Reduce weight if overweight

Referral to smoking cessation services

Long-term risk factor management will be undertaken by GP

DVLA advice as regards driving a taxi (class 2 for black cab, class 1 for private hire taxi – see DVLA guidelines)

## Addressing concerns/answering questions
- *Have I had a heart attack?* We need to do some blood tests and several heart tracings to find out, and then can plan further treatment with this information.
- *What can I do to prevent having a heart attack in the future?* It is important to reduce the risks of heart disease, and so it is really important to stop smoking completely, lose weight (if overweight) and control cholesterol levels and high blood pressure.
- *Can I drive my cab for the last few months before I retire?* You will need to inform the DVLA and don't drive the taxi cab until this is sorted out – you will need to meet certain criteria before relicensing. You shouldn't drive your private car either until your symptoms are controlled.

## Discussion with examiners
The examiners may ask you to clarify details of the above diagnosis and ask questions about your planned investigations and management.

A possible question includes:
- *How would you risk-stratify patients following an episode of, e.g., unstable angina?* Scoring systems to predict the outcomes following unstable angina and non-ST elevation MI include GRACE and TIMI.

    Global Registry of Acute Coronary Events (GRACE) estimates the risk of in-hospital and six-month mortality in patients with acute coronary syndrome. Variables include age, heart rate, systolic blood pressure, creatinine, presence and class of heart failure, cardiac arrest on admission, ST-segment deviation, and whether cardiac biomarkers were elevated.

    The Thrombolysis In Myocardial Infarction (TIMI) score correlates significantly with increased risk of events at/by day 14 (all-cause mortality, new or recurrent MI, or severe recurrent ischaemia requiring coronary revascularization). Variables include age ≥65, having at least three risk factors for coronary heart disease, previous coronary stenosis of ≥50%, ST segment deviation on admission ECG, ≥ 2 episodes of angina in the previous 24 hours, elevated cardiac biomarkers, use of aspirin in the previous 7 days.

**Examiners' information and requirements**

The candidate should:

1. Identify key features from the history: chest pain on exertion, eased by rest. Past history of angina diagnosed by GP. Risk factors for cardiac disease
2. Identify key examination findings: examination may well be completely normal
3. Outline a sensible management plan, including assessing risk and planning inpatient versus outpatient investigations, management of risk factors. Be aware of GRACE and TIMI scores
4. Give a clear explanation to the patient of your diagnosis and plan, address his concerns and answer his questions; include the key areas to be explained (DVLA, issues as regards taxi driving)

**Further reading/resources**

Chest pain of recent onset – NICE guidance (2011): www.nice.org.uk/nicemedia/live/12947/47938/47938.pdf

Guidelines on the management of stable angina pectoris: www.escardio.org/guidelines-surveys/esc-guidelines/Pages/stable-angina-pectoris.aspx

GRACE score: www.outcomes-umassmed.org/grace/acs_risk/acs_risk_content.html

TIMI risk score: www.timi.org/ *and* www.mdcalc.com/timi-risk-score-for-uanstemi/

DVLA rules: www.dft.gov.uk/dvla/medical/ataglance.aspx

# Scenario 33 | Palpitations ?atrial fibrillation

## Candidate's information

**Your role:** you are an ST2 in the MAU and a local GP has referred to you Mr Rowley, a 40-year-old bank manager, following an episode of palpitations and shortness of breath. BP 125/75, pulse 70, temperature 37.3°C on arrival at the MAU.

**Your task:** to assess the patient's problems and address any questions or concerns raised by him.

## Patient's information

**You are:** Paul Rowley, age 40 years, a bank manager.

**Your problem:** you are usually well but over the past few months you've noticed episodes of a brief racing of your heart lasting seconds, particularly at night. These episodes have become a little more frequent over the past 6 months, and you had attributed this to stress.

You had a longer episode today, lasting an hour, and it felt different from usual. You felt your pulse and counted the rate at 120 per min. Your pulse felt irregular too. You were a little short of breath with the palpitations but you had no chest pain. It all went away just before you arrived at the hospital and before you had the heart tracing. You can usually walk for miles without problems (you walk your dog several times a week). Your heart rate feels normal now.

No weight loss, diarrhoea or abdominal pain.

### Past medical history and drug history:
- No past history of note
- Drinks 2–3 L/day of Diet Coke. Doesn't drink tea or coffee, and doesn't take any alternative medicines or illicit drugs
- No regular medications
- No drug allergies

### Social history:
- Alcohol: usually two or three glasses of wine per week, had a few more than usual last night (one bottle of wine over dinner and the rest of the evening)
- Non-smoker

### Other issues including family history:
- Father had an irregular heart beat after his heart attack in his 70 s; lived until 85 but needed to take warfarin. He had a few problems with the warfarin, bleeding from one nose-bleed was so much that he needed to have a blood transfusion in hospital

## Your questions for the candidate:
- *What's causing this?*
- *Have I had a heart attack?*
- *Will I need to take warfarin?*

---

## Candidate

### History/key questions
Palpitations: onset, length of episodes

How many episodes, and when was the first (recent versus lifelong/chronic symptoms)?

Speed and rhythm of palpitations (patient taps out rate/rhythm): did the patient feel/count their own pulse during the episode?

Any associated symptoms (chest pain, shortness of breath, sweating, syncope/dizziness)

Any triggers noticed (alcohol, caffeine) or relieving factors (e.g. Valsalva)

Ask about thyroid dysfunction: weight loss, heat intolerance, tremor, diarrhoea

Cardiovascular symptoms, including chest pain and those of cardiac failure

Any signs of infection: ask about chest, urinary symptoms, fever

Exercise tolerance: what does he usually have to do to get breathlessness?

### Drug history
Any current medications including β-blockers, β2-agonists, levothyroxine, carbimazole, propylthiouracil

Any drug allergies

Over-the-counter medicines

Illicit drug use such as amphetamines, cocaine or ecstasy

### Past medical history
Any cardiovascular risk factors: smoking, diabetes, raised cholesterol, hypertension, obesity, etc.

### Social history
Alcohol history; caffeine intake (coffee, tea, stimulant drinks)

Smoking history

Driving licence?

### Other issues including family history
Any history of cardiac disease or sudden death

## Address patient's questions and concerns
- *Have you had any thoughts about what is going on?*
- *Is there anything in particular you're concerned about?*
- *Do you have anything you would like to ask?*

## Key areas for examination
A list of what to look for (in examination order; describe findings on examination)

Overall inspection

Respiratory rate; any chest pain

Signs of hyperthyroidism (tremor, tachycardia, sweating, eye signs)

Pulse (rate, rhythm, volume, collapsing, etc.)

CVS: BP, JVP, standard cardiac examination (apex beat/heaves/thrills, HS, murmurs)

Ask to see observation charts, resting ECG, blood results (including thyroid function) and PA erect CXR

Examination in this patient is normal (likely to be an actor) with normal resting ECG (sinus rhythm), and blood tests including troponins are normal

## Differential diagnosis
Paroxysmal arrhythmia, e.g. SVT or paroxysmal atrial fibrillation (PAF). Dietary trigger – excess of alcohol, caffeine

Ventricular arrhythmia: either ventricular ectopics or non-sustained VT

Non-cardiac cause of symptoms (e.g. anxiety, gastro-oesophageal reflux)

## Discussion with patient
Explain diagnosis

Explain plan, including investigations and management

Address patient's concerns/answer their questions

You've had intermittent short-lived palpitations over several months but the ones today lasted a lot longer. You're in normal rhythm now. We need to do some tests to see if we can determine the cause. There are a few possibilities so we need to ensure you get the correct treatment. It may be that you have the same condition as your father and you will need warfarin. There are no signs of a heart attack from the tracings or the blood tests.

## Investigations

Basic tests including U&E, TFT, Mg, calcium, phosphate

Troponins (if any chest pain or concerns, i.e. cardiac ischaemia)

Resting ECG

CXR

ECG monitoring: 7-day event recorder (24 h tapes will often miss significant events as only pick up events which happen in that 24 h period; 7-day event monitoring is more helpful)

ECHO to exclude structural heart disease, e.g. mitral valve disease (common) or ASD as cause for late-onset AF (rare)

Cardiology referral

## Management

Lifestyle advice – reduce caffeine and alcohol

Treatment of arrhythmia if seen on tape: bear in mind single prolonged episode with SOB

If PAF, can then discuss role of medications and anti-coagulation; CHA2DS2-**VASc** scoring system

Nocturnal symptoms could be ectopics; role of anxiety in interpreting symptoms

### Addressing concerns/answering questions

• *What's causing this?* See explanation above. The heart tracing today showed a normal heart rhythm. We need to find out the cause of your symptoms, and can arrange a portable heart rhythm monitoring device for either one or seven days with leads stuck to your chest to see what the heart rhythm and rate is when you have these episodes. If we identify any runs of irregular heart beat on the tests, we will need to consider further medications (depending on the type of abnormal heart rhythm found), including warfarin for particular heart rhythms (AF).

• *Have I had a heart attack?* There's no signs of a heart attack on the heart tracing or blood tests.

• *Will I need to take warfarin?* Not at the moment, as we need to see what the heart rate and rhythm is during these episodes. If we identify any runs of irregular heart beat on the tests, we will need to consider further medications (depending on the type of abnormal heart rhythm found), including warfarin for particular heart rhythms (AF) as this reduces the risk of complications associated with this particular heart rhythm.

## Discussion with examiners

The examiners may ask you to clarify details of the above diagnosis and ask questions about your planned investigations and management.

A possible question includes:
*How do you decide who needs anticoagulation for AF?* Use the CHA2DS2-VASc score (Table H33.1), which uses risk factors to guide choice between no therapy, antiplatelet therapy and anticoagulant therapy.

**Table H33.1** The CHA2DS2-VASc score

| Feature | Score |
| --- | --- |
| Congestive cardiac failure /LV dysfunction | 1 |
| Hypertension | 1 |
| Age over 75 years | 2 |
| Age between 65 and 74 years | 1 |
| Stroke/TIA/thromboembolic event | 2 |
| Vascular disease (previous MI, peripheral arterial disease or aortic plaque) | 1 |
| Diabetes mellitus | 1 |
| Female | 1 |

Adjusted stroke rates are reported in the European Society of Cardiology guidelines: 1.3% per year if score 1, 2.2% with a score of 2, 3.2% score 3, up to 15.2% if score 9.

Scores of 2 or more – anticoagulation with warfarin is indicated, and needs to be discussed with the patient.

Score of 1 is intermediate risk, and aspirin / antiplatelet therapy or anticoagulation should be considered, and discussed with the patient. Oral anticoagulation is preferred (see European Society of Cardiology guidelines).

Score of 0 is low risk. Options include aspirin or no anticoagulation/antiplatelet therapy. No therapy is preferred option.

See also Vol. 1, Station 3, Cardiovascular, Case 8.

**Further reading/resources**

NICE guidance on atrial fibrillation: www.nice.org.uk/CG36

ACCF/AHA/HRS Focused Update on the Management of Patients With Atrial Fibrillation (2011): www.circ.ahajournals.org/content/123/1/104.extract

European Society of Cardiology AF guidelines: www.escardio.org/guidelines-surveys/esc-guidelines/pages/atrial-fibrillation.aspx

# Scenario 34 | Breathlessness/ congestive cardiac failure

## Candidate's information

**Your role:** you are an ST2 in the general medical clinic. A GP has referred Mrs Brice to the clinic with a 3-month history of breathlessness on exertion and ankle oedema. A resting ECG was normal in the surgery, and FBC, U&E and TFT were normal a month ago.

**Your task:** to assess the patient's problems and address any questions or concerns raised by her.

## Patient's information

**You are:** Joan Brice, a 75-year-old woman.

**Your problem:** you are short of breath on exertion, even if walking about 200 yards. Previously (up to about 3 months ago), you were able to walk about a mile. Your breathing gets worse when lying flat in bed so now you sleep on three pillows. You don't wake with breathlessness, and you haven't noticed any coughing at night. You've noticed some ankle swelling. It's all progressively developed over the past 3 months – it's crept up on you.

You have no chest pain, palpitations, fever, cough or sputum. You can sometimes hear a bit of a wheeze if you've walked too fast.

### Past medical history and drug history:
- Diabetes for 10 years; also hypertension, high cholesterol
- Your doctor mentioned that your heart tracing (ECG) suggested you might have had a heart attack in the past – you don't remember having one
- Current medications include metformin 1 g bd; simvastatin 40 mg nocte; ramipril 2.5 mg od; aspirin 75 mg od

### Social history:
- Smoking: 5/day for past 6 months (previously 20/day for 30 years) – you also cut down a few years ago as you heard that it would help with the diabetes
- Alcohol: 2 glasses of wine per week

### Other issues:
- Shortness of breath interfering with ability to go shopping – previously able to walk down to shops and go round without a problem. Now need to take a taxi down, and to rest regularly on the way round the supermarket

### Family history
- Nil of note

### Your questions for the candidate:
- *Have I had a heart attack?*
- *Can you get my breathing back to normal?*
- *Is my smoking to blame?*

# Candidate

## History/key questions

Exercise tolerance: try to quantify change, e.g. unlimited walking changing to climbing stairs

Orthopnoea, paroxysmal noctural dyspnoea (suggest cardiac failure)

Chest pain, eased by rest or GTN: think of ischaemic heart disease

Ask about palpitations, rate/rhythm and whether associated with SOB

Respiratory causes: smoking history in pack-years and occupational history, cough, wheeze, sputum (daily compared to intermittent; productive [infective, chronic bronchitis], dry [asthma, interstitial lung disease])

Weight loss, fever, chest pain, stridor

Haemoptysis (TB, neoplasia, PE, can be in CCF)

Oedema (CCF, cor pulmonale due to COPD)

Any long-haul flights or other thromboembolic risk factors?

### Drug history

Check list of regular medications: already on treatment for heart failure? (diuretics, ACE inhibitor, β-blocker)

Any changes to medicines over past 6 months

Any negative inotropes

Allergies?

### Past medical history

Check not already known to have asthma, IHD, COPD

Causes of heart failure: any IHD, valvular problems already known about

Cardiac risk factors: diabetes, raised cholesterol, hypertension, smoking history, family history of IHD, obesity

### Social history

Smoking and alcohol history

## Address patient's questions and concerns

• Have you had any thoughts about what is going on?
• Is there anything in particular you're concerned about?
• Do you have anything you would like to ask?

## Key areas for examination

A list of what to look for (in examination order; describe findings on examination)

Focused examination regarding CCF (remember in the exam that the patient will have been treated so you are looking for signs of compensated heart failure, e.g. peripheral oedema with a normal or near normal JVP, unlikely to have 3rd heart sound but may have 4th (providing she is not in AF, of course)

Listen carefully for mitral regurgitation and assess the pulmonary component of the 2nd heart sound to determine secondary pulmonary hypertension)

Look for signs of recent peripheral oedema (wrinkled skin, etc.)

Signs of fluid retention:
  Poor peripheral perfusion
  BP – low
  Elevated JVP
  Apex beat – displaced
  RV heave

Heart sounds/any murmurs, 3rd/4th heart sounds, gallop rhythm if tachycardic. Functional mitral regurgitation or tricuspid regurgitation

Chest examination: bibasal crackles, wheeze, pleural effusions

Tender hepatomegaly and ascites can also be present

Check for peripheral oedema

Ask to see the blood results, resting ECG and a PA erect chest X-ray. Ask for the ECHO result if available

## Differential diagnosis

Congestive cardiac failure: causes include ischaemic cardiomyopathy, valvular heart disease, arrhythmia, severe hypertension, other cardiomyopathies

(Severe anaemia has been excluded by GP's recent normal FBC)

## Discussion with patient

Explain diagnosis

Explain plan, including investigations and management

Address patient's concerns/answer their questions

One of the possible causes for your breathlessness is narrowing of the arteries to the heart leading to weakening of the heart muscle, rather than a single event like a heart attack. We need to carry out investigations to look at how well the heart is pumping, and the valves in the heart. Other tests may be needed depending on the results of the investigations. The treatment aims to take the fluid off the lungs, which is causing your breathlessness, and we will give you other tablets to strengthen the heart. Smoking will have been part of the reason for the heart arteries narrowing and it is very important to stop smoking. I can refer you to our hospital team to help you to stop smoking.

## Investigations

History and examination consistent with cardiac failure (SOB on exertion, orthopnoea, oedema)

Need to investigate to find out cause, and reduce symptoms/improve prognosis

Basic tests: FBC, U&E, LFT, TFT to exclude causes (hypothyroidism) and associated diseases (e.g. renal impairment) including metabolic causes (haemochromatosis, anaemia, etc.)

CXR

ECG: resting

ECHO to assess LV ejection fraction, and whether due to cardiomyopathy (global impairment) and/or regional wall abnormalities (IHD). Is it systolic or diastolic heart failure?

## Management

Management with diuretics, ACEI, spironolactone, β-blockers if systolic heart failure – symptomatic management if diastolic

Manage cardiac risk factors

Referral to smoking cessation services in hospital/community

If ECG shows LBBB and ejection fraction <35%, consider cardiac resynchronization therapy (plus implantable cardiac defibrillator [ICD] if IHD)

## Addressing concerns/answering questions

- *Have I had a heart attack?* One of the possible causes for your breathlessness is narrowing of the arteries to the heart leading to weakening of the heart muscle, rather than a single event like a heart attack. We need to carry out investigations to look at how well the heart is pumping, and the valves in the heart. Other tests may be needed depending on the results of these investigations.

- *Can you get my breathing back to normal?* The treatment aims to take the fluid off the lungs, which is causing your breathlessness, and we will give you other tablets to strengthen the heart. It is important to stop smoking too (see below).

- *Is my smoking to blame?* Smoking will have been part of the reason for the heart arteries narrowing and can also cause breathlessness through its effects on the lungs too, so it is very important to stop smoking. I can refer you to our hospital team to help you stop smoking.

## Discussion with examiners

The examiners may ask you to clarify details of the above diagnosis and ask questions about your planned investigations and management.

A possible question includes:

- *What are the recommended therapies for symptomatic (class II–IV) heart failure and why?* According to 2012 European Society of Cardiology guidelines, ACE inhibitors, beta-blockers and mineralocorticoid receptor antagonists:

   'ACE inhibitor is recommended in addition to a beta-blocker for all patients with ejection fraction ≤40% to reduce the risk of heart failure hospitalization, and the risk of premature death.'

   'Beta-blocker is recommended in addition to ACE inhibitor (or angiotensin receptor blocker) for all patients with ejection fraction ≤40% to reduce the risk of heart failure hospitalization, and the risk of premature death.'

   'Mineralocorticoid receptor antagonist is recommended for all patients with persisting symptoms (NYHA class II–IV) and an ejection fraction ≤ 35% despite treatment with an ACE inhibitor (or an ARB if an ACE is not tolerated) and a beta-blocker to reduce the risk of heart failure hospitalization, and the risk of premature death.'

---

### Examiners' information and requirements

The candidate should:

1. Identify key features from the history: reduced exercise tolerance due to breathlessness, orthopnoea, oedema, with several cardiac risk factors, and recent normal FBC, U&E and TFT excluding anaemia, hyper- and hypothyroidism, renal impairment as causes

2. Identify key examination findings including signs of CCF

3. Outline a sensible management plan, being clear that evidence-based therapies are only applicable to systolic heart failure

4. Give a clear explanation to the patient of your diagnosis and plan, address her concerns and answer her questions. Consider involvement of heart failure nurse specialist (if available) for further education and advice

---

## Further reading/resources

Chronic heart failure – guidelines from the British Society for Heart Failure: www.bsh.org.uk/

ESC guidelines for the management of acute and chronic heart failure: www.escardio.org/guidelines-surveys/esc-guidelines/pages/acute-chronic-heart-failure.aspx

2010 focused update of ESC guidelines on device therapy in heart failure: www.escardio.org/guidelines-surveys/esc-guidelines/pages/device-therapy-heart-failure.aspx

# Scenario 35 | Syncope/aortic stenosis

## Candidate's information

**Your role:** you are an ST2 in elderly care. Mrs Fortescue has been referred to you by the emergency department following a collapse. BP 95 systolic at the scene, now 105/78. GCS has been 15/15 since the ambulance arrived.

**Your task:** to assess the patient's problems and address any questions or concerns raised by her.

## Patient's information

**You are:** Cybil Fortescue, a 75-year-old woman.

**Your problem:** you collapsed whilst out shopping alone. This is the second time that this has happened. You stopped driving on the advice of your GP after the first episode about 8 weeks ago. You didn't have any investigations after your collapse. Your GP said she'd think about it if another one happened.

This time you were sitting down having lunch in a café, and remember waking up with passers-by and a paramedic talking to you.

You have noticed slight breathlessness whilst out shopping or climbing stairs which is new over the past 3 months. You have felt dizzy on exertion but no chest pain. You have been feeling more tired than usual over the past few months as well. Gardening has been a little harder than usual.

The previous episode occurred at home, and you found yourself lying half off the sofa. You couldn't remember what had happened, and you were alone at home at the time.

### Past medical history and drug history:
- Recently started on ramipril 2.5 mg od for high blood pressure
- Atenolol had given you lethargy

### Social history:
- You live with your husband, and until recently you have used the car to shop, etc., as no other local support – your family live some distance away and your husband doesn't drive any more following the stroke he had three years ago. He needs your help with washing and dressing, and you do all the shopping and cooking
- Non-smoker, no alcohol

### Other issues including family history:
- Brother died suddenly aged 82 years

### Your questions for the candidate:
- *Will it happen again?*
- *Will I need an operation?*
- *When can I start driving again? My husband needs to get to his appointments.*

# Candidate

## History/key questions

Overall history similar to the other syncope cases above

Collateral history essential

Bystanders (in person or over the phone)

Paramedics who can verbally pass on information gained from bystanders; need to see their transfer sheet (notes, observations [BP, pulse, SaO$_2$, etc.] and some history, less detailed than narrative handed over in person)

Ask how she felt immediately before the collapse (any warning symptoms or signs such as dizziness, visual changes, nausea; aura may suggest seizure; sudden-onset headache [SAH]); rash, fever, headache, photophobia (meningitis); chest pain, palpitations, dizziness, SOB (cardiac/arrhythmia); any associated chest pain, SOB, palpitations

What was she doing immediately before the collapse? Provides clues as to cause: exercise-induced need to exclude cardiac causes; postural hypotension (e.g. standing from sitting position); vasovagal (hot rooms, anxiety/upset); seizure activity (known triggers include lack of sleep, drugs including illicit drugs, alcohol, illness, hunger, strobe lights); hypoglycaemic (history of diabetes, fasting). Passing urine (micturition syncope)

Any previous episodes and their precipitants?

What happened during the episode?

Does she remember collapsing/hitting the floor (helps differentiate from fall)?

Did she lose consciousness? Duration of LOC

Any signs consistent with a seizure (patients who have a vasovagal syncope may twitch a little)

Ask how she felt after the collapse. Ask about confusion, incontinence, headache, photophobia

Speed of recovery important: fast in vasovagal compared to more prolonged following a seizure, often with postictal confusion/headache or transient limb weakness (Todd's paresis)

Associated symptoms: any tongue-biting, urinary incontinence or weakness in arms or legs after the event?

### Drug history

Prescribed medications including β-blockers, BP medications, ACEI; oral hypoglycaemic drugs/insulin; α-blockers for prostate (in males)

Any recent additions/alterations in medication

Over-the-counter medications

Drugs which prolong QT

Illicit drugs including amphetamine, cocaine, ecstasy, any performance-enhancing drugs

### Past medical history

Previous episodes?

Diabetes: autonomic neuropathy

Any IHD, epilepsy

### Social history

Effects on the patient; effects of not being able to drive

Alcohol history

Does she drive? Or swim?

Ask about effects of collapse on life/ADL/confidence/ independent living

Unexplained syncope: see DVLA guidelines

### Family history

Any family history of sudden death (ask about siblings and rest of family), epilepsy, IHD

### Address patient's questions and concerns

- *Have you had any thoughts about what is going on?*
- *Is there anything in particular you're concerned about?*
- *Do you have anything you would like to ask?*

## Key areas for examination

A list of what to look for (in examination order; describe findings on examination)

Overall inspection

Evidence of urinary incontinence

GCS/AMT: exclude confusion

Rash: inspect carefully

Neck stiffness: Kernig's

Look for signs of tongue-biting

CVS examination:

Pulse; slow-rising in AS

BP

Apex beat

Heart sounds

Murmurs: manoeuvres to accentuate the murmurs

Signs of aortic stenosis (regular, slow-rising pulse, low volume/narrow pulse pressure, undisplaced apex beat)

First heart sound normal; 2nd soft; harsh ejection systolic murmur in the aortic area. Look for a systolic thrill over the aortic area which would signify severe aortic stenosis (AS). Radiation to carotids

Ask to see blood glucose reading, blood results, transfer sheet from paramedics including any ECG rhythm strips, resting ECG – usually shows LVH in significant AS; L/S BP

This patient has clinical signs of AS

## Differential diagnosis

Syncope due to AS

Differentials to consider include arrhythmias, orthostatic hypotension; consider wider causes of syncope

## Discussion with patient

Explain diagnosis

Explain plan, including investigations and management

Address patient's concerns/answer their questions

Our aim is to investigate the cause of your collapse. Examination of your heart suggests a narrowing of a heart valve, but further tests are required to confirm this. Please don't drive whilst we carry out these investigations to find the cause. If the cause is found and treated, then you need to hold off driving for at least 4 weeks, but if it is not possible to find and treat the cause, then you will need to stop driving for a minimum of six months. We will be able to review the situation in clinic with the results of your investigations.

## Investigations

FBC, U&E: exclude anaemia as cause of reduced exercise tolerance

ECG: to assess LV hypertrophy ± LV strain pattern, ST changes, LAD, conduction delays (1st-degree AV block, LBBB)

ECHO: to assess area of valve, LV size, degree of hypertrophy and LV function (assess severity of aortic stenosis)

## Management

If considering AS, stop ACEI (recently started)

Surgical treatment is indicated for symptomatic patients or valve gradient >50 mmHg (await ECHO) – risk of sudden death in symptomatic patients with severe AS

## Addressing concerns/answering questions

- *Will it happen again?* We need to carry out tests to find out why you collapsed. There is a risk of having another collapse as one of your heart valves looks to be narrowed. I suggest stopping the ramipril blood pressure tablet that you've been taking as this will help reduce the risk of it happening again.
- *Will I need an operation?* We need to carry out some investigations including a scan of the heart to look at the valves in detail, and can discuss the available options with these results. If the collapse is thought

to be due to narrowing of the aortic valve, then an operation may well be indicated.

- *When can I start driving again? My husband needs to get to his appointments.* Our aim is to investigate the cause of your collapse. Examination suggests a narrowing of a valve in the heart, and further tests are required. For unexplained collapse but with clinical evidence of a structural heart cause, the DVLA rules state that no driving is allowed for 4 weeks if the cause is treated, or 6 months revoked if not. We need to review your situation in clinic with the results of the investigations. We would advise no driving until tests are completed and we can be clear on whether the 'cause has been treated'.

## Discussion with examiners

The examiners may ask you to clarify details of the above diagnosis and ask questions about your planned investigations and management.

A possible question includes:

- *What are the complications of aortic stenosis?* Complications of AS include LV impairment, arrhythmias and heart block, sudden death, pulmonary hypertension, infective endocarditis, haemolysis; complications of embolization, Heyde's syndrome (iron deficiency anaemia due to acquired von Willebrand factor deficiency).

See also Vol. 1, Station 3, Cardiovascular, Case 5.

---

### Examiners' information and requirements

The candidate should:

1. Elicit a clear history of syncope and differentiate between the different causes
2. Correctly identify the murmur of aortic stenosis
3. Outline a management plan including appropriate investigations (ECG, ECHO)
4. Give a clear explanation to the patient of your diagnosis and plan, address her concerns and answer her questions; identify the risk of sudden death in symptomatic patients with severe AS

---

## Further reading/resources

DVLA – At a glance guide to the current medical standards of fitness to drive: www.dft.gov.uk/dvla/medical/ataglance.aspx

# Scenario 36 | Syncope (orthostatic)

## Candidate's information
**Your role:** you are an ST2 in the acute medical unit. You are asked to look at Mr Sloley, a 75-year-old man with a history of collapse. The ED notes report that he collapsed in a restaurant after standing up to go to the toilet. Bystanders noticed some twitching of his arms and legs, but he was back to normal within 5 min.

**Your task:** to assess the patient's problems and address any questions or concerns raised by him.

## Patient's information
**You are:** Stephen Sloley, a 75-year-old man.

**Your problem:** you were out dining with friends at one of your regular restaurants. You remember standing up to go to the bathroom, felt dizzy and then collapsed. You woke up on the floor and felt normal after about 5–10 min. You weren't that concerned as you thought that you had simply fainted but your friends persuaded you to go to hospital with the paramedics. You haven't been incontinent of urine and you haven't bitten your tongue. Your friends reported to the ED team that you knew where you were almost immediately afterwards and you were just a little embarrassed.

You have felt a little dizzy on standing up, usually in the morning, over the past 6 months – you just get up slowly and the dizziness settles in a few minutes. You've been eating and drinking normally, with no diarrhoea or vomiting.

### Past medical history and drug history:
- Alfusozin for prostate (BPH)
- Bendroflumethiazide 2.5 mg once per day
- No past history of collapses or seizures

### Social history:
- You live with your wife and neither of you drive. She's well and is on her way to the hospital to see you

### Other issues including family history:
- No family history of illness – both parents died in their 90s of old age

### Your questions for the candidate:
- *Have I had a seizure?*
- *Do I have to stay in hospital?*

# Candidate

## History/key questions

Consider the different causes of syncope

Did the patient lose consciousness? Does he remember hitting the floor (fall > LOC/syncope)?

Symptoms pre-collapse: history of dizziness on standing with rapid recovery on sitting (e.g. symptoms on getting up in the morning/dizziness on rising from bed in morning); suggests postural hypotension

Speed of onset and recovery important: sudden syncope without warning likely to be due to arrhythmia; consider structural heart disease, e.g. HOCM, in young with sudden collapse on exertion without warning

Symptoms post-collapse, e.g. speed of recovery, any evidence of postevent confusion. Post-event confusion, urinary and/or faecal incontinence, tongue-biting suggest seizure but are not diagnostic

Ask about associated chest pain; was collapse related to exertion?

Any associated breathlessness, haemoptysis, pleuritic chest pain (symptoms suggestive of PE)

Known angina or symptoms consistent with new diagnosis of angina: consider cardiac cause

Any triggers (provocative factors) identified? These include exertion, emotion, heat, coughing, vomiting, swallowing (vagal surge), standing for prolonged duration, micturition, defaecation – situational syncope. Neck movements – carotid sinus hypersensitivity

Previous episodes: describe events including above details. Ask about the frequency, any previous investigations; any triggers identified?

Ask about headache, limb weakness, speech problems (dysphasia, dysarthria): consider neurological causes such as SAH

Ask about any pain or injuries from the fall/syncopal episodes

Any information from the passers-by: ask about length of time of reduced consciousness, confusion, etc. Ask about pallor, drowsiness, nausea ± vomiting – consistent with vasovagal syncope. They may also be able to provide useful information about limb movements (slight twitches in vasovagal versus full seizure). They may have felt the patient's pulse during the episode (absent [cardiac arrest], slow, fast, irregular versus regular)

### Past medical history

Ask about diabetes, known cardiac disease, neuropathy or epilepsy

### Drug history

Ask about regular medicines: is he on antihypertensive, antiarrhythmic or antianginal medications; α-blockers for prostatism?

### Social history

Any family history of sudden death or collapse

Does the patient drive, and what vehicles

## Address patient's questions and concerns

- *Have you had any thoughts about what is going on?*
- *Is there anything in particular you're concerned about?*
- *Do you have anything you would like to ask?*

## Key areas for examination

A list of what to look for (in examination order; describe findings on examination)

CVS examination

Pulse: rate, rhythm, character

Heart sounds, any murmurs, e.g. aortic stenosis, HOCM. The outflow murmurs of HOCM increase with the Valsalva manoeuvre (aortic outflow obstruction and mitral regurgitation), and reduce with squatting

BP

L/S BP – ask for the results

ECG: rate, rhythm; QTC; heart blocks/interventricular conduction delays; δ-waves in WPW

Blood glucose

Drug chart/medication list

Say that you would like to carry out a complete neurological examination to exclude a neurological event

## Differential diagnosis

In the elderly, most likely causes are:

Orthostatic hypotension

Reflex syncope (e.g. carotid sinus hypersensitivity)

Cardiac disease (including brady- and tachyarrhythmias)

Unexplained

PE

## Discussion with patient

Explain diagnosis

Explain plan, including investigations and management

Address patient's concerns/answer their questions

Your collapse sounds like it is due to your blood pressure dropping when you stand up, and this can cause you to black out/lose consciousness. It doesn't sound like a seizure, but we need the results of some tests to help work out why you had the collapse. I will arrange some tests now (blood tests, X-rays) and a heart scan as an outpatient, to find out the cause. I don't think we'll need to keep you in hospital, but I will arrange for you to see the consultant in clinic once the results are back.

## Investigations

Blood tests: exclude severe anaemia

ECG

Blood glucose

Drug chart/medication list: looking for drugs which can cause syncope or exacerbate causative conditions

Consider (and explain what they may show/what you are looking for):

Carotid sinus massage

ECHO (structural heart disease/valvular lesions, e.g. severe aortic stenosis, LV dysfunction, HOCM, cardiac tamponade, tumour or thrombus, aortic dissection)

Tilt table: to differentiate between reflex syncope and orthostatic hypotension. Forms of reflex syncope include vasovagal syncope, situational syncope and carotid sinus syncope

Cardiac monitoring: various options; start with 24 h tape (Holter monitoring). Later options include an event recorder (7 days) or an implantable loop recorder

## Management

Stop any drugs which are either causing or exacerbating the problems

## Addressing concerns/answering questions

• *Have I had a seizure?* Your collapse is due to your blood pressure dropping when you stand up causing you to black out. It doesn't sound like a seizure. We need the results of some basic tests to help work out why you had the collapse and we can arrange some of those now – blood tests, X-rays, and I'll arrange some other tests as an outpatient to find out the cause.

• *Do I have to stay in hospital?* I don't think we'll need to keep you in hospital, but I'll come back and let you know when all the results are back from today's tests.

## Discussion with examiners

The examiners may ask you to clarify details of the above diagnosis and ask questions about your planned investigations and management.

A possible question includes:

• *The history sounds like postural hypotension – what would a tilt-table test add?* Provides hard evidence of susceptibility to vasovagal syncope (and helps confirm this as the diagnosis); can help guide further management depending on the pattern seen.

---

**Examiners' information and requirements**

The candidate should:

1. Identify key features from the history: episode of syncope consistent with orthostatic hypotension
2. Identify key examination findings including normal examination findings; need for L/S BP
3. Outline a sensible management plan, including advice on driving, outpatient investigations
4. Give a clear explanation to the patient of your diagnosis and plan, address his concerns and answer his questions

---

# Scenario 37 | Chronic obstructive pulmonary disease (COPD)

## Candidate's information

**Your role:** you are an ST2 in the general medical clinic. You have been asked by a GP to see this 50-year-old man with known COPD regarding his weight loss. He has also noticed a recent deterioration in his exercise tolerance.

**Your task:** to assess the patient's problems and address any questions or concerns raised by him.

## Patient's information

**You are:** Trevor Bailey, a 50-year-old man.

**Your problem:** you've had chronic chest problems for the past 10–15 years. Your breathing has got noticeably worse over the past 4 months and you have had to stop working as a cleaner because of your breathing. You used to be able to climb stairs and go shopping without having to stop due to breathlessness, but now you have to stop two or three times when climbing the stairs to go to bed.

You've had a daily cough for years, producing brown/grey mucus. Your wheeze gets worse when you walk but improves with inhalers. You have been needing antibiotics frequently from your GP over this past 4 months or so, after you start coughing up green sputum.

Your bowels are regular and you have no rectal bleeding, no heartburn and no tummy pain. Swallowing is fine.

You've had a poor appetite and weight loss over the past 4 months (6 kg weight loss). The weight loss has been unintentional – you haven't been dieting. You have not been coughing up blood. Generally feeling weak and unwell.

### Past medical history and drug history:
- COPD
- No history of cardiac disease, hypertension, diabetes mellitus
- Salbutamol inhaler as needed
- Tiotropium 18 µg inh once per day
- Seretide 250 2 puffs twice per day

### Social history:
- Worked as a cleaner for past 30 years. Never been on building sites and no known contact with asbestos. Never been a miner, potter or welder
- Born in the UK, last in Europe 3 years ago, never travelled to Asia or Africa
- Smoker: 30–40 cigarettes per day for past 35 years
- Occasional alcohol (1 or 2 glasses of wine per week for past 10 years, less since you have been losing weight)

### Other issues including family history:
- No family history of TB or other lung conditions

**Your questions for the candidate:**
- *Have I got cancer?*
- *Is it worth stopping smoking now? Isn't it just too late?*

## Candidate

### History/key questions

Ask about the key respiratory symptoms:

Breathlessness – ask about triggers, current and previous exercise tolerance

Cough, sputum, fever, chest pain, haemoptysis, stridor

Any weight loss – quantify

Change in sputum produced – colour, consistency, volume

Ask about other causes of weight loss (consider non-chest causes too)

Ask about appetite, nausea or vomiting

Any change in bowel habit, rectal bleeding, dysphagia or new dyspepsia

Any fever

### Drug history

Current medications including inhalers, nebulizers

Any use of oxygen (PRN cylinder or long-term oxygen therapy)

### Past medical history

Any operations in the past

What investigations has the patient had for their lungs – spirometry, pulmonary function tests, scans, bronchoscopies, pleural biopsies, chest drains? What has been diagnosed?

### Social history

Smoking history: quantify using pack-years (20 cigarettes per day for 1 year = 1 pack-year)

Rolling tobacco: quantify in ounces per week

Ask about occupational history: asbestos exposure, coal mining, potteries, welding, and other sources of occupational dust; farming

Pets

Any family history of TB, any known TB contacts

Birthplace (area endemic for TB?)

Are you in an area endemic for TB (particularly PACES exams outside UK)?

Foreign travel in the past and where to? Any travel to Africa, India/Pakistan, Asia

### Address patient's questions and concerns

- *Have you had any thoughts about what is going on?*
- *Is there anything in particular you're concerned about?*
- *Do you have anything you would like to ask?*

## Key areas for examination

A list of what to look for (in examination order; describe findings on examination)

Overall inspection

Signs of weight loss; muscle wasting (generalized) with loose skinfolds

Respiratory rate and use of accessory muscles of breathing

Chest shape, scars on chest/drain sites/puncture wounds from biopsies

Hands: tar staining of fingers, finger clubbing, wasting of small muscles of the hand (unilateral with Pancoast tumour), $CO_2$ retention flap

Look for Horner's syndrome

Mouth/tongue: cyanosis, angular cheilitis, pursed lips

Lymphadenopathy: supraclavicular, cervical

Trachea: position/?central; hyperexpanded chest leading to tracheal tug

JVP elevated in cor pulmonale or simply due to increased intrathoracic pressures

Expansion: hyperexpanded chest

Percussion: look for signs of effusion/consolidation

Auscultation: may be normal or prolonged expiration or wheeze. Later, reduced breath sounds, crackles. Listen for signs of effusion/consolidation including bronchial breathing

Say that you would like to examine abdomen to complete your assessment for causes of weight loss

Ask to see a recent chest X-ray, blood results, medication list, spirometry, sputum culture and sensitivity

Examination in this patient – hyperexpanded chest, prolonged expiration

## Differential diagnosis

Chronic cough productive of sputum, consistent with chronic bronchitis; recurrent symptoms consistent with LRTI. Given multiple courses of antibiotics, need to consider malignancy and atypical infection including TB (patient with chronic lung disease, weight loss, extensive smoking history)

## Discussion with patient

Explain diagnosis

Explain plan, including investigations and management

Address patient's concerns/answer their questions

You have had a chronic lung problem for some time but this has got worse over the past months with weight loss. This needs to be investigated, and so we'll start with some blood tests, a sputum sample to look for infection and a chest X-ray. We will also refer you for more detailed scans of your chest and arrange an appointment to see a chest specialist who may arrange further investigations.

## Investigations

Routine bloods for FBC, ESR, CRP, U&E, TFT, TTG (exclude other causes of weight loss)

Arterial blood gas

ECG: p pulmonale (RA hypertrophy), signs of RV hypertrophy

Lung function tests

Sputum for microscopy, culture and sensitivity; may include acid-fast bacilli (AFB) and TB culture

CT chest (HRCT) ± staging CT chest for cancer

ECHO if clinical suspicion of pulmonary hypertension, CCF or cor pulmonale

## Management

Treatment depends on cause; treat any infection, diagnose/treat any malignancy found

Stop smoking and refer to smoking cessation services (combination of counselling and medical therapy)

Use of pulmonary rehabilitation

Supplements, e.g. nutritional supplements such as Fortisip/Fortijuice/Ensure, etc.

Referral to dietitians

Respiratory referral for consideration of further investigations based on results of the above tests, e.g. bronchoscopy to exclude obstructing lesion

## Addressing concerns/answering questions

- *Have I got cancer?* There are several different possible causes for becoming more breathless and also losing weight. These vary from less serious problems such as infections through to more serious problems including the most serious. Cancer is one of the serious causes, but we need to carry out these tests to find out what is causing your problems.
- *Is it worth stopping smoking now? Isn't it just too late?* It is worth stopping smoking as it reduces the ongoing damage to your lungs (it slows the decline in lung function [FEV$_1$]). We will arrange referral to the smoking cessation clinic to help you stop.

## Discussion with examiners

The examiners may ask you to clarify details of the above diagnosis and ask questions about your planned investigations and management.

Other possible questions include:
- *What is the MRC dyspnoea scale?* According to NICE guidance, this scale grades the degree of breathlessness related to activities:
  1. Not troubled by breathlessness except on strenuous exercise
  2. Short of breath when hurrying or walking up a slight hill
  3. Walks slower than contemporaries on level ground because of breathlessness or has to stop for breath when walking at own pace
  4. Stops for breath after walking about 100 metres or after a few minutes on level ground
  5. Too breathless to leave the house, or breathless when dressing or undressing.
- *Who should be assessed for supplemental oxygen (long-term oxygen therapy) at home?* According to NICE guidance, anyone with:
  - Severe outflow obstruction (FEV$_1$ <30% predicted)
  - Cyanosis
  - Polycythaemia
  - Peripheral oedema
  - Raised JVP
  - O$_2$ saturations of ≤92% breathing air

See also Vol. 1, Station 1, Respiratory, Case 3.

---

### Examiners' information and requirements

The candidate should:
1. Identify key features from the history: chronic SOB and daily sputum production consistent with chronic bronchitis; anorexia and marked weight loss; significant smoking history
2. Identify key examination findings including evidence of chronic lung disease and signs of weight loss
3. Provide a list of differential diagnoses, which includes COPD, neoplasia, TB
4. Outline a sensible management plan including the investigations outlined above
5. Give a clear explanation to the patient of your diagnosis and plan, address his concerns and answer his questions

---

## Further reading/resources

BTS/NICE COPD guidelines, updated 2010: www.guidance.nice.org.uk/CG101

GOLD www.goldcopd.org

# Scenario 38 | Asthma

## Candidate's information

**Your role:** you are the medical registrar on-call in the MAU. A 25-year-old woman has been referred by A&E with an acute asthma attack: the wheeze didn't resolve with inhalers only. She has since settled following 2 × 2.5 mg nebulized salbutamol. Observations on arrival to A&E 3 hours ago were pulse 95, RR 20, peak expiratory flow rate 300.

**Your task:** to assess the patient's problems and address any questions or concerns raised by her.

## Patient's information

**You are:** Sarah Atley, a 25-year-old woman.

**Your problem:** you have had asthma for 10 years or so. You've had a runny nose for the past 5 days. You've felt wheezy for the past 2 days and short of breath climbing stairs. No chest pain, coughing up blood or weight loss. Not feverish.

You kept using your blue inhaler until it ran out today – it didn't help a great deal today, whereas usually it does. Your GP did prescribe a brown inhaler 3 or 4 months ago but you didn't notice any difference after taking it intermittently when you felt wheezy, so you stopped it about a month ago. For the past month, you've been using the blue inhaler 3–4 times per day – this settles the feeling of wheezing and you can climb the stairs OK. Your usual PEFR is 400, and you can't remember getting much higher than this.

### Past medical history and drug history:
- Hayfever in the summer
- No eczema
- Salbutamol inhaler. No drug allergies

### Social history:
- Smoked 10/day for past 8 years
- No pets at home

### Other issues including family history:
- Usually activities are not limited – takes inhaler before playing football
- Works in IT

### Your questions for the candidate:
- *Can you give me an inhaler that works?*
- *Will the steroids/brown inhaler make me fat?*
- *Do I need to stay in hospital?*

## Candidate

### History/key questions

Symptoms of respiratory infection and asthma; ask about wheeze, chest tightness, breathlessness, cough, sputum, fever, haemoptysis

Do inhalers improve symptoms, e.g. cough, wheeze?

What makes symptoms worse: triggers include exercise, infection, allergens, drugs (β-blockers, NSAIDs), emotional upset

Patient's usual asthma control; daytime symptoms, night-time symptoms, effects on ADLs/does it stop her doing anything?

Time off school or work due to asthma

Frequency of blue inhaler use (salbutamol); patient's rating of control

Last course of oral steroids

Ever been admitted to hospital (how many times in past year?)

Ever been admitted to ICU, ever ventilated

Elicit medication list, and how often (and whether) using them. Do you ever have days when you're busy and you miss some of the doses?

Local side-effects, e.g. hoarse voice, oral thrush, taste of steroids, lack of perceived benefit

Is she using a spacer/washing mouth after steroid inhalers?

Who usually follows up her asthma – practice nurse at GP surgery or GP?

Need to elicit the patient's understanding of asthma, their use of the different types of inhalers, and the role of smoking

#### Social history

Smoker? (tobacco – quantify in pack-years; cannabis, crack cocaine)

### Address patient's questions and concerns

- *Have you had any thoughts about what is going on?*
- *Is there anything in particular you're concerned about?*
- *Do you have anything you would like to ask?*

### Key areas for examination

A list of what to look for (in examination order; describe findings on examination)

No wheeze audible on examination

Overall inspection: respiratory rate, use of accessory muscles, speaking sentences (full sentences/split sentences/unable to speak)

Chest shape; trachea position (central versus displaced)

Pulse

BP

Chest examination: expansion, percussion, auscultation, vocal resonance

Observations including $SaO_2$, temperature, PEFR on arrival and now

PEFR (actual and expected/predicted); PEFR technique

CXR

Inhaler technique: do you have your inhalers with you? I would like to check your technique (PEFR is now 350 over one hour after initial treatment)

Examine the sputum pot

### Differential diagnosis

Asthma: poor control/limited understanding/concordance (preferred term rather than 'compliance') with medications

Viral, bacterial, occupational exacerbation

Contribution of smoking

Need to consider whether this is a severe or life-threatening exacerbation of asthma?

### Discussion with patient

Explain diagnosis

Explain plan, including investigations and management

Address patient's concerns/answer their questions

Asthma is an inflammatory condition of the airways which leads to narrowing of the airways and wheeze. The blue inhaler is a reliever that you can use to open the airways when you feel wheezy, whereas the brown inhaler is a preventer used to keep the airways settled and keep the wheeze away. The reliever only works if you keep taking it regularly, and it will reduce your need for the blue inhaler. It is important to stop smoking as it can make your asthma worse

### Investigations

Blood tests including FBC, U&E, CRP

PEFR versus usual and expected PEFRs

CXR: BTS guidelines suggest not routinely recommended in absence of suspected pneumothorax, pneumomediastinum, consolidation, life-threatening asthma, failure to respond to therapy

ABG if indicated (for severe or life-threatening)

### Management

Grade severity of asthma on presentation: BTS guidelines (see *BNF*)

Smoking cessation essential

Other triggers: housedust mite, pollen, cat dander, etc.

Education about inhalers (relievers and preventers)

Does she already have a written asthma plan from her GP? PEFR machine at home?

Provide information on what to do if the condition doesn't settle on increased inhalers in the future

Asthma/respiratory specialist nurse input would be helpful, either in MAU or in the community (practice nurse)

## Addressing concerns/answering questions

• *Can you give me an inhaler that works?* You need to be on a combination of short- and long-acting inhalers. Brown inhalers work to prevent flare-ups of the asthma, and need to be taken morning and night every day, seven days per week, and it may take some time for you to notice the improvement. The blue inhaler is a reliever, to reduce the wheeze. After taking the inhalers correctly, you should notice that you don't need to use the blue one as much. If this is not the case, your GP can increase your treatment.

• *Will the steroids/brown inhaler make me fat?* No, only tiny amounts are absorbed. The vast majority of the steroids you inhale are not absorbed into the blood stream, and therefore won't cause weight gain.

• *Do I need to stay in hospital?* No, your peak flow is nearly back to your usual level, and you look to have settled on the treatment from the ED. We will need to give you a course of steroids and liaise with your GP to arrange an appointment within two days to review your progress. We will ask the respiratory team to see you in about a month's time.

## Discussion with examiners

The examiners may ask you to clarify details of the above diagnosis and ask questions about your planned investigations and management.

A possible question includes:

• *What is the definition of acute severe asthma and life-threatening asthma in terms of clinical presentation?* Acute severe asthma (according to BTS/SIGN guidelines): PEFR 33–50% of best or predicted; Respiratory rate ≥25/minute, heart rate ≥110/minute, inability to complete sentences in one breath.

Life threatening: PEFR <33% of best or predicted. $SpO_2$ <92%, $paO_2$ <8 kPa, 'normal' $paCO_2$. Clinical signs include altered consciousness level, exhaustion, arrhythmia, hypotension, cyanosis, silent chest, poor respiratory effort.

---

### Examiners' information and requirements

The candidate should:

1. Identify key features from the history: non-severe asthma attack; not requiring admission
2. Identify causes for poor asthma control, patient's understanding of asthma and inhaler use
3. Outline a sensible management plan including correct inhaler technique, explanation of inhaler use, smoking cessation
4. Give a clear explanation to the patient of your diagnosis and plan, address her concerns and answer her questions

---

### Further reading/resources

British Thoracic Society/SIGN guidance regarding asthma (2012): www.brit-thoracic.org.uk/guidelines

*British National Formulary* (BNF) 64. BMJ Publishing Group Ltd and Royal Pharmaceutical Society (2012). See asthma section (BTS guidelines on the management of acute and chronic asthma)

# Scenario 39 | Pleural effusion

## Candidate's information

**Your role:** you're one of the doctors in the MAU. A GP has referred a patient with gradual onset of shortness of breath over the past 2 months.

**Your task:** to assess the patient's problems and address any questions or concerns raised by her.

## Patient's information

**You are:** Florence Lewis, a 65-year-old woman.

**Your problem:** you have experienced increased shortness of breath over the past 2–3 months; it gradually came on and you put it down to the smoking. Slight right chest ache in the past month, worse on deep breathing. Weight loss of 8 lb over the past few months. Feeling of breathing being restricted. No cough, sputum or coughing up blood. No ankle swelling.

You saw your GP with a cough and some breathlessness two months ago, and you were prescribed some antibiotics. You felt a little better afterwards, but then the breathing got gradually worse again. You haven't seen your GP since, but saw her today and you were referred to hospital.

### Past medical history and drug history:
- Breast cancer 5 years ago (right-sided, treated by wide local excision) – doctors gave the all-clear 2 years ago, and are due to see you again in a few months' time

### Social history:
- Smoked 20/day for past 45 years. Never really considered giving up – you've been told in the past that you should
- Alcohol: a brandy at weekends only
- You have never worked with asbestos, or worked in mines or potteries

### Other issues including family history:
- Father has coeliac disease
- No known TB contacts

### Your questions for the candidate:
- *Is it serious? Is it the cancer back?*
- *Can't you just drain off the fluid?*
- *Why didn't my GP tell me about this 2 months ago when he examined me? I'd seen him with a chest infection.*

## Candidate

### History/key questions

Standard respiratory questions

Fever (acute versus chronic; any night sweats suggestive of TB)

Pleuritic chest pain (infection, PE, malignancy)

Cough, sputum, haemoptysis. Any change in sputum produced – colour, consistency, volume

SOB, change in exercise tolerance

Weight loss (quantify)

Stridor

Ask about other causes of weight loss (consider non-chest causes too): ask about appetite, any change in bowel habit, rectal bleeding, dysphagia or new dyspepsia

Any fever, lymphadenopathy

Ask if patient has noticed any lumps or bumps in the breasts or any of the glands (lymph nodes)

Questions to differentiate between neoplasia and other causes such as cardiac failure, parapneumonic, empyema, TB

### Past medical history

Any history of heart problems (IHD, heart failure), TB, breast cancer, RA, SLE, lymphoma

### Social history

Smoking and industrial history (express smoking history in pack-years)

Foreign travel to areas endemic for TB (Asia, Africa, India/Pakistan, etc.)

Any friends or relatives with TB

Born in UK or area endemic for TB

### Address patient's questions and concerns

• *Have you had any thoughts about what is going on?*
• *Is there anything in particular you're concerned about?*
• *Do you have anything you would like to ask?*

## Key areas for examination

A list of what to look for (in examination order; describe findings on examination)

Overall inspection: signs of weight loss

Respiratory rate and use of accessory muscles of breathing

Hands: tar staining of fingers, finger clubbing, wasting of small muscles of the hand (unilateral with Pancoast tumour), $CO_2$ retention flap

Look for Horner's syndrome

Evidence of RA or SLE (butterfly rash)

Mouth/tongue: cyanosis, angular cheilitis, pursed lips

Lymphadenopathy: supraclavicular, cervical, axillary (given history of breast cancer)

Trachea: position/central (trachea deviates away from side of large effusions)

JVP elevated in heart failure and in cor pulmonale

Chest examination:

  Breast examination/signs of a mastectomy

  Chest shape, scars on chest/drain sites/puncture wounds from biopsies/radiation burns

  Expansion – reduced on the side of the effusion

  Percussion – stony dull over effusion

  Auscultation – reduced breath sounds, bronchial breathing above effusion. Listen for wheeze and fine basal end-inspiratory crackles of pulmonary oedema

Look for evidence of peripheral oedema

This case: reduced chest expansion right base, reduced breath sounds right base with reduced vocal resonance; clubbing

## Differential diagnosis

Right basal pleural effusion. Need to exclude malignancy given the history, e.g. lung pathology/neoplasia given smoking history and clubbing, and consider metastatic breast cancer

Wide potential differential diagnosis list for pleural effusions, e.g. CCF, neoplasia (primary or secondary), infective/pneumonia, mesothelioma – long list of possible causes (see questions section below)

## Discussion with patient

Explain diagnosis

Explain plan, including investigations and management

Address patient's concerns/answer their questions

Some fluid is collecting around your right lung and we need to find out why this has happened as this is making you breathless. We're also concerned about your unintentional weight loss and will need to consider the full range of causes given the weight loss, history of breast cancer in the past and your smoking history. We will organize some blood tests and scans of your chest and will refer you for an urgent outpatient appointment with the respiratory physicians.

## Investigations

Routine blood tests

PA erect CXR

Diagnostic tap of fluid (ultrasound guidance) (samples for MCS, protein, albumin, LDH, cytology [to confirm malignancy, successful in about 60%]). Use of ultrasound guidance reported to increase likelihood of successful aspiration and reduce risk of organ perforation/puncture/other complications

Other tests may be required on the pleural fluid:

Glucose – very low (<1.6 mmol/L) in RA-associated effusion

pH – if empyema suspected. If less than 7.2, tube drainage of the fluid is required

Ziehl–Nielsen staining and TB culture may be indicated as part of microbiological investigations

Triglycerides and cholesterol help differentiate chylothorax

Amylase levels in pancreatitis-associated effusions

Haematocrit if haemothorax

Further investigations following respiratory review including:

Staging CT chest – review imaging at MDT meeting; further review at either breast or lung MDT depending on the cause (or both)

Pleural biopsy

Thoracoscopy or video-assisted thoracoscopic surgery (indicated if exudative effusion but has had non-conclusive diagnostic tap and malignancy still thought present)

Bronchoscopy only if haemoptysis or bronchial obstructing lesion thought present

## Management

Depends on cause: transudate versus exudate

Review of imaging at MDT

Decide on follow-up

### Addressing concerns/answering questions

- *Is it serious? Is it the cancer back?* There are various different causes for the fluid collecting round the lung. These vary from a reaction to having had an infection in the lung, through to more serious problems which can include cancer. It is important to carry out some tests to find out what is going on.
- *Can't you just drain off the fluid?* We will take some fluid off to analyse it, and this will help determine the cause of the fluid collection. The treatment of the fluid collection does depend on identifying and treating the underlying cause.
- *Why didn't my GP tell me about this 2 months ago when he examined me? I'd seen him with a chest infection.* The fluid collection may not have been there two months ago, and you received antibiotics for a chest infection. We can compare the X-rays from when you needed the antibiotics with the latest films to see how things have changed over time.

## Discussion with examiners

The examiners may ask you to clarify details of the above diagnosis and ask questions about your planned investigations and management.

Other possible questions include:

- *What are the causes of exudate (effusion fluid protein concentration >30g/L)?* Common causes include infection (pneumonia [parapneumonic]/ empyema [pH < 7.3]), TB, neoplasia (bronchial carcinoma, mesothelioma, secondaries/metastases from GI tract, breast, ovary and pancreas), lymphoma, pulmonary embolism/infarction, connective tissue disorders (RA, SLE), reactive, e.g. to pancreatitis, subphrenic collection or hepatic abscess, post CABG, post MI/ Dressler's, benign asbestos effusion. Rare causes include drugs – methotrexate, amiodarone, phenytoin, nitrofurantoin, β-blockers. Other causes include chylothorax, yellow nail syndrome and oesophageal perforation.
- *What are the causes of a transudate (effusion fluid protein concentration <30g/L)?* Common causes include congestive cardiac failure, cirrhosis (ascites crossing diaphragm to cause hepatic hydrothorax). Less common causes include hypoalbuminaemia, nephrotic syndrome, hypothyroidism, peritoneal dialysis. Rare causes include constrictive pericarditis and Meig's syndrome (ascites, pleural effusion with ovarian fibroma).

See also Vol. 1, Station 1, Respiratory, Case 5.

**Examiners' information and requirements**

The candidate should:

1. Identify key features from the history: pleural effusion in a 65-year-old woman with a recent history of lower respiratory tract infection treated with antibiotics, and a past history of breast cancer and a 45 pack-year smoking history
2. Identify key examination findings including right pleural effusion, clubbing
3. Outline a sensible management plan as detailed above including tests to determine the cause of effusion, imaging and urgent referral to the respiratory physicians
4. Give a clear explanation to the patient of your diagnosis and plan, address her concerns and answer her questions

**Further reading/resources**

British Thoracic Society Pleural Disease Guideline 2010: www.brit-thoracic.org.uk (management of pleural effusions)

# Scenario 40 | Short of breath ?pulmonary embolism

## Candidate's information

**Your role:** you are the ST2 in the MAU, and a local GP has referred a 30-year-old woman with a 4-day history of chest pain, worse on inspiration. SaO$_2$ 92% on room air, BP 130/90, pulse 110 on arrival at the MAU.

**Your task:** to assess the patient's problems and address any questions or concerns raised by her.

## Patient's information

**You are:** Vicky Rawlinson, a 30-year-old woman.

**Your problem:** you have had 4 days of right-sided chest pain, worse on coughing and deep breathing. Initially you thought that this was a muscle strain. You have become short of breath on exertion over the past few days; you've just started to get breathless climbing stairs. You thought this was because the pain was limiting your breathing. No recent long journeys or air travel. No pain in calf or swelling. No cough or haemoptysis.

You gave birth to a healthy baby boy 10 days ago (vaginal delivery, no tears or stitches). You were on enoxaparin (heparin) injections daily in the late stages of pregnancy because of your history of three previous miscarriages. You were advised to continue after you gave birth, but you haven't taken any since you left hospital.

### Past medical history and drug history:
- No previous admissions to hospital other than for the birth. No operations previously
- No past history of DVT or PE
- On oral contraceptive pill prior to pregnancy – Dianette (third-generation OCP)
- One child (recently born)

### Social history:
- Smokes 5/day
- Alcohol: 3 pints of lager on Friday and Saturday nights usually. None for past 7 months since found out about pregnancy
- Works in sales (desk job)

### Other issues including family history:
- Sister had several clots in her legs during her 20s – now on long-term warfarin
- You plan to have more children

**Your questions for the candidate:**
- *Can I still stay on the pill?*
- *How long is the treatment if it is a clot?*
- *Can I try for more children whilst on warfarin?*
- *Can I still breastfeed while I have the injections or if taking warfarin?*
- *Can I go home tonight to be with my baby?*

---

## Candidate

### History/key questions

Examination normal – reports chest pain on deep inspiration and coughing only

Full respiratory questions

SOB: onset, what makes her SOB (e.g. at rest, walking upstairs, walking 1 mile)?

Cough, sputum, any haemoptysis. What's her usual baseline exercise tolerance?

Pleuritic chest pain: site, onset, exacerbants

Wheeze?

Ask for features suggestive of an alternative to PE as the cause of pain, e.g. any recent heavy lifting or trauma to suggest musculoskeletal pain; cough productive of sputum, rigors/fevers

Any syncopal episodes or history consistent with postural hypotension

Any calf pain, swelling

Any vaginal bleeding / how much vaginal bleeding post-birth – should have slowed or nearly stopped by 10 days. Ask about other sources of bleeding if considering full dose anticoagulation or potentially needing thrombolysis – breathlessness could be due to anaemia as a consequence of blood loss peripartum

Risk factors for DVT/PE: recent operation(s), long journeys/prolonged immobility or reduced mobility, neoplasia, pregnancy

Any known thrombophilia (factor V Leiden, protein C and protein S deficiency: AT III)

If female, any recurrent miscarriages suggestive of antiphospholipid syndrome (this is the likely indication for her needing enoxaparin in pregnancy)

Anyone in the family ever had a clot in the legs or lungs, etc., and does any clotting problem run in the family?

#### Drug history

Including use of oral contraceptive pill, any inhalers

Any allergies to medications

#### Past medical history

Any previous DVT, PE or arterial thrombi

Any history of respiratory problems such as asthma

#### Social history

Smoking and alcohol history

NB: must think about the newborn baby too – is mother breastfeeding? Who is looking after the baby at the moment? If breastfeeding and V/Q or CTPA planned, will need to express milk before either scan. Then will need to discard milk until able to restart breastfeeding 8 h after CTPA, 12 h after V/Q or Q scanning (check hospital's local protocols)

Some obstetric units will look after new mothers and newborn babies whilst awaiting inpatient investigations, e.g. for PE, particularly when the baby is only a few days old

Aim to keep baby and mother together – bonding important

Does she have her midwife's contact details and the name of her obstetrician? Does she have any letters regarding her previous investigations, and the indication for enoxaparin? If at same hospital, check electronic patient record. Contact the obstetric registrar on-call for advice

### Address patient's questions and concerns
- *Have you had any thoughts about what is going on?*
- *Is there anything in particular you're concerned about?*
- *Do you have anything you would like to ask?*

### Key areas for examination

A list of what to look for (in examination order; describe findings on examination)

Any chest pain or SOB?

Respiratory rate and use of accessory muscles of breathing

CVS: pulse, BP, $SaO_2$

Hands and peripheral perfusion/any cyanosis

Mouth/tongue: cyanosis, angular cheilitis, pursed lips

Lymphadenopathy: supraclavicular, cervical, axillary

Respiratory: trachea – position/central

JVP: elevated in heart failure, cor pulmonale and in massive PE (can be associated with acute RV failure – increased JVP, parasternal heave)

Chest wall inspection/chest shape:

Expansion

Percussion

Auscultation

May have a pleural rub with PE or pneumonia; wheeze can be heard in acute PE

Look for clinical evidence of DVT or oedema

Ask to see ECG, ABG results and a CXR if already performed

## Differential diagnosis

Pulmonary embolism is the key differential which needs to be excluded given her presentation in the immediate post-partum period and her risk factors (probable antiphospholipid syndrome and family history of recurrent VTE requiring lifelong warfarin)

Musculoskeletal pain

Pneumonia: but no fever, cough or sputum, and chest clear on examination

The most common symptoms of PE are SOB, pleuritic chest pain, cough, calf or leg swelling, and signs can include tachycardia, tachypnoea, clinical signs of DVT; hypotension is less common but massive PE can lead to right ventricular failure (raised JVP, parasternal heave and S3 – pulmonary component of S2)

Given her recent pregnancy, need for enoxaparin (presumed antiphospholipid syndrome) and now pleuritic chest pain with hypoxia, need to exclude PE

## Discussion with patient

Explain diagnosis

Explain plan, including investigations and management

Address patient's concerns/answer their questions

You report chest pain worse on breathing in or coughing shortly after giving birth and this means that we need to exclude a clot in the lung. It is likely that the obstetricians were giving you blood-thinning injections during your pregnancy for something called the antiphospholipid syndrome. This condition leads to the recurrent miscarriages that you have had in the past and also makes clots more likely even though you have been having the injections. We plan to give you a full

dose of the injection to thin the blood and carry out a scan to confirm the presence of a clot.

## Investigations

Stratification of probability of PE based on history, examination, investigations and two-level Wells score

ECG: most common ECG findings are a normal ECG or sinus tachycardia. Look for signs of right heart strain. Can also see non-specific changes in T-waves and ST segments

CXR: can be normal. Look for small effusions, segmental or subsegmental collapse

ABG may be normal: check alveolar-arterial (A-a) gradient as may indicate V/Q mismatch

NICE advise use of the two-level Wells Score for PE (Table H40.1)

**Table H40.1** Two-level Wells score

| Clinical feature | Points |
|---|---|
| Clinical signs and symptoms of DVT (minimum of leg swelling and pain on palpation of the deep veins) | 3 |
| An alternative diagnosis is less likely than PE | 3 |
| Heart rate > 100 beats per minute | 1.5 |
| Immobilization for more than 3 days or surgery in the previous 4 weeks | 1.5 |
| Previous DVT/PE | 1.5 |
| Haemoptysis | 1 |
| Malignancy (on treatment, treated in the last 6 months, or palliative) | 1 |

Clinical probability simplified scores

| | |
|---|---|
| PE *likely* | More than 4 points |
| PE *unlikely* | 4 points or less |

If PE *likely* according to Wells score, NICE recommend CT pulmonary angiogram. If CTPA contraindicated (allergy to contrast media, renal impairment, or those in whom the radiation risk would be too high) then VQ scan indicated. If this test (CTPA or VQ) is negative, and DVT is suspected, arrange a Doppler ultrasound of the leg to confirm/exclude DVT

If two-level Wells score is *unlikely* PE, NICE advises to check D-dimer. If positive, arrange CTPA. If negative, excludes PE, but patient needs to be aware of the symptoms and signs of PE, and when to return to hospital (safety-netting)

NICE advises to consider alternative diagnoses if:

• Patients with an *unlikely* two-level PE Wells score and **either** a negative D-dimer test **or** a positive D-dimer test and a negative CTPA

- Patients with a *likely* two-level PE Wells score and **both** a negative CTPA **and** no suspected DVT

D-dimer is however unlikely to be helpful in this patient as it is likely to be elevated with recent childbirth and she has a high clinical probability of PE

Arrange CTPA (scores 4+ as heart rate > 100, alternative diagnosis less likely than PE). NB breastfeeding advice above

If unstable (massive PE/shock), urgent CTPA but if too unstable for CT, then bedside ECHO to look at right heart (assess for RV dysfunction/dilation [RV overload]) and consider thrombolytic therapy (note contraindications and relative contraindications to thrombolysis)

Role of thrombophilia screen whilst unanticoagulated: lupus anticoagulant in the meantime

## Management

Admit

Low molecular weight heparin/anticoagulation: give in this case at treatment dose (e.g. enoxaparin 1.5 mg/kg sc od)

Consider ambulatory care of PE only if low-risk presentation and protocols are in place for this at your institution (check local arrangements/protocols)

Arrange for care of mother and baby/liaise with midwife and on-call O&G team

## Addressing concerns/answering questions

- *Can I still stay on the pill?* If you are found to have a clot, we would advise against continuing the combined oral contraceptive pill due to the increased risk of clotting. You can't take this during breastfeeding (affects milk supply). Your GP will be able to advise you further about contraception, and it is possible to go onto the progesterone-only pill whilst breastfeeding and it is better in terms of clot risk. Other alternative contraceptives are available including coils, implants and injections.
- *How long is the treatment if it is a clot?* This does depend on whether you have any predisposing reasons for developing clots. We need more information about why you were on the heparin injections as this will affect the length of time you need the warfarin. You will need warfarin for at least 6 months, but you may need longer term anticoagulation and we will ask the haematologist to see you in clinic to advise about this. They will be able to decide how long they think you will need the warfarin.
- *Can I try for more children whilst on warfarin?* We strongly advise you to use an effective form of con-

traception whilst on warfarin as this medicine can affect the unborn child/foetus causing birth defects. If, after seeing the haematologists, they decide that you need to be on warfarin long-term, then we would need to plan future pregnancies with the help of medical obstetricians and the haematologists, as a switch to enoxaparin injections would be required rather than the warfarin.

- *Can I still breastfeed while I have the injections or if taking warfarin?* Neither cross the placenta, so you can breastfeed on enoxaparin or warfarin.
- *Can I go home tonight?* The answer to this question depends on whether there are ambulatory care pathways in place for PE, and which criteria are used. In the interim, I would advise staying in and having the scan as an inpatient. We are getting in touch with the obstetricians to see if you can be admitted to their ward and keep your baby with you.

## Discussion with examiners

The examiners may ask you to clarify details of the above diagnosis and ask questions about your planned investigations and management

Investigations and management:

Family history of thromboembolic disease and gives history consistent with antiphospholipid syndrome (recurrent miscarriage/arterial and venous thrombosis) requiring enoxaparin pre-delivery. She now presents with pleuritic chest pain and hypoxia in the postpartum period; need to anticoagulate and exclude PE.

Other possible questions include:

- *What are the side-effects of enoxaparin?* Haemorrhage, thrombocytopenia, osteoporosis, hyperkalaemia (inhibition of aldersterone), injection site reactions, allergic reactions including anaphylaxis.
- *Please discuss the administration of warfarin/enoxaparin in pregnancy and breast-feeding.* Warfarin doesn't cross into breast milk in significant amounts and is reported to be safe. Low molecular weight heparin molecules are too large to cross into breast milk. Warfarin can cross the placenta so it is essential for the patient to use a reliable form of contraception due to risks of warfarin on the foetus (nasal hypoplasia, stippled epiphyses, choanal stenosis due to warfarin use in the first trimester. Risk of bleeding in foetus in later pregnancy/third trimester). Stillbirth/foetal death is more common in warfarin-treated mothers). Low molecular weight heparin does not cross the placenta and is not known to be harmful.

- *Is a D-dimer going to be helpful?* As the two-level Wells PE score is 4 or above (recent pregnancy/PE most likely diagnosis = score of at least 4.5) then imaging is required without the need for a D-dimer. It would probably be elevated due to the recent pregnancy and isn't indicated in a patient with high clinical probability of PE.

---

### Examiners' information and requirements

The candidate should:

1. Identify key features from the history: post-partum, family history of DVT, recurrent miscarriages → enoxaparin given during pregnancy, presents with history consistent with PE
2. Identify key examination findings including normal examination but pleuritic pain (on coughing/breathing in)
3. Outline a sensible management plan; includes appropriate investigation and treatment for PE; giving low molecular weight heparin as treatment for PE whilst awaiting scans
4. Give a clear explanation to the patient of your diagnosis and plan, address her concerns and answer her questions

### Further reading/resources

Agnelli G. Current concepts: acute pulmonary embolism. NEJM 2010;363:266–74.

Royal College of Obstetricians and Gynaecologists' guideline on thromboembolic disease in pregnancy/peripartum period: www.rcog.org.uk

NICE guidelines on PE (2012) – includes Wells scores and flowcharts for DVT and PE: www.guidance.nice.org.uk/CG144

# Scenario 41 | Rheumatoid arthritis/ breathlessness

## Candidate's information
**Your role:** you are working in the general medical clinic, and have been referred a 65-year-old woman with a chronic dry cough and breathlessness. Her rheumatoid arthritis is well controlled.

**Your task:** to assess the patient's problems and address any questions or concerns raised by her.

## Patient's information
**You are:** Lina Thomas, a 65-year-old woman.

**Your problem:** you have had rheumatoid arthritis for the past 18 years. Your hands and wrists were the main problem but they have settled down over the past few years. You've been able to go back to work full time, and have been feeling well with no problems with your joints. You took methotrexate weekly for 4 years.

You have had a dry cough for the past six months, thought by your GP to be due to acid reflux. No improvement with the antiacid medication omeprazole. You're not coughing up any mucus. No nocturnal cough or wheezing. You have no haemoptysis, wheezing, fever or chest pain. Your weight is stable.

You have been gradually feeling more breathless on exertion. A year ago, you were able to walk as far as you wanted. Now you get a little short of breath at about 500 yards or if you climb your stairs too fast at home. You have only really begun to notice this over the past few months.

You last went abroad 2 years ago to Spain. You've never been to Africa, Asia or outside Europe.

You've never met anyone with TB and no-one in the family has TB. One of your friends was reading on the internet and suggested you ask the specialist about TB. You've been worried since, as you could then have passed it on to your family,

If asked, you did have some breathing tests before going onto methotrexate – you were told that these were normal.

## Past medical history and drug history:
- Rheumatoid arthritis
- Never had any operations, and never admitted to hospital
- Never had gold injections for your arthritis

## Social history:
- Ex-smoker, 10/day for 10 years. Stopped 10 years ago
- No pets (cats, birds, etc.)
- Works in an office – not been to any farms. Never worked in the mines, potteries, etc.

**Other issues including family history:**

Nil of note

**Your questions for the candidate:**
- *What's making me so breathless?*
- *Will I have to stop the methotrexate? It's helped me so much.*
- *Is it TB? I have been reading about it on the internet.*
- *Can you treat it?*

---

# Candidate

## History/key questions

Ask about breathlessness, particularly on exertion, and any changes in recent months/years

Current exercise tolerance and premorbid exercise tolerance, e.g. 6 months ago before the breathlessness began

Cough, and whether dry or productive of sputum. Any nocturnal cough?

Sputum: dry cough versus thick, purulent sputum in bronchiectasis

Chest pain: pleuritic, heaviness, ache

Weight loss, change in appetite

Wheeze, haemoptysis, fever

Any exacerbants noticed?

Any history of foreign travel, TB contacts/family history of TB

Birthplace: was she born in an area endemic for TB?

### Past medical history

Any known lung disease: asthma, COPD, past neoplasia

Any history of radiotherapy, e.g. for breast cancer

### Drug history

Drug causes of pulmonary fibrosis: gold injections (fibrosis can be reversible); methotrexate; list includes amiodarone, bleomycin, nitrofurantoin, sulphasalazine

### Social history

Smoking history

Any pet birds/pigeons, etc. Any other pets

Occupational history including exposure to asbestos, mining, potteries, welding, farming

## Address patient's questions and concerns

- *Have you had any thoughts about what is going on?*
- *Is there anything in particular you're concerned about?*
- *Do you have anything you would like to ask?*

# Key areas for examination

A list of what to look for (in examination order; describe findings on examination)

Overall inspection: signs of weight loss

Respiratory rate and use of accessory muscles of breathing

Hands: symmetrical deforming arthropathy of RA

Tar staining of fingers, finger clubbing (bronchiectasis), wasting of small muscles of the hand (unilateral with Pancoast tumour), $CO_2$ retention flap

Look for rheumatoid nodules on extensor aspect of elbows

Face: look for Horner's syndrome; evidence of SLE (butterfly rash)

Mouth/tongue: cyanosis, angular cheilitis

Lymphadenopathy: supraclavicular, cervical

Trachea: position

JVP

Chest examination: includes inspection for radiation burns, radiotherapy tattoos, scars on chest/drain sites/puncture wounds from biopsies. Shape of chest including any evidence of hyperexpansion

Signs of a previous mastectomy (tattoos and skin changes from previous radiation): if so, say you would do breast examination

Expansion

Percussion: can be reduced

Auscultation: air entry can be reduced in fibrosis. Listen for fine end-inspiratory crackles, including at axilla. Signs may be basal or apical

Look for other respiratory manifestations of RA including pleural effusion

Ask to see the observation chart including $SaO_2$, RR, pulse and BP; medication lists, spirometry, recent CXR

This patient has fine basal crackles that don't clear with coughing.

## Differential diagnosis

Interstitial lung disease such as pulmonary fibrosis: either as consequence of methotrexate therapy (basal) or as rheumatoid lung (apical or basal fibrosis).

## Discussion with patient

Explain diagnosis
Explain plan, including investigations and management
Address patient's concerns/answer their questions

Your cough and shortness of breath may be due to some inflammation or scarring in your lungs. We need to carry out some tests to find out why this is happening. It can happen with the rheumatoid arthritis or because of the methotrexate. We need to find out the answer so that the rheumatologists can decide whether to continue with the methotrexate or switch you to a different medicine. I'll arrange some X-rays and blood tests, and ask the chest doctors to see you urgently in their clinic.

## Investigations

Basic bloods including FBC, ESR, CRP
CXR
HRCT
Full pulmonary function tests including TLCO (and then compare to baseline tests pre-methotrexate)
Respiratory referral ± further investigations as indicated, e.g. bronchoscopy

## Management

Review of methotrexate with the results of the above investigations – stop the drug now and review in clinic.

The investigations will need to be urgent, and she will need review by the rheumatologist responsible for her care. Will need to let her rheumatology specialist nurses know about this new development, and the plans for referral/investigation. They will be able to arrange appropriate rheumatology follow-up, and are likely to be the clinicians responsible for monitoring and/or prescribing the methotrexate currently.

## Addressing concerns/answering questions

- *What's making me so breathless?* There is a wide range of causes for breathlessness and we need to arrange some tests to find out why. Your cough and shortness of breath may be due to some inflammation or scarring in your lungs. It can happen with the rheumatoid arthritis or because of the methotrexate.
- *Will I have to stop the methotrexate? It's helped me so much.* Methotrexate is one possible cause of your breathlessness, but we need to find out the actual cause(s) so that the rheumatologists can decide whether to continue with the methotrexate or switch you to a different medicine.
- *Is it TB? I have been reading about it on the internet.* I don't think you have TB as your symptoms aren't suggestive of TB, and you are at low risk given your lack of foreign travel, no TB contacts, etc.
- *Can you treat it?* Treatment depends on the cause, which can range from simply stopping methotrexate, through to medications such as steroids.

## Discussion with examiners

The examiners may ask you to clarify details of the above diagnosis and ask questions about your planned investigations and management.

Other possible questions include:
- *What are the other respiratory manifestations of RA?* Pleural effusions (exudates), pleural nodules, interstitial lung disease, pneumonitis, bleeding, Caplan's syndrome, bronchiectasis, bronchiolitis obliterans, pulmonary hypertension, pulmonary vasculitis.
- *What are the causes of pulmonary fibrosis?* Causes can be categorized into disease groups – connective tissue disorders/rheumatological disorders, drugs, extrinsic allergic alveolitis, granulomatous diseases (TB, sarcoid), industrial dust diseases, post radiation, cryptogenic fibrosing alveolitis.

See also Vol. 1, Station 1, Respiratory, Case 6 and Section I, Station 5, Locomotor, Case 1.

---

**Examiners' information and requirements**

The candidate should:
1. Identify key features from the history: dry cough, progressive SOB in patient with RA, and taking methotrexate
2. Identify key examination findings including evidence of RA (hands ± nodules), and bilateral fine basal crackles on chest examination
3. Differential diagnosis to include interstitial lung disease/pulmonary fibrosis due to rheumatoid arthritis or methotrexate
4. Outline a sensible management plan, including a multidisciplinary approach to management, involving the patient, rheumatology and respiratory physicians
5. Give a clear explanation to the patient of your diagnosis and plan, address her concerns and answer her questions

# Scenario 42 | Haemoptysis

## Candidate's information

**Your role:** you are an ST2 in the MAU and you've been referred Mr Gillingham, a 60-year-old man who reports several episodes of haemoptysis. He has been treated for a lower respiratory tract infection, but symptoms persist.

**Your task:** to assess the patient's problems and address any questions or concerns raised by him.

## Patient's information

**You are:** Gary Gillingham, a 60-year-old man.

**Your problem:** you've coughed up blood once or twice a day for the past 3 weeks. Initially there were only little streaks in your spit every time, but this week you've been coughing up a little more; today was a teaspoon-full of blood, so you thought that it was time to come to hospital.

Two weeks ago, you went to your GP who thought that it could all be due to a chest infection so prescribed a 5-day course of amoxicillin, but this didn't help. You saw a different GP today and she referred you up here. You have not had a chest X-ray yet.

You usually cough up greeny-white sputum every morning; you call this your 'smoker's cough'.

You've lost 5 kg in weight over the past 2 months and your appetite is slightly reduced. No chest pain, wheeze, fever or night sweats.

Your exercise tolerance is unchanged – able to walk at least a mile on the flat.

### Past medical history and drug history:
- No current medications
- No allergies known
- Never had TB, not known to have kidney problems

### Social history:
- Smoking: 20 cigarettes per day for the past 40 years
- You live alone with your puppy, Buster, who can't be left alone for long as he wrecks the house
- Born in the UK
- Last foreign travel 6 months ago to Spain, never been outside Europe

### Other issues including family history:
- No-one in the family has been unwell
- No history of TB or cancer
- Both parents died in their sleep in their 70s

**Your questions for the candidate:**

- *Is it cancer?*
- *Do I have to stay in hospital?*

---

## Candidate

### History/key questions

Ask patient to describe the events. Need to be clear that it is haemoptysis that's being reported rather than haematemesis

Onset, duration and frequency of haemoptysis

Appearances of blood, volume (e.g. clots, large cupful versus streaks in sputum)

Sputum: colour, change from normal

Any evidence of infection: fever, sputum. Any chronic lung disease?

Ask about respiratory symptoms including breathlessness, wheeze, chest pain, weight loss, cough and sputum

Any known medical conditions (Ehlers–Danlos); any kidney problems in the past (Goodpasture's, Wegener's granulomatosis)?

Ever had TB in the past?

Any recent procedures (bronchoscopy, lung biopsy)

Ask about foreign travel (PE)

Any foreign body ingestion: choking episodes prior to the onset of haemoptysis?

### Drug history

Anticoagulant, antiplatelet use

Any cocaine use

### Social history

Smoking history in pack-years

Alcohol use

### Address patient's questions and concerns

- *Have you had any thoughts about what is going on?*
- *Is there anything in particular you're concerned about?*
- *Do you have anything you would like to ask?*

## Key areas for examination

A list of what to look for (in examination order; describe findings on examination)

Overall inspection: signs of weight loss

Respiratory rate and use of accessory muscles of breathing

Hands: tar staining of fingers, finger clubbing, wasting of small muscles of the hand (unilateral with Pancoast tumour), $CO_2$ retention flap

Look for Horner's syndrome

Mouth/tongue: cyanosis, angular cheilitis, pursed lips

Lymphadenopathy: supraclavicular, cervical, axillary

Trachea: position

Chest examination:

Chest shape, scars on chest/drain sites/puncture wounds from biopsies/radiation burns

Hyperexpanded chest/signs of chronic lung disease

Expansion/percussion/auscultation: any evidence of collapse/consolidation/effusion

Look for oedema/DVT

Ask to see observations chart including oxygen saturations, chest X-ray, routine blood tests, sputum culture if available

## Differential diagnosis

Haemoptysis and weight loss in a 40 pack-year smoker without symptoms of respiratory infection: top differential diagnosis is bronchial neoplasia but important to exclude TB and pulmonary infection, vasculitis/Wegener's/Goodpasture's

Haemoptysis can be caused by airways disease, pulmonary parenchymal or vascular diseases

## Discussion with patient

Explain diagnosis

Explain plan, including investigations and management

Address patient's concerns/answer their questions

Coughing up blood is concerning and we need to look for causes for this in the breathing pipes. I'll arrange a chest X-ray and blood tests here now and then we can discuss the results. I think we'll need to arrange a scan of your chest as an outpatient, and refer you to the chest doctors for further investigations which may include a camera test looking into the airways. It's important to stop smoking – I can refer you to the smoking cessation clinic.

## Investigations

Bloods including U&E, FBC, CRP, ESR, INR, calcium, anti-GBM antibody

Urinalysis (Goodpasture's, Wegener's)

CXR

HRCT chest/staging CT as neoplasia suspected

Sputum culture/MCS and AFB

## Management

Urgent respiratory referral (rapid access pathway/2-week wait clinic)

Bronchoscopy

Referral to smoking cessation service

### Addressing concerns/answering questions

• *Is it cancer?* We need to look for all the different causes for you coughing up blood, ranging from infection to more serious problems, which includes cancer. We are waiting for an X-ray today here and some blood tests but it's likely that we will need to arrange an urgent scan of your chest, and referring you to the chest doctors who will see you in clinic; they may well arrange a special camera test to look into the breathing tubes to find out the cause of the bleeding.

• *Do I have to stay in hospital?* We need to wait and see what the results show, but it's likely that we can arrange any necessary scans as an outpatient, and follow-up in the respiratory clinic.

## Discussion with examiners

The examiners may ask you to clarify details of the above diagnosis and ask questions about your planned investigations and management.

A possible question includes:
• *What are the causes of haemoptysis to consider?* Pneumonia, neoplasia (lung cancer), tuberculosis, pulmonary embolism, bronchiectasis, vasculitis and pulmonary haemorrhage (Goodpasture's).

---

### Examiners' information and requirements

The candidate should:

1. Identify key features from the history. These include weight loss, smoking history, haemoptysis

2. Identify key examination findings including signs of weight loss, tar staining, clubbing

3. Provide a list of differential diagnoses including neoplasia and TB

4. Outline a sensible management plan, including appropriate referrals for investigations and smoking cessation, and to respiratory clinic

5. Give a clear explanation to the patient of your diagnosis and plan, address his concerns and answer his questions

---

# Other reported respiratory cases

- Patient with haemoptysis and Ehlers–Danlos syndrome
- Chronic cough
- Pulmonary TB

# Scenario 43 | Headache: progressive/ memory issues

## Candidate's information

**Your role:** you are the SHO in the Medical Assessment Unit. Mr Johnstone is a 55-year-old man referred by his GP with a history of headache and poor concentration. He has presented to the MAU with his wife who provides the bulk of the history.

**Your task:** to assess the patient's problems and address any questions or concerns raised by him and his wife.

## Patient's information

**You are:** Jacob Johnstone, a 55-year-old right-handed accountant.

**Your problem:** you have had 6–8 weeks of dull, constant, right-sided headaches, which you attributed to stress at work and poor sleep. The headaches have gradually got worse/more frequent over this period and have been a little worse at night, and you thought that they have been waking you up.

Over the past few weeks, you've noticed difficulty reading, particularly the start of sentences, and colleagues have noticed that your writing isn't as neat as before. You are an ardent fan of the *Times* crossword but have found it much harder than usual over the past 4 weeks at least. You've been intermittently forgetful. You work as an accountant and are the sole income earner for the household. You have no weakness in the arms or legs. No unsteadiness whilst walking. No double vision. No fever, cough, shortness of breath. No weight loss, change in bowel or bladder. Your wife has noticed that you've been a little aggressive at times at home, getting angrier quickly.

No history of epilepsy or seizures. No episodes of loss of consciousness or collapses. You are experiencing reduced appetite, and perhaps feeling a little nauseated at times.

### Past medical history and drug history:
• No relevant previous history and on no medication

### Social history:
• Lives with wife
• Ex-smoker: 25/day for 20 years
• No recent foreign travel

### Other issues including family history:
• No illnesses run in the family

### Your questions for the candidate:
• *Is it a brain tumour? I've been reading up on the internet.*
• *Is it because I smoked?*

## Candidate

### History/key questions

History may well be mainly provided by his wife, particularly if he is confused or disorientated

The combination of headache and change in cognitive function points towards a structural space-occupying lesion but other differential diagnoses need to be considered, including subacute meningitis, e.g. TB or malignant meningitis, chronic subdural haematoma. Also headache and cognitive blunting can rarely be a presentation of giant cell arteritis

Ask about:

Headache

Nausea/vomiting

Seizures or episodes of loss of consciousness/collapse

Cognitive dysfunction, change in personality

Speech disturbance

Visual disturbance/change in visual fields

Scalp tenderness

Consider TB meningitis and other subacute meningitides, e.g. cryptococcus, lymphoma or primary non-bacterial meningitis (causes include inflammatory, neoplastic, paraneoplastic, granulomatous disease)

Ask about night sweats, fevers and constitutional symptoms, such as weight loss, anorexia

Also enquire about recent travel and any possible contacts with TB or infectious diseases

Right- or left-handed in order to assess likelihood of dysphasia

Any falls or history of head injury (even if thought trivial)

### Drug history

Any new medicines: ask about the use of opiates/codeine for headache, use of sedatives such as benzodiazepines

### Past medical history

Any known neoplasia in the past including brain, lung, melanoma, renal cell cancer, breast or colorectal cancer

### Social history

Alcohol intake (consider Wernicke's encephalopathy in differential diagnosis for memory impairment)

Smoking history in pack-years

Anyone else in the family unwell, e.g. partner also suffering from carbon monoxide poisoning?

Any recent foreign travel?

### Address patient's questions and concerns

• *Have you had any thoughts about what is going on?*

• *Is there anything in particular you're concerned about?*

• *Do you have anything you would like to ask?*

## Key areas for examination

A list of what to look for (in examination order; describe findings on examination)

Assess AMT (MMSE ideally, although clear time constraints); at the very least, check orientation to time, place and person. Briefly assess receptive language function by asking patient to perform simple commands, e.g. 'Could you close your eyes, please?', 'Could you show me your right hand?'. Be careful not to gesture and so give non-verbal clues

Also check expressive language function by asking patient to name common objects, e.g. a pen, a watch and a key

The CNS is the focus but there won't be time for a full neurological examination

Cranial nerves; pupils (ensure equal); look for diplopia/ VI palsy

Fundoscopy: look for signs of papilloedema

Visual fields: also look for features of inattention, which may be present even when visual fields are full

Tenderness over temporal arteries

To complete the examination, you would like to formally assess all the cranial nerves and perform a full examination of the peripheral nervous system. The changes may well be subtle, e.g. unilateral slight pupil asymmetry or unilateral pronator drift, even if the patient hasn't reported limb weakness

Ask the patient to walk to assess for ataxia and gait apraxia which is commonly seen in disorders of the periventricular white matter, e.g. normal pressure hydrocephalus and small vessel cerebrovascular disease

Examination of the chest and abdomen would be appropriate to look for features of pleural effusion or mass lesion but if not possible (likely given time constraints), this should at least be mentioned as a necessary part of the examination in clinical practice

## Differential diagnosis

Progressive neurological problem: symptoms consistent with cerebral tumour/space-occupying lesion in the absence of other clues but other conditions to consider would include:

Subacute meningitides, e.g. TB, primary non-bacterial meningitis, lymphoma or cryptococcus: unlikely in the absence of other clues, such as constitutional symptoms; previous malignancy; history of TB or HIV exposure

Cerebral vasculitis or granulomatous angiitis of the CNS – rare but treatable but less likely in the absence of other features of vasculitis systemically

Chronic subdural haematoma – more likely in the elderly but has to be considered

An atypical presentation of giant cell arteritis – cognitive symptoms are rare but can occur but other focal neurological signs might well be present, e.g. cranial nerve palsies

Depression and functional headache – an important differential as this combination is common and potentially treatable

Metabolic causes such as hyponatraemia or hypercalcaemia or hypothyroidism, worth mentioning

## Discussion with patient

Explain diagnosis

Explain plan, including investigations and management

Address patient's concerns/answer their questions

We need to find out what is causing these problems. Our main concern is that something is wrong in the brain – causes can range from minor to the most serious, including tumours. We will need to do some investigations, starting with blood tests. You may also need a chest X-ray and some brain scans. We would advise you not to drive until the investigations have been completed and in due course the DVLA may need to be informed.

### Investigations

Symptoms suggestive of progressive structural neurological problem: headache (worse overnight), with features of raised intracranial pressure, visual issues, memory and concentration

TFT, U&E (exclude hyponatraemia/metabolic problems, uraemia)

CXR

CT with contrast or MRI

### Addressing concerns/answering questions

- *Is it a brain tumour? I've been reading up on the internet.* We need to carry out tests to find out what is causing the headaches and memory problems. I plan to do a scan of the brain which would tell us whether there are signs of, e.g. bleeding in the brain or a growth or tumour but there are several other possible causes too.

- *Is it because I smoked?* Smoking in the past may be relevant but it is difficult to say without the results of the investigations.

## Discussion with examiners

The examiners may ask you to clarify details of the above diagnosis and ask questions about your planned investigations and management.

Other possible questions include:

- *If the imaging (CT/MRI) is normal, what's your next step?* If there's no space-occupying lesion, we will need to consider further investigations such as lumbar puncture.

- *If the CT scan shows a tumour, then what?* The scans will need to be sent over to the local neurosurgical referral centre, and the case discussed with the on-call team. The tumour may be a primary or metastastic / secondary tumour. If the appearances are consistent with metastases the patient will need a chest X-ray and a CT abdomen / pelvis / chest with contrast to look for the primary tumour / source of the metastases. Cerebral oedema round the tumour can be treated with dexamethasone with PPI; may also need a prophylactic anticonvulsant (check with neurosurgeons). Neurosurgical MDT (including oncology) will guide further management.

---

**Examiners' information and requirements**

The candidate should:

1. Identify key features from the history. Symptoms suggestive of progressive structural neurological problem: headache (worse overnight), with features of raised intracranial pressure, visual issues, memory and concentration

2. Identify key examination findings including neurological examination/fundoscopy/ AMT ± gait

3. Outline a sensible management plan: CT ± MRI head

4. Give a clear explanation to the patient of your diagnosis and plan, address his concerns and answer his questions

---

### Further reading/resources

Larner A. Not all morning headaches are due to brain tumours. Pract Neurol 2009;9:80–4.

# Scenario 44 | Headache: migraine

## Candidate's information
**Your role:** you are an ST2 in the acute medical unit. A patient has been referred in by her GP with 'recurrent headaches, worse today with photophobia. Please exclude serious causes'.

**Your task:** to assess the patient's problems and address any questions or concerns raised by her.

## Patient's information
**You are:** Antonia Tillman, a 30-year-old woman.

**Your problem:** you've been having right-sided headaches on and off for 6 months in the front/right of your head. Each usually lasts 3–4 h and you go to bed and the headache settles overnight. Once it took 48 h to settle down. You can see sparkly lights in your right eye when the pain's at its worst. You have noticed that the headaches can be worst premenstrually. This headache started last night and was still there this morning. It got a little worse after breakfast and was only on the right side of your head and eye. It felt throbbing and you score it 7/10. Your usual headaches are similar in intensity, but it was painful to look into bright lights today so you attended your GP. There were the usual sparkling lights in your right eye and your vision was a little blurred but this has now settled. You have vomited once. The headache has improved since you were admitted.

### Past medical history and drug history:
- You take ibuprofen and paracetamol for your headache and have never tried anything else
- No drug allergies known

### Social history:
- You smoke 10/day, and have done so for the past 15 years

### Other issues including family history:
Nil of note

### Your questions for the candidate:
- *Is it a brain tumour?*
- *Do I need any tests?*
- *Are there any other medicines I could try?*

# Candidate

## History/key questions

Ask about the headache and the associated symptoms

Site: unilateral versus bilateral headache; often unilateral throbbing headache in migraine

Character: throbbing; any diurnality; worse with coughing or straining

Onset: gradual, sudden

Duration of headache episodes, and when did they start?

Frequency of headaches

Associated features: auras (often visual but can be sensory, verbal or motor; blurring of vision, fortification spectra, dysphasia); nausea, photophobia, phonophobia, disequilibrium (migrainous vertigo), hemiparesis

Exacerbating and relieving factors: e.g. common triggers for migraine – lack of sleep/sleep deprivation, hormones in women, starvation, dietary precipitants, caffeine, alcohol, cheese, exercise

Ascertain whether the headache is of recent onset or whether there is a long-standing pattern of episodic headache, and if so, at what age headaches first started (migraine typically starts around the menarche)

Which approaches has she already tried for migraine – hot towels, basic simple analgesia

### Drug history

Medications

Important: what is the regular analgesia usage pattern? Is the patient taking regular opiates, codeine, etc.? Analgesic overuse headache is likely if painkillers are being taken more frequently than 12 days per month

Is there any history of contraceptive use?

### Past medical history

Enquire about previous malignancy or other serious systemic illness, e.g. arthritis (to suggest SLE)

### Social history

Tobacco use

Alcohol intake per week

Consider possible risk factors for HIV exposure

## Address patient's questions and concerns

• *Have you had any thoughts about what is going on?*
• *Is there anything in particular you're concerned about?*
• *Do you have anything you would like to ask?*

# Key areas for examination

A list of what to look for (in examination order; describe findings on examination)

Overall impression: in pain, evidence of photophobia?

Rash: look for petechial/purpuric rash of meningococcal septicaemia or malar rash of lupus

Neck stiffness, Kernig's sign

Cranial nerves, particularly visual fields (migraine-related stroke can present with isolated hemianopia)

Pupils: think of Horner's syndrome

Fundoscopy: exclude papilloedema

If time permits, examine for local sources of pain, e.g. temporomandibular joint, cervical spine tenderness or restricted movement, greater occipital nerve tenderness

Explain that you would like to examine the peripheral nervous system: given time constraints, the examiners are likely to stop you

# Differential diagnosis

Migraine with aura seems the likeliest primary diagnosis, but can only be confidently diagnosed when there is an established pattern of episodic headache with typical features. The International Headache Society criteria require at least five attacks of headache with unilateral throbbing quality and associated nausea or photophobia or phonophobia (see Further reading/resources below)

Additionally it seems likely that this patient is suffering analgesic rebound or overuse headache

The acute presentation with visual aura should raise suspicion of other causes of acute headache, particularly cerebral venous sinus thrombosis or posterior cerebral circulation ischaemia

Migraine can be symptomatic or secondary, for example as a manifestation of the antiphospholipid antibody syndrome

Acute causes of headache, e.g. SAH or meningitis, seem less likely in the light of the clinical scenario but are worth mentioning as important but improbable differentials

**Key facts/areas to consider** (including information available in scenario summary before station starts): the patient has been referred by a GP colleague who must therefore have significant concerns that this is more than 'just another headache' and the patient also will have high levels of anxiety. Care must therefore be taken to analyse the history carefully. The issue of analgesic rebound headache does need to be carefully discussed, and also do explore the role of hormonal treatments, e.g. combined oral contraceptive in particular

## Discussion with patient

Explain diagnosis
Explain plan, including investigations and management
Address patient's concerns/answer their questions

Your history is consistent with migraine. There are no alarm features and nothing concerning on examination. We will start with NSAIDs and you should take the medicines early in the headache. An antiemetic is also advisable to improve analgesic absorption. You should avoid things that bring on the headache and avoid analgesic overuse. We will probably not need to do a CT/MRI as all your symptoms fit with migraine.

## Investigations

Consider differential diagnosis of severe headache:
  Migraine
  Cluster headache
  Musculoskeletal/cervical spondylosis
  Space-occupying lesion
  Sinusitis
  Ears – otitis media
  Dental pain, particularly temporomandibular joint dysfunction
  Trigeminal neuralgia

## Management

Non-steroidal anti-inflammatory or paracetamol combined with an antiemetic first (evidence indicates there is benefit from antiemetics even with no nausea as the problem is one of gastrostasis that hinders absorption of analgesics)
Then consider triptans if poor response to NSAID or combination analgesics
Watch out for medication overuse headache

No need for CT/cross-sectional imaging if history consistent with migraine and diagnostic criteria fulfilled and there are no concerning features on examination
Discuss the option of prophylactic treatments for migraine and caution in using the combined oral contraceptive when there is a history of migraine with aura. (Difficult discussion as regards use of OCP in women of child-bearing age: generally considered to be contraindicated where there are focal neurological features in the aura or if there are other cerebrovascular risks.)

### Addressing concerns/answering questions

- *Is it a brain tumour?* Your history is consistent with migraine. There are no alarm features and nothing concerning on examination so a brain tumour is highly unlikely.
- *Do I need any tests?* We won't need to carry out a scan at this stage as your symptoms fit with migraine.
- *Are there any other medicines I could try?* We will start with anti-inflammatory medications (NSAIDs) and you should take the medicines early in the headache (e.g. soon after it starts). An anti-sickness tablet (antiemetic) is also advisable to improve absorption of the painkillers. You should avoid things that bring on the headache (dietary triggers, avoid overtiredness) and avoid analgesic overuse.

## Discussion with examiners

The examiners may ask you to clarify details of the above diagnosis and ask questions about your planned investigations and management.

A possible question includes:
- *When would scans be indicated?* Imaging only required when criteria for migraine not clearly met or there are new Red Flag features. Imaging in this case is debatable in view of the acute presentation and lack of clear history of established headache pattern.

## Examiners' information and requirements

The candidate should:

1. Identify key features from the history: a history of recurrent headache attacks over time. Headaches have lateralized, throbbing quality and are associated with nausea or photophobia or phonophobia. 'Red Flag' symptoms are excluded, e.g. diurnality, symptoms of raised intracranial pressure and symptoms of constitutional illness or focal neurological disease

2. Identify key examination findings including normal fundoscopy, normal visual fields and other cranial nerve examination. Excluded localized causes of head and neck pain, e.g. TMJ dysfunction with targeted examination

3. Outline a sensible management plan: recognize migraine, treat symptomatically. Discuss imaging/need for further investigations. Imaging only required when criteria for migraine not clearly met or there are new Red Flag features. Imaging in this case is debatable in view of the acute presentation and lack of clear history of established headache pattern. Discuss use of analgesics and antiemetics and prophylactic treatment in migraine as well as the role of analgesic overuse in propagating chronic daily headache

4. Give a clear explanation to the patient of your diagnosis and plan, address her concerns and answer her questions. Reassurance about the likely benign nature of the condition. The need to avoid analgesic overuse and the management of risk factors for migraine. Prompt use of analgesic and antiemetic, indications for prophylaxis; regular meals and avoid overfatigue. Difficult discussion as regards use of OCP in women of child-bearing age: generally considered to be contraindicated where there are focal neurological features in the aura or if there are other cerebrovascular risk factors

## Further reading/resources

Weatherall M. Chronic daily headache. Pract Neurol 2007;7:212–21.

British Association for the Study of Headache guidelines: www.bash.org.uk

# Scenario 45 | Subarachnoid haemorrhage

## Candidate's information
**Your role:** you are an ST2 in MAU. A 30-year-old woman, Ms Frampton, with a history of severe headache has been referred to you by the ED. CT head in the ED has been reported as normal. The ED charge nurse mentions to you that the patient has told him that she wants to go home.

**Your task:** to assess the patient's problems and address any questions or concerns raised by her.

## Patient's information
**You are:** Josie Frampton, a 30-year-old woman.

**Your problem:** whilst getting ready for work earlier today, you had a sudden severe headache; it came on out of the blue. It felt like someone had smacked you in the back of the head. Your speech felt a bit muddled afterwards. The headache lasted about 4 h and eased a bit whilst you were in the ED. You still have a headache, in the back of your head.

It was your worst ever headache. You don't normally get headaches. The headache wasn't made better by anything, and wasn't worse with coughing or bending over. You vomited a couple of times at home. Your eyes felt sore, worse in bright light.

You think you'd be fine at home as the headache has eased whilst you've been in the medical unit. You can take painkillers at home. The charge nurse mentioned that you'd need a lumbar puncture, and this scares you. Your best friend had a painful epidural during her recent childbirth, and needles have always made you feel a bit sick. You fainted the last time you had a vaccination.

You have no fever or rash.

### Past medical history and drug history:
- Never been in hospital
- Not on any medications

### Social history:
- Lives with partner of 3 years
- Non-smoker, drinks alcohol once a week (a few small glasses of wine)

### Other issues including family history:
- No-one in your family has had any problems with bleeding in the brain

### Your questions for the candidate:
- *Can't I go home? The A&E staff told me that the CT scan was normal.*
- *I'm afraid of having a lumbar puncture – do I really need one?*

# Candidate

## History/key questions

Headache: onset (gradual versus sudden), site, character, global rather than lateralized (migraine is typically lateralized)

Severity is key: severe sudden-onset pain is consistent with SAH, 'worst headache I've ever had'

May be associated with syncope

Duration

Photophobia, neck stiffness

Any previous headaches and their frequency, character, etc.

Associated features: auras, nausea, photophobia, hemiparesis

Exacerbating and relieving factors: ask about posture (lying flat), effects of simple analgesia

Common triggers for migraine: lack of sleep/sleep deprivation, hormones in women, starvation, dietary precipitants, caffeine, alcohol, cheese, exercise

### Drug history

Any history of analgesic overuse, e.g. >12 days per month

### Past medical history

Any history of hypertension, renal disease (think: polycystic kidney disease) or any history of joint hypermobility (to suggest Ehlers–Danlos syndrome)

### Social history

Smoking: a significant risk factor for SAH

### Other issues including family history

Check for family history of brain haemorrhage; SAH can be familial

## Address patient's questions and concerns

- *Have you had any thoughts about what is going on?*
- *Is there anything in particular you're concerned about?*
- *Do you have anything you would like to ask?*

## Key areas for examination

A list of what to look for (in examination order; describe findings on examination)

Is patient in pain? Any photophobia?

Inspection: any rash?

Assess speech, cognition during conversation: GCS, AMT

Assess neck stiffness/Kernig's sign

Cranial nerves including fundoscopy

You would like to examine the peripheral nervous system: unlikely to have time to do this

Check the blood pressure

Look for features of joint hypermobility and connective tissue disorders, e.g. Marfan's or Ehlers–Danlos

## Differential diagnosis

After a negative CT scan, the risk of SAH is around 2% (see Further reading/resources below)

Other important diagnoses include cerebral venous sinus thrombosis, arterial dissection, reversible cerebral vasoconstriction syndrome, colloid cyst of the third ventricle and early meningitis. There is an 8% risk of diagnoses in this group. Other innocuous causes of thunderclap headache include 'blitz' migraine, cough headache and coital cephalalgia

Need to exclude SAH given history of sudden-onset headache (possible sentinel bleed)

**Key facts/areas to consider** (including information available in scenario summary before station starts): the risk of recurrent haemorrhage in the next week is circa 30%. There is a 50% mortality following rebleeding and 50% of survivors will be left permanently disabled. SAH is therefore not a diagnosis to miss. The combination of CT and a lumbar puncture taken at least 12 h after symptom onset, if normal, excludes SAH as a cause for the symptoms

## Discussion with patient

Explain diagnosis

Explain plan, including investigations and management

Address patient's concerns/answer their questions

CT is only part of the assessment/one of several investigations required to exclude serious causes of headache, including bleeding in the brain. We need the combination of a scan and a lumbar puncture to properly rule out the more serious causes of your severe headache.

You need to explain the importance of staying in hospital for an LP, and the results, as this will exclude a serious bleed in the brain/explain consequences of this being untreated (death, disability).

You need to address possible needle phobia; careful explanation of the practicalities of LP. Lying on side, curled up. Clean up the skin, freeze skin with local anaesthetic (will sting then go numb) and then pass a small thin needle to take some fluid out. She will feel some pushing and prodding, and it can be uncomfortable.

Explain the LP procedure, including risks and benefits. Side-effects may include post-LP headache in 30% of cases which can be severe in around 5% of cases. Low back pain following LP is common initially but is persistent in less than 2% of cases. Very rarely, patients may develop postprocedure subdural haematoma but this is extremely unlikely in a young person. Local nerve root irritation at the time of the procedure is common but the risk of nerve injury is negligible.

If a bleed is confirmed, then you will need to discuss this with the brain surgeons at the local referral centre, and likely to need to transfer patient to them for ongoing management.

### Investigations
Non-contrast head CT sensitivity: 98% in first 24 h

Needs LP with measurement of opening pressure, samples for MCS, protein, glucose and xanthochromia

Paired serum sample for glucose

NB: the CSF specimen for proteins, glucose and xanthochromia should be transported to the lab immediately shielded from light (to prevent photodegradation of oxyhaemoglobin) and one specimen should be immediately centrifuged down for spectrophotometry. SAH is confirmed only if bilirubin is found on spectrophotometry. The presence of oxyhaemoglobin alone does not confirm SAH

### Management
Hourly monitoring of GCS, pupils, BP, pulse, RR.

### Addressing concerns/answering questions
- *Can't I go home? The A&E staff told me that the CT scan was normal.* We think you may have had a small bleed in the brain called a subarachnoid haemorrhage. This is not always visible on a CT scan. In some cases a small bleed can be a warning sign that can allow us to investigate, find a cause and treat before further bleeds occur. It is important to be sure whether there has been a bleed or not, as we would need to arrange further tests and treatment for you to reduce the risk of a further bleed in the future.
- *I'm afraid of having a lumbar puncture – do I really need one?* Yes – we need the combination of the CT scan and a lumbar puncture to make the diagnosis. If

the sample from the lumbar puncture shows the presence of blood in the spinal fluid you have had a bleed and will need further investigation. If the fluid is clear then you have not had a bleed in the brain, and then we would be looking to discharge you home as the pain has improved.

## Discussion with examiners
The examiners may ask you to clarify details of the above diagnosis and ask questions about your planned investigations and management.

A possible question includes:
- *What happens if xanthochromia is positive?* You would refer the patient to your local neurosurgical centre to review CT scan images, discuss immediate medical management including nimodipine treatment, and request their advice regarding the need for further inpatient tests, and/or transfer to the neurosurgical centre.

---

**Examiners' information and requirements**

The candidate should:
1. Identify key features from the history: sudden-onset severe headache with associated confusion
2. Identify key examination findings including presence or absence of rash, neck stiffness
3. Subarachnoid haemorrhage needs to be major differential diagnosis
4. Outline a sensible management plan, including deferring the LP until 12 h post symptom onset and ensure that CSF is examined for xanthochromia by spectrophotometry
5. Provide a clear plan for referral to neurosurgeons if xanthochromia is positive
6. Give a clear explanation to the patient of your diagnosis and plan, address her concerns and answer her questions

---

### Further reading/resources
Van Gijn J, Rinkel G. How to do it – investigate the CSF in a patient with a sudden headache and a normal CT brain scan. Pract Neurol 2005;5:362–5.

# Scenario 46 | Transient ischaemic attack: loss of vision

## Candidate's information

**Your role:** you are an ST2 in the MAU and you have been asked to review a 56-year-old woman who has been referred by her GP after having just had a short episode of visual loss.

**Your task:** to assess the patient's problems and address any questions or concerns raised by her.

## Patient's information

**You are:** Jane Williams, aged 56 years.

**Your problem:** you went to your GP after the episode at 9am today. It all came on suddenly whilst you were walking to work, like shutters coming down on your right eye. Your vision went black in your right eye for about 20 minutes. Your vision then gradually returned over about 5 minutes and your manager sent you to your GP. You didn't have any weakness of your arms or legs. You didn't have any headache, change in your speech or loss of consciousness. You've never had anything like this before.

### Past medical history and drug history:
- Diagnosed with diabetes 1 year ago, treated with metformin 1 g twice per day. Also taking simvastatin 40 mg at night and enalapril once per day for high blood pressure diagnosed at the same time
- No past history of heart disease and no previous strokes/TIAs

### Social history:
- Smoked 20/day for the past 25 years, but have given up today
- Been working in a shop selling carpets for the past 10 years
- Live with husband and adult son

### Other issues including family history:
- No-one in the family has ever had a stroke or brain tumour

### Your questions for the candidate:
- *Have I had a stroke?*
- *Why has this happened to me and why now?*
- *Do I need to stay in hospital?*
- *Will it happen again?*

## Candidate

### History/key questions

Obtain a clear history of the event (visual loss in this case): speed of onset; extent of visual changes – was it loss, blurring or other changes? Was visual loss complete or quadrantic?

Was the visual loss truly monocular or was it homonymous?

Duration of loss of vision. Single or multiple episodes?

Ever happened before, and if so did she get it investigated (and if she did, what was the final diagnosis)?

Any associated limb weakness, dysarthria, dysphasia, dysphagia or diplopia

Any associated headache, jaw claudication (temporal arteritis), disorientation or confusion

Ask about vascular risk factors including diabetes, hypertension, raised cholesterol, smoking (in pack-years) and obesity

Any past strokes, mini-strokes or event similar to today's

Any other vascular events, e.g. MI, claudication

Ever had an irregular heart beat and/or been on warfarin

#### Drug history

Is patient on aspirin or other antiplatelet agents such as clopidogrel, dipyridamole?

Ever been intolerant of any of these in the past (e.g. dyspepsia, GI bleeds)

### Address patient's questions and concerns

• *Have you had any thoughts about what is going on?*
• *Is there anything in particular you're concerned about?*
• *Do you have anything you would like to ask?*

## Key areas for examination

A list of what to look for (in examination order; describe findings on examination)

Inspection: alert, any pain/headache?

Cranial nerves (including fundoscopy, pupils and visual fields)

Heart sounds/murmurs and bruits (including carotids)

Is the patient in AF?

BP (reported as 120/75)

ECG

Say that you would wish to carry out a full examination of the peripheral nervous system (time won't allow this)

Ask to see resting ECG, blood results, blood glucose

## Differential diagnosis

Transient ischaemic attack, amaurosis fugax is the likeliest diagnosis. The presence of multiple vascular risk factors would support this

Acephalgic migraine (migraine accompagnée) is a common differential diagnosis in a woman of this age group but it is a diagnosis of exclusion and would not be favoured in the presence of multiple vascular risk factors

Cardioembolic causes need to be considered, and a search for valvular heart disease or bacterial endocarditis should be considered (with or without AF)

**Key facts/areas to consider** (including information available in scenario summary before station starts). The ABCD2 score stratifies the risk of stroke following TIA. You should have a working knowledge of this scoring system (see below). NICE recommends that all patients with an ABCD2 score of 4 or above should be investigated and treated within 24 h and those with a score of 3 or less within 7 days

### Discussion with patient

Explain diagnosis

Explain plan, including investigations and management

Address patient's concerns/answer their questions

You should advise the patient that the loss of vision in her eye raises the possibility of disturbance of the blood supply to the eye and that investigation of the circulation is advisable.

### Investigations

ABCD2 score to guide decision about admission (inpatient investigations) versus discharge with outpatient investigations and TIA clinic follow-up: see below. Her score is 2 (duration of symptoms and known to have diabetes)

FBC, U&E, glucose, ESR, cholesterol/lipids

ECG (look for AF) – sinus rhythm in this case

CXR

Carotid Dopplers: as soon as possible for low-risk TIA and within 24 hours if high-risk TIA, and certainly within 7 days according to NICE guidance

CT/MRI (to look for evidence of multiple infarcts/cerebrovascular disease)

ECHO: only if there are signs of valve disease or endocarditis

• **ABCD2 score** consists of:
  A – age: 60 years of age or older, *1 point*
  B – blood pressure at presentation: BP systolic 140 and/or 90 diastolic mmHg or greater, *1 point*

C – clinical features: unilateral weakness, *2 points*; speech disturbance without weakness, *1 point*

D – duration of symptoms: 60 min or longer, *2 points*; 10–59 min, *1 point*

D – presence of diabetes: *1 point*

- Role of scoring system is to triage patients into high risk (specialist assessment, investigations and management within 24 h) or low risk (rapid-access TIA clinic): check local protocols as there will be some local variations (including out-of-hours access to advice/review from stroke physicians on-call)
- Two-day risk of stroke based on ABCD2 score:
  Score 6–7: 8.1%
  Score 4–5: 4.1%
  Score 0–3: 1%
- Admit for inpatient monitoring/investigations/management if:
  Crescendo TIAs (two or more events in past 7 days)
  Lateralizing signs on examination, fluctuating symptoms, or haven't yet resolved
- Urgent specialist review and imaging (<24 h) if ABCD2 score is 4 or more (patient at higher risk for early stroke) or if chronic or paroxysmal AF, patient on warfarin, prosthetic valve or young (<50) with neck pain. Start aspirin 300 mg od, book carotid Dopplers. Advise patient not to drive until advised to restart by the stroke consultant; they then may need to inform the DVLA
- If ABCD2 score is 0–3 or episode >7 days ago: low risk of TIA – needs to be referred to rapid-access TIA clinic, to be seen within 1 week

## Management

Stop smoking/referral to smoking cessation

Antiplatelet agent: aspirin 300 mg od for 2 weeks then 75 mg od thereafter. Dipyridamole 200 mg bd SR to be added in also as per NICE guidance for TIA

Manage risk factors (diabetes, smoking, hypertension, hyperlipidaemia, obesity)

Referral to vascular surgeons for carotid endarterectomy if carotid stenosis >70%

## Addressing concerns/answering questions

- *Have I had a stroke?* The symptoms are classed as a 'TIA' or mini-stroke. The chances of this event leading to a major stroke at this time are low but risk factors for stroke must be looked for and addressed.
- *Why has this happened to me and why now?* You have significant risk factors for vascular disease, chief of which is smoking which you need to try and stop immediately.

- *Do I need to stay in hospital?* No, you can go home and be seen in TIA clinic for further investigations in the next week (as your ABCD2 score is <4).
- *Will it happen again?* There is a risk of further events of about 1% a year but this can be reduced by continuing to stop smoking and controlling your diabetes and other cardiovascular risk factors.

## Discussion with examiners

The examiners may ask you to clarify details of the above diagnosis and ask questions about your planned investigations and management.

Other possible questions include:
- *Can she drive her car?* Driving after a TIA – say that you would refer to the DVLA 'At a Glance' booklet to ensure up-to-date advice. Also see www.cks.nhs.uk. For private car drivers (group 1), no driving for at least 4 weeks but they may resume driving after this period if clinical recovery is satisfactory. There is no need to notify the DVLA unless there is a residual neurological deficit 1 month after the episode.
- *What is the role of scoring systems in triaging patients into high risk (within 24 h or may need inpatient assessment) or low risk (rapid access TIA clinic)?* Use the ABDC2 score as outlined above.
- *If you diagnosed her with paroxysmal atrial fibrillation (currently in sinus rhythm, confirmed on ECG, but earlier ECGs showed AF) why is this significant, and how would you decide on further management?* Atrial fibrillation is a significant risk factor for stroke and I would use the CHA2DS2-VASc score for atrial fibrillation stroke risk to calculate her risk of stroke and help guide the decision about starting warfarin. The CHA2DS2-VASc score uses the criteria shown in Table H46.1.

Table H46.1 The CHA2DS2-VASc score criteria

| Feature | Score |
| --- | --- |
| Congestive cardiac failure / LV dysfunction | 1 |
| Hypertension | 1 |
| Age over 75 years | 2 |
| Age between 65 and 74 years | 1 |
| Stroke/TIA/thromboembolic event | 2 |
| Vascular disease (previous MI, peripheral arterial disease or aortic plaque) | 1 |
| Diabetes mellitus | 1 |
| Female | 1 |

Scores of 2 or more – anticoagulation with warfarin is indicated, and needs to be discussed with the patient.

Score of 1 is intermediate risk, and aspirin / antiplatelet therapy or anticoagulation should be considered, and discussed with the patient. Oral anticoagulation is preferred (see European Society of Cardiology (ESC) guidelines).

Score of 0 is low risk. Options include aspirin or no anticoagulation / antiplatelet therapy. No therapy is preferred option.

This patient scores 5, a 6.7% per year stroke risk (Lip et al 2010 stroke study, and the ESC guidelines) and oral anticoagulation would be indicated if she was in AF or had PAF.

---

### Examiners' information and requirements

The candidate should:

1. Elicit a clear history from patient of TIA, and single episode of visual loss
2. Define risk factors for TIA/vascular disease and be able to calculate the ABCD2 score for this patient
3. Perform a targeted neurological examination
4. Explain the diagnosis of TIA to the patient including investigations and management (including vascular risk factors/smoking cessation)
5. Quote the ABCD2 score and outline a management plan based on this, including the need for cerebral imaging and carotid Dopplers, antiplatelet agents, management of risk factors, smoking cessation and referral to the stroke team
6. Give a clear explanation to the patient of your diagnosis and plan, address her concerns and answer her questions

---

### Further reading/resources

Diagnosis and initial management of acute stroke and TIA. NICE Clinical Guideline CG68, July 2008: www.guidance.nice.org.uk/CG68

European Society of Cardiology AF guidelines: www.escardio.org/guidelines-surveys/esc-guidelines/GuidelinesDocuments/guidelines-afib-FT.pdf

Lip GY, Nieuwlaat R, Pisters R, Lane DA, Crijns HJ. Refining clinical risk stratification for predicting stroke and thromboembolism in atrial fibrillation using a novel risk factor-based approach: the Euro Heart Survey on Atrial Fibrillation. Chest 2010;137:263–272.

# Scenario 47 | Left-sided weakness in a young woman

## Candidate's information

**Your role:** you are the SHO on call for medicine. A 20-year-old woman has been admitted by ambulance to the Emergency Department after she developed left-sided weakness whilst at the hairdressers. GCS 15/15 throughout. BP 125/70, pulse 90 on arrival.

**Your task:** to assess the patient's problems and address any questions or concerns raised by her.

## Patient's information

**You are:** Maura Donnelly, a 20-year-old woman.

**Your problem:** you were at the hairdressers this morning, in preparation for your sister's 21st birthday party tonight. You were tired as you were out on the town last night, had poor sleep overnight, and you've been having headaches on/off. Whilst having your hair washed, you started having a headache; it was in the centre/right side of forehead moving round to the side. The headache was similar to your usual migraine, just a little more severe. The staff got you a cup of tea and you found that you couldn't lift up the cup of tea. You could move your arm but it was very weak. You reluctantly allowed your hairdresser to phone for an ambulance and by the time the ambulance arrived, the weakness had all gone, perhaps 10 min later.

You didn't notice any changes in your vision, and no sparkling lights were seen. Your speech was normal. You didn't try to stand up as the staff told you to stay in the chair. This has never happened before.

### Past medical history and drug history:
• On oral contraceptive pill – past 5 years

### Social history:
• Lives with boyfriend
• No plans to start a family
• Smokes 5/day
• Drinks half bottle of wine 5 nights per week, sometimes more at weekends

### Other issues including family history:
• Mother had a stroke age 55; now on warfarin

### Your questions for the candidate:
• *Have I had a stroke?*
• *Can I stay on the pill?*

## Candidate

### History/key questions

Ask about the headache and the associated symptoms. Same as usual migraine or different?

Site, unilateral versus bilateral headache; often unilateral throbbing headache in migraine

Character: lateralized? Throbbing?

Onset: gradual or sudden

Duration of headache episodes, and when did they start?

Frequency of headaches

Associated features: auras (often visual but can be sensory, verbal or motor; blurring of vision, fortification spectra, dysphasia); nausea, photophobia, hemiparesis

Exacerbating and relieving factors, e.g. common triggers for migraine – lack of sleep/sleep deprivation, hormones in women, starvation, dietary precipitants, caffeine, alcohol, cheese, exercise

### Drug history

Tried which approaches for migraine: hot towels, basic simple analgesia

Important: what is the regular analgesia? Is the patient taking regular opiates, codeine, etc.? (Analgesic withdrawal headaches)

### Past medical history

Any past medical history

### Social history

Tobacco use

Alcohol intake per week

### Address patient's questions and concerns

• *Have you had any thoughts about what is going on?*
• *Is there anything in particular you're concerned about?*
• *Do you have anything you would like to ask?*

## Key areas for examination

A list of what to look for (in examination order; describe findings on examination)

Overall impression: in pain, evidence of photophobia?

Rash: look for petechial/purpuric rash of meningococcal septicaemia

Neck stiffness, Kernig's

Cranial nerves

Pupils: look for Horner's syndrome – carotid dissection may declare itself in this way

Fundoscopy: exclude papilloedema

Be sure to check eye movements for nystagmus or strabismus/dysconjugate eye movements to suggest a brainstem syndrome

Look for evidence of motor deficit in the limbs: look particularly for cerebellar features which might indicate a posterior circulation ischaemic event

Check the BP and pulse and indicate you would like to listen to the heart for valvular heart disease

Explain that you would like to examine the peripheral nervous system and also look for evidence of joint hypermobility syndrome (which can predispose to arterial dissection): given time constraints, the examiners are likely to stop you

Blood glucose

Observation charts

## Differential diagnosis

Migraine with hemiparesis, so-called complex migraine, is the lead differential. A TIA is less likely but not impossible

In the light of onset at the hairdressers during neck extension, carotid and vertebral dissection should both be considered. The lack of other brainstem symptoms is somewhat against a posterior circulation disorder due to vertebral dissection. Horner's syndrome (carefully look for it in all cases of 'stroke') would be a major pointer to carotid dissection (see Vol. 1, Station 3, CNS, Case 41, Footnote)

Causes of stroke and TIA in the young need to be considered, particularly:

Antiphospholipid antibody syndrome

Valvular heart disease including endocarditis

Vasculitides including SLE, Sjögren's

Hyperlipidaemia

AF

Paradoxical embolism due to PFO or ASD (but very controversial and only really implicated as a cause of stroke where there is a proven thrombophilia present with a PFO)

**Key facts/areas to consider** (including information available in scenario summary before station starts): migraine and the oral contraceptive are independent risk factors for stroke, albeit causing only a small increase in the absolute relative risk. Arterial dissection is one of the most common causes of stroke in the young

## Discussion with patient

Explain diagnosis

Explain plan, including investigations and management

Address patient's concerns/answer their questions

The cause of your symptoms is probably migraine but, in view of the unusual features, we need to carry out further investigations. You need to stop taking the oral contraceptive pill to reduce the risk of stroke and you should stop smoking.

## Investigations

MRI imaging to look for evidence of multifocal cerebrovascular disease and carotid/vertebral artery dissection (best seen on fat-saturated axial scans of the neck)

Screening for hereditary hyperlipidaemias and antiphospholipid antibody syndrome, SLE and other vasculitides, e.g. ANA, ESR and CRP

## Management

Smoking cessation

Reduce alcohol intake: currently 25+ units per week

The oral contraceptive pill and migraine: see above. Suggest alternative methods of contraception – the progestogen-only pill, implant or injection would be reasonable alternatives or an IUD could be considered

Referral to neurologists or stroke physician as outpatient

Discuss with patient the risks and benefits of antiplatelet agents. If all investigations are reassuring, aspirin is unlikely to confer any proven benefit but some clinicians may still offer antiplatelet agents as prophylaxis

## Addressing concerns/answering questions

- *Have I had a stroke?* Most likely diagnosis is hemiplegic migraine, migraine which causes one-sided weakness not a stroke.
- *Can I stay on the pill?* You should change from the combined pill to either a progesterone-only contraceptive (pill, injection, implant or Mirena coil) or a copper IUD. Use of combined oral contraceptive pills in migraine can increase the risk of developing a stroke.

## Discussion with examiners

The examiners may ask you to clarify details of the above diagnosis and ask questions about your planned investigations and management.

Other possible questions include:

- *What are some of the common triggers of migraine?* Lack of sleep/sleep deprivation, hormones in women, starvation, dietary precipitants, caffeine, alcohol, cheese, exercise.
- *How does carotid dissection (see Vol. 1, Station 3, CNS, Case 41, Footnote) present?* Headache or neck pain, amaurosis fugax, focal weakness, reduced sensation of taste, partial Horner's syndrome (ptosis and miosis), neck swelling, pulsatile tinnitus or audible bruit, migraine-like symptoms reported. The first manifestation of carotid dissection may be a TIA or stroke due to a carotid embolus breaking off from the clot forming at the site of the dissection.

See also Vol. 1, Station 3, CNS, Case 8 and Case 41, Footnote.

---

### Examiners' information and requirements

The candidate should:

1. Identify key features from the history: history consistent with migraine; consider differentials of TIA and vertebral artery dissection; history of oral contraceptive pill use, smoking
2. Identify key examination findings including no focal neurology
3. Outline a sensible management plan, including imaging, stopping smoking, switch of oral contraceptive pill
4. Give a clear explanation to the patient of your diagnosis and plan, address her concerns and answer her questions

---

# Scenario 48 | Parkinson's disease/falls in an elderly woman

## Candidate's information

**Your role:** you are an ST2 in a general medical 'falls' clinic. Mrs Gardner's GP has referred her to the clinic as she has been falling recently and he's asked for your help with identifying why.

**Your task:** to assess the patient's problems and address any questions or concerns she raises.

## Patient's information

**You are:** Isabel Gardner, a 75-year-old woman.

**Your problem:** you have been finding it harder to get around at home, and have had a couple of falls at home. You remember tripping over the edge of the carpet in the dining room twice – this has never been a problem before. For the past few months you have been finding the steps inside and outside the house difficult. Your daughter is buying an extra rail to help you on the steps. Your handwriting is a bit more spider-like than before, and your grandchildren have complained about not being able to read your writing.

Your GP suggested that you see the specialist at the hospital to find out what's going on. You have noticed that your left hand has been shaky for the past 6–12 months, but you had put that down to old age and perhaps the medications you've been on for your blood pressure. You have no memory problems, your bowels are regular, no swallowing problems and your weight is stable. Your daughter usually comes with you to all your outpatient appointments but she is away in Spain on holiday so you've come alone.

### Past medical history and drug history:

- High blood pressure: practice nurse says that it has been fine at the GP surgery; you're also on aspirin to prevent heart attacks – GP thought it wise
- Bisoprolol 2.5 mg od, aspirin 75 mg od

### Social history:

- You live alone in a bungalow but with several steps inside the house (into kitchen, up into bathroom) and to get into the property (front and back doors) which you are finding harder to cope with. No rail in bathroom. You use a bath seat, but struggle to get in and out of the bath
- Daughter visits daily to help with the cleaning, washing clothes and she takes you out shopping

### Other issues including family history: Nil of note

**Your questions for the candidate:**
- *Can you get me better? I want to stay in my own house.*
- *What causes Parkinson's disease?* (if mentioned by the doctor)

---

## Candidate

### History/key questions

Parkinson's disease (PD) is defined as an extrapyramidal syndrome manifesting 3 out of the following 5 features: bradykinesia, tremor, rigidity, postural instability and gait disorder

Early symptoms include daytime somnolence and reduced sense of smell

Ask about onset of motor signs: typically asymmetrical. Patients may notice a loss of dexterity when performing familiar tasks, such as doing buttons or cleaning

Patients typically notice gait disorder with tripping or falls and reduced walking speed and stiffness, especially in routine tasks like turning in bed or getting in or out of the bath

The tremor is of low 4–6 Hz frequency and 'pill rolling' in type in the upper limb, more noticeable / pronounced at rest

Micrographia (small handwriting) is a common complaint if sought for

Associated symptoms can include fatigue, constipation, impaired sleep

Impaired dressing/co-ordination

Swallowing: dysphagia, drooling saliva

Constipation

Ask specifically about symptoms of autonomic dysfunction, postural hypotension and bladder symptoms which might suggest multiple system atrophy as a cause for the parkinsonism rather than true idiopathic PD

Also enquire about visual hallucinations and cognitive problems which might suggest diffuse Lewy body disease

Ask about vascular risk factors which might suggest 'vascular PD' or small vessel cerebrovascular disease

### Drug history

Check current drug history and any recent changes in medicines. Particularly enquire about the use of neuroleptics or antiemetics which may have extrapyramidal side-effects

### Past medical history

Any stepwise deterioration consistent with multiple strokes

Any history of vascular disease (stroke, TIA, MI, IHD, intermittent claudication, etc.)

### Social history

Important to understand the social issues/environmental factors which will be contributing to recurrent falls

### Address patient's questions and concerns
- *Have you had any thoughts about what is going on?*
- *Is there anything in particular you're concerned about?*
- *Do you have anything you would like to ask?*

## Key areas for examination

A list of what to look for (in examination order; describe findings on examination)

Mask-like facies (expressionless), hypersalivation/dribbling, so-called hypomimia/reduced blinking

Peripheral CNS:

Unilateral rest tremor

Rigidity (leadpipe or cogwheeling – tremor and increased tone). Remember to test tone with and without contralateral limb tapping – the so-called 'activation phenomenon' – it is often astonishingly effective

Bradykinesia: test by asking the patient to tap their index finger on their thumb quickly in both hands simultaneously. Also ask the patient to rapidly pronate and supinate the hands. These manoeuvres usually admirably demonstrate asymmetry of movement and bradykinesia

Micrographia, worth eliciting if time permits

Soft voice without intonation worth looking for and commenting on without labouring the point with formal assessment

Postural instability: imbalance and loss of righting reflexes. Best assessed by the 'pull test': the candidate stands behind the patient in standing and gently pulls backwards on the patient's shoulders, warning the patient that they may lose their balance but that they will not be allowed to fall. Patients with PD lose balance and stagger backwards often requiring support. Unaffected individuals just sway

Gait: essential to assess this; short shuffling steps, may exhibit some freezing

Other signs of extrapyramidal syndromes:

Lying and standing BP for postural drop which might suggest multiple system atrophy

Vertical gaze palsy: patient cannot move eyes vertically upwards in pursuit but the eyes do deviate upwards with vestibular ocular reflex when the neck is flexed downwards with the patient fixating on a point in front of them, i.e. 'doll's eyes reflex'. This would be suggestive of progressive supranuclear palsy (PSP)

## Differential diagnosis

Idiopathic Parkinson's disease: most likely if other features are absent and history suggests insidious asymmetrical onset

Drug-induced parkinsonism: the most common alternative differential diagnosis suggested by a history of neuroleptic or antiemetic use

Vascular PD refers to the presence of extrapyramidal features in the presence of cerebrovascular disease. Cognitive impairment may be more prominent with gait apraxia, i.e. 'sticky feet' rather than the festinant gait of idiopathic PD

PSP is suggested by truncal instability and vertical gaze palsy

Multiple system atrophy may present with pure autonomic failure, cerebellar ataxia or parkinsonism (known as striatonigral degeneration). The parkinsonism doesn't respond well to treatment and autonomic features are usually prominent

Diffuse Lewy body disease (DLBD) is characterized by dementia and prominent visual hallucinations with parkinsonism

Essential tremor is probably the most common cause of diagnostic confusion and misdiagnosis of PD. It is a postural tremor that is fine and somewhat quicker than the PD pill-rolling phenomenon. Ask patient to hold hands out in front of them and the tremor will manifest, whereas PD tremor is more marked at rest

**Key facts/areas to consider** (including information available in scenario summary before station starts):

PD is a clinical diagnosis. Although DaTscan isotope brain scanning can be helpful in differentiating essential tremor from isolated PD tremor, this is rarely necessary unless the clinical signs are very limited. The isotope-labelled-DaTscan compound binds to the

dopamine transporter in the brain. The transporters are then detected using SPECT, which measures the amount and location of the radioactive isotope in the brain. The PD mimics (multiple system atrophy, PSP and DLBD) do not respond well to dopamine replacement therapy. Idiopathic PD is much more likely to be asymmetrical than symmetrical

## Discussion with patient

Explain diagnosis

Explain plan, including investigations and management

Address patient's concerns/answer their questions

Your movement disorder is due to an impairment of 'automatic movements' which we all take for granted, and this is due to some degeneration (age-related changes) in the brain. There are various causes and includes Parkinson's disease. Typically, idiopathic Parkinson's disease responds well to treatment. The disease is not uncommon and there is good support from specialist nurses and patient groups.

### Investigations and management

Referral to movement disorders clinic

• Consider a trial of dopaminergic therapy if symptoms severe and disabling (L-dopa with dopa decarboxylase inhibitors)

MDT approach to reducing risk of falls (environmental factors include issues with rugs/carpet, steps)

• Occupational therapy (assess environmental factors and provide equipment including rails to improve safety / aid mobility)

• Physiotherapy (improve gait and balance, provide walking aids and also help you develop ways to get up if you fall)

• Social work (help with personal care)

Support groups

### Addressing concerns/answering questions

• *Can you get me better? I want to stay in my own house.* In terms of the Parkinson's we can consider starting medication and we will need to see how you respond to these. There are ways of reducing the risk of falls, and maintaining your independence: professionals such as the occupational therapists assess environmental factors and provide equipment including rails, for example, which will help you stay in your house. Physiotherapists can help you improve your gait and balance, provide walking aids and help you develop ways to get up if you fall. If you need more help with washing and dressing, a package of care can be provided.

- *What causes Parkinson's disease?* Parkinson's is caused by the degenerative loss of certain nerve cells in the brain leading to reduced dopamine levels. This causes slowing of movement, tremor and rigidity.

## Discussion with examiners

The examiners may ask you to clarify details of the above diagnosis and ask questions about your planned investigations and management.

Investigations and management:

PD is a clinical diagnosis (see key facts above)

Differential diagnosis of falls in the elderly includes extrapyramidal disorders, postural hypotension, cardiac syncope, normal pressure hydrocephalus, diffuse small vessel cerebrovascular disease

Clinical signs of PD: cardinal features include resting tremor, rigidity, bradykinesia, postural instability, unilateral cogwheeling

Associated conditions: constipation, dysphagia, dementia

Other possible questions include:

- *Describe your management of this condition.* See investigations and management. MDT approach, including neurology, physiotherapy and occupational therapy.
- *What treatment would you suggest – and when to start?* Dopamine – L-dopa with dopa decarboxylase inhibitors. Dopamine agonists (don't forget the uncommon but important side-effects of sudden-onset sleep and pathological gambling and hyper-sexuality with some of these agents). The argument about early and delayed use of L-dopa is unresolved but most specialists agree that where there are marked symptoms, L-dopa should not be withheld. Enzyme inhibitors: both MAO-B and COMT inhibitors are now available and offer useful smoothing and pro-longation of L-dopa effects. Procyclidine for drug-induced PD if need to stay on drug.

- *What environmental causes are there for the falls?* Potential causes for falls identified include steps inside and outside the bungalow, possible loose carpet edges/rugs and lack of rail in bathroom.
- *What changes would you suggest to her environment?* Assessment by occupational therapy and physiotherapy in her home; equipment such as rails for steps and in the bathroom; fitting the carpets and removal of rugs to avoid raised edges which could lead to falls.

See also Vol. 1, Station 3, CNS, Case 3.

---

### Examiners' information and requirements

The candidate should:

1. Identify key features from the history: gait disorder, features of tremor and rigidity and bradykinesia and a search for cognitive impairment, autonomic dysfunction, cerebrovascular disease and drugs that cause extrapyramidal side-effects. Identify possible environmental causes for falls
2. Identify key examination findings including signs of untreated PD, eye movement disorder, postural hypotension, features of cerebrovascular disease and cognitive impairment
3. Outline a sensible management plan: referral to movement disorders clinic and consider a trial of dopaminergic therapy if symptoms severe and disabling; MDT approach to reducing risk of falls
4. Give a clear explanation to the patient of your diagnosis and plan, address her concerns and answer her questions

---

### Further reading/resourses

Parkinsons UK: www.parkinsons.org.uk
NICE: www.nice.org.uk/CG35

# Scenario 49 | Cranial nerve VI palsy: sudden onset

## Candidate's information

**Your role:** you are an ST2 in the acute medical unit. Mr Parker has been referred by his GP with sudden-onset double vision. He is known to have diabetes and hypertension.

**Your task:** to assess the patient's problems and address any questions or concerns he raises.

## Patient's information

**You are:** Keith Parker, a 62-year-old man.

**Your problem:** you noticed double vision on waking up yesterday morning – it was slight but seemed to slowly worsen during the day. You notice the double vision when looking to the left and only when looking with both eyes. You have not noticed any drooping of your eyelids. You also have a mild persistent headache on the right side of your head, which came on at the same time as the double vision. The headache is not associated with nausea, photophobia or phonophobia. You haven't noticed any weakness or sensory disturbance in your arms or legs. You have no problem with walking or balance. No falls or confusion. No blurring or loss of vision. Your vision is similar today to last night. Your memory seems normal. No problem with dizziness, speech, hearing, swallowing or breathing. No weight loss. You've never had these problems before.

### Past medical history and drug history:
- Diabetes: managed on diet initially, then started on metformin 4 years ago
- TIA about 2 years ago (briefly had slurred speech): investigated and nothing found – felt likely to be related to diabetes
- Mildly raised cholesterol: on simvastatin
- Cough with BP tablets: stopped them recently (haven't been back to GP)

### Social history:
- Non-smoker
- 6–8 pints of lager per week

### Other issues including family history:
- No family history of stroke, heart attack
- Father died of colorectal cancer in his 90s

### Your questions for the candidate:
- *Have I had a stroke?*
- *Will this go away?*
- *Can I still drive?*

# Candidate

## History/key questions

Onset of diplopia: monocular or binocular (ophthalmological/functional versus true neurological disorders)

Horizontal versus vertical

Which areas does he see double in (e.g. going downstairs [CN IV], lateral gaze [VI], at rest [III])?

Any drooping of the eyelid (ptosis in CN III, neuromuscular junction disorders [NMJ], myopathy, autoimmune, e.g. Miller-Fisher's, Guillain–Barré syndrome [GBS])

Any associated headache (acute or chronic), character of headache (worse on lying down, worse on sneezing or coughing to suggest raised intracranial pressure [ICP])

Any associated visual loss (central scotoma or reduced visual acuity suggesting optic nerve/disc involvement in raised ICP)

Any hearing symptoms (tinnitus or deafness), nausea, vomiting, vertigo (brainstem pathology)

Any signs of fatigability (better after resting eyes for few hours, worse when trying to focus, e.g. watching TV)

Ask about bulbar symptoms: speech difficulties (dysarthria, dysphagia, shortness of breath). Any suggestions of fatigability (inflammatory brainstem lesion, postinfectious autoimmune variant of GBS, NMJ, e.g. myasthenia gravis [MG])

Weakness or sensory disturbance in upper and lower limbs

Difficulty with gait and balance (sensory ataxia in Miller-Fisher's syndrome, Wernicke's)

Weight loss, night sweats (raised ICP from SOL)

Preceding history of memory disturbance, change in behaviour

Ask about risk factors for cerebrovascular disease: hypertension, diabetes, cholesterol, smoking history as per TIA checklist

Questions to discriminate between causes:

1. Fatigability is suggestive of NMJ, e.g. myasthenia gravis (onset likely to be gradual rather than acute)

2. Weight loss, night sweats, symptoms of raised ICP suggest cerebral space-occupying lesion, causing false localizing sign (onset of diplopia itself can be sudden but other associated symptoms can precede diplopia by weeks or months)

3. Recent flu/diarrhoeal illness or associated ataxia may suggest acute inflammatory demyelinating neuropathy (Miller-Fisher's, variant of GBS; triad of ataxia, ophthalmoplegia, areflexia)

4. High vascular risk factors may point towards microvascular cause as the most likely diagnosis

5. Preceding higher function disturbance including memory might suggest additional CNS involvement such as SOL including lymphoma, inflammatory causes, e.g. vasculitis, neurosarcoidosis, infective, e.g. tuberculosis, Lyme disease

### Drug history

?On antiplatelets, anticoagulants

Any antihypertensives, which diabetes treatment, cholesterol?

### Past medical history

Previous strokes/MI/vascular events? Known to have IHD, peripheral vascular disease?

Recent flu symptoms or diarrhoea?

### Social history

Smoking history (quantify in pack-years) and alcohol history

## Address patient's questions and concerns
- *Have you had any thoughts about what is going on?*
- *Is there anything in particular you're concerned about?*
- *Do you have anything you would like to ask?*

## Key areas for examination

A list of what to look for (in examination order; describe findings on examination)

Assess speech (bulbar, pseudobulbar, staccato) and orientation to time/place/person. Simple 1-step and 2-step commands, name objects (pen, watch and their function)

Examine all the cranial nerves (particularly CN II, III, IV, VI), trying to elicit only the key signs

Failure of the affected eye to abduct past the mid-line in VI nerve palsy

Look for ptosis and existing complex ophthalmoplegia (myopathy in thyroid disorder, Wernicke's, NMJ in MG, inflammatory in GBS, vascular in patient with risk factors)

Look for broken pursuit or abnormal saccades (indicating brainstem pathology), nystagmus or internuclear ophthalmoplegia (cerebellar involvement in MS)

Pupil size (Horner's), relative afferent pupillary defect in optic nerve atrophy (MS), visual field defect (cerebrovascular event), visual acuity (NB: in papilloedema visual acuity is preserved until very late, c.f. optic neuritis)

Fundoscopy examination for papilloedema (raised ICP), optic atrophy, DM and hypertensive retinopathy

Temporal artery tenderness (GCA)

Screen gait for ataxia and Romberg's (cerebellar, upper motor neurone lesions, GBS, Wernicke's)

Explain that you would like to complete the examination by examining the upper and lower limbs for long tract signs or peripheral nerve involvement, and check for organomegaly and lymphadenopathy to look for evidence of malignancy

Urinalysis: protein (vasculitis, connective tissue disease; we already know patient is diabetic)

Blood pressure

ECG (AF)

On examination in this patient, there is an isolated left VI nerve palsy, no other focal neurology

## Differential diagnoses

Autoimmune: connective tissue disease (Sjögren's, SLE, RA, Behçet's), MG, GBS

Vascular: microvascular, thromboembolic, R cavernous sinus or superior orbital fissure lesion, MCA aneurysm

Infiltrative: amyloidosis

Infective: Lyme, TB, viral (HIV, human T-lymphotrophic virus [HTLV] in immunocompromised)

Other: thyroid, Wernicke's encephalopathy

Neurological causes for binocular diplopia are due to problems with the extraocular muscles (myopathy), their innervation (cranial nerves and their nuclei in the brainstem) or interactions between the nerve and muscles (NMJ disorders) causing dysconjugate eye movements

The onset is acute so the likely diagnoses are either vascular or inflammatory. This patient's strong risk factors favour a vascular event as the most likely aetiology (microvascular, thromboembolic; diabetic neuropathy being the most common)

Consider tumours (posterior fossa tumour, cerebellopontine angle lesion, lymphoma), MS (although expect younger onset), inflammatory (GCA, vasculitis, neurosarcoidosis)

NB: VI nerve palsy from pontine stroke would leave quadriparesis and bilateral small pupils. A unilateral CN VI nucleus lesion will cause ipsilateral lateral gaze palsies (failure of ipsilateral eye abduction and contralateral eye adduction due to lesion of ipsilateral paramedian pontine reticular formation and contralateral medial longitudinal fasciculus, and possible CN VII involvement)

## Discussion with patient

Explain diagnosis

Explain plan, including investigations and management

Address patient's concerns/answer their questions

A nerve affecting the movement in the eye has weakened, either due to your diabetes, a stroke or a different cause. We need to carry out some investigations to find out why it's happened. Then we will wait and see what happens as there may be a degree of natural recovery. We will treat any medical conditions that are putting you at risk of this (e.g. manage any risk factors). You should not drive for at least 1 month.

## Investigations

Basic 'stroke' investigations and referral to stroke/neurology

Urinalysis

Bloods including ESR ± vasculitis screen, ECG, blood glucose

Imaging: CT ± MRI/diffusion-weighted imaging (MRI with contrast and DWI sequence would be helpful as better visualization of infarction [old and new], meningeal enhancement, brainstem lesions including parenchymal inflammation)

± Lumbar puncture: protein, glucose, cytology (depending on the MRI findings)

Dopplers/ECHO

Ophthalmology as regards prisms in VI CN palsy

### Addressing concerns/answering questions

- *Have I had a stroke?* Most likely it is nerve damage from the toxic effect of the diabetes but stroke is a possibility so we need to exclude this by doing further investigations, including imaging of your brain.
- *Will this go away?* It is usually transient (ranges from days to 4–6 weeks, sometimes up to 6 months or more). It is important to control or treat risk factors.
- *Can I still drive?* Anyone with suspected stroke has to inform the DVLA and their car insurance company. They are not able to drive for at least a month.

## Discussion with examiners

The examiners may ask you to clarify details of the above diagnosis and ask questions about your planned investigations and management.

Other possible questions include:
- *What is the differential diagnosis of CN VI palsy?* See differential diagnosis list above.

- *What is the management of CN VI palsy secondary to diabetes?* Secondary prevention with antiplatelet agents, treat hypertension and cholesterol, stop smoking, and aim for HbA1C <6.5%. The condition may resolve itself.
- *What are the differential diagnoses if the onset is gradual?* Primary tumour causing direct infiltration or nerve stretching from raised ICP, chronic meningitis (TB or malignant), inflammatory (vasculitis, sarcoidosis).
- *How would you investigate this patient?* MRI with contrast followed by LP.
- *How would MRI help?* Parenchymal lesion, infarction, meningeal enhancement in leptomeningeal carcinomatosis or granulomatous disease, demyelination, aneurysm (MRA or CTA).
- *What would you see in the CSF?* High protein and positive oligoclonal bands isolated only in CSF in neuroinflammatory lesion; low glucose and high lymphocytes in TB meningitis or lymphoma, low glucose and high protein in malignancy.

See also Vol. 1, Station 3, CNS, Case 16.

---

**Examiners' information and requirements**

The candidate should:

1. Identify key features from the history: acute history of diplopia associated with mild headache; vascular risk factors including diabetes, raised cholesterol, hypertension and previous TIA
2. Identify key examination findings including right VI nerve palsy, no papilloedema/may have signs of diabetic retinopathy
3. Outline a sensible management plan including investigations and referral to stroke/neurology
4. Give a clear explanation to the patient of your diagnosis and plan, address his concerns and answer his questions

# Scenario 50 | Blackout: first fit

## Candidate's information

**Your role:** you are an ST2 in acute medicine and the A&E registrar has asked you to see Mr Appleby, a 45-year-old truck driver who suffered a collapse earlier in the day.

**Your task:** to assess the patient's problems and address any questions or concerns he raises.

## Patient's information

**You are:** Garth Appleby, a 45-year-old lorry driver.

**Your problem:** you collapsed suddenly whilst shopping. You remember walking into the supermarket and smelling something strange, but then woke up in the ambulance on arrival at the hospital. The passers-by told the paramedics that you suddenly fell to the floor next to the freezer cabinet, started shaking, and they couldn't rouse you for about 4–5 min; a passing nurse told the paramedics that after the shaking stopped you were drowsy and confused for half an hour; you started to improve only when you were in the ambulance on the way to hospital. You bumped your head and have a slight headache, and felt a bit muddled for a few hours after it all happened. You didn't have any incontinence of urine; you think you bit your tongue as it feels a little swollen on the left side.

### Past medical history and drug history:
- No previous episodes
- No associated chest pain or SOB
- No regular medications and never taken illicit drugs (cocaine, etc.)

### Social history:
- You work as a self-employed truck driver, supporting your wife and two children
- Alcohol: 2–3 pints of 3.8% lager on Friday and Saturday nights

### Other issues including family history:
- No family history of seizures or collapses

### Your questions for the candidate:
- *What happened?*
- *Will it happen again?*
- *What about driving and my job?*
- *Can you prevent this from happening again?*

# Candidate

## History/key questions

Key points: (i) pre-event, (ii) during event, (iii) post-event

NB: collateral history is essential – bystanders (in person or over the phone), paramedics (verbally pass on information gained from bystanders and see their transfer sheet [handover sheet contains notes, a less rich source of information]). Basically use every source available to provide information to help you (and subsequent doctors) decide between a fit or other cause – important consequences for patient

### Pre-event/prodrome

Ask how he felt immediately before the collapse, e.g. warnings/aura

Events preceding a seizure can include aura: somato-sensory (olfactory, auditory or visual hallucinations), autonomic or 'psychic'

Other warning symptoms or signs, e.g. dizziness, visual changes, nausea; sudden-onset headache (SAH)

Other symptoms for clue to diagnosis: rash, fever, headache, photophobia (meningitis), chest pain, palpitations, dizziness, SOB (cardiac/arrhythmia/PE)

NB: migrainous headache can have visual aura, e.g. fortification spectra, unformed flashes of white and/or black images, but rarely multicoloured (c.f. occipital seizure)

What was he doing immediately before the collapse (provoking factors/triggers)? Provides clues as to cause:

  Cardiogenic/vasovagal – exercise-induced; postural hypotension (e.g. standing from sitting position); vasovagal (hot rooms, anxiety/upset); passing urine, cough (micturition and stress syncope)

  Seizure – ask for common triggers, e.g lack of sleep; drugs including illicit drugs; alcohol and herbal or alternative therapies; any recent illness (fever, neck stiffness, rash); hunger; strobe lights; hypoglycaemia (history of diabetes, fasting)

Any previous episodes? Were these ever investigated? Any precipitant identified? If known seizure, ask about compliance with antiepileptic medications

### During event

Does he remember collapsing/hitting the floor? (helps differentiate syncope from simple fall)

Did he lose consciousness? Duration of LOC

Any signs consistent with a seizure (patients who have a vasovagal syncope may twitch a little)

Collateral history from bystanders/witness (if available):

  How did the patient look prior to event? (pale, cyanosed, appeared 'vacant', sweating profusely, confused/irritable?)

  Did the patient lose consciousness? If yes, what was the duration?

  Was anything else seen/heard? (groaning noises, stiffness, twitching and jerking of limbs, eyes both closed/opened, eyes rolled back, twitching of face)

  Duration of event and the side of involvement (left/right/both)

### Post-event

Ask how he felt after the collapse. Ask about confusion, incontinence, tongue-biting, headache, photophobia, lethargy, weakness in arms or legs after the event

NB: speed of recovery is important – fast in vasovagal compared to more prolonged (30 min to hours) following a seizure, often with postictal confusion/headache or transient limb weakness (Todd's paresis)

Obtain information from bystanders/witnesses regarding speed of recovery

### Drug history

If known to have epilepsy – any missed doses or new medicines (with potential effects on metabolism of anticonvulsants)

Prescribed medications including β-blockers, BP medications, ACE inhibitors, oral hypoglycaemic drugs, insulin

Over-the-counter medications, herbal and alternative medicines

Drugs which prolong QT interval

Illicit drugs including amphetamine, cocaine, cannabis, ecstasy, any performance-enhancing drugs

### Past medical history

Previous episodes?

History of seizure/epilepsy (since birth to present)

Previous history of head injury, history of malignancy or brain tumour, cerebrovascular disease

Any history of febrile convulsion, childhood central nervous system infection, e.g. encephalitis, meningitis or birth trauma (childhood asphyxia)

Diabetes: autonomic neuropathy; immunocompromised?

Any IHD, cardiac arrhythmias

### Social history

Alcohol history: important to consider alcohol withdrawal seizure; quantify alcohol intake in units per week

Lifestyle (sleep hygiene, frequent nights out in clubs with stroboscopic lights)

Any family history of sudden death (ask about siblings and rest of family), epilepsy, IHD, arrhythmias, pacemakers

Ask about occupation, driving

### Address patient's questions and concerns

• *Have you had any thoughts about what is going on?*
• *Is there anything in particular you're concerned about?*
• *Do you have anything you would like to ask?*

## Key areas for examination

A list of what to look for (in examination order; describe findings on examination)

Any congenital anomalies (Sturge–Weber's, neurofibromatosis, tuberous sclerosis)

Other causes of epilepsy: look for learning disabilities, mobility/wheelchair bound; cerebral palsy and other syndromic epilepsy disorders

GCS, pupils, visual fields (any hemianopia?), ophthalmoplegia, look for facial hemisensory loss, facial asymmetry, tongue deviation (also look for signs of bitten tongue)

Upper and lower limb neurological screening: gait, check for tone (spasticity), power, reflexes including both plantars, and clonus, cerebellar signs

Look for a petechial rash

Neck stiffness/Kernig's sign

Ask to see the observations including temperature, lying and standing BP, blood glucose, ECG (AV block, QT interval, WPW syndrome, ischaemic changes) from both paramedics and hospital records

Mention that you would like to examine the peripheral nervous system fully, including fundoscopy to look for papilloedema, optic atrophy, diabetic eye changes, full cardiovascular examination (unlikely to be time for this)

## Differential diagnosis

Syncope: cardiogenic – dysrhythmia, vasovagal
Hypoglycaemia
Seizure (epileptic)
Non-epileptic disorder
Transient ischaemic attack

Seizure is the most likely diagnosis – history is consistent with generalized seizure (supported by the history of possible olfactory aura, history from bystanders in terms of the description during the event and long duration of postictal confusion, LOC and no recollec-

tion of event from patient. Doesn't sound like vasovagal, cardiogenic or hypoglycaemic attacks but they need to be excluded by simple first-line investigations

## Discussion with patient

Explain diagnosis
Explain plan, including investigations and management
Address patient's concerns/answer their questions

The history of your symptoms is consistent with a seizure. This is likely to be a first epileptic fit but this needs to be properly investigated and we will need specialists to look at your need for medications and the impact this will have on your job and your driving licence.

### Investigations

Bloods including inflammatory markers

CT/MRI: inpatient versus outpatient. CT head is usually done as inpatient if space-occupying lesion is suspected. If patient is well with no evidence of infection and has no further seizure with normal CT head, he can be discharged with urgent outpatient MRI scan and neurology follow-up (ideally within 2 weeks)

EEG: interictal recording commonly normal in patients with epilepsy (50%), and normal EEG doesn't exclude patient having epilepsy. EEG plays a role in supporting the diagnosis, when combined with good history and clinical examination and associated imaging findings. It also plays a role in seizure classification, especially in neonatal/childhood/juvenile epilepsy to aid treatment with appropriate group of antiepileptic drugs

### Management

Outpatient neurology/epilepsy and 'first fit' clinic referral: often rapid access pathway available. Admit depending on the aetiology (e.g. suspected CNS infection, space-occupying lesion, high risk of recurrence, significant comorbidities that might endanger patient upon discharge). Important to seek specialist advice as diagnosis has significant consequences – driving, employment, lifestyle changes, etc.

DVLA advice for truck driving (UK driving licensing) – see www.dvla.gov.uk

Advice leaflet on 'first fit'

### Addressing concerns/answering questions

• *What happened?* From the information we have at the moment, it is most likely that you have had an epileptic seizure.
• *Will it happen again?* Depends on age, aetiology, combined with EEG and neuroimaging findings.

Overall risk of seizure recurrence after first unprovoked seizure is 50%; risk is much reduced if no aetiology is identified including normal EEG and neuroimaging findings (14% at 1 year and 24% at 2 years). Patients with structural lesions on CT or MRI scans have a risk of recurrence up to 65% at 2 years.

- *What about driving and my job?* This depends on the type of lorries you are driving, the licence you have, when you obtained it and the results of the investigations planned. You have a legal obligation to inform the DVLA to explain the situation and they will assess when you can drive. If you drive before they have declared you fit you will not be covered by your insurance. With a Group 1 licence you would need to avoid driving until the results of the investigations are available. You would need a minimum of 6 months off driving from the date of the seizure, longer (12 months) if there are clinical factors or investigation results which suggest the risk of another seizure is 2% or greater per year. (NB if the group 1 licence was obtained before 1997, group 1 licence holders also able to drive lorries between 3.5–7.5 tonnes but not larger lorries or buses. This has implications/opportunities for your future employment.)

With a Group 2 HGV licence you would need a minimum of 5 years off driving if all the invesigations are normal, you have not taken any antiepilepsy medication during this time and the assessing neurologist feels the risk of further seizures is less than 2% a year. If the risk is greater than 2% or there are structural changes on the investigations DVLA epilepsy guidance applies: regulations require a driver to 'remain seizure-free for 10 years since the last attack without anticonvulsant medication'.

- *Can you prevent this from happening again?* The planned investigations, CT scan and EEG will help us to give you more information about whether you are likely to have further seizures. If they suggest that you are at risk of more seizures we can start medication to reduce your seizures. This will be followed up in the epilepsy clinic.

## Discussion with examiners

The examiners may ask you to clarify details of the above diagnosis and ask questions about your planned investigations and management.

Other possible questions include:
- *Would you start an antiepileptic drug?* No if it is the first fit and there is no specific aetiology, and EEG and neuroimaging findings are normal.
- *What is the management of status epilepticus?* Definition: recurring seizures, without patient regaining consciousness between attacks, for ≥30 min. Failure of appropriate management to terminate the attack may result in significant cerebral anoxia and permanent brain damage or death. ABCD, secure airway, inform anaesthetist for urgent review. Treatment – IV lorazepam 4 mg bolus (alternative diazepam, clonazepam), IV phenytoin loading dose 18 mg/kg with cardiac monitoring, then 300 mg IV/po od. If condition continues despite treatment, will need anaesthetic drugs such as propofol or thiopentone, intubation and ventilation and transfer to ICU. Urgent investigations: CT head, EEG (to confirm status), check for contributory factors, e.g. electrolyte imbalance (Mg, U&E, calcium), sepsis (inflammatory markers, blood cultures, CXR), lumbar puncture if necessary (in suspected CNS infection). Measurement of blood levels of antiepileptic drugs (AEDs) is helpful in patients known to be on them (to check concordance and help physicians to adjust treatment). Instigate usual AEDs regime in patients known to have epilepsy. NB: recurrent focal seizures: carbamazepine, lamotrigine, levetiracetam, topiramate, gabapentin, lacosamide. Recurrent generalized seizures – sodium valproate, lamotrigine, levetiracetam. Know common side-effects for counselling, especially in young women who still want to conceive.
- *Name some predisposing factors for seizures.* Alcohol, poor sleep hygiene, CNS stimulant drugs, interactions with usual antiepileptic drugs, stress, non-concordance to medication, brain injury, cerebrovascular disease, structural brain lesion, CNS infection and systemic sepsis, metabolic, hypoxia, electrolyte imbalance.

**Examiners' information and requirements**

The candidate should:

1. Identify seizure as the probable cause of syncopal episode: LOC with clinical features suggestive of epilepsy
2. Outline a clear management plan including appropriate specialist referrals
3. Organized outpatient management: 'first fit' clinic with appropriate urgent outpatient investigations, e.g. EEG and MRI (epilepsy sequence)
4. Give a clear explanation of your diagnosis and plan to the patient; address the patient's concerns and explain DVLA guidance. Reassure him as this may well be an isolated event

**Further reading/resources**

DVLA: www.dvla.gov.uk

NICE guidance on epilepsy: www.guidance.nice.org.uk/CG137

Epilepsy Action: www.epilepsy.org.uk/info/

International League Against Epilepsy UK (ILAE): www.ilae.org/

# Scenario 51 | Essential tremor

## Candidate's information

**Your role:** you are an ST2 in the Care of the Elderly medical clinic. You have been asked by a GP to see this 70-year-old man with a long history of tremor. The patient is concerned that he may have Parkinson's disease, and hadn't wanted to try any medications from his GP without a specialist review.

**Your task:** to assess the patient's problems and address any questions or concerns raised by him.

## Patient's information

**You are:** Albert Soames, a 70-year-old man.

**Your problem:** you have a tremor in both hands. It's been there for probably 5–6 years, and hasn't changed a great deal over the past couple of years. It gets worse when you're anxious or when giving a talk at the local Neighbourhood Watch meeting that you chair every month. You've not tried any medicines but the tremor settles after a few drinks (beer). The reason you went to your doctor is that your friends had noticed a new tremor affecting your head over the past 6 months or so and mentioned it to you, and you saw a programme on TV about Parkinson's disease.

You're walking OK and no differently from before. Your speech and writing are also pretty much the same as before. No change in bowel habit or swallowing.

### Past medical history and drug history:
- No other past medical problems
- Never been into hospital

### Social history:
- Non-smoker
- You drink about 10 units alcohol/week

### Other issues including family history:
- Your father had a slight tremor in the last years of his life – died age 90
- A family friend in his 70s died from dementia linked to Parkinson's disease – it was very upsetting for everyone involved

### Your questions for the candidate:
- *Do I have Parkinson's disease?*
- *Will it get worse?*
- *Do you have any treatments for it?*

# Candidate

## History/key questions

When did tremor start? How has it changed over this period?

Unilateral versus bilateral. If bilateral, which side starts first? Or about the same time?

Head and neck involvement (titubation)?

Does the tremor occur at rest (resting tremor, e.g. PD)/ during change in posture (postural tremor)/during movement or approaching a target (kinetic tremor/ intention tremor, e.g. cerebellar disease)/all the time (drugs, metabolic, physiological)?

Exacerbants: emotion, being watched, stress/anxiety, exercise, fatigue, alcohol

Relieving factors: essential tremor often eased by alcohol

NB: PD tremor occurs at rest, usually starts off as uni-lateral and asymmetrical. PD tremor usually affects the hands but can involve lower limbs, but not the head and neck. It is exacerbated by stress, infection or anxiety and improves with action

Any changes in gait, handwriting. See old hand-writing samples

Any change in voice. Difficulty swallowing. Drooling of saliva

Any double vision (tremor from Parkinson's plus syn-drome of supranuclear palsy)

Any cramps in the hands or feet, or turning of the head (dystonia)

Any postural dizziness, sphincter disturbance, palpita-tions (autonomic symptoms in Parkinson's plus syndrome, e.g. Shy–Drager syndrome)

Any deterioration in cognitive function (dementia)? Or hallucinations (Lewy body dementia)

### Drug history

Ask about drugs which can cause tremor, e.g. β-adrenergic agonists, SSRIs, TCA, theophylline, caf-feine, valproate, lithium

Drug withdrawal can also cause tremor – alcohol, ben-zodiazepines, morphine/opiates

### Past medical history

Any history of thyroid problems (thyrotoxicosis)/goitre

CVA (basal ganglia)

### Social and family history

Any family history of tremor? Parkinson's? Early-onset dementia?

Occupational history – mercury

## Address patient's questions and concerns

- *Have you had any thoughts about what is going on?*
- *Is there anything in particular you're concerned about?*
- *Do you have anything you would like to ask?*

## Key areas for examination

A list of what to look for (in examination order; describe findings on examination)

Signs of PD: drooling saliva, mask-like (expressionless/ hypomimia) face

Monotonous speech: slurring/quiet/husky/ monoto-nous (in PD), staccato (cerebellar)

Check for eye movement (failure of upward gaze ini-tially in PSP), nystagmus (cerebellar in Parkinson's plus syndrome)

Signs of thyroid eye disease (see Section I, Station 5, Eyes, Case 1)

Head and neck involvement (jaw and tongue can be involved in PD, not whole head), any palatal tremor (lesions in dentato-rubro-olivary pathways)

Comment about character of tremor (coarse/fine, resting/kinetic/action)

Lift both arms outstretched and observe tremor

NB: essential tremor is seen in hands and arms, when arms are outstretched and at the end of a task-directed action, e.g. drinking liquid from a glass; can be unilateral or bilateral

NB: PD patients have slow, fine resting tremor (3–6 Hz), pill-rolling (hands) in character, usually unilateral or asymmetrical. Note PD triad of bradykinesia/rigidity/ resting tremor (See Vol. 1, Station 3, CNS, Case 3)

Check for bradykinesia: See Vol. 1, Station 3, CNS, Case 3.

Tone: constant rigidity throughout the range of move-ment (leadpipe), cogwheeling on testing of tone at wrist (due to rigidity being superimposed by tremor)

Look for other cerebellar signs (dysdiadochokinesia, ataxia, intention tremor); dystonia

Gait: problem with initiation (freezing), festinant/ stooped/poor arm swing/small shuffling steps 'as if trying to keep up with his own centre of gravity'/ falling backward on retropulsion/poor turning in PD; broad-based and difficulty with tandem walking in cerebellar ataxia

Get patient to write (micrographia)

Pulse: exclude AF, tachycardia (thyroid)

## Differential diagnosis

Essential tremor: symmetrical, exacerbating and reliev-ing factors, especially better with alcohol. No other

Red Flag signs to suggest parkinsonism or any cerebellar signs or symptoms

PD: unlikely: symmetrical/bilateral, head tremor, not characteristic of resting tremor, improves with alcohol, no other hard signs of parkinsonism, e.g. bradykinesia, rigidity, parkinsonian gait

Psychological

Other differential diagnoses include cerebellar/Parkinson's plus syndrome, orthostatic, MS (rubral tremor), basal ganglia, stroke (unlikely bilateral) and drug-induced

NB: essential tremor is called familial tremor if there is a family history (50% autosomal dominant pattern). It is usually called benign essential tremor if sporadic

## Discussion with patient

Explain diagnosis

Explain plan, including investigations and management

Address patient's concerns/answer their questions

What you have is 'essential tremor' which is benign and it is not PD; it is worse when you are anxious or under stress and better with alcohol. It commonly involves the hand, usually in a symmetrical manner bilaterally. It runs a fairly benign course and rarely progresses or involves the head, voice, tongue, leg or trunk. It is usually absent on resting.

We will give you a trial of a medication that helps to reduce or possibly abolish the tremor (β-blockers such as propranolol). We will see whether the tremor improves as we follow you up in our clinic.

### Investigations

Check thyroid function test, liver function tests, B12, serum copper and caeruloplasmin in younger patient (to exclude Wilson's disease)

MRI brain only needed if structural lesion or cerebrovascular disease in basal ganglia is suspected

### Management

Reassurance: head tremor not seen in PD. History suggestive of essential tremor and no Red Flag signs of Parkinson's plus syndrome

Propranolol (crosses blood–brain barrier) in low dose and then titrate up

### Addressing concerns/answering questions

- *Do I have Parkinson's disease?* Very unlikely. We will see how you respond to the β-blockers. You have no features of Parkinson's disease.

- *Will it get worse?* Some run a benign course and some slowly progress to become more coarse or involve other parts of the body.

- *Do you have any treatments for it?* Mild symptoms: physical (using weights) and psychological measures, lifestyle changes (e.g. reduce caffeine intake or stimulants), propranolol 40 mg 2–3 times daily, alternatively primidone initially 50 mg od, others include benzodiazepines, calcium channel blockers, gabapentin. Thalamotomy or thalamic deep brain stimulation can be tried in very severe and debilitating cases.

## Discussion with examiners

The examiners may ask you to clarify details of the above diagnosis and ask questions about your planned investigations and management.

Other possible questions include:

- *Do you know any test to diagnose essential tremor?* Mostly from tremor history, including family history, age of onset, clinical findings and response to β-blockers. Electromyography or tremographic accelerometer can be used to assess the frequency, amplitude and rhythmicity of the tremor. Severity and response to treatment can be assessed by functional assessment, Tremor Scale and using Archimedes spirals (getting patient to draw smooth spiral on a piece of paper).

- *Do you know of any tests to exclude PD?* Good history-taking and examination skills are paramount. If suspect PD or in atypical tremor, DaTscan (ioflupane I-123 injection) can help to differentiate between essential tremor and parkinsonian syndrome. It detects dopamine transporters using single photon emission computed tomography (SPECT). It measures the amount and location of radioactive ioflupane I-123 in the brain. However, this test cannot differentiate between idiopathic Parkinson's disease and multisystem atrophy or PSP. The test is normal in essential tremor. The scan can be used as an adjunct to clinical examination.

See also Vol. 1, Station 3, CNS, Case 3.

**Examiners' information and requirements**

The candidate should:

1. Identify key features from the history: chronic history, bilateral tremor, recent head tremor. Exacerbated by stress/anxiety, eased by alcohol
2. Identify key examination findings including bilateral tremor, no cerebellar signs, no signs of PD/cogwheeling
3. Make the diagnosis of essential tremor rather than PD and outline a sensible management plan
4. Give a clear explanation to the patient of your diagnosis and plan, address his concerns and answer his questions

**Further reading/resources**

www.wemove.org/

# Scenario 52 | Temporal arteritis

## Candidate's information
**Your role:** you are an ST2 in the MAU. A 70-year-old woman has been referred by her GP with headache and blurred vision.

**Your task:** to assess the patient's problems and address any questions or concerns raised by her.

## Patient's information
**You are:** Amelia Maudsley, a 70-year-old woman

**Your problem:** you have a 1-week history of dull right-sided headache which has become much more severe over the past 24h. You have also had 3 days of pain in the right jaw just below the ear which has been worse on chewing. Also painful to brush hair on that side of the head. In the past six hours, you have had slight blurring of vision in your right eye – now cleared.

You have no arm or leg weakness, or speech change noticed by you or your family. No rash. You have felt generally lethargic/fatigued over the past week or so. You haven't been eating as normal – just lost your appetite.

**Past medical history and drug history:**
- High blood pressure and raised cholesterol, both of which GP says are well controlled by diet and tablets
- Takes aspirin 75 mg once per day, perindopril and simvastatin 40 mg
- Attends practice nurse for BP checks – last needed to see GP about 6 months ago after a fall

**Social history:**
- Independent, lives alone
- Son visits and helps out with jobs round the house
- Retired accountant

**Other issues including family history:**
- Nothing runs in the family

**Your questions for the candidate:**
- *Have I had a stroke?*
- *How serious is this?*
- *How do you take a biopsy? Do I need a general anaesthetic?*

# Candidate

## History/key questions

Multiple symptoms reported in GCA/temporal arteritis

Onset can be rapid, but may be insidious

Ask about low-grade fever (can be high in 15%), myalgia, fatigue, anorexia, weight loss; these may be present for weeks or months before presentation

Headache occurs in approximately two-thirds, and early. Classic description is of temporal headache but it can be diffuse

Scalp sensitivity (washing or brushing hair)

PMR symptoms in approximately 40%

Arteritis causing jaw claudication (chewing food or talking) in half of patients

Visual symptoms include partial or complete loss of vision in one or both eyes (reported in 20%). If untreated, second eye likely to become involved in 1–2 weeks. Urgent treatment essential to reduce the risk of visual loss. Other symptoms include diplopia

Ask about evidence of arteritis elsewhere, e.g. intermittent claudication, angina, bruits

Ask about weight loss (occurs in 14%)

## Address patient's questions and concerns

• *Have you had any thoughts about what is going on?*
• *Is there anything in particular you're concerned about?*
• *Do you have anything you would like to ask?*

## Key areas for examination

A list of what to look for (in examination order; describe findings on examination)

Patient's temperature

Look for aching/stiffness/tenderness of upper limbs consistent with PMR (40%)

Palpate temporal/occipital arteries: tenderness (scalp tenderness in 50%), thickening, reduced pulsation; overlying skin can be red

Assess visual acuity, visual fields, fundoscopy: pallor/oedema of optic disc; cotton wool patches and small haemorrhages can also be seen

Full CNS examination (if sufficient time)

Look for signs of vascular disease elsewhere (or say you would), including left and right arm BPs (differential BPs may be a result of large vessel vasculitis), peripheral pulses and listen for bruits

Check for proximal muscle tenderness (myalgia). Failure of shoulder abduction in PMR is due to pain rather than true weakness

Say that you would like to carry out full examination of peripheral nervous system (insufficient time) as can see neurological signs in 30% (mononeuropathy or polyneuropathy of arms/legs)

Ask to see blood results if available, particularly ESR, CRP, FBC, alkaline phosphatase

## Differential diagnosis

GCA/temporal arteritis is the key differential diagnosis

Vasculitis of different sorts

Cerebrovascular disease: given transient blurring/visual loss, need to consider TIA

**Key facts/areas to consider** (including information available in scenario summary before station starts): empirical treatment important before biopsy as potential consequences of delay, e.g. visual loss, are preventable/avoidable

American College of Rheumatology Criteria for giant cell arteritis: three or more of the following (three or more is reported to have both sensitivity and specificity greater than 90% for giant cell arteritis):

Onset at 50 years of age or older

New type of headache

Clinically abnormal temporal artery: thickened, tender or nodular, with decreased pulsation

ESR 50 mm/h or greater

Abnormal arterial biopsy showing necrotizing arteritis with mononuclear infiltrate or granulomatous inflammation, usually with multinucleated giant cells

## Discussion with patient

Explain diagnosis

Explain plan, including investigations and management

Address patient's concerns/answer their questions

You have inflammation of an important artery. We need to give you steroids to settle this down, whilst arranging for a small sample of this blood vessel to be taken to confirm the diagnosis. Explain the procedure for temporal artery biopsy, including potential side-effects. Procedure usually performed under local anaesthetic. Potential complications include bleeding, infection, damage to nerve branches (facial / auriculotemporal nerves), hair loss around scar line, non-diagnostic sample.

## Investigations

Blood tests including ESR

Review by ophthalmology if visual disturbance

Biopsy of temporal artery within 3 days (70% get positive histology with 2 cm segment of artery) – can have skip lesions so a normal biopsy doesn't exclude GCA/temporal arteritis. Can be up to 2 weeks into steroid course

## Management
Steroids: start immediately with prednisolone at a dose of 60–80 mg od if visual disturbance, 40 mg od if not; 40 mg weeks 1–4, 30 mg weeks 5–6, and 20 mg weeks 7–8. Some will treat with IV initially. Reduce down to 5–7.5 mg then slower beyond this guided by clinical symptoms. Expected duration = 2 years
PPI
Bone protection: high risk of osteoporosis with prolonged steroids
Advice on driving depends on presence of visual disturbance (diplopia, changes in visual acuity and visual fields): see DVLA guidelines

## Addressing concerns/answering questions
- *Have I had a stroke?* Your symptoms are due to inflammation of some blood vessels rather than a stroke which is a clot in an artery in the brain.
- *How serious is this?* It is potentially serious if left untreated as the blood vessels in your eyes can be affected causing problems with your vision. The steroids settle the inflammation and reduce the risk of complications, initially a high dose and then gradually reducing it down.
- *How do you take a biopsy? Do I need a general anaesthetic?* The procedure is usually performed under local anaesthetic. Potential complications include bleeding, infection, damage to nerve branches (facial / auriculotemporal nerves), hair loss around scar line, taking a non-diagnostic sample.

## Discussion with examiners
The examiners may ask you to clarify details of the above diagnosis and ask questions about your planned investigations and management.

A possible question includes:
- *Would you start treatment or wait for confirmation of diagnosis by biopsy?* The consequences of delay or waiting, inadequate management or missing this diagnosis include permanent visual loss (central retinal artery occlusion). Manage by starting steroids immediately and then obtaining a tissue sample shortly after, and this helps reduce the risk of visual loss but still potentially allows us to obtain diagnostic tissue sample. Discuss steroid dose and duration, and need for PPI cover. Immunosuppression and use of steroid-sparing agents – less effective than steroids.

---

**Examiners' information and requirements**

The candidate should:

1. Identify key features from the history: headache, jaw claudication, painful to brush hair and visual disturbance
2. Identify key examination findings including palpation of temporal arteries (visual fields) and fundoscopy
3. Need to provide diagnosis of temporal arteritis and outline a sensible management plan including the need for steroids now and then arranging a biopsy; long-term steroids required
4. Give a clear explanation to the patient of your diagnosis and plan, address her concerns and answer her questions

---

## Further reading/resources
www.cks.nhs.uk
www.cks.nhs.uk/giant_cell_arteritis/

# Scenario 53 | Carpal tunnel syndrome

## Candidate's information
**Your role:** you are an ST2 in the general medical clinic. A GP has referred a 55-year-old woman with pain in the hands and fingers, worse after exercise.

**Your task:** to assess the patient's problems and address any questions or concerns raised by the patient.

## Patient's information
**You are:** Kay Holton, a 55-year-old personal assistant to a local businessman.

**Your problem:** you are experiencing tingling in the fingers in both hands, worse on the right than the left, particularly at the end of the day. This has slowly become more noticeable in the past 3 months. You work as a secretary and it does interfere with your job as your hands can feel a little weaker than usual by the end of a full day's work. It's less of an issue at the weekends or on holiday. You've noticed that your thumb and first two fingers are affected; the tingling is worse at night and eased by shaking your wrists/hands. You're worried about keeping your job, as typing seems to bring it all on. You have experienced weight gain of 1 stone over the past year.

**Past medical history and drug history:**
- Known hypothyroidism with a stable dose of levothyroxine over the past few years

**Social history:**
- Your mother has rheumatoid arthritis and is very disabled by it – you're keen to avoid this

**Other issues including family history:**
- Nil of note

**Your questions for the candidate:**
- *Have I got rheumatoid arthritis?*
- *Will it go away without treatment?*
- *How long does it take to recover from the surgery?*

# Candidate

## History/key questions

Symptoms of carpal tunnel syndrome: predominantly nocturnal pain, paraesthesiae and tingling in fingers in the median nerve distribution (first 3½ fingers – thumb, index finger, middle finger and half of the ring finger), but can affect the whole hand in a glove distribution

Symptoms can wake the patient up during the night; eased by shaking/wringing the hand or by running under hot water. It can recur in the day after use or after rest. Exacerbated by activities which extend the wrist, e.g. typing, driving, using phone, continuing with arm/wrist in same position for prolonged periods of time, including sleep

Contributing factors include endocrine diseases (hypothyroidism, Cushing's, acromegaly); fluid retention in pregnancy, menopause and chronic liver disease; diabetes; rheumatoid arthritis; obesity; amyloidosis. Also wrist trauma (local swelling or direct nerve injury); dialysis; lifestyle/occupation (typist, handling vibrating tools); idiopathic

Motor involvement in more severe cases can lead to functional problems (such as clumsiness or weakness – unable to open jar lids, problems holding objects)

## Address patient's questions and concerns

• *Have you had any thoughts about what is going on?*
• *Is there anything in particular you're concerned about?*
• *Do you have anything you would like to ask?*

## Key areas for examination

A list of what to look for (in examination order; describe findings on examination)

Aim to identify a cause of the symptoms (e.g. carpal tunnel syndrome) and look for signs of underlying medical conditions exacerbating the condition, such as acromegaly, pregnancy, RA, myxoedema, DM, gout, previous fractures of radius

Hands/upper limbs: test all motor and sensory function in the upper limbs, but put extra focus on the hands given the history consistent with carpal tunnel syndrome

Inspection: look for scars of previous surgery; thenar and lumbricals I and II wasting (late sign suggesting chronic problems); dialysis fistula (current and previous sites); gouty tophi; RA hands; size of the hands (acromegaly), dry skin (hypothyroid); blood glucose monitoring scars on fingers (diabetes)

NB: the median nerve supplies the five intrinsic muscles of the hand (LOAF – 1st and 2nd Lumbricals, Opponens pollicis, Abductor pollicis brevis, Flexor pollicis brevis). It gives out a branch called the anterior interosseous nerve just below the elbow, supplying flexor digitorum profundus I and II, flexor pollicis longus and pronator quadratus

Motor findings: weakness in thumb abduction (abductor pollicis brevis), opposition of the thumb by touching the base of the little finger (opponens pollicis), flexion of thumb at proximal phalanx (flexor pollicis brevis). Weakness in thumb and index finger opposition (making a tight circle) usually suggests that the aetiology is proximal to the carpal tunnel region itself, e.g. pronator teres syndrome. Also quickly check for other intrinsic nerve involvement to rule out more proximal lesions, i.e. finger extensors (radial nerve) and index finger and little finger abduction (ulnar nerve to first dorsal interosseus and abductor digiti minimi respectively)

Sensory findings: ask patient to draw/map out area with reduced sensation (thumb, index and middle fingers, and half of her ring finger). Check for pinprick and light touch. NB: palmar sensory branch leaves the median nerve proximal to the tunnel, hence thenar sensory loss usually suggests a severe carpal tunnel compression or a more proximal lesion in the forearm

Phalen's: ask patient to keep both wrists in full palmar flexion for 1 min – may bring on symptoms in the median nerve distribution in the affected side

Tinel's: tapping over the course of the median nerve at the wrist causes tingling in the median nerve distribution

Check for upper limb reflexes, especially C6 (biceps and supinator) to differentiate between pure median nerve pathology and C6 radiculopathy

Quick look for acromegalic, Cushing's or hypothyroid facial features, insulin injection sites on the abdominal wall, peritoneal dialysis scars or renal transplant scars

Say that to complete your examination, you would do a full peripheral nerve examination looking for signs of peripheral neuropathy or mononeuritis multiplex, including cranial nerves. You would also want to perform fundoscopy to look for signs of diabetic retinopathy, check blood sugar and check urine for glucose.

## Differential diagnosis

C6/C7 or C8/T1 radiculopathy
Brachial plexopathy (lateral chord)

Mononeuritis multiplex

Peripheral neuropathy

Reflex sympathetic dystrophy following insult or trauma (complex regional pain syndrome)

The characteristic history and the median nerve distribution of symptoms and signs, sparing other muscles supplied by different nerve territories (the anatomy and localization make radiculopathy or plexopathy unlikely)

## Discussion with patient

Explain diagnosis

Explain plan, including investigations and management

Address patient's concerns/answer their questions

Carpal tunnel syndrome is a condition that affects the median nerve that runs down your arm all the way to your hand, which has been compressed at the wrist as it passes beneath a tendon in your wrist. This irritates the nerves which causes the tingling sensation. If the compression progresses, there is a high chance that the nerve can be further damaged, causing numbness and weakness in the hand. There are a few factors that contribute to this condition and having an underactive thyroid is one of them. It can also be made worse by being a little bit overweight. We will carry out tests to confirm what I found today, and we can then discuss what the next step would be. This may include adjustment of your thyroid medications, weight loss, wearing a wrist splint, steroid injection or surgery if the pressure on the nerve needs to be released.

## Investigations

Check TSH, fasting blood glucose, blood pressure, rheumatoid factor, ESR and hand X-ray (if suspect RA)

Nerve conduction studies are helpful to support the diagnosis and grade the severity before surgical procedures. The role of EMG is to exclude plexopathy or radiculopathy. However, mild carpal tunnel syndrome might reveal normal nerve conduction studies and focal demyelination might appear later on as the disease progresses. Parameters in nerve conduction studies include slowing of median nerve sensory conduction velocity and onset latency across the wrist and, as the compression worsens, the motor nerve will be affected, causing delayed distal motor latency and, in severe cases, attenuation of motor amplitude.

## Management

Treat any exacerbating or predisposing conditions (weight loss in obesity / await delivery if pregnant / treat hypothyroidism or other endocrine diseases)

Practical advice: rest, wrist splint or braces at night, referral to occupational therapist

Medication: for neuropathic pain – amitriptyline, gabapentin, pregabalin, local steroid injection, NSAIDs, diuretics

Consider surgical decompression or corticosteroid injection if severe or constant symptoms, severe sensory and / or motor disturbance; if no improvement with conservative treatment within 3 months; if condition progressive (motor or sensory deficit)

Poor prognostic indicators following conservative treatment:

Disease >10 months

Age >50

Positive Phalen's >30 sec

Prolonged motor and sensory latency on electrophysiological study

Constant paraesthesiae

Two-point discrimination >6 mm

### Addressing concerns/answering questions

- *Have I got rheumatoid arthritis?* Your symptoms and the reduced sensation and power on examination fit with a condition called carpal tunnel syndrome. There are no signs of joint inflammation to suggest that you have rheumatoid arthritis.
- *Will it go away without treatment?* The condition may resolve by itself depending on the cause but some simple measures can help speed the recovery or prevent further deterioration, e.g. wearing a splint at night or at times during the day.
- *How long does it take to recover from the surgery?* It depends on the severity of the damage to the nerve. In mild-to-moderate cases, you may regain motor function followed by sensory improvement. In severe cases, i.e. significant motor involvement, muscle wasting, there will be residual symptoms. With successful surgery, recurrence is rare and, if so, the initial diagnosis then needs to be reconsidered.

## Discussion with examiners

The examiners may ask you to clarify details of the above diagnosis and ask questions about your planned investigations and management.

Other possible questions include:

- *Explain the median nerve innervations.* The median nerve originates from C6/T1 roots, lateral cord of the brachial plexus. It branches out at the antecubital fossa to supply pronator teres, flexor carpi radialis, palmaris longus and flexor digitorum profundus.

Compression at this site can cause pronator teres syndrome. It branches out just below the antecubital fossa as the anterior interosseous nerve which supplies flexor digitorum profundus I and II, flexor pollicis longus and pronator quadratus. It supplies the hand muscles distally which are the lumbricals I and II, opponens pollicis, abductor pollicis brevis and flexor pollicis brevis (LOAF). Most proximal muscles are from C6/C7 and distal muscles from C8/T1.

- *Would a normal nerve conduction study make you doubt your diagnosis – and would you still recommend surgery?* Carpal tunnel syndrome is a clinical diagnosis based on clinical symptoms and signs. Nerve conduction study is helpful to support the diagnosis but might miss very mild disease. As a general rule, the test itself has a sensitivity of >85% and specificity of >95%. In mild cases, surgical treatment is not warranted. Patients with very severe symptoms and a normal electrodiagnostic study or symptoms disproportionate to the electrophysiological findings will need reassessing and the diagnosis reconsidered, e.g. imaging of the cervical spine looking for radiculopathy. The use of ultrasound in assessing the diameter of the median nerve at the wrist is currently under evaluation.

See also Vol. 1, Station 3, CNS, Case 33.

---

**Examiners' information and requirements**

The candidate should:

1. Identify key features from the history: pain at night, eased by wringing/shaking, exacerbated by work (typing)
2. Identify key examination findings with a focused examination: characteristic motor and sensory changes of carpal tunnel syndrome; use of Phalen's and Tinel's signs to reinforce diagnosis. Looking for signs of other associated conditions, e.g. diabetes, acromegaly, etc.
3. Outline a sensible management plan including conservative measures, referral for nerve conduction studies and referral to surgeons for consideration of operation if carpal tunnel syndrome confirmed
4. Give a clear explanation to the patient of your diagnosis and plan, address her concerns and answer her questions

# Scenario 54 | Multiple sclerosis/diplopia

## Candidate's information

**Your role:** you are one of the doctors on-call in the MAU. You have been asked to see this 62-year-old man who has presented with double vision.

**Your task:** to assess the patient's problems and address any questions or concerns raised by him.

## Patient's information

**You are:** Bill Wheeldon, a 62-year-old man.

**Your problem:** your main problem is double vision, which started about a week ago, and your vision has been blurred at times. The double vision is worse when you look to either side. There has been no loss of vision during this episode. This blurring of vision seems to be worse when you're taking a hot bath. Apart from the double vision, you have no other complaints. No arm or leg weakness, no numbness or pins and needles noticed. No change in bladder or bowel function. No swallowing or speech difficulty. No headache. No problem with your walking. You don't get any 'tingling/electrical' feeling shooting down your spine when you bend your neck forward.

You remember having similar symptoms about 2 years ago in the summer, which lasted about 3 weeks, and it settled on its own. You then had painful loss of vision in your left eye, which lasted for a few hours, and the vision in your left eye remained blurry for about a week. Your vision then gradually improved but you remained seeing double. You had no loss of vision in the right eye. You were still able to work and drive. After a couple of weeks it hadn't settled so you went to see your GP who advised you to go and see an optician. You didn't get time to go and it all settled a week or so later. Your blood sugar had been checked and it was normal.

You've come to hospital now after seeing your GP for the second time, who told you in no uncertain terms to come and get assessed.

### Past medical history and drug history:
- Never been in hospital. Last visit to GP was for blurred vision (as above) 2 years ago
- No regular medications

### Social history:
- You smoke 10/day and have done for the past 30 years

### Other issues including family history:
- Mother had multiple sclerosis and needed a wheelchair by the age of 40 and was bedbound by 50, needing carers daily. She died of pneumonia a few years later

**Your questions for the candidate:**
- *Will I lose my sight?*
- *Have I got MS like my mum?*
- *Will I end up in a wheelchair like my mother?*
- *Why has this happened?*

---

## Candidate

### History/key questions

Ask about the onset of the double vision/diplopia. Length of each episode

Are you seeing double all the time or only on looking in certain directions?

Does the double vision disappear when you close one eye (monocular versus binocular to differentiate between neurological and ophthalmological causes; is this internuclear ophthalmoplegia or lateral rectus palsy)?

Is your vision compromised? If yes, in what way (general blurring, central scotoma, total loss)?

Is it painful (to suggest inflammatory process of optic neuritis)? Left/right/both eyes? Did your vision ever improve, back to your baseline? How about colour vision?

Any other similar episodes in the past? (ask using similar questions above)

Any headache? (autoimmune, inflammatory, vascular causes)

Any other neurological symptoms:

Speech disturbance (dysarthria); swallowing difficulties (dysphagia)

Motor – upper or lower limb weakness; stiffness; spasms; gait; clumsiness; tremor (intention); lethargy

Sensory – altered sensation (paraesthesiae/numbness/tingling); sensory and cerebellar ataxia (gait disturbance or instability with or without eyes closed or in the dark); Lhermitte's and Uthoff's phenomena

Autonomic system – most commonly bladder symptoms in women, impotence in men; postural dizziness; syncope; palpitations; facial flushing; altered bowel habit

Changes in mood and cognition can also occur early: ask about mood/euphoria or depression, impaired memory, dementia

### Drug history

Including allergies

### Past medical history

Ask about any previous episode(s) of paresis; loss of vision; sphincter dysfunction

### Other issues including family history

Family history of MS, demyelinating disease (e.g. neuromyelitis optica), neurological disorders

### Social history

Occupation (impact on job, etc.)

### Address patient's questions and concerns

- *Have you had any thoughts about what is going on?*
- *Is there anything in particular you're concerned about?*
- *Do you have anything you would like to ask?*

### Key areas for examination

A list of what to look for (in examination order; describe findings on examination)

Cranial nerves: full examination including:

Pupils: size, RAPD (optic neuropathy)

Visual fields (typically central scotoma) and visual acuity (Snellen chart if available)

Eye movements and patient-reported diplopia – look carefully for any III, IV, VI cranial nerve lesions; look for internuclear ophthalmoplegia, nystagmus

Look for pink, swollen optic disc (optic neuritis) or atrophy – its absence might suggest retrobulbar disease if history is highly suggestive

Note speech character while talking to patient

Observe gait for broad-based, tandem walking, spasticity and Romberg's

Examine for past-pointing, intention tremor and dysdiadochokinesis

Examine tone for spasticity, reflexes for hyperreflexia and clonus

Examine both plantars for Babinski's reflex

Mention that if time permits, you would like to examine cranial nerves, peripheral motor for pyramidal weakness and sensory modalities. You would also like to check for colour vision using bedside Ishihara plates (colour desaturation, in particular red, can occur in optic neuritis)

This patient has internuclear ophthalmoplegia (INO). Nystagmus is ataxic in that the abducting eye has greater nystagmus than the adducting eye. With this there is dissociation of conjugate eye movements due to failure of adduction of the affected eye. There may be a divergent strabismus at rest. On looking to contralateral side of the lesion, e.g. right, the right eye abducts with nystagmus and there is impairment of adduction of the left eye. When the abducting eye is covered, the medial movement of the other eye occurs normally. The divergent strabismus causes diplopia

INO is caused by a lesion in the medial longitudinal fasciculus (MLF) in the mid-brain, which leads to failure of ipsilateral eye adduction and contralateral nystagmus. This can be due to demyelinating/inflammatory disease, cerebrovascular, space-occupying lesion, etc.

## Differential diagnosis

MS: two episodes of neurological symptoms (blurring 2 years ago which settled, then subsequent acute episode of double vision). The initial symptoms were probably due to optic neuritis and INO and the most recent is due to INO with a MLF lesion. He has a risk factor of positive family history

Other differential diagnoses:

Inflammatory – neuromyelitis optica (also known as Devic's disease, positive aquaporin 4 antibody, optic neuritis with spinal cord lesions extending over three or more segments); sarcoidosis; chronic relapsing inflammatory optic neuritis

Autoimmune – vasculitis; lupus; Behçet's

Vascular – ischaemic neuropathy

## Discussion with patient

Explain diagnosis

Explain plan, including investigations and management

Address patient's concerns/answer their questions

Your eyes are not moving in sync like they should, and we need to find out why. There are several causes for this, and in view of the two separate attacks over a few years, this can be caused by inflammatory damage to nerves and the brainstem. The painful loss of vision that you had 2 years ago is again probably due to damage to the nerve in the left eye. One of the possible causes for this is MS. However, we need to carry out some scans of the head and eyes, and possibly a lumbar puncture to draw some fluid from your spine. This is better done as an inpatient. It is likely that we might adopt a 'watch-and-wait' approach while waiting for these investigations to come back and then most likely

offer you treatment with high-dose steroids (preferably intravenously) and observe the response. We will also refer you to our neuro-ophthalmology team (if available within the trust) for more detailed eye assessment and advice.

You will need to inform the DVLA that you are currently under investigation for visual disturbance and possible MS. You will be sent a questionnaire and will need your vision rechecked before you can drive again. This will be explained to you by the DVLA.

## Investigations

NB: diagnostic criteria for MS needs evidence of dissemination of lesions in time and space and exclusion of other diagnoses

Bloods (to exclude other diagnoses): autoimmune screen for connective tissue disease (ANA, dsDNA, ENA, ESR), vasculitic screen (ANCA), serum ACE (sarcoidosis), aquaporin-4 antibody (for neuromyelitis optica if normal MRI brain, but presence of optic neuritis, brainstem and cord disease)

Imaging: MRI brain, brainstem and spinal cord (with gadolinium (Gd)-enhancing sequence): periventricular lesions in 95% of patients with MS, white matter abnormalities in 90%. Most recent revised McDonald's MRI criteria were published in 2010 (see Further reading/resources):

Dissemination of lesion in space: ≥1 T2 lesion in at least 2 of 4 areas of the CNS (periventricular, juxtacortical, infratentorial, spinal cord)

Dissemination of lesion in time: a new T2 and/or Gd-enhancing lesion(s) on follow-up MRI scan, with reference to a baseline scan; simultaneous presence of asymptomatic Gd-enhancing and non-enhancing lesions at any time (silent lesions)

Visual evoked potentials: may show delay of central conduction time in visual pathways due to demyelination. It provides further evidence of demyelination and dissemination in space

Lumbar puncture: isolated CSF oligoclonal bands (sample sent together with paired serum electrophoresis) present in 90% patients (and not present in serum)

Referral to neurologist: multidisciplinary approach from neurologists, neuro-ophthalmologist, MS specialist nurses, physiotherapist, occupational therapists, dietitians, GP

## Management

Referral to neurologists/involve MS specialist nurse/MDT care

Four components of management:

*Acute relapse (shorten the duration of episode):* if MS confirmed → high-dose IV steroids (methylprednisolone 0.5–1.0 g IV od for 3–5 days – see NICE guidance). If severe relapse unresponsive to corticosteroid, plasma exchange can be tried (total of 5× exchanges per treatment)

*Prevention of new lesions or further relapse:* disease-modifying therapy (usually only for relapsing-remitting course): interferon-β1a (Avonex, Rebif), interferon-β1b (betaseron), glatiramer acetate (Copaxone), mitoxantrone (Novantrone), natalizumab (Tysabri) and first oral agent fingolimod (Gilenya). First line (see NICE guidelines) would be interferon-β but need to fulfil criteria. More severe disease may benefit from natalizumab infusion

Criteria for interferon-β treatment for relapsing/remitting MS:
  **1.** ≥2 clinically significant relapses in last 2 years
  **2.** able to walk 10 m or more (preferably 100 m or more, Expanded Disability Status Scale ≤5.5)
  **3.** not pregnant or attempting conception
  **4.** ≥18 years and no contraindications to the use of interferon-β

Criteria for natalizumab in relapsing/remitting MS:
  for rapidly evolving severe disease: ≥2 disabling relapses in 1 year and ≥1 Gd-enhancing lesions on brain MRI or a significant increase in T2 lesion load compared to previous MRI

*Symptomatic treatment:* neurogenic bladder care (anticholinergic drugs: oxybutynin, tolteradine, intermittent self-catherization if postmicturition residual volume >100 mL, urologist/incontinence clinic referral, botulinum toxin); spasticity (baclofen, tinazidine, benzodiazepines, botulinum); neuropathic pain (gabapentin, pregabalin, amitryptiline); diet modification ± PEG, mood/psychodepression (antidepressants, cognitive behavioural therapy, referral to psychiatrist); crectile impotence (sildenafil)

*Rehabilitation* to promote function and information on MS Society

### Addressing concerns/answering questions

- *Will I lose my sight?* Most optic neuritis will get better after 3–4 weeks (sometimes up to a year or longer) but steroids (either oral or intravenous) can help accelerate the recovery. Depending on the result of the MRI and lumbar puncture, steroids can also help speed up the recovery of the lesion in the brainstem that causes the INO. However, the full recovery is variable and does not rely on steroid treatment. Some people might still complain of subtle defects such as colour or depth perception or blurring of vision. Similarly, if the brain lesion resolves, the double vision may improve. Some people might find that the eye symptoms worsen in hot weather/taking hot bath (Uthoff's phenomenon), or when they are tired or under emotional or physical stress.

- *Have I got MS like my mum?* There are various causes for these symptoms but given that you have had two attacks within the last 2 years, the history is highly suggestive that there is a problem in your brain and nerves. MS frequently presents like this but we need to confirm this by imaging your brain and spinal cord, and also testing the nerve function in your eyes.

- *Will I end up in a wheelchair like my mother?* The ability to walk depends on the severity, frequency of the relapses and the type of MS. Relapsing/remitting MS has a better outlook, as patients will have complete or near-complete recovery (70–80% patients) after a few months. However, some patients might have residual disability after subsequent relapses. The frequency of these relapses can be reduced with disease-modifying treatment. Primary progressive MS (10–20% patients) has a slightly poorer outlook as the disability progresses with minimal recovery, if any, and it does not respond to disease-modifying therapies. Ten percent of patients follow a benign course where after a few relapses, the disease remains in remission for many years. It is premature to predict the course of the disease at this stage or to determine which type of MS you have. However, with the information that I have at present, it seems that you have a relapsing/remitting type.

- *Why has this happened?* The aetiology is still unknown but many working hypotheses have been tested. It is thought that the inflammatory process or damage to the nerve and brain cells is due to an immune response caused by environmental factors and genetic susceptibility. However, we currently do not have enough evidence to pinpoint which exact factors are to blame.

## Discussion with examiners

The examiners may ask you to clarify details of the above diagnosis and ask questions about your planned investigations and management.

Other possible questions include:
- *What are the criteria for diagnosing MS?* Revised McDonald's criteria (2010).

- *What are the types of MS?* Relapsing/remitting, secondary progressive, primary progressive.
- *What is the most significant complication of natalizumab treatment?* Progressive multifocal leucoencephalopathy (PML), a rare opportunistic infection of the CNS caused by reactivation of the human polyomavirus JC virus (overall incidence 1.4 cases per 1000 patients).
- *Who is at higher risk?* Patients with serum-positive JC virus antibody; increased duration of treatment (>24 months); previous exposure to immunosuppressants. Some centres use a 3–4 months drug holiday after 1 year of treatment due to the risk of PML but this increases the risk of immune reconstitution syndrome.

See also Vol. 1, Station 3, CNS, Cases 10, 16 and 32.

---

**Examiners' information and requirements**

The candidate should:

1. Identify key features from the history: previous painful visual loss, two discrete episodes of diplopia, with internuclear ophthalmoplegia demonstrated on this occasion
2. Identify key examination findings including internuclear ophthalmoplegia, optic atrophy and lack of cerebellar signs
3. Outline a sensible management plan including appropriate investigations and onward referral to a neurologist/ophthalmologist
4. Give a clear explanation to the patient of your diagnosis and plan, address his concerns and answer his questions

---

**Further reading/resources**

Polman CH et al. Diagnostic criteria for multiple sclerosis: 2010 revisions to the McDonald criteria. Ann Neurol 2011;69:292–302

www.mssociety.org.uk/

www.nationalmssociety.org/index.aspx

NICE guidance: www.guidance.nice.org.uk/

# Scenario 55 | Peripheral neuropathy

## Candidate's information

**Your role:** you are an ST2 in the neurology clinic. You have been asked to see this 55-year-old woman who presents with pain and numbness in her hands and feet; she was diagnosed with colorectal cancer a year ago and underwent an operation. Her recent CT and colonoscopy were clear. Her colorectal surgeon has referred her to you regarding the numbness.

**Your task:** to assess the patient's problems and address any questions or concerns raised by her.

## Patient's information

**You are:** Janice Hales, a 55-year-old woman.

**Your problem:** you have a 9-month history of numbness in your hands and feet. The symptoms have not progressed during this time. You feel a bit clumsy and struggle with fine control. You sometimes struggle with doing up small buttons. You've not noticed any weakness in your arms or legs.

You had chemotherapy after an operation to remove a cancer from the right side of the colon. This numbness started during your chemo with capecitabine and oxaliplatin, on about the fifth cycle, and although it used to improve on your weeks off, towards the end it just didn't change. You didn't have your last chemo as you didn't feel well. The numbness has slightly improved since that was cancelled, but only a little.

You've also been getting some diarrhoea; your stools don't flush away easily. This has started over the past 6 months or so. Your GP sent off a stool sample which was fine.

### Past medical history and drug history:
- Pernicious anaemia; on vitamin B12 replacement with 2–3 monthly injections (2-monthly if you feel tired before the 3 months is up). GP occasionally tests the levels and says that these are fine
- Not known to have diabetes mellitus
- Never had these kind of problems before

### Social history:
- Smoked 10 per day, stopped since just before the operation
- Alcohol: used to drink a couple of glasses of wine per night, perhaps a couple of bottles per week maximum as a student. Never drunk more than this. Never had a problem with alcohol and never been criticized about drinking. No morning stiffeners. Since the cancer operation you just have the occasional glass of wine

### Other issues including family history:
- Mother had diabetes when she was older, i.e. early 70s

**Your questions for the candidate:**

- *What's causing the numbness?*
- *I thought it may be the chemo, but it was doing me good. Would switching chemo have helped?*
- *Does the cancer cause this?*

---

## Candidate

### History/key questions

What changes did patient notice? Motor, sensory or both?

Character of the sensory symptoms? Negative symptoms, e.g. numbness, inability to feel texture, inability to feel hot/cold; positive symptoms, e.g. tingling, burning, pins and needles, itching, crawling, hypersensitive; try to elicit the nature of the neuropathy whether it is purely large fibre, small fibre or both, or pure dorsal column or sensory neuronopathy or ganglionopathy as this helps to narrow down the causes to some extent. If it is a burning sensation, does she have to remove the blanket off her legs at night?

Any problem with balance? If there is, is the instability made worse with both eyes closed or in the dark (try to differentiate balance problem due to sensory ataxia or non-sensory, e.g. weakness or cerebellar pathology)?

Motor/muscle symptoms if any: negative symptoms, e.g. weakness, lethargy, heaviness, gait abnormality; positive symptoms, e.g. tremors, cramps, muscle twitching (fasciculations) or quivering of the muscles (myokymia); myalgia; spasms; fine motor dexterity (dropping things, using cutlery)

Over what period did the symptoms develop (acute <4 weeks, subacute 4–8 weeks, chronic >8 weeks)?

What pattern are the symptoms (glove and stocking, symmetrical, asymmetrical, unilateral, ascending/descending suggesting peripheral neuropathy, mononeuritis multiplex, mononeuropathy)?

Ask about autonomic symptoms and sphincter disturbance (postural hypotension, constipation, atonic bladder or neurogenic bladder – ask about recurrent UTI, urinary incontinence, difficult micturition), erectile dysfunction, looking for autonomic neuropathy

Ask about any bulbar symptoms

How have symptoms changed over this period (e.g. have the symptoms improved since the chemotherapy was stopped, suggesting iatrogenic toxic cause)?

What effect is this having on her, and her ability to do day-to-day tasks?

### Drug history

Drug causes: ask about the type of chemotherapy drugs used (see differential diagnosis below), long-term antibiotics, anti-TB therapy, antiretrovirals, etc.

### Past medical history

Is patient known to have diabetes, B12 deficiency, alcohol dependency, malignancy or connective tissue disorder?

### Social history

Does anyone in the family have similar problems with the nerves in their hands or feet?

Occupational history: any exposure to organophosphate poisoning, heavy metals

### Address patient's questions and concerns

- *Have you had any thoughts about what is going on?*
- *Is there anything in particular you're concerned about?*
- *Do you have anything you would like to ask?*

## Key areas for examination

A list of what to look for (in examination order; describe findings on examination)

Look for signs of muscle wasting in upper and lower limbs (especially the lumbricals and interosseous muscles in the hands and extensor digitorum brevis in the feet); pes cavus and claw hands (long-standing neuropathy); fasciculations

Look for possible clues to the aetiology: insulin injection sites, insulin pump, vasculitic purpuric rash, bruises (liver disease from, e.g. alcohol), leuconychia (poor nutrition), AV fistula/dialysis catheter (renal failure)

Look for signs of ulceration on the feet (neuropathic, diabetes – punched-out ulcers; peripheral vascular disease)

Given the history, start with sensory examination: assess fine touch, proprioception, vibration, temperature difference/hot versus cold differentiation, fine/blunt discrimination (map out in dermatomes). If time is running out check at least one dorsal column (vibration/proprioception) and one small fibre (pinprick)

Test for power and reflexes: upper and lower limbs, is it a proximal or distal distribution or both?

PNS: palpate for thickened nerves (diabetes, sarcoidosis, amyloidosis) although this can be omitted if time is running out. Tone is usually normal

Test for Romberg's sign and quickly assess gait looking for sensory ataxia (positive Romberg's, heavy heel strike, stomping gait, slightly broad-based with absence of cerebellar signs)

## Differential diagnosis

Peripheral sensory neuropathy as evidenced by symmetrical impairment of sensation in a glove-and-stocking distribution; likely to be due to chemotherapy agent(s). Platinum analog chemotherapy such as oxaliplatin and vinca alkaloids such as vincristine and vinblastine are commonly associated with peripheral neuropathy (predominantly sensory in the former). Capecitabine is not commonly associated with neuropathy although there are cases reported in the literature

Differential diagnosis for predominantly sensory neuropathy (needs confirmation from nerve conduction study):

Metabolic – pyridoxine intoxication or B12 deficiency

Autoimmune – Sjögren's syndrome

Drugs – chemotherapy agents, chloramphenicol, metronidazole, phenytoin

Paraneoplastic (especially with anti-Hu antibody but usually associated with small cell lung cancer)

Infection – HIV

Hereditary

Important to consider diabetes (common cause in developed world), leprosy (worldwide)

## Discussion with patient

Explain diagnosis

Explain plan, including investigations and management

Address patient's concerns/answer their questions

The nerves in your hands and feet are less sensitive than they should be, and could be partially damaged due to a range of causes. We need to exclude diabetes, a common cause, but drugs such as chemotherapy can cause this. In order to confirm this, we need to arrange for nerve conduction testing to be done. This basically means using minor electrical pulses to test the function of your nerves. We need to wait and see how it recovers, as the main treatment is removal of the cause (stopping the chemo). We would also arrange for some blood tests to further help us in looking for the cause of this.

Diarrhoea is likely to be bile acid diarrhoea due to having an operation which removed the right side of the colon and the last bit of the small bowel. A drug called cholestyramine can be used to manage this.

## Investigations

Neuropathic blood screen: renal and liver functions, vitamin B12, TFT, ESR, paraneoplastic antibodies (particularly anti-Hu)

Other blood tests that can be done: serum ANCA (vasculitis), serum electrophoresis, urine Bence Jones protein (paraproteinaemia)

Urinalysis: exclude glycosuria

Nerve conduction studies (looking for distribution and type of neuropathy)

## Management

Stop the offending agent, e.g. chemotherapeutic agent

Observe

## Addressing concerns/answering questions:

- *What's causing the numbness?* The nerves in your hands and feet are not working normally which gives you the numbness in your fingers. There are many possible causes for this but it looks likely to be related to the chemotherapy you had. We will arrange tests to confirm that the nerves are affected and to rule out other causes.

- *I thought it may be the chemo, but it was doing me good. Would switching chemo have helped?* The effects on the nerves vary between different people, and reducing the dose of the chemo or switching to a different drug can help. The effects of the chemo on the nerves can also gradually build up over time. We will need to wait and see how the nerves respond to stopping the chemotherapy, as you have reported some improvement since the last chemotherapy.

- *Does the cancer cause this?* It looks like it's the chemotherapy rather than the cancer itself that has caused this. Certain chemotherapy medications have been known to cause this, and your recent CT scan and colonoscopy were fine.

## Discussion with examiners

The examiners may ask you to clarify details of the above diagnosis and ask questions about your planned investigations and management.

A possible question includes:
- *What do you think the cause is? If you think it's the chemotherapy, how could you find out?* Most likely cause is chemotherapy. It can occur as acute neurotoxicity or chronic cumulative sensory neuropathy. This can be minimized with dose modification or stopping the chemotherapy entirely. Symptoms are reversible in majority of patients usually less than 6–12 months. Some centres have also tried neuromodulatory agents, e.g. Ca/Mg infusion or supplement for acute neurotoxicity. Explanation and patient education are paramount.

  Causes for peripheral neuropathy: metabolic – diabetes, pyridoxine toxicity, B12, niacin and thiamine deficiency, uraemia, myxoedema, thyrotoxicosis; inflammatory – GBS, chronic inflammatory demyelinating polyneuropathy, sarcoidosis, Sjögren's, SLE, vasculitis; infection – leprosy, Lyme disease, HIV, diphtheria, HSV, HTLV, CMV, amyloidosis; malignancy – multiple myeloma, paraneoplastic; drugs/toxins – alcohol, antiretroviral, anti-TB (isoniazid), organophosphates, heavy metals, chemotherapy medications, nitrofurantoin, amiodarone, phenytoin, metronidazole.

See also Vol. 1, Station 3, CNS, Case 1.

---

### Examiners' information and requirements

The candidate should:
1. Identify key features from the history: glove-and-stocking neuropathy, following chemotherapy, sensory symptoms
2. Identify key examination findings including evidence of sensory neuropathy in symmetrical glove-and-stocking distribution (peripheral neuropathy)
3. Outline a sensible differential diagnosis and management plan, including nerve conduction studies
4. Give a clear explanation to the patient of your diagnosis and plan, address her concerns and answer her questions

---

### Further reading/resources

Saif MW, Reardon J. Management of oxaliplatin-induced peripheral neuropathy. Ther Clin Risk Man 2005;1(4): 249–58

Neuropathy: www.neuromuscular.wustl.edu/index.html

# Scenario 56 | Urinary tract infection: male/sexual history

## Candidate's information

**Your role:** you are an ST2 in the MAU clinic. A 28-year-old man has been referred with dysuria by his GP.

**Your task:** to assess the patient's problems and address any questions or concerns raised by him.

## Patient's information

**You are:** Harry Green, a 28-year-old man.

**Your problem:** you've noticed a burning sensation when you pass urine, and you're passing urine a bit more often. You have been having to go at night over the past few weeks (1/night). Your main concern, though, is the intermittent white creamy discharge from your penis for the past 3 weeks, which started 3 days after sex on holiday. About 6 months ago, you split from your long-term partner, with whom you had unprotected intercourse.

Whilst on a recent trip abroad (a month ago) with friends, you had unprotected intercourse with two partners, both female. Vaginal intercourse, no anal. No sex with men. No idea of their backgrounds or sexual history. Both were UK holidaymakers in Spain and you're not in contact with them.

You have had 14 sexual partners in total, all protected except for the recent two and your long-term partner, Jackie, whom you've just got back together with. You had unprotected intercourse with her last night. She's unaware of your urine problems, and the discharge.

You noticed a faint red, lacy rash over your wrist last week which has now gone away.

### Past medical history and drug history:
- Never admitted to hospital, no operations
- No current medications and no allergies

### Social history:
- Lives alone
- Non-smoker
- Occasional alcohol (on holiday)

### Other issues including family history:
- No family history of any medical conditions
- Both parents well. No siblings

**Your questions for the candidate:**
- *I think I've caught something from the sex on holiday. Have I caught venereal disease (VD)?*
- *How do I tell Jackie?*

## Candidate

### History/key questions

Given the urinary symptoms in a young male: need to exclude UTI and sexually transmissible infection (STI)

Need to take full sexual health history

Symptoms: dysuria, urethral discharge, skin problems, oral and perianal symptoms

Any eye symptoms (e.g. gritty or red eyes) and/or arthropathy consistent with sexually acquired reactive arthritis (previously called Reiter's)

Reasons for attendance (patient may mention that he's concerned about the white discharge starting shortly after episode(s) of unprotected sexual intercourse)

Bridging questions: tactful ways of linking general health questions to more specific sexual health questions (easier if already identified that patient is concerned about possible STI)

Last sexual intercourse: which gender; type of sexual intercourse (oral, anal, vaginal); condom use/barrier contraception – used throughout and remained intact?

Relationship with partner (long term, ?duration, casual sexual contacts – traceable versus non-traceable)

Partner's health, any symptoms

Previous partner(s) in last 3 months: questions as above for each including the nationality/country of birth for the sexual partners (part of risk assessment process)

If no partners in last 3 months, when was last time?

All men should be asked if they have had sex with another man in the past

Is current partner aware of his symptoms, had recent sexual health check, or known to have any previous or current STI?

Is partner with him today?

Risk assessment:

Any previous STIs

Ever had any testing in the past (genitourinary medicine (GUM) clinic, GP, hospital) for HIV or STI

Any vaccination history for hepatitis B

Ever had sex abroad other than with partner with whom he was travelling

Medical treatment abroad

Ever exchanged money in return for sex (UK or abroad)

Ask about medications and any drug use (injecting drug use, sharing of needles, syringes, drug preparation equipment)

### Address patient's questions and concerns
- *Have you had any thoughts about what is going on?*
- *Is there anything in particular you're concerned about?*
- *Do you have anything you would like to ask?*

### Key areas for examination

A list of what to look for (in examination order; describe findings on examination)

Overall inspection

Look for rash (petechial, lacy rash of gonococcus; maculopapular rash can be seen in HIV seroconversion)

Eyes: any evidence of redness/conjunctival injection

Abdominal: look for suprapubic/renal angle tenderness (UTI)

Genitourinary: examination of testes, penis/external genitalia; any evidence of discharge (if so, say you would swab this for MCS); look for balanitis/epididymitis

Any arthropathy (sexually acquired reactive arthritis)

Ask to see urinalysis results, any previous swabs/microbiology tests and results of blood tests

### Differential diagnosis

STI (important to use this terminology and not 'sexually transmitted disease', VD, etc.)

Urinary infection (although discharge not consistent with UTI)

### Discussion with patient

Explain diagnosis

Explain plan, including investigations and management

Address patient's concerns/answer their questions

The combination of discharge and burning in a young man makes us concerned about a sexually transmissible infection, particularly given your recent unprotected intercourse with new partners. We need to test the discharge and also carry out a full check-up, including checking for possible infections including chlamydia and trichomonas. We would recommend blood tests for hepatitis B, C, syphilis, HIV (now a treatable infection, considered a chronic disease, particularly if diagnosed early).

## Investigations
Full sexual history

Diagnostic testing: may be more appropriate to do this in GUM setting, but opportunistic testing is encouraged – will need HIV serology, syphilis serology, hepatitis B

GUM clinic attendance (advise attend clinic with partner). Advise open and honest approach (consequences of untreated pelvic inflammatory disease in female/fertility; reinfection). Provide contact details for GUM clinics as many offer walk-in clinics as well as prebooked

Diagnostic testing (some tests can be carried out in MAU, but others may be best carried out in the setting of a sexual health [genito urinary medicine] clinic): swab discharge (90–95% sensitivity for gonorrhoea if discharge present); nucleic acid amplification tests on urine (better than swab if asymptomatic/no discharge); also test for chlamydia (high rate of coinfectivity); may need specialist swabs for intraurethral culture, viral culture if concerns about herpes

## Management
Counsel regarding testing for STIs including HIV – both patient and his current partner (treatable infections/part of full sexual health MOT) – remember will need to recheck in 3 months if HIV negative

Abstain from sexual intercourse until a week after both partners have completed treatment

Discharge, rash, dysuria suggestive of gonococcus – current treatment ceftriaxone 500 mg IM single dose, with azithromycin 1 g po as single dose

MSSU (exclude coexistent UTI) – if proven UTI in a male need urology referral (ultrasound kidneys, ureter, bladder, and cystoscopy)

Contact tracing

Advice about protected sexual intercourse with future new sexual partners (e.g. outside current relationship)

## Addressing concerns/answering questions
• *I think I've caught something from the sex on holiday. Have I caught venereal disease (VD)?* I think that the combination of the discharge from your penis and burning when you pass urine is likely to be a sexually transmissible infection, particularly given your recent unprotected intercourse with new partners. We need to test the discharge and also to carry out a full check-up, including checking for possible infections including chlamydia and trichomonas. We would recommend blood tests for hepatitis B and C, syphilis, HIV (now a treatable infection, considered a chronic disease, particularly if diagnosed early). We can give treatment for the most likely infection once the swabs have been sent.

• *How do I tell Jackie?* Honest approach best. I suggest that you explain to Jackie that you had a sexual partner whilst separated from her, and your doctors think you've caught an infection from this partner on holiday. I suggest that you explain to her that the doctors have given you treatment and advise that she gets a full check-up. Explain that it is important that she does get a check-up and receives any necessary treatment as there are potential risks to her future fertility if certain infections are left untreated.

## Discussion with examiners
The examiners may ask you to clarify details of the above diagnosis and ask questions about your planned investigations and management.

A possible question includes:
• *Would you carry out all the tests yourself?* All of the tests could be carried out in the Sexual Health clinic as they have the skills and equipment to ensure that all the tests are carried out properly, and some results will be available on the day. They also have the most robust systems for contact tracing. It is, however, important to carry out opportunistic screening and provide advice and treatment on this visit as well as facilitating onward referral, as there is a risk that he won't attend a second clinic. Some clinics will allow you to make an appointment online with the patient, or over the telephone. Others have walk-in clinics. It is a strictly confidential service and the patient's GP won't be informed automatically.

For notes on HIV, see discussion in Section I, Station 5, Skin, Case 36 and Station 5, Eyes, Case 20.

## Examiners' information and requirements

The candidate should:

1. Identify key features from the history: dysuria and discharge in young male with recent history of unprotected sexual intercourse with untraceable casual partners. Diagnosis is STI until proven otherwise
2. Identify key examination findings including nil of note likely in this case
3. Outline a sensible management plan including sexual health check (history, examination, investigations including diagnostic testing for STI, HIV; facilitate GUM attendance)
4. Give a clear explanation to the patient of your diagnosis and plan, address his concerns and answer his questions

## Further reading/resources

British Association of Sexual Health and HIV: www.bashh.org. Includes 2011 guidelines for the management of gonorrhoea in adults; BASHH 2006 national guidelines – consultations requiring sexual history taking; guidelines on other STIs, including post-HIV exposure prophylaxis

# Scenario 57 | Swollen calf in a young woman

## Candidate's information

**Your role:** you are one of the doctors on-call in the MAU. A local GP has referred this 25-year-old woman who complains of right calf swelling after flying home from a holiday in Thailand.

**Your task:** to assess the patient's problems and address any questions or concerns raised by her.

## Patient's information

**You are:** Katy Brigham, a 25-year-old woman.

**Your problem:** your upper right calf has been sore and perhaps a little swollen for the past 4 days. You had been away for 2 weeks in Thailand (beach and watersports at Koh Samui), and flew home 3 days ago. You've had a good holiday with watersports activities and partying, and have now come home for a rest.

Today you noticed pain in your calf so you went to your doctor as someone at work suggested that it could be a clot in your leg from the long flight, and mentioned the risk of then getting clots in the lung. You have had no shortness of breath, chest pain, cough or coughing up blood. No fever. You don't remember having any insect bites recently, even whilst away camping. Looking at your leg now, it doesn't seem as swollen as it was after the flight. It was a long flight followed by a few hours in a car home. It still feels a little sore when you walk on it.

### Past medical history:
• Never been in hospital, no operations

### Drug history:
• You've been taking the pill for 4 years without any problems
• Occasional paracetamol
• No drug allergies

### Social history:
• Smoked 10/day for the past 6 years
• Alcohol: drink 3 pints of lager on the weekend

### Other issues including family history:
• No-one in your family has ever had clots in their legs or lungs

### Your questions for the candidate:
• *Do I need to stay in hospital?*
• *Is it safe to stay on the pill?*

## Candidate

### History/key questions

Ask questions regarding the swollen leg:

Any history of trauma

How long has the leg been swollen for, gradual or sudden onset

Ask about pain, swelling, increased temperature of leg, fever, change in colour/redness of leg

Unilateral or bilateral lower limb swelling; extent (ankle versus calf versus whole leg including thigh)

Ask about thrombotic risk factors: immobility, recent operation/surgery, prolonged bedrest or long journey (coach, air travel, car, etc.)

Any known thrombophilia, any known neoplasia

Use of oral contraceptive pill/HRT/tamoxifen

Ask about symptoms of PE: chest pain, breathlessness, cough, haemoptysis

Any known joint problems including RA, OA (in case Baker's cyst) or venous insufficiency

Any history of trauma

Any family history of DVT, PE

### Past medical history

Ask about general health

Is patient pregnant?

Any medical problems which could suggest DVT secondary to conditions such as malignancy (weight loss) or inflammatory bowel disease (diarrhoea, weight loss, rectal bleeding, abdominal pain), thrombophilia (recurrent miscarriages in antiphospholipid syndrome)

### Drug history

Ever injected drugs (anywhere, including groin) in the past or currently

Wells' score often forms part of clinical assessment (usually as a structured proforma for patients with possible DVTs): see below

### Address patient's questions and concerns

- *Have you had any thoughts about what is going on?*
- *Is there anything in particular you're concerned about?*
- *Do you have anything you would like to ask?*

## Key areas for examination

A list of what to look for (in examination order; describe findings on examination)

Examine lower limbs

First check with patient whether any pain/tenderness prior to examining

Adequate exposure of lower limbs (at least to groin)

Inspection: compare left with right. Look for obvious size differential between the legs

Look for presence, extent and location of swelling (measure left and right legs with measuring tape 10 cm below level of tibial tuberosity)

Look for:

Erythema, distended superficial veins

Bruising or injury

Rash; delineated erythema consistent with cellulitis and/or tracking of cellulitis up to groin

Any crusting/discharge

Any wounds, ulcers or abrasions

Tinea pedis in toe interspaces – potential source of cellulitis/entry points

Injection sites/sinuses in groin L/R over femoral veins

Palpation: leg soft (normal), firm or pitting oedema

Feel temperature of both legs and compare L/R

Determine where the tenderness is: is it over superficial veins (phlebitis), diffuse or localized?

Any change in sensation

Palpate for tenderness in the popliteal fossa (Baker's cyst)

Look for evidence of knee pathology: any effusion, tenderness over joint, increased temperature?

Active and passive ROM in knee

Peripheral pulses

Abdominal examination: exclude abdominal/pelvic masses

Check the observation chart for temperature (fever in cellulitis), oxygen saturations, pulse and BP

In this patient, calf measurements are equal. Non-tender, soft calf. No tenderness in popliteal fossa. No clinical signs of DVT or ruptured Baker's cyst

## Differential diagnosis

Probable dependent oedema due to prolonged flight/travel – now improved

Differential diagnosis includes musculoskeletal pain (strained muscle)

Other differential diagnosis to consider and exclude (clinical examination ± investigations as needed):

Ruptured Baker's cyst (but non-tender popliteal fossa/no calf tenderness)

No clinical evidence of DVT based on examination today

## Discussion with patient

Explain diagnosis

Explain plan, including investigations and management
Address patient's concerns/answer their questions

People's legs often get swollen on long flights, and then settle, as yours have. The pain on walking looks like muscle and bone pain/strains, perhaps due to the watersports on holiday. There are no signs of a clot in the leg, which is reassuring.

## Investigations
Clinical assessment including use of the two-level Wells score – this patient scores −2
The two-level Wells score is used to estimate the probability of DVT based on clinical assessment (history and examination) and is usually on the DVT proforma available in MAUs.

Score 1 point each for:
Active cancer (e.g. receiving treatment or cancer within previous 6 months or receiving palliative care)
Paralysis, paresis or recent plaster immobilization of the lower extremities
Recently bedridden for 3 days or more, or major surgery requiring general or regional anaesthetic within the previous 12 weeks
Localized tenderness along the distribution of the deep venous system
Entire leg swollen
Calf swelling >3 cm compared with asymptomatic leg (measure each leg 10 cm below tibial tuberosity)
Pitting oedema confined to the symptomatic leg
Collateral superficial veins (non-varicose)
Previous documented DVT

Score minus 2 points for:
Alternative diagnosis at least as likely as DVT

Probability of DVT based on two-level Wells score:
2 points or more – DVT likely
1 point or less – DVT unlikely

Bloods: basic bloods including FBC, U&E, CRP
If score is 2 or over, arrange US Doppler of leg. If US Doppler is positive, diagnose and treat for DVT. If US Doppler is negative, check D-dimer
If D-dimer is positive, repeat US Doppler 6-8 days later. If D-dimer is negative, DVT is not likely; consider other diagnoses
If Wells score is low risk, 0 or less, then carry out D-dimer
If D-dimer negative, then explain to the patient that DVT is not likely; consider other diagnoses

If D-dimer is positive, then arrange US Doppler scan: if US Doppler is positive, diagnose and treat as DVT. If negative, explain to the patient that DVT is not likely
If US Doppler arranged, prescribe anticoagulation with low molecular weight heparin until patient reviewed with scan result, and then can decide on further management
Ambulatory care as per local protocol
Decide on further management, e.g. need for warfarin if proven DVT when results of US Doppler available

## Management
For this patient, D-Dimer is negative
Management of musculoskeletal pain is analgesia, continue to mobilize
Reassurance
Discharge to care of GP with discharge letter

### Addressing concerns/answering questions
• *Do I need to stay in hospital?* No. You can go home with some painkillers but remain active.
• *Is it safe to stay on the pill?* Yes.

## Discussion with examiners
The examiners may ask you to clarify details of the above diagnosis and ask questions about your planned investigations and management.

Other possible questions include:
• *What are the features of a ruptured Baker's cyst?* A Baker's cyst is a popliteal synovial cyst, and these can rupture causing pain, erythema, increased temperature, swelling, tenderness and bruising in the lower leg. Rupture of asymptomatic cysts can occur in patients with no previously recognized chronic joint disease. Management includes analgesia and rest. Baker's cysts can also enlarge into the calf below the knee, causing erythema and oedema and can present in a similar fashion to a DVT.
• *What do you do if the first US scan is indeterminate or negative when the patient has a high clinical probability of DVT?* Continue anticoagulation with low molecular weight heparin and arrange a repeat Doppler ultrasound scan in a week. US also needs to look for a ruptured Baker's cyst.

See also Section I, Station 5, Other, Case 2.

## Examiners' information and requirements

The candidate should:

1. Identify key features from the history – swollen calf after recent flight; no other risk factors for DVT
2. Identify key examination findings – normal examination in this case with no evidence of DVT. Use the two-level Wells score
3. Outline a sensible management plan including mobilising analgesia
4. Give a clear explanation to the patient of your diagnosis and plan, address her concerns and answer her questions

## Further reading/resources

NICE guidance on venous thromboembolic disease, management of venous thromboembolic diseases and role of thrombophilia testing, including Wells scores and flowcharts for DVT and PE (2012): www.guidance.nice.org.uk/CG144.

# Scenario 58 | Deep venous thrombosis (DVT) secondary to neoplasia: elderly patient

## Candidate's information

**Your role:** you are on-call in the MAU. You have been asked by a GP to see this 75-year-old man with a swollen left calf.

**Your task:** to assess the patient's problems and address any questions or concerns raised by him.

## Patient's information

**You are:** Patrick Tompkins, a 75-year-old retired postmaster.

**Your problem:** you've had a swollen, tender left calf for the past week. It has gradually got a bit worse and is now painful to walk on. No fever, shortness of breath, chest pain. Never had this problem before.

For the past 3–4 months, you have been losing weight (4 kg in total), your appetite has been poor, and you have been passing 3–4 loose bowel motions per day. You previously opened your bowels once per day. You get a little bit of lower tummy pain just before you need to open your bowels. No rectal bleeding. You sometimes need to rush to open your bowels. Never been incontinent.

Your main concern is the diarrhoea, and the calf is just a nuisance. No mouth ulcers or joint pains. Feeling a little tired/lethargic. No cough, sputum, wheeze, chest pain, shortness of breath or coughing up blood.

### Past medical history and drug history:
- Not on any medicines
- Never been in hospital

### Social history:
- Lives with wife. She's well but away with her friends on a weekend hill-walking holiday
- Used to smoke 20/day for 30 years, none for 10 years

### Other issues including family history:
- No-one in your family has had clots in their legs or lungs
- No family history of inflammatory bowel disease or colon cancer

### Your questions for the candidate:
- *Why are my bowels causing me such trouble?*
- *Can I go home? I need to feed the cats as my wife is away.*

## Candidate

### History/key questions

Ask questions regarding the swollen leg: any history of trauma

How long has the leg been swollen for? Gradual or sudden onset

Ask about pain, swelling, increased temperature of leg, fever, change in colour/redness of leg

Unilateral or bilateral lower limb swelling; extent (ankle versus calf versus whole leg including thigh)

Ask about thrombotic risk factors: immobility, recent operation, prolonged bedrest or long journey (coach, air travel, car, etc.), any known thrombophilia, any known neoplasia

Ask regarding symptoms of PE: chest pain, breathlessness, cough, haemoptysis

Any known joint problems including RA, OA (in case Baker's cyst)

Need to identify whether any underlying neoplasia/conditions predisposing to thromboembolic disease (TED):

Ask about weight loss, general health

Ask about change in bowel habit, rectal bleeding, abdominal pain, urgency (colonic neoplasia, IBD) as well as dysphagia, dyspepsia, reflux symptoms

Respiratory symptoms including cough, sputum, wheeze, chest pain, shortness of breath, haemoptysis

Ask about urinary symptoms including dysuria, discharge, frequency, nocturia, hesitancy, poor stream

Any known prostate problems?

### Drug history

Any changes in medicines to account for diarrhoea, e.g. recently started on lansoprazole or, if newly diagnosed diabetic, has he been started on metformin?

Any drug allergies?

### Past medical history

Ever been in hospital?

Had any investigations for his change in bowel habit yet (e.g. any blood tests, colonoscopy/lower GI endoscopy, barium enema, CT)?

### Social history

Smoking history (in pack-years)

Alcohol history (in units per week)

### Other issues including family history

Ask whether any of his blood relatives have ever had colon cancer or inflammatory bowel disease

Any family history of DVT or PE

### Address patient's questions and concerns

· *Have you had any thoughts about what is going on?*
· *Is there anything in particular you're concerned about?*
· *Do you have anything you would like to ask?*

## Key areas for examination

A list of what to look for (in examination order; describe findings on examination)

Examine lower limbs: check with patient whether any pain/tenderness first

Inspection: compare left with right. Look for extent of swelling (measure diameter of both legs with tape measure 10 cm below the level of tibial tuberosity); any erythema, distended superficial veins; bruising or injury; rash; delineated erythema consistent with cellulitis

Any crusting/discharge

Any wounds, ulcers or abrasions, any tinea pedis in toe interspaces – potential source of cellulitis/entry points

Palpation: leg soft, firm and/or pitting oedema. Feel temperature and compare L/R. Determine where the tenderness is – is it over superficial veins (phlebitis), diffuse or localized?

Any change in sensation

Palpate for tenderness in the popliteal fossa

Peripheral pulses

Abdominal examination: exclude abdominal masses

Check the observation chart for temperature (fever in cellulitis), oxygen saturations, pulse and BP

Say that you would like to complete the examination by carrying out a digital rectal examination (rectal cancer, prostate cancer)

For this case: swollen firm left calf with slight erythema, tender on deep palpation; increased temperature compared to the right side. Abdominal examination normal

## Differential diagnosis

Unilateral firm, tender, warm swollen leg, non-tender popliteal fossa and no history of trauma

DVT main differential diagnosis for leg swelling

The main differential for the change in bowel habit with weight loss would be colonic neoplasia but could be due to inflammatory bowel disease (second peak incidence in the elderly)

**Key facts/areas to consider** (including information available in scenario summary before station starts): important to ask about trauma – a painful swollen calf after trauma raises the differential diagnosis of compartment syndrome (tense swelling with neurovascular deficit – no pulses, reduced sensation) – orthopaedic emergency

## Discussion with patient

Explain diagnosis
Explain plan, including investigations and management
Address patient's concerns/answer their questions

Find out what he thinks is happening – he may already suspect something serious causing his weight loss.

There are various possible causes for the swelling in your leg, including a clot in the veins in the leg. We will need to give you a daily injection to thin the blood whilst we wait for a scan of the veins in the next few days. This can all be carried out as an outpatient, and we have specialist nurses who run a clinic for this. We do however also need to look into the problems you have been having with your bowels, and the weight loss. There are various causes for this ranging from the less serious to most serious and I would recommend that we carry out some tests.

We will send some blood tests today, and arrange either an urgent appointment to see the gastroenterologists (directly booked from the MAU) or direct booking of an outpatient colonoscopy (it may be possible to get a gastroenterology opinion today on the unit to facilitate this).

To explain the colonoscopy: it is an endoscopy test to look round the bowels for causes of the diarrhoea. The colonoscopy requires laxatives the day before the test to clear out the bowels, then you come into hospital for a morning or an afternoon. They will give you sedation and painkillers, or 'gas and air' (Entonox) to make the procedure more comfortable. The camera is flexible and about the size of my little finger, and is passed around the colon. It allows the endoscopist to take pictures and tissue samples, and carefully remove any polyps that we may see. Polyps are benign mushroom-like growths from the bowel which would be carefully removed. The department will send out an information leaflet with details of the possible risks – these include pain/discomfort, rare reactions to the medications, a 1 in 20 risk of an incomplete procedure requiring a repeat colonoscopy on a different day or a different test (CT scan), bleeding (rarely requiring observation, blood transfusion, a repeat colonoscopy or an operation), and rarely a perforation (leak of air and bowel contents requiring an operation to fix).

## Investigations

FBC (anaemia in colorectal cancer and IBD), U&E, TFT, ESR, CRP (inflammatory response in IBD), TTG (in view of weight loss, need to exclude coeliac disease but not a cause of his DVT), LFT, INR, PSA
CXR – ex-smoker (30 pack-years)
Clinical assessment including use of the two-level Wells score (see previous case for two-level Wells score) to assess the probability of DVT – this patient scores 2 based on the leg swelling (>3 cm) and tenderness.
2 points or more – DVT likely
1 point or less – DVT unlikely
If score 2 or over, arrange US Doppler of leg
If US Doppler is positive, diagnose and treat for DVT. If US Doppler is negative, check D-dimer
If D-dimer is positive, repeat US Doppler 6–8 days later. If D-dimer is negative, DVT is not likely; consider other diagnoses
If Wells score is low risk, 0 or less, then carry out D-dimer
If D-dimer is negative, then explain to the patient that DVT is not likely; consider other diagnoses
If D-dimer is positive, then arrange US Doppler scan. If US Doppler is positive, diagnose and treat as DVT. If D-dimer is negative, then explain to the patient that DVT is not likely
If USS arranged, prescribe anticoagulation with low molecular weight heparin until patient reviewed with scan result, and then can decide on further management
Ambulatory care as per local protocol
Decide on further management, e.g. need for warfarin if proven DVT when results of USS Doppler available; will need to let gastroenterology know he's on warfarin if considering colonoscopy

## Management

Enoxaparin 1.5 mg/kg SC once per day until scan performed and patient reviewed post scan to decide on further management
Need to manage anticoagulation carefully, and be aware of more complex patients (anaemia, malignancy, liver disease) as well as patients with higher bleeding risk (recent peptic ulcer, coagulopathy, thrombocytopenia, recent eye or brain surgery, uncontrolled hypertension)

Ambulatory care: involve the DVT clinic – usually have protocols for investigations/management and ongoing ambulatory care

Will also need to refer for urgent (fast-track) gastroenterology review/colonoscopy (to exclude colonic cancer or IBD) given his weight loss and altered bowel habit

## Addressing concerns/answering questions

• *Why are my bowels causing me such trouble?* We need to arrange some investigations to find out why you have lost weight and started having diarrhoea. Your leg looks likely to have a clot in the veins and this is causing the swelling and pain. Some bowel conditions can cause clots in the leg. The bowel could be inflamed, or possibly a more serious condition is present and, as discussed, blood tests and a colonoscopy camera test will help us diagnose the cause.

• *Can I go home? I need to feed the cats as my wife is away.* Yes, we can arrange these investigations as an outpatient. We need to ensure that you get the blood thinning injection every day, and the appointment for a scan of the leg. We'll need to give you details of when to come back to the unit for the injections, and for the ultrasound scan.

## Discussion with examiners

The examiners may ask you to clarify details of the above diagnosis and ask questions about your planned investigations and management.

Other possible questions include:

• *How do you decide if the patient is fit for a colonoscopy?* The patient needs to be able to take the bowel preparation and tolerate the laxatives' effects as well as the procedure itself (which can be uncomfortable, and carries potential risks including bleeding and perforation requiring an operation). He needs to be mobile enough to take the laxative preparation and

be able to get to the toilet (multiple loose bowel motions); need to ensure that the patient's comorbidities are taken into account, e.g. renal impairment, heart failure, anticoagulation and diabetes.

• *What follow-up would you arrange and with whom?* As above – either review by gastroenterology on the MAU or a rapid access referral (2 weeks) given the weight loss, altered bowel habit and now probable left-sided DVT.

See also Section I, Station 5, Other, Case 2.

---

### Examiners' information and requirements

The candidate should:

1. Identify key features from the history: acute swelling of calf, change in bowel habit with weight loss

2. Identify key examination findings including clinical signs of DVT

3. Outline a sensible management plan, including investigations to confirm diagnosis of DVT and referral to appropriate specialists for ongoing investigations of altered bowel habit and weight loss (gastroenterology/colonoscopy)

4. Give a clear explanation to the patient of your diagnosis and plan, address his concerns and answer his questions

---

### Further reading/resources

2012 NICE guidelines on venous thromboembolic diseases: the management of venous thromboembolic diseases and the role of thrombophilia testing: www.guidance.nice.org.uk/CG144 includes Wells scores and flowcharts for DVT and PE.

# Scenario 59 | Deterioration in renal function

## Candidate's information

**Your role:** you are an ST2 covering the medical wards on-call. You've been asked to see this 65-year-old woman with diabetes and hypertension who was admitted 3 days ago with a urinary tract infection, but the nurses are concerned about her poor urine output. BP 100/75, pulse 96. Today's blood tests have shown U&E 20, creatinine 160, eGFR 30.

**Your task:** to assess the patient's problems and address any questions or concerns raised by her.

## Patient's information

**You are:** Dina Salmon, a 65-year-old woman.

**Your problem:** you were admitted 3 days ago with a urine infection. You had burning pain on passing urine, going two or three times at night, and lots of times in the day for about 3 days; then you started getting pain in your lower right back where your doctor says your kidneys are. You hadn't got better on the tablets your GP prescribed (cefalexin) and the pain worsened so you came to hospital. You felt a bit better on the antibiotics given in the MAU but had some fever and sweats overnight and started feeling sick and vomiting last night. You can't drink because of the nausea, and the intravenous fluid drip was stopped yesterday morning.

### Past medical history and drug history:
- Came into hospital a few years ago with pain in the same kind of place – the doctors were wondering about kidney stones but a CT scan was OK with no stones, and everything settled down after a course of antibiotics
- Type 2 diabetes mellitus
- High blood pressure
- Preadmission medicines ramipril 5 mg twice per day, metformin 1 g bd and occasional paracetamol for arthritis

### Social history:
- Live alone
- Daughters live nearby
- Independent
- Retired bank clerk
- Non-smoker
- No alcohol

### Other issues including family history:
- Mother died from a stroke age 75
- No family history of diabetes

- (If told that the doctor is going to stop the BP tablets, even temporarily) *I'm worried about my blood pressure. My mum had a stroke which the doctors put down to her blood pressure. Don't I need these tablets?*
- *Will my kidneys recover? Will I need dialysis?*

---

## Candidate

### History/key questions

Ask about symptoms leading up to admission: dysuria, frequency, nocturia, haematuria, fever, back pain, any syncopal episodes/postural hypotension

Acute history versus chronic (NB: ask for old results: creatinine normal on admission): ask about chronic symptoms including nausea, loss of appetite

Since admission: ask about oral intake, nausea, vomiting, diarrhoea

Rash (petechial rash of streptococcal infection or ITP)

#### Past medical history

Any past problems with the kidneys. Ever needed dialysis or renal biopsy. Any idea what her last urine dipstick showed (any signs of protein in the kidneys?). Does she see a kidney doctor?

Ask about risk factors for renal disease: diabetes, hypertension, vascular disease (ask about history of strokes/TIA, angina/MI, peripheral vascular disease)

Any recent instrumentation of urinary tract (increased risk of urinary tract infection/potentially different organisms)

#### Drug history

Ask about NSAIDs, aspirin, nephrotoxic drugs, e.g. diuretics, ACE inhibitors, angiotensin II inhibitors, statins, recent courses of antibiotics

#### Social history

Ask about smoking history (pack-years) and alcohol intake

#### Other issues including family history

Anyone in the family had problems with the kidneys, needed dialysis or transplant?

### Address patient's questions and concerns

- *Have you had any thoughts about what is going on?*
- *Is there anything in particular you're concerned about?*
- *Do you have anything you would like to ask?*

## Key areas for examination

A list of what to look for (in examination order; describe findings on examination)

GCS/consciousness level: any drowsiness or confusion (uraemia)

Respiratory rate/pattern, e.g. Kussmaul respiration due to acidosis

Temperature, pulse, BP (apyrexial, pulse 80, 110/70 in this patient at the time of your assessment)

Assess fluid balance and decide whether hypovolaemic, euvolaemic or fluid overloaded:

Assess circulation: pulse, capillary refill/peripheral perfusion, BP

Assess JVP at 45°

Look for nailfold infarcts (vasculitis), rash (petechial rash in streptococcal sepsis; vasculitis/Henoch–Schönlein purpura rash)

Listen to lungs: any evidence of pulmonary oedema

Abdominal examination: look for signs of abdominal tenderness (suprapubic/renal angle); is bladder palpable?

Look for oedema (ankles/lower leg, sacrum)

Ask to see observation charts: check current observations – any evidence of shock requiring vigorous fluid resuscitation and the Sepsis 6 bundle (see Further reading/resources below)

Have there been prolonged periods of hypotension (e.g. due to sepsis/systemic inflammatory response syndrome) leading to acute tubular necrosis? Has her fever settled on IV antibiotics?

Blood glucose results

Urinalysis

Blood results from before and during this admission: the results available from the examiners are from the day of admission (urea 7, creat 75, eGFR 71) and today (48 h later) with urea 20, creat 160, eGFR 30

Results of blood and urine cultures sent on admission:

*E. coli* grown on the blood cultures, sensitivities awaited

MSSU outstanding; no microscopy available but admission urinalysis showed 2+ blood, 2+ protein and 3+ leucocytes

Fluid balance chart: received 2 L per day of IV and oral fluids for first 24 h, but no IV fluids in the past 24 h (drinking less than a litre with poor oral intake due to nausea, and vomited at least three times in past 24 h)

Current drug chart and checklist of the medicines on admission (looking for nephrotoxic drugs – ACEI, NSAIDs): she has remained on the ramipril (missed today's dose as vomiting/nausea) and has been taking PRN naproxen 500 mg once or twice per day for pain (last dose 24 h ago, as has been vomiting). Check which antibiotics she has been on (stat dose of 5 mg/kg gentamicin on admission then coamoxiclav 1.2 g IV tds since – as per trust protocol for acute pyelonephritis)

CXR

## Differential diagnosis

Acute kidney injury:

Urinary sepsis / pyelonephritis (*E. coli*) in combination with dehydration (reduced intake, increased losses through vomiting), use of NSAIDs and ACE inhibitor

Consider possible chronic renovascular disease due to diabetes or hypertension (although baseline results normal)

**Key facts/areas to consider** (including information available in scenario summary before station starts): some information available in summary: urinary tract infection mentioned, as is her past history of diabetes and hypertension (both risk factors for chronic renal impairment), and current U&E results showing kidney injury

## Discussion with patient

Explain diagnosis
Explain plan, including investigations and management
Address patient's concerns/answer their questions

You've been on treatment for an infection in your urine, which is more common in people with diabetes, but the blood results show that your kidneys aren't working now as well as they were. This is likely to be due to a combination of things – the infection, losing fluid through vomiting, not eating and drinking as much as normal, and also the BP medications. We need to continue to treat the infection but also give you some fluids through the veins, anti-sickness injections and stop

some of your medicines temporarily to allow your kidneys to recover back to normal. I'll also request a scan to check that the kidneys are draining properly.

## Investigations

Check MSSU/BC results (ensure on correct antibiotics by checking sensitivities)

ABG including lactate

CXR to exclude pneumonia (another source of infection)

Repeat bloods including ESR, CRP, FBC, CK (U&E already done today)

Renal screen including ANA, ANCA, immunoglobulins, C3/4, protein electrophoresis

Urine for urinalysis and Bence Jones protein (exclude vasculitis, myeloma)

Need to exclude obstruction (urgent renal ultrasound to assess renal size, exclude hydronephrosis/hydroureter, exclude bladder outflow obstruction/residual volume)

## Management

Stop NSAID and ACEI

Rehydrate IV with crystalloid

Ensure on correct antibiotics for urinary sepsis

Antiemetics

Say that you would check all drugs in BNF/renal drug handbook to see whether you need to adjust dose for renal impairment

Urinary catheter; monitor urine output; exclude urinary retention (obstructive uropathy)

Referral to renal physicians

### Addressing concerns/answering questions

• *I'm worried about my blood pressure. My mum had a stroke which the doctors put down to her blood pressure. Don't I need these tablets?* At the moment your BP is actually low. We will monitor your blood pressure and your blood results to see how the kidneys improve with treatment – we can restart blood pressure medications if you need them once your kidneys have improved. Kidneys often get affected by urine infections and dehydration, and medicines like ramipril can also affect the kidneys. We are treating the infection with antibiotics, rehydrating you with fluids through the veins, and will give you medicines for nausea so that you can eat and drink.

• *Will my kidneys recover? Will I need dialysis?* I expect your kidneys to improve over the next few days and we will keep you informed of progress. Rarely, people's kidneys don't improve as expected and need to be supported with dialysis. I think that your kidneys will improve with the treatment we are giving as they were working normally when you came into hospital but we will need to keep a close eye on you.

## Discussion with examiners

The examiners may ask you to clarify details of the above diagnosis and ask questions about your planned investigations and management.

Other possible questions include:
- *What is the management of obstructive uropathy?* Obstructive uropathy is kidney injury due to blockage of the urinary tract; locations of blockage range from prostatic / bladder outflow, bladder pathology (ureterovesical junctions), to ureteric and renal obstruction. Stones, prostatic pathology (benign prostatic hyperplasia or cancer) and pelvic/retroperitoneal malignancies are the most common causes. Relieving the obstruction reduces the pressure on the affected kidney(s), e.g. with a catheter in the case of BPH, and allows the kidneys to recover. Risks of obstruction include infection. Obstruction can be relieved by catheter, nephrostomy or ureteric stent depending on the location of the obstruction. Investigation and management of the underlying cause is then required. There will be a polyuric phase following relief of the obstruction which can lead to marked hypovolaemia, and strict fluid balance is required.
- *What are the components of the Sepsis 6 bundle (Surviving Sepsis Campaign) and why are the severe sepsis bundles advocated?* Reducing mortality due to severe sepsis requires an organized process that guarantees early recognition and consistent application of evidence-based practices. The Severe Sepsis Bundles are a series of therapies that, when implemented together, achieve better outcomes than when implemented individually. The resuscitation bundle is a combined evidence-based goal that must be completed within 6 hours for patients with severe sepsis, septic shock and/or lactate >4 mmol/L (36 mg/dL). The goal is to perform all indicated tasks 100% of the time within the first 6 hours of identification of severe sepsis. The tasks are:

Measure serum lactate

Obtain blood cultures prior to antibiotic administration

Administer broad-spectrum antibiotic within 3 h of ED admission and within 1 h of non-ED admission

In the event of hypotension and/or a serum lactate > 4 mmol/L, (a) deliver an initial minimum of 20 mL/kg of crystalloid or an equivalent; (b) apply vasopressors for hypotension not responding to initial fluid resuscitation to maintain mean arterial pressure (MAP) >65 mmHg

In the event of persistent hypotension despite fluid resuscitation (septic shock) and/or lactate > 4 mmol/L, (a) achieve a central venous pressure (CVP) of ≥8 mmHg; (b) achieve a central venous oxygen saturation ($ScvO_2$) ≥70% or mixed venous oxygen saturation (SvO) ≥65%.

Quoted directly from: www.survivingsepsis.org/Bundles/Pages/SepsisResuscitationBundle.aspx

---

### Examiners' information and requirements

The candidate should:

1. Identify key features from the history: admitted with infection; vomiting and reduced intake overnight; continued ACE inhibitor and NSAID use, and acute kidney injury on blood tests. Identify key past history including diabetes and hypertension
2. Identify key examination findings including euvolaemic but negative fluid balance on chart
3. Outline a sensible management plan as detailed above; must include correct antibiotics, stopping offending drugs, rehydrating and excluding obstruction with an ultrasound
4. Give a clear explanation to the patient of your diagnosis and plan, address her concerns and answer her questions

---

### Further reading/resources
www.survivingsepsis.org

# Scenario 60 | Fever in the returning traveller

## Candidate's information

**Your role:** you are an ST2 on the medical admissions unit. You have been asked to see this man who has been feeling unwell and feverish since returning from holiday last week.

**Your task:** to assess the patient's problems and address any questions or concerns raised by him.

## Patient's information

**You are:** Kim Lake, a 52-year-old marketing manager for an engineering firm (valves in industrial machines).

**Your problem:** you have been feeling unwell for the past week or so, with fever, muscle aches and slight headache. The headaches eased after paracetamol but the fever was particularly bad last night, disturbing your sleep, and you couldn't go to work today. You attended A&E as your GP is closed this afternoon. You have not felt like this before – feels a little different to flu as you feel relatively well in between the high temperatures.

You went abroad on business to Gambia 3 months ago, returning 2 weeks ago. You felt a little unwell in the last few days there but you thought that this was due to the food as several other people were unwell, and your tummy felt a bit upset. You had diarrhoea a couple of times in the first week after you got back. No diarrhoea in the past week. No rash, photophobia or jaundice. No abdominal pain or rectal bleeding. No swimming when you were away. Only a couple of insect bites near the start of your time in Gambia, and they settled quickly.

You went to your GP before you flew to Gambia and she talked to you about vaccinations and about taking antimalarial tablets this time. You had some vaccinations and she prescribed antimalarial tablets for you, but you never picked up the prescription as you had been to Africa before without having any problems (you're a regular traveller to Gambia) and you didn't see any mosquitoes the previous times. The tablets were also pretty expensive, and as you didn't think you actually needed to take them, you didn't waste the money buying them.

You've had no unprotected sex with anyone except your wife with whom you travelled (she fundraises in the UK for a church project in Gambia and helps teach there while you're working). No other sexual partners since you married 25 years ago.

### Past medical history and drug history:
• No regular medications
• No drug allergies

**Social history:**

• Non-smoker

• Drinks a couple of pints of beer, 2–3 times per week

**Other issues including family history:**

• Wife well. She had treatment for malaria a few years ago when you visited Kenya together but you were fine

**Your questions for the candidate:**

• *Should I have taken the antimalarials?*

• *Do I have to stay in hospital? I've got a big contract coming up.*

---

## Candidate

### History/key questions

Generic questions about fever to find out source:

Duration of symptoms – in one series 80% of falciparum malaria patients presented within a month of returning home, compared to 36% of vivax malaria patients. Falciparum malaria is most likely to occur within three months of the patient's return from an endemic area

Non-specific symptoms such as myalgia, arthralgia, fatigue, lethargy, chills/hot and cold, nausea ± vomiting, headache

Respiratory symptoms – cough, sputum, breathlessness/exercise tolerance, haemoptysis, chest pain, weight loss

Gastroenterological symptoms – diarrhoea, abdominal pain, rectal bleeding, anorexia, nausea, vomiting

Lymphadenopathy/sore throat

Headache, rash, photophobia – differential diagnosis includes meningitis

Ask about travel-associated infection (main differential in someone recently returned from Gambia): symptoms whilst away and since return

Think destination, setting and activities

Area(s) travelled to is particularly important: may be multiple regions or countries, each with their own specific risks. You wouldn't be expected to know the exact risks for each and every specific area but malaria is particularly common in sub-Saharan Africa and you should be aware of this potential risk in this patient. Other important information includes locations of stop-overs and types of travel

Where did he stay whilst in Gambia?

Duration of travel important (e.g. 1 week in a city compared to 3 months out in the countryside of the country)

Ask about details of immunizations including antimalarials, and whether these were taken as per the instructions, e.g. most antimalarials, such as mefloquine and doxycycline, need to be taken for a period before and after the trip

### Drug history

Current medications, any drug allergies, any new medicines

### Past medical history

Any known medical conditions, particularly those that may cause symptoms or predispose to infections

### Social history

Smoking, alcohol history

### Address patient's questions and concerns

• *Have you had any thoughts about what is going on?*

• *Is there anything in particular you're concerned about?*

• *Do you have anything you would like to ask?*

## Key areas for examination

A list of what to look for (in examination order; describe findings on examination)

GCS

Examine for lymphadenopathy, rashes, bites

Any signs of anaemia or jaundice (sclera or skin): both can occur in *Falciparum malariae* infection

Oropharynx

Chest, heart, abdominal examination. Exclude hepatosplenomegaly

Request temperature chart, list of medications, any available blood results and to view a CXR

Say that you would like to carry out an examination of the genitals/exclude inguinal lymphadenopathy

Examination normal – only abnormality was temperature 37.9°C on the temperature chart

## Differential diagnosis

Key differential given the above history is malaria, and this needs to be the primary target of investigations. No obvious diarrhoeal, respiratory causes. With malaria, 40% may not have fever at time of presentation, and examination can be entirely normal

Differential diagnoses include other travel-associated infections: typhoid fever, hepatitis, dengue fever, avian influenza, severe acute respiratory syndrome, HIV, meningitis/encephalitis, viral haemorrhagic fever (according to British Infection Society guidelines)

Other differential diagnosis includes mononucleosis (due to Epstein–Barr virus or cytomegalovirus)

## Discussion with patient

Explain diagnosis
Explain plan, including investigations and management
Address patient's concerns/answer their questions

The likely cause for your fever and feeling unwell is an infection caught whilst abroad. Given the area you travelled to, it is very important that we look carefully for malaria, and give you treatment as needed. We're also going to send off tests looking for other causes of your symptoms. Depending on the type of malaria, and how significant the infection is, we can advise on whether you need to come into hospital and have the medication through the veins rather than tablets.

## Investigations

Basic blood tests – FBC, INR, U&E, LFT, ESR, CRP (may show mild anaemia, thrombocytopenia, coagulopathy and renal impairment in malaria)

Blood cultures (for typhoid and/or other bacteraemia)

Urine dipstick (haemoglobinuria)

Faeces for microscopy, culture, cysts and parasites if diarrhoea

Urgent thick and thin films on three consecutive days + rapid diagnostic testing (RDT) for malaria, irrespective of whether antimalaria prophylaxis has been taken or not. Send to lab immediately, and ask for result within 1 hour

NB: malaria prophylaxis may delay the onset of symptoms and obscure the microscopic diagnosis. Stop the chemoprophylaxis on admission to hospital as this may interfere with parasite detection

Although almost as sensitive as expert malaria prophylaxis for falciparum malaria, RDT is less sensitive for non-falciparum malaria (as it cannot give the additional information of parasite count, maturity, presence of mixed species, RDT is an adjunct not a replacement for microscopy)

Urine cultures

CXR to rule out community-acquired pneumonia

Hepatitis A, B, C, E serology if jaundice or hepatitic changes on liver tests

HIV serology: explain it is part of the routine work-up for patients with fever (a treatable condition, and picking it up early is important as treatment can be started)

## Management

Depends on the results (need to identify cause, and for malaria, which type, level of parasitaemia)

If malaria confirmed, need to know the type/parasitaemia level, and refer to local malaria guidelines, British Infection Society guidelines on malaria (UK), involve local microbiology specialists and/or local infectious diseases referral centre to advise on therapy

If falciparum, mixed infection or species unclear: admit

If falciparum: need to know parasite count, as it is one of several criteria which will guide management

If severe/complicated falciparum infection (see the British Infection Society criteria below, and their malaria guidelines for further information): involve critical care team/consider admission to ICU. Seek help from specialist infection/tropical medicine unit. Give oxygen. Careful fluid balance. Monitor blood glucose closely. ECG monitoring (particularly during quinine IV); 4 hourly obs including GCS. Daily FBC, INR, U&E, LFT, parasite count. If shock, treat for gram-negative sepsis

If complicated falciparum or patient vomiting: IV quinine loading dose, then 8 hourly with po doxycycline (see guidelines for details) or artesunate

If uncomplicated falciparum: oral treatment

If non-falciparum malaria (vivax, ovale, malariae) then outpatient therapy is usually appropriate depending on clinical judgement, availability of follow-up, etc.

'If in doubt ask for help': say that you would ask for advice from your local referral centre for infectious diseases. They will be able to guide you on the likely infective agents depending on the areas visited, and may take the patient if severe/complicated falciparum malaria (e.g. needs exchange transfusions, etc). Further advice would certainly be required if the malaria investigations are negative and other causes need to be excluded

Adherence to antimalarials doesn't exclude malaria

Notify all cases to local Health Protection Agency

### Addressing concerns/answering questions

- *Should I have taken the antimalarials?* We do advise taking the antimalaria tablets to reduce the risk of malaria which can be a very serious infection, and can be life-threatening. Let's focus on finding and treating what's making you unwell now, and we can deal with future travel later. Once I've got more information I will let you know.
- *Do I have to stay in hospital? I've got a big contract coming up.* I would advise waiting until the results are back, and I can then explain the plan including whether we would advise you to stay in hospital based on these results. As discussed above.

## Discussion with examiners

The examiners may ask you to clarify details of the above diagnosis and ask questions about your planned investigations and management.

Other possible questions include:
- *How would you assess the severity of malaria?* Using the British Infection Society (BIS) criteria for malaria below:

Major features of severe or complicated falciparum malaria (as per BIS guidelines) = one or more of:
- Impaired consciousness or seizures
- Hypoglycaemia
- Parasite count equal to or greater than 2% (lower counts do not exclude severe malaria)
- Haemoglobin equal to or less than 8 g/dL
- Spontaneous bleeding/disseminated intravascular coagulation
- Haemoglobinuria (without G6P deficiency)
- Renal impairment or electrolyte/acid–base disturbance (pH <7.3)
- Pulmonary oedema or ARDS
- Shock (BP <90/60) (algid malaria) may be due to gram-negative bacteraemia

- *What are the possible complications of severe 'complicated' malaria?*
  'Cerebral malaria' – altered consciousness / coma +/– seizures
  Hypoglycaemia – common complication
  Acute Respiratory Distress Syndrome (ARDS) / non-cardiogenic pulmonary oedema
  Shock / circulatory collapse (algid malaria)
  Metabolic acidosis
  Acute kidney injury; fluid and electrolyte abnormalities

Hepatic dysfunction (jaundice due to haemolysis; cholestasis due to falciparum)
Coagulopathy +/– disseminated intravascular coagulation
Severe anaemia or massive intravascular haemolysis; haemoglobinuria ('blackwater fever')
Sepsis from other sources (e.g. gram-negative sepsis causing marked hypotension / shock)
Splenic rupture (falciparum)
- *Why check for 6GP deficiency if primaquine is being considered as treatment for non-falciparum malaria?* G6PD deficiency has been shown to offer protection against severe life-threatening infection in these individuals, but drug treatment with primaquine in these individuals can cause severe haemolytic anaemia.

---

### Examiners' information and requirements

The candidate should:
1. Identify key features from the history (3-month stay in area of high malaria prevalence, no use of antimalarials, presenting with fever in returning traveller)
2. Identify key examination findings including normal examination but fever on chart
3. Outline a sensible management plan including essential urgent blood films to make the diagnosis of malaria, and appropriate treatment of malaria once confirmed. This includes referring to the local and/or national guidelines, calling local infectious disease centre for advice; admitting as necessary; treatment will be guided by clinical condition, confirmation of malaria and parasitaemia level, amongst other factors
4. Give a clear explanation to the patient of your diagnosis and plan, address his concerns and answer his questions

---

### Further reading/resources

British Infection Society (www.britishinfection.org) has published guidelines on:
1. Management of malaria in the UK, 2007 (flowchart and paper)
2. Fever in returned travellers presenting in the United Kingdom: recommendations for investigation and initial management, 2008

# Other reported miscellaneous cases

- Marfan's/lens dislocation (see Section I, Station 5, Locomotor, Case 9)
- Elderly care, recurrent falls; environment/patient factors, etc.
- Ehlers–Danlos syndrome (see Section I, Station 5, Skin, Case 29)
- Loss of libido
- Lymphoedema (see Section I, Station 5, Other, Case 8)
- Familial hypercholesterolaemia with tendon xanthomas (see Section I, Station 5, Skin, Case 7)
- Cervical rib
- Wegener's granulomatosis (see Section I, Station 5, Locomotor, Case 10)
- Lymphadenopathy/breast cancer
- Pyrexia of unknown origin ± lymphadenopathy
- Renal transplant/rejection (see Vol. 1, Station 1, Abdominal, Case 1)
- UTI/pyelonephritis

# Section I
# Short Case *Records*

*'Be professional in presentation. I agree it's an easy exam – it's easy to fail'.**

These books exist as they are because of many previous candidates who, over the years, have completed our surveys and given us invaluable insight into the candidate experience. Please give something back by doing the same for the candidates of the future. For all of your sittings, whether they be a triumphant pass or a disastrous fail . . .
**Remember to fill in the survey at www.ryder-mrcp.org.uk**

THANK YOU

In the third edition of this book, the skin, locomotor, endocrine and eye short cases were presented in the same section as the respiratory, abdominal, cardiovascular and central nervous system short cases with no great distinction made between them. As discussed in the Introduction to this volume of *An Aid to the MRCP PACES*, the Colleges have in their own words:

'*no plan to remove skin, locomotor, endocrine, and eye problems from the clinical issues that may be assessed in the new Station 5. Candidates must prepare to be examined in these areas as they do now*'.

However, in our communications with the Colleges, they also stated with regard to the old Station 5:

'*However, the format of Station 5 does need to change for reasons that have been described in various communications to all PACES examiners. Many of the cases used now are unsuitable – they are "spot diagnoses" which are followed by a viva examination relating to the subject and this is not appropriate as knowledge is tested already and more appropriately in the written papers. Many of the cases follow a well-worn formula for which candidates prepare and clinical thinking is not tested well. The frequent exhibition of chronic plaque psoriasis, simple goitre, or mutilating rheumatoid hands has little relevance to the skills of a Core Medical Trainee. In the end, the marks at (the old) Station 5 contribute little to the discrimination of candidate ability in comparison to the other stations and so something better is required*'.

And:

'*New Station 5 opens the opportunity to test integrated clinical thinking about a range of clinical problems from the curriculum in a way that junior doctors practise every day – including skin, locomotor, endocrine, and eye problems as well as others*'.

In the third edition of this book, we presented all the skin, locomotor, endocrine and eye short cases that have ever occurred in the MRCP clinical exam over the years according to our surveys, and we presented them in the same format as for Stations 1 and 3. This format has served candidates well over the years with regard to preparing for the various short cases that have occurred and in line with the Colleges' advice that 'Candidates must prepare to be examined in these areas as they do now'; it therefore seems reasonable to leave them in the format which has served well in the past. Nevertheless, we suggest you consider with each the new format of the exam as discussed in the Introduction to this volume and in Section H, as well as the seven skills being tested, and *think through the ways in which scenarios could be created for the short cases concerned*. This exercise in itself will be very valuable preparation. For example, in the old Station 5, the candidate might have been presented with a patient with acromegaly and would have first been required to spot the diagnosis and then examine relevant systems – visual fields, hands for size and carpal tunnel syndrome, etc., and then the candidate might be invited to ask the patient relevant questions – headache, vision, sweating, shoe size – and then management might be discussed.

In the new Station 5, all these components would still be present but dealt with in the new integrated clinical assessment format. The main differences are that in the old format, only what could be dealt with in 5 minutes would be covered, whereas in the new format all of this has to be covered and all within 10 minutes. And whereas in the old format, the examiner could take the lead in determining which aspects would be covered, in the new format the candidate is left to ensure that all is covered that can be in 8 minutes, with just 2 minutes being led by the examiners. For the example of acromegaly, Ed Fogden in Section H has chosen headache and vision problems for the scenario. Even though at first sight you might think 'spot diagnosis' is no longer as prominent in the new Station 5, the candidate would nevertheless ideally 'spot' the acromegaly early in order to direct the rest of the case accordingly.*
Ed Fogden's case of course represents the newly presenting acromegaly patient with a pituitary macroadenoma causing headache through pressure effects and bitemporal hemianopia through the tumour impinging on the optic chiasm. In reality, such patients go for transsphenoidal surgery relatively quickly which means that the majority of acromegalic patients appearing in the exam have already been treated, often years before. Some will have residual bitemporal hemianopia. Time will tell how often such patients have a scenario made up for them to act as if they were newly presenting with acromegaly and how often there will be clinical scenarios more aligned with problems associated with acromegaly which was treated years before – there may still be residual visual problems, problems from imperfectly treated, associated hypopituitarism or from carpal tunnel syndrome (see Vol. 2, Section F, Experience 14). We share these thoughts with you so that with each short case, you may think through the possible scenarios that might be made up around the case concerned, as well as those that might be real for the actual patient with the condition concerned in its current state of treatment and disease progression.

With regard to the short cases in the skin, locomotor, endocrine and eye subspecialties, all are there, common and rare. Should we reduce the number? The problem is – which would we cut out? We know that picking and choosing between cases to prepare for can be a tricky business – see footnote on central nervous system short case number 44 in Volume 1. On the one hand, one has to consider whether an MRCP exam host would not allow in an unusual skin case that came his way when he sat the MRCP years before; on the other hand, it does seem increasingly likely that the rarer cases in the past will become even rarer in the new Station 5.† We have elected not to leave out any but leave you to decide what level of risk you are prepared to take!

For general introductory comments with regard to the *aides-mémoire* (clinical descriptions for presentation to the examiner), otherwise known as short case *records*, which we present in this section, we refer you to the introductory paragraphs of Vol. 1, Section C of the fourth edition of *An Aid to the MRCP PACES*.

---

*See Vol. 2, Section F, Experience 13, Station 5, Case 1 for an example of where spotting the diagnosis early in the new Station 5 helped. Possibly also Vol. 2, Section F, Experience 5, Station 5, Case 1.

†However, see Vol. 2, Section F, Experience 12, Station 5. Yellow nail syndrome appearing in the new Station 5! Evidence that rare cases may still occur.

# Station 5
# Skin

| Short case | Checked and updated as necessary for this edition by |
|---|---|
| **1** Systemic sclerosis/CREST syndrome | Dr Shireen Velangi* |
| **2** Neurofibromatosis (von Recklinghausen's disease) | Dr Malobi Ogboli* |
| **3** Osler–Weber–Rendu syndrome | Dr Malobi Ogboli and Dr Brian Cooper* |
| **4** Psoriasis | Dr Malobi Ogboli* |
| **5** Rash of uncertain cause | Dr Shireen Velangi* |
| **6** Dermatomyositis | Dr Malobi Ogboli* |
| **7** Xanthomata | Dr Shireen Velangi and Professor Elizabeth Hughes* |
| **8** Vitiligo | Dr Shireen Velangi and Professor Hugh Jones* |
| **9** Adenoma sebaceum in tuberous sclerosis complex | Dr Malobi Ogboli* |
| **10** Pseudoxanthoma elasticum | Dr Malobi Ogboli* |
| **11** Lichen planus | Dr Shireen Velangi* |
| **12** Yellow nail syndrome | Dr Shireen Velangi* |
| **13** Gouty tophi | Dr Shireen Velangi* |
| **14** Alopecia areata | Dr Shireen Velangi* |
| **15** Eczema | Dr Shireen Velangi* |
| **16** Pretibial myxoedema | Dr Malobi Ogboli* |
| **17** Clubbing | Dr Malobi Ogboli and Dr Omer Khair* |
| **18** Necrobiosis lipoidica diabeticorum | Dr Shireen Velangi * |
| **19** Lupus pernio | Dr Shireen Velangi and Dr Omer Khair* |
| **20** Tinea | Dr Malobi Ogboli* |
| **21** Koilonychia | Dr Shireen Velangi* |
| **22** Raynaud's phenomenon | Dr Malobi Ogboli* |
| **23** Erythema nodosum | Dr Shireen Velangi* |
| **24** Sturge–Weber syndrome | Dr Malobi Ogboli* |
| **25** Purpura | Dr Shireen Velangim and Dr Chris Fegan* |
| **26** Peutz–Jeghers syndrome | Dr Malobi Ogboli and Dr Brian Cooper* |
| **27** Vasculitis | Dr Shireen Velangi* |
| **28** Ehlers–Danlos syndrome | Dr Malobi Ogboli* |
| **29** Livedo reticularis | Dr Shireen Velangi* |
| **30** Pemphigus/pemphigoid | Dr Shireen Velangi* |
| **31** Radiation burn on the chest | Dr Omer Khair* |
| **32** Herpes zoster | Dr Shireen Velangi* |
| **33** Henoch–Schönlein purpura | Dr Malobi Ogboli* |
| **34** Mycosis fungoides | Dr Shireen Velangi* |
| **35** Morphoea | Dr Malobi Ogboli* |

| Short case | Checked and updated as necessary for this edition by |
|---|---|
| **36** Kaposi's sarcoma (AIDS) | Dr Shireen Velangi and Dr Kaveh Manavi* |
| **37** Porphyria | Dr Malobi Ogboli* |
| **38** Lupus vulgaris | Dr Malobi Ogboli* |
| **39** Dermatitis herpetiformis | Dr Malobi Ogboli* |
| **40** Urticaria pigmentosa (mastocytosis) | Dr Malobi Ogboli* |
| **41** Palmoplantar keratoderma (tylosis) | Dr Shireen Velangi* |
| **42** Secondary syphilis | Dr Malobi Ogboli* |
| **43** Ectodermal dysplasia | Dr Malobi Ogboli* |
| **44** Partial lipodystrophy | Dr Shireen Velangi and Dr Fouad Albaaj* |
| **45** Fabry's disease | Dr Malobi Ogboli* |
| **46** Reiter's syndrome/reactive arthritis/ keratoderma blennorrhagica | Dr Shireen Velangi* |
| **47** Malignant melanoma | Dr Shireen Velangi* |
| **48** Acanthosis nigricans | Dr Malobi Ogboli* |
| **49** Keratoacanthoma | Dr Malobi Ogboli* |
| **50** Pyoderma gangrenosum | Dr Malobi Ogboli and Dr Brian Cooper* |
| **51** Psychogenic/factitious | Dr Malobi Ogboli* |

*All suggested changes by these specialty advisors were considered by Dr Bob Ryder and were either accepted, edited, added to or rejected with Dr Ryder making the final editorial decision in every case.

Dr Malobi Ogboli, Consultant Dermatologist, City Hospital, Birmingham, UK
Dr Shireen Velangi, Consultant Dermatologist, City Hospital, Birmingham, UK
Dr Brian Cooper, Consultant Gastroenterologist, City Hospital, Birmingham, UK
Dr Omer Khair, Consultant Chest Physician, City Hospital, Birmingham, UK
Dr Chris Fegan, Consultant Haematologist, University Hospital of Wales, Cardiff, UK
Dr Fouad Albaaj, Consultant Nephrologist, City Hospital, Birmingham, UK
Professor T Hugh Jones, Consultant Physician and Endocrinologist and Honorary Professor of Andrology, Barnsley Hospital and University of Sheffield, UK
Professor Elizabeth Hughes, Consultant Chemical Pathologist and West Midlands Regional Postgraduate Dean, Sandwell General Hospital, West Bromwich, UK
Dr Kaveh Manavi, Consultant in GU/HIV Medicine, University Hospitals Birmingham NHS Foundation Trust, Birmingham, UK

# Case 1 | Systemic sclerosis/ CREST syndrome

**Frequency in survey for 3rd edition:** main focus of a short case in 15% of attempts at PACES Station 5, Skin. Additional feature in a further 1%.

**Survey note:** mixed connective tissue disease has also occurred.

Systemic sclerosis/CREST syndrome is dealt with in Station 5, Locomotor, Case 3.

# Case 2 | Neurofibromatosis (von Recklinghausen's disease)

**Frequency in survey for 3rd edition:** main focus of a short case in 13% of attempts at PACES Station 5, Skin. Additional feature in a further 4%.

**Survey note:** occurred as either a spot diagnosis, with or without a mention of the associated features, or as a case with an associated nerve pressure effect (such as one with an associated ulnar nerve/T1 lesion).

## Record

There are multiple *neurofibromata* and *café-au-lait spots* (normal person allowed up to five of the latter). The diagnosis is neurofibromatosis.*

*or*

There are multiple skin lesions: *sessile* and *pedunculated* cutaneous *fibromata*, as well as neurofibromata which are both *soft* and *firm*, *single* and *lobulated*, and felt both as mobile subcutaneous lumps† and *nodules* along the course of peripheral nerves. There are *café-au-lait* spots (especially in the axillae – axillary freckling occurs in two-thirds of affected individuals). The diagnosis is neurofibromatosis.*

---

Autosomal dominant.
The condition is usually asymptomatic.

### Complications

Kyphoscoliosis
Pressure effects of the neurofibromata on peripheral nerves and cranial nerves, especially:
  (a) acoustic neuroma (?Vth, VIth, VIIth, VIIIth nerve lesions, nystagmus and cerebellar signs; may be bilateral; see Vol. 1, Station 3, CNS, Case 25)*
  (b) Vth nerve neuroma
Spinal nerve root involvement which may cause:
  (a) cord compression

  (b) muscle wasting
  (c) sensory loss (Charcot's joints may occur)
Sarcomatous or other malignant change (5–16%)
Lung cysts (honeycomb lung)
Pseudoarthrosis and other orthopaedic abnormalities
Plexiform neuroma‡

**Other intracranial tumours which can occur** in this condition are:
Gliomata (optic nerve and chiasma; cerebral)
Meningiomata*
Medulloblastomata

---

*The phakomatoses or neurocutaneous syndromes are characterized by disordered growth of neurocutaneous tissues. More than 20 syndromes have been described, the most important of which are *neurofibromatosis 1 (von Recklinghausen's* – chromosome 17), neurofibromatosis 2 (chromosome 22), tuberous sclerosis (see Station 5, Skin, Case 9) and Sturge–Weber disease (see Station 5, Skin, Case 24). *Neurofibromatosis 2*, often called *central neurofibromatosis*, is rare and characterized by bilateral acoustic neuromata and often other intracranial tumours such as meningiomata or ependymomata. A few *café-au-lait* spots are present in about 40% of cases. At-risk family members should be screened regularly with hearing tests, etc.

†Neurofibromatosis should not be confused with lipomatosis with its characteristic soft subcutaneous lumps. In Dercum's disease (usually middle-aged women) subcutaneous lipomata may be painful and associated with marked obesity. These are easily recognized because, unlike neurofibromata, they are subcutaneous, soft, rounded or lobulated nodules that are moveable against the overlying skin.
‡An entire nerve trunk and all its branches are involved in diffuse neurofibromatosis with associated overgrowth of overlying tissues leading to gross deformities (temporal and frontal scalp are favourite sites but it may occur anywhere); may grow to lemon or even melon size.

## Other features of neurofibromatosis

An association with phaeochromocytoma – 5% of cases
(?blood pressure)

Nodules of the iris – these are small, circular, pigmented
hamartomata of the iris (Lisch nodules)

Hamartomata of the retina
Rib notching
Mental deficiency
Epilepsy
Renal artery stenosis

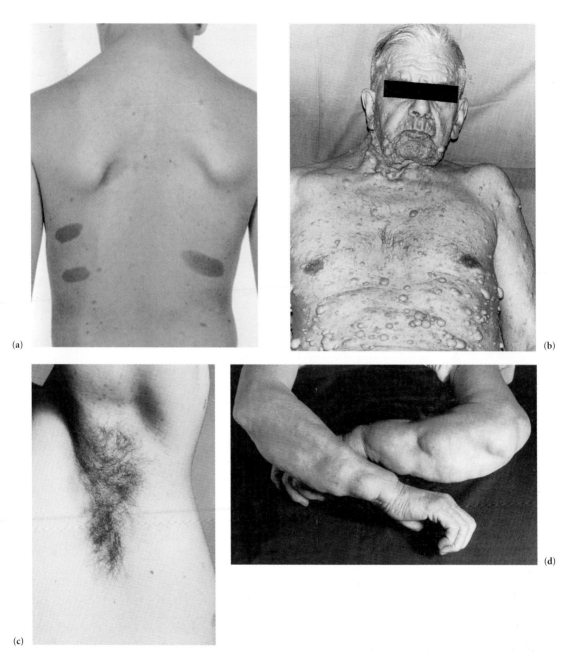

(a)

(b)

(c)

(d)

**Figure I5.1** (a) *Café-au-lait* spots: multiple small and three large (>1 cm) dark macules with well-demarcated margins. (b) Myriad skin-coloured and darkish neurofibromata. (c) Axillary freckling. (d) Lipomatosis: multiple, soft, easily moveable, subcutaneous nodules.

# Case 3 | Osler–Weber–Rendu syndrome

**Frequency in survey for 3rd edition:** main focus of a short case in 11% of attempts at PACES Station 5, Skin.

## Record

There is *telangiectasia* on the face, around the *mouth*, on the lips, on the *tongue* (look under the tongue), the buccal and nasal mucosa and on the fingers, of this (?clinically anaemic) patient (who has none of the features of systemic sclerosis; see Station 5, Locomotor, Case 3).

The diagnosis is Osler–Weber–Rendu syndrome (hereditary haemorrhagic telangiectasia). The lesions may occur elsewhere, especially in the gastrointestinal tract, and may bleed. Patients may present with *epistaxis* (the most common and sometimes the only site of bleeding), *gastrointestinal (GI) haemorrhage*, chronic iron deficiency *anaemia* and occasionally with haemorrhage elsewhere (e.g. haemoptysis).

---

Usually considered to be autosomal dominant. In fact, it is a family of disorders caused by mutations in various genes.

The telangiectasia consists of a localized collection of non-contractile capillaries and shows a prolonged bleeding time if punctured. The disease is frequently heralded by recurrent epistaxis in early childhood. In some cases, it presents as anaemia due to chronic blood loss from GI telangiectasia. In some variants (the pattern in individual families tends to be constant), pulmonary arteriovenous aneurysms are common and increase in frequency (as do the telangiectasia) with advancing age. These cases may have *cyanosis* and *clubbing,* and *bruits* over the lung fields. The neurological complications include haemorrhage and the formation of bland or mycotic aneurysms. In the eye there may be bloody tears (conjunctival telangiectasia); retinal haemorrhage or detachment may occur. Cirrhosis* (due to telangiectasia or multiple transfusions) and massive intrahepatic shunting may occur.

### Treatment

Chronic oral iron therapy may be required. Oestrogens (inducing squamous metaplasia of the nasal mucosa) may be helpful if epistaxis is the main symptom. Also for epistaxis, a low dose of the antifibrinolytic agent tranexamic acid may be successful but should not yet be considered the standard approach. Individual lesions should not be cauterized. Pulse dye laser may be used to destroy cutaneous and accessible mucosal lesions.

*See Vol. 2, Section F, Experience 40.

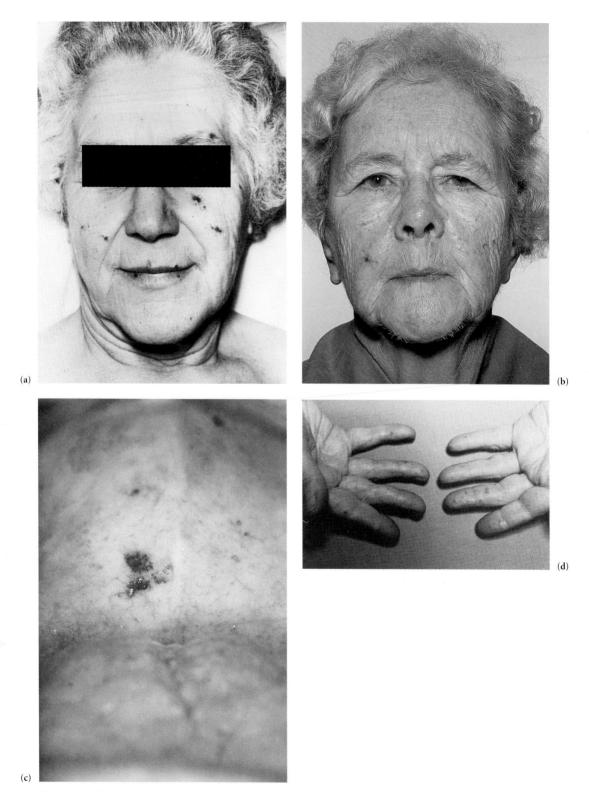

(a)

(b)

(c)

(d)

**Figure I5.2** (a,b) Facial telangiectasia. (c) Palatal telangiectasia. (d) Multiple, 1–2 mm, discrete, red macular and papular telangiectasia on the fingers.

# Case 4 | Psoriasis

**Frequency in survey for 3rd edition:** main focus of a short case in 11% of attempts at PACES Station 5, Skin. Additional feature in a further 1%.

## Record

There are patches of psoriasis over the *bony prominences*, particularly the *elbows* and *knees*, and also on the *trunk* and *scalp* and in the *intragluteal cleft* (the latter two areas are frequently overlooked). The plaques are circular with well-defined edges and they are *red* with a *silvery scaly* surface.

The patient has psoriasis.

I note also that there is an *asymmetrical arthropathy* involving mainly the *terminal interphalangeal joints*. There is *pitting* of the fingernails and *onycholysis*. Some of the nail plates (say which) are thickened and there is a thick scale (*hyperkeratosis*) under them.

The patient also has psoriatic arthropathy.*

## Treatment

Treatments for the skin lesions include sunlight, phototherapy (narrowband UVB, psoralen and UVA light [PUVA]), coal tar, dithranol, local steroids, calcipotriol (and other vitamin D analogues). Systemic treatment with acitretin (a retinoid), antimetabolites (methotrexate, azathioprine, hydroxyurea), cyclosporin or biological therapies (infliximab, etanercept, adalimimab, ustekinumab), because of their side-effects, should be reserved for severe widespread disease unresponsive to topical measures. Analgesic anti-inflammatory agents are used for the pain of the arthropathy. Sulphasalazine, methotrexate and the biological therapies have become established as effective agents for the treatment of psoriatic arthropathy. Leflunomide, cyclophosphamide and mycophenolate are used as second- or third-line agents. Chloroquine is contraindicated as it may exacerbate the skin lesions (it can even cause exfoliative dermatitis). Intra-articular steroids are useful for a single inflamed troublesome joint, but risk exacerbating the skin lesions.

## Incidence

One to 5% of Caucasians in north-western Europe and USA. Uncommon among Japanese, North American Indians and Afro-Americans.

See also Station 5, Locomotor, Case 2.

---

*There is no evidence of a link between the activity of the skin lesions and the arthropathy.

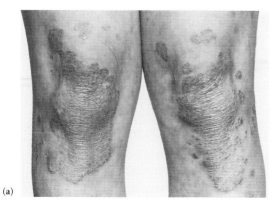 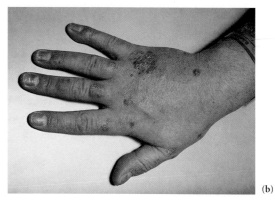

(a) (b)

**Figure I5.3** (a) Psoriasis: typical plaques. (b) Psoriasis with nail pitting.

# Case 5 | Rash of uncertain cause

**Frequency in survey for 3rd edition:** main focus of a short case in 6% of attempts at PACES Station 5, Skin.

It was already clear from our initial PACES survey that being faced with a rash of uncertain cause was not an uncommon situation for a candidate in the old PACES, Station 5. It was also clear that it is not necessarily a reason to fail. To prepare for this, we suggest you study the Examination *routines* 'Examine this patient's rash' (see Section G, Examination *routine* 17) and 'Examine this patient's skin' (see Section G, Examination *routine* 16). Describe the rash using appropriate terms, commenting on distribution and symmetry, and discuss appropriate differential diagnoses, giving points in favour or against each. In other words, demonstrate your knowledge of the dermatological conditions that you do know about even if you are uncertain about the case before you. Mention how you might proceed to investigate, in particular by taking skin scrapings, swabs or a diagnostic biopsy.

Consider discussing how you might treat the patient whilst awaiting confirmation of the diagnosis, including stopping unnecessary drugs, rehydration, treating bacterial superinfection and using soap substitutes and emollients for comfort.

The following are three anecdotes from our PACES survey.

## Anecdote 1: Look at this patient

This man's skin was really red. There were no plaques or scales but I said he had psoriasis. The examiners asked me how I would manage this man if it was a Friday night at 5.30 p.m. and I was in the accident and emergency department and I could not get in touch with a dermatologist. I said that I would rehydrate, that I would treat any infection aggressively and that I would use simple aqueous creams. I passed the exam but on reflection, I thought that I should have said that he had a drug rash and as I was walking away, the examiners said, 'Did you really think it was psoriasis?' and I said, 'No!'. They smiled!

## Anecdote 2: Take a look at this lady's rash

She had a widespread, macular, erythematous rash and the examiners told me that the dermatologists did not know the diagnosis! I described the rash and explained that I would take a full history, including a drug history, and if in doubt I would do some blood tests and biopsy the lesion. They did not ask me any questions.

## Anecdote 3: This patient has a rash which is congenital – what is the cause?

The patient had dysmorphic features and an old tracheostomy scar. There were also bilateral small scars over the carotids/jugular veins. There was a papular rash over the neck and shoulders. I had no idea what it was. I felt the examiners were after a specific syndrome.* I expected to fail this station but got a clear pass from both examiners for Station 5.

---

*?Pseudoxanthoma elasticum or Ehlers–Danlos syndrome.

# Case 6 | **Dermatomyositis**

**Frequency in survey for 3rd edition:** main focus of a short case in 3% of attempts at PACES Station 5, Skin.

## *Record*

There is a *heliotrope* * *rash* over the *eyelids* and *periorbital* areas and the *backs* of the *hands,* especially around the *knuckles* (Gottron's papules) and *fingernails* (prominent nailfold telangiectasia is characteristic). It is (may be) also present over the extensor surfaces of the elbows and knees. There is subcutaneous oedema (mainly around the eyes and due to a transient increase in capillary permeability). There is (may be) *proximal muscle weakness* and tenderness. The diagnosis is dermatomyositis.

---

Male to female ratio is 2:1.

## Other features of dermatomyositis

Features and associations similar to polymyositis (see Vol. 1, Station 3, CNS, Case 45)

Association with malignancy (the current recommendation is that patients over 40 years of age with dermatomyositis should be investigated for an associated malignancy particularly in the breasts, ovary, lungs and GI tract; see Footnote, Vol. 1, Station 3, CNS, Case 45)

Overlap with rheumatic fever, rheumatoid arthritis, scleroderma, lupus erythematosus and other connective tissue diseases may occur (steroid responsiveness more likely)

Signs of other connective tissue diseases more common than in pure polymyositis

Dysphagia due to upper oesophageal involvement

Raynaud's and arthralgia are frequent

Subcutaneous and intramuscular calcifications may occur

Helpful investigations include serum muscle enzymes (CPK and aldolase), urinary creatine, electromyography (EMG) (fibrillation, polyphasic action potentials and in some patients high-frequency bizarre repetitive discharges) and muscle biopsy. The erythrocyte sedimentation rate (ESR) is often normal despite active disease

The mainstay of treatment is steroids (initially in high doses). High-dose intravenous immunoglobulin may be effective in refractory cases. Immunosuppressive agents, such as azathioprine, may be used to control the condition with a reduced steroid dose

May present with pseudohaematuria due to myoglobulinaemia

There is a juvenile form occurring in the first decade. Myopathy is severe, healing occurs with contractures and calcification in the skin and muscles, but Raynaud's is rare. There is no association with malignancy.

---

*From the shrub *Heliotropium* which has fragrant purple flowers. The characteristic rash is a purple/violet/lilac colour. The skin changes may be subtle and easily overlooked. The classic heliotrope rash is diagnostic of the condition and though it is most commonly seen in the childhood form, it also occurs in the adult form. Other skin manifestations include *local and diffuse erythema, erythema nodosum-like lesions, eczema, exfoliating dermatitis, blisters and scaling* and *maculopapular eruptions.* The skin lesions may occasionally ulcerate.

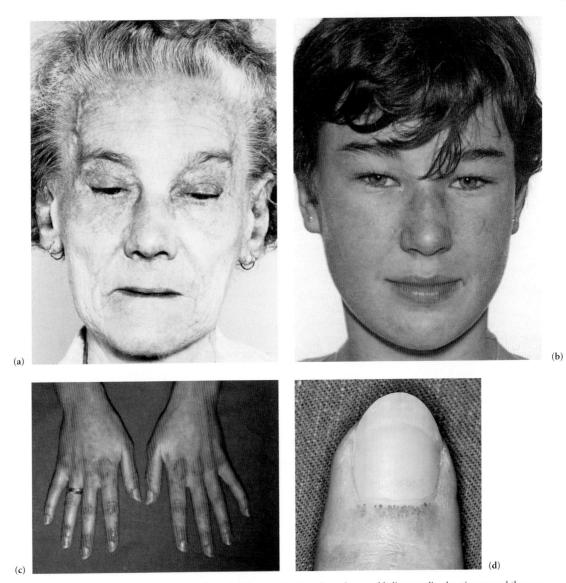

**Figure I5.4** (a) Note the characteristic distribution of the rash. (b) Note the oedema and heliotrope discoloration around the eyes. (c) Gottron's papules: flat-topped, violaceous papules over the knuckles and interphalangeal joints. (d) Nailfold telangiectasia is characteristic.

# Case 7 | **Xanthomata**

**Frequency in survey for 3rd edition:** main focus of a short case in 2% of attempts at PACES Station 5, Skin. Additional feature in a further 2%.

## *Record* 1

There are *tendon xanthomata** (?corneal arcus, xanthelasma) in the *extensor tendons* on the back of the *hand*, and on the *Achilles* and *patella* tendons (can occur in other tendons). They suggest *familial hypercholesterolaemia*. (In this condition raised and nodular *tuberous xanthomata** may also occur in the homozygous form, usually symmetrically, over the *extensor aspects of the joints* and on the *buttocks*. They may be several millimetres to several centimetres in size.)

## *Record* 2

There are (orange or) *yellow papules* (up to 5 mm in diameter) on the *extensor surfaces*, particularly over the *joints*, on the *limbs* and on the *buttocks* and *back*. They are (sometimes) surrounded by a rim of erythema (and may be tender and/or itchy). This is *eruptive xanthomatosis** (?lipaemia retinalis on fundoscopy. There is often abdominal pain and there is a risk of acute pancreatitis. It suggests severe *hypertriglyceridaemia* – plasma triglycerides of the order of 20–25 mmol/L – 'milky plasma' syndrome).†

---

Xanthomata can develop due to altered lipid metabolism or as a result of local cell dysfunction.

Familial hypercholesterolaemia is associated with premature development of vascular disease. Familial hypertriglyceridaemia does not appear to be an important risk factor for atherosclerosis but equivalent hypertriglyceridaemia due to familial combined hyperlipidaemia‡ is associated with an increased risk. Multivariate analysis suggests that the associated low levels of high-density lipoprotein (HDL) with hypertriglyceridaemia are related to a significantly increased risk of ischaemic heart disease.

### Familial hypercholesterolaemia

NICE 2008: consider this possibility if total cholesterol more than 7.5 mmol/L, especially with personal or family history of cardiovascular disease (CVD). In such a patient the Simon Broome criteria§ should be used. Prescribe a high-intensity statin to achieve more than 50% reduction in low-density lipoprotein (LDL).

### Order of priorities in treating hyperlipidaemia¶

1 Primary prevention:** NICE guidance 2008 (updated 2010) indicates that statin therapy is recommended as

---

*Tendon xanthomata take years to resolve and may persist indefinitely. Eruptive xanthomas resolve within weeks of starting systemic treatment for the hypertriglyceridaemia. Tuberous xanthomas take months to resolve.

†This level of hypertriglyceridaemia is usually due to overproduction of triglycerides occurring at the same time as hindrance of removal. For example, the coexistence of familial hypertriglyceridaemia (type IV), diabetes and/or alcohol consumption. Treatment of the secondary cause usually leads to a dramatic reduction in triglyceride levels and greatly reduces the risk of acute pancreatitis which is the main threat of this condition.

‡Affected family members show a combined rise in plasma cholesterol and triglycerides, or hypercholesterolaemia alone, or hypertriglyceridaemia alone.

§Simon Broome diagnostic criteria for individuals (probands). See www.nice.org.uk/nicemedia/live/12048/41707/41707.pdf or type Simon Broome, NICE into a search engine.

¶NB: The screening and treatment of families with hypercholesterolaemia.

**Guidelines for treatment are changed from time to time. Candidates are advised to check the current guidelines before going for the exam.

part of the management strategy for the primary prevention of CVD for adults who have a 20% or greater 10-year risk of developing CVD. This level of risk should be estimated using an appropriate risk calculator (including Framingham). Or by clinical assessment for people for whom an appropriate risk calculator is not available or appropriate (e.g. older people, people with diabetes or people in high-risk ethnic groups). Treatment for the primary prevention of CVD should be initiated with simvastatin 40 mg.

2 Secondary prevention:**People with acute coronary syndrome should be treated with a high-intensity statin (e.g. atorvastatin 80 mg).†† Treatment for secondary prevention of CVD should achieve total cholesterol targets of less than 4 mmol/L and LDL of less than 2 mmol/L.

3 Identify and treat any causes of secondary hyperlipidaemia such as:
  (a) diabetes mellitus (?Medic-Alert band, fundi)
  (b) alcoholism (may be the occult underlying cause of treatment failure)
  (c) nephrotic syndrome (?generalized oedema)
  (d) myxoedema (?facies, pulse, ankle jerks)
  (e) cholestasis (?icterus)
  (f) myelomatosis
  (g) oral contraceptives.

4 Dietary treatment to lose weight in obesity (in particular low saturated fat).

## Treatment

Every effort should be made to reduce total cholesterol below 4.0 mmol/L and the fasting triglyceride level to 2.0 mmol/L. To begin with, all patients should be started on a low-fat diet, which may reduce total cholesterol and triglyceride by around 20% in patients with polygenic hyperlipidaemia and hypertriglyceridaemia.

Patients with familial hypercholesterolaemia are less responsive to diet alone. Alcohol consumption should be reduced. Some patients with hypertriglyceridaemia are particularly sensitive to alcohol, and their livers produce excess very low-density lipoprotein (VLDL) particles, even from a modest alcohol intake. Smoking must be stopped.

Patients with combined hyperlipidaemia and hypertriglyceridaemia (without hypercholesterolaemia) respond well to diet, exercise and fibrates. Patients with hypercholesterolaemia require a diet and a lipid-lowering agent. Treatment with statins (HMG co-A reductase inhibitors) lowers serum cholesterol substantially and has been shown to reduce mortality and morbidity from cardiovascular and CVD in many controlled trials.

## Types of hyperlipidaemia simplified
### Comparatively common

Type IIa (e.g. familial hypercholesterolaemia) – raised cholesterol only

Type IIb (e.g. familial combined hypercholesterolaemia) – raised cholesterol and triglycerides

Type IV (e.g. familial hypertriglyceridaemia) – raised triglycerides

### Rare

Type I – raised chylomicrons, very high triglycerides, eruptive xanthomata

Type III – an inherited defect in apolipoprotein E synthesis (mostly intermediate-density remnants) and triglycerides to an equal extent. It is characteristically associated with palmar and tuberous xanthomata and is very responsive to fibrates

Type V – raised chylomicrons and triglycerides

††Recently (2011) an increased risk of diabetes has been associated with high-dose statin use. One possible mechanism for this could be through the statin side-effect of myopathic pain which becomes more likely as the dose is increased. Such pain in some individuals may limit exercise and hence lead to increased weight and diabetes. Myopathic side-effects should always be actively sought and, if found, the possibility of reducing the statin dose considered.

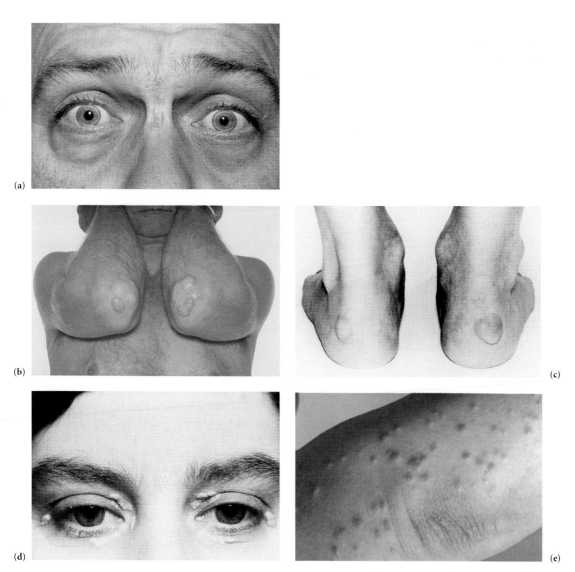

(a)

(b)

(c)

(d)

(e)

**Figure I5.5** (a) Arcus senilis. (b,c) Tendon xanthomata on the elbows and Achilles of the same patient. (d) Xanthelasma. (e) Eruptive xanthomata.

# Case 8 | Vitiligo

**Frequency in survey for 3rd edition:** main focus of a short case in 2% of attempts at PACES Station 5, Skin.

## *Record*

There are areas of *depigmentation* around the eyes and mouth, on the knees and on the dorsum of the feet (the hands, axillae, groins and genitalia are the other commonly affected areas).

The patient has vitiligo.

---

Vitiligo affects up to 2% of the population. The incidence is equal in both sexes, although females present in dermatology clinics for cosmetic reasons. There is a family history in about one-third of the patients.

Sites subject to friction and trauma are often affected and Koebner's phenomenon (a lesion appearing at the site of skin damage) is common. Vitiligo is usually symmetrical but occasionally the depigmentation can be unilateral and follow the pattern of a dermatome. It is a multifactorial polygenic disorder and individuals are usually otherwise healthy. Halo naevi (hypopigmented rings surrounding dark naevi), leucotrichia, premature greying of the hair and alopecia areata as well as vitiligo may all be associated with any of the **organ-specific autoimmune diseases:**

Myxoedema (?pulse, ankle jerks, facies; see Station 5, Endocrine, Case 5)

Hashimoto's disease (?goitre; see Station 5, Endocrine, Case 5)

Graves' disease (?exophthalmos, fidgety, goitre, tachycardia, etc; see Station 5, Endocrine, Case 3)

Pernicious anaemia (?pallor, spleen, subacute combined degeneration of the cord [SACD]; see Station 5, Other, Case 6)

Atrophic gastritis associated with iron deficiency anaemia

Addison's disease (?buccal, skin crease, scar and general pigmentation, hypotension, etc; see Station 5, Endocrine, Case 7)

Idiopathic hypoparathyroidism (Chvostek's and Trousseau's signs, tetany, paraesthesiae and cramps, cataracts, ectodermal changes, moniliasis, mental retardation, psychiatric disturbances, bradykinetic rigid syndrome, epilepsy)

Premature ovarian failure

Diabetes mellitus (?fundi)

Renal tubular acidosis

Fibrosing alveolitis (?basal crepitations; see Vol. 1, Station 1, Respiratory, Case 1)

Chronic active hepatitis (?icterus, etc.)

Primary biliary cirrhosis (?xanthelasma, pigmentation, icterus, scratch marks, etc; see Vol. 1, Station 1, Abdominal, Case 17).

The organ-specific autoimmune diseases tend to occur in association with each other (*polyglandular autoimmune disease*) so that patients with one have an above normal chance of developing another. Some patients are prone to extensive mucocutaneous candidiasis* (candidiasis-endocrinopathy syndrome) and from this two distinct syndromes emerge. The clinical features of the syndromes are compared in Table I5.1.

Vitiligo, the cutaneous marker of organ-specific autoimmune disease, may occur in the non-organ-specific autoimmune disease systemic sclerosis.†

---

*The mucocutaneous candidiasis is associated with hypergammaglobulinaemia, IgA deficiency and anergy to *Candida albicans*.
†Rarely there is an overlap between the organ-specific and non-organ-specific autoimmune diseases. Sjögren's syndrome occupies an intermediate position, being associated with rheumatoid arthritis on one hand and autoimmune thyroiditis on the other.

Primary biliary cirrhosis is another condition which bridges the gap. It is associated with Sjögren's syndrome, Hashimoto's thyroiditis and renal tubular acidosis on one hand, and systemic sclerosis, CREST syndrome, rheumatoid arthritis, coeliac disease, dermatomyositis and mixed connective tissue disease on the other.

**Table I5.1** Comparison of the clinical features of the major syndromes characterized by multiple endocrine gland hypofunction

|  | Multiple endocrine deficiency syndrome (Schmidt's syndrome) | Polyglandular deficiency with mucocutaneous candidiasis |
|---|---|---|
| Hypoadrenalism | Common | Common |
| Hypothyroidism | Common | Rare |
| Diabetes mellitus (type I) | Common | Rare |
| Gonadal failure | Less common | Less common |
| Hypoparathyroidism | Rare | Common |
| Pituitary insufficiency | Rare | Rare |
| Autoantibodies to endocrine tissues and gastric parietal cells | Often present | Often present |
| Sex distribution | Strong female predominance | Female preponderance about 4:1 |
| Inheritance | Usually 'sporadic' but susceptibility related to HLA haplotype and may be inherited as autosomal dominant | Generally inherited as autosomal recessive; no apparent HLA association; siblings characteristically affected |
| Time of onset | Usually becomes evident during adult life | Typically becomes evident during childhood preceded by chronic mucocutaneous moniliasis |
| Other associated 'autoimmune' diseases and characteristics | Pernicious anaemia; hyperthyroidism; coeliac disease; alopecia; vitiligo; myasthenia gravis; isolated red cell aplasia | Pernicious anaemia; malabsorption; alopecia; vitiligo; IgA deficiency; hypergammaglobulinaemia; chronic active hepatitis; proliferative glomerulonephritis |

From *Cecil's Textbook of Medicine*, 19th edn, 1992, p. 1389.

## Treatment

Affected subjects asking for help should be referred to those dermatologists who have a special interest in this condition, who can select the appropriate options for treatment, and who can be persistent until desirable cosmetic improvement is achieved. No single therapy for vitiligo produces good responses for all patients, so treatment should be individualized with the risks and benefits taken into account.

Education, referral to patient support groups, cosmetic camouflage and sunscreens are very important. Potent topical steroids and topical tacrolimus ointment are useful in early localized disease. Systemic phototherapy (narrowband UVB 311 nm, 8-methoxypsoralen + UVB and PUVA) can be effective in up to 70% of patients with early extensive disease, but many treatments may be required and hands and feet may be resistant to treatment.

The excimer laser is effective but expensive and prolonged treatment may be required. Surgical treatment (grafts) can only be used in selected inactive cases.

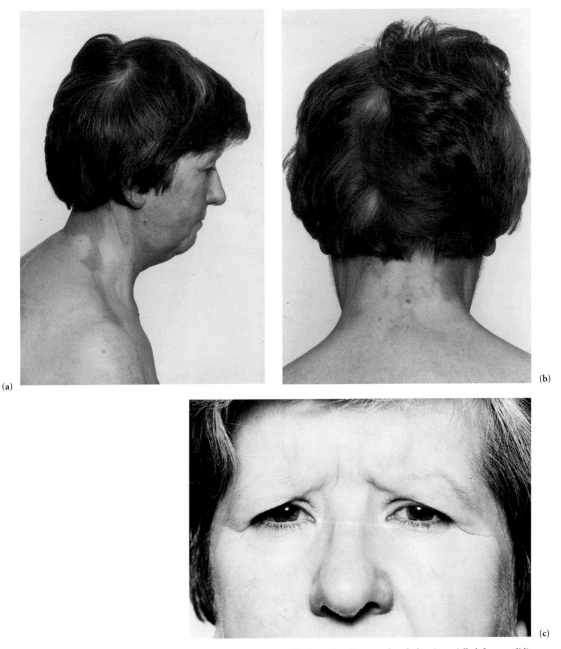

**(a)**

**(b)**

**(c)**

**Figure I5.6** (a–c) Note the areas of vitiligo and alopecia areata, including loss of eyebrows and eyelashes (especially left upper lid), in this patient with diabetes mellitus.

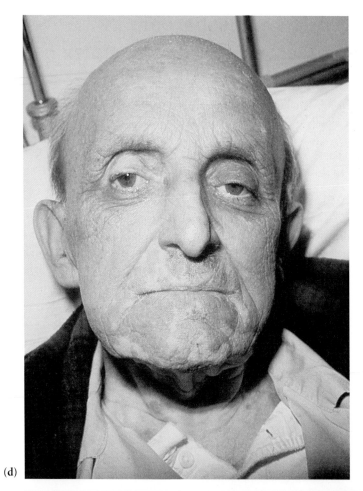

(d)

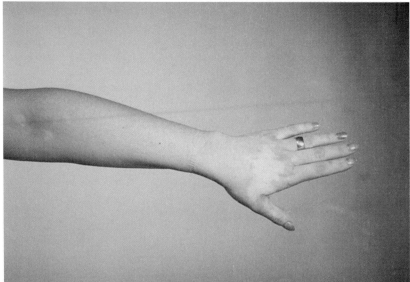

(e)

**Figure I5.6** (*Continued*) (d) Vitiligo. (e) Vitiligo of the hand.

# Case 9 | Adenoma sebaceum in tuberous sclerosis complex

**Frequency in survey for 3rd edition:** main focus of a short case in 2% of attempts at PACES Station 5, Skin.

**Survey note:** candidates were asked to look at the face; the clue was usually given that the patient had epilepsy or 'funny turns'.

## Record

There is a *papular, salmon-coloured* eruption on the centre of the face (over the *butterfly* area), especially in the *nasolabial* folds. These angiomatous, glistening papules are called adenoma sebaceum (check for *periungual fibromata* and *shagreen patches*).

There may be a history of *epilepsy* and *mental deficiency** which together with *adenoma sebaceum* make up the triad associated with tuberous sclerosis (epiloia).

---

Tuberous sclerosis is a phakomatosis (see also Footnote, Station 5, Skin, Case 2). Autosomal dominant but 80% are sporadic due to new mutations.† The gene is on chromosomes 16p13 and 9q34.

### Hamartomata

Tuberous sclerosis is characterized by the development of hamartomata of the skin, central nervous system, kidneys, retina, heart, lungs and bone. Hamartomata consist of excessive overgrowth of mature, normal cells and tissues in an organ.

### Skin lesions

A number of hamartomatous lesions of the skin are seen. The term *adenoma sebaceum* is a misnomer; the lesions are actually angiofibromata. They usually appear around the age of 4 and become more prominent after puberty. The leathery *shagreen patches* (flesh-coloured lumpy plaques which resemble studded leather) over the lower back and ungual *fibromata* (firm pink periungual papules which appear at puberty) growing out from the nailbeds of the fingers and toes are seen in perhaps 40% of cases. *Hypopigmented macules* (in an oval or *mountain ash leaf* configuration, rounded at one end and tapered at the other), especially on the trunk or buttocks, are present from birth in *nearly all patients*; they are easier to see in fair-skinned patients with a Wood's lamp. Intraoral fibromata and hyperplastic gums are also seen and there may be increased pigmentation as manifest in bronzing of the skin and *café-au-lait* macules.

### Other organs

Cerebral hemispheres contain multiple hamartomata or tubers (calcified lesions are well seen on computed tomography [CT] scans but uncalcified ones may show up better on magnetic resonance imaging [MRI]). Epilepsy occurs in 80% of cases; it usually starts below the age of 5 and is often difficult to control. The diagnosis may be missed and subtle skin lesions should be sought even in adults presenting with epilepsy

Renal hamartomata (angiomyolipomata) in two-thirds of patients (may cause pain or bleeding). There may be polycystic kidneys

---

*May be mild or severe. One-third have normal, or even superior, intelligence.

†Before concluding that an affected child of apparently normal parents is the result of a new mutation, the parents should be examined with a Wood's lamp for the presence of *ash leaf macules*, which may be the only manifestation of the disease.

They should also be examined by an ophthalmologist for *retinal phakomata* and pigmentary changes, which are present in 50% of patients.

Retinal hamartomata‡ (phakomata), which appear yellow, in 50% (also occur in neurofibromatosis; see Station 5, Skin, Case 2)

Cardiac hamartomata (rhabdomyomata) in 30% (may cause dysrhythmias or congestive cardiac failure)

Cystic lung disease due to hamartomatous lesions composed of smooth muscle cells in 1% (mostly women over 20 years; may cause pneumothorax, breathlessness, cyanosis and cor pulmonale)

## Treatment

For cosmetic reasons, adenoma sebaceum may be destroyed by electrodesiccation or laser surgery but they tend to recur.

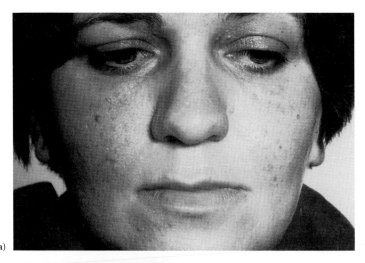

(a)

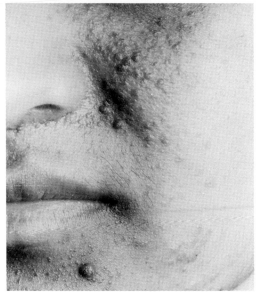

(b)

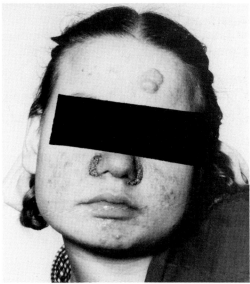

(c)

**Figure I5.7** (a) Angiofibroma papules in butterfly distribution. (b) Skin-coloured papules in the nasolabial fold. (c) Clusters of angiofibromata in the nasolabial folds.

‡See also Station 5, Eyes, Case 18; optic disc drusen may also occur.

# Case 10 | **Pseudoxanthoma elasticum**

**Frequency in survey for 3rd edition:** main focus of a short case in 2% of attempts at PACES Station 5, Skin.

## Record

There is *loose skin* mainly over the *neck, axillae, antecubital fossae* and *groins*, in which there are seen yellow, chamois-coloured papules, coalescing to form larger *yellow pseudoxanthomatous plaques* (there may be *redundant folds of lax skin*). There is a *'plucked chicken skin'* appearance because of the clear margins around the hair follicles.

This patient has pseudoxanthoma elasticum.

---

It is inherited in an autosomal recessive pattern and is due to mutations in the *ABCC6* gene on chromosome 16p13.1. It is characterized by progressive calcification and fragmentation of elastic fibres in the skin, retina and cardiovascular system. Angina, myocardial infarction, claudication, decreased visual acuity in a young person, haematemesis and melaena are some of the presenting features. Asymptomatic skin lesions usually appear by the age of 30 years but may go undetected until old age. Steroids should be avoided and the diagnosis is confirmed by skin biopsy.

### Other features which may occur

Angioid streaks* in the retina (60% have eye changes)
Blue sclerae

Macular degeneration – diminished visual acuity, blindness
Loose-jointedness
Hypertension due to renovascular disease (50%)
Gastrointestinal (10%), genitourinary or respiratory haemorrhage
Coronary artery disease
Peripheral vascular disease (weak or absent pulses, claudication, often vascular calcification)
Mitral incompetence
Hypothyroidism (?due to involvement of thyroid vasculature)
Miscarriages

---

*The triad of skin lesions, angioid streaks of the retinae and vascular abnormalities is called the *Grönblad–Strandberg syndrome*. Other causes of angioid streaks (poorly defined, greyish streaks radiating across the fundus, which represent the rupture of Bruch's membrane secondary to an elastic fibre defect) include Ehlers–Danlos syndrome, Paget's disease of the bone, sickle cell anaemia and hyperphosphataemia.

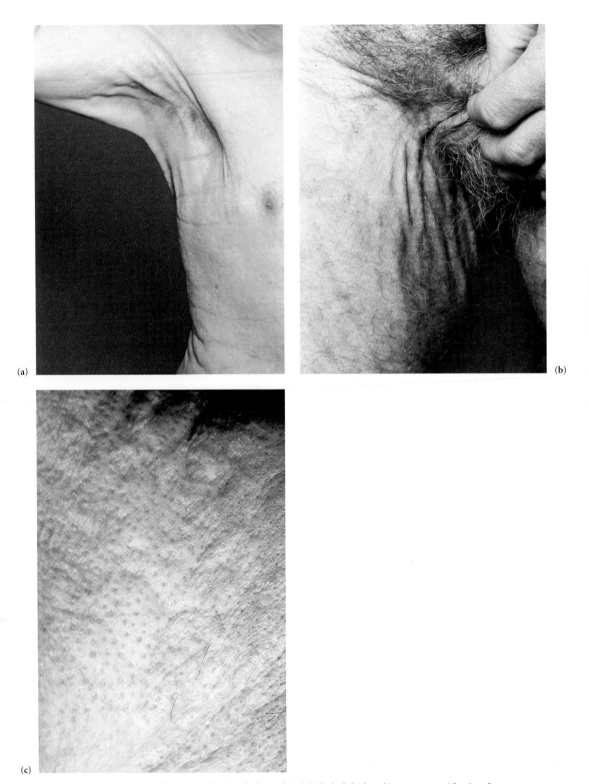

**Figure I5.8** Pseudoxanthoma elasticum. (a,b) Note the loose skin. (c) Plucked chicken skin appearance. (*Continued*)

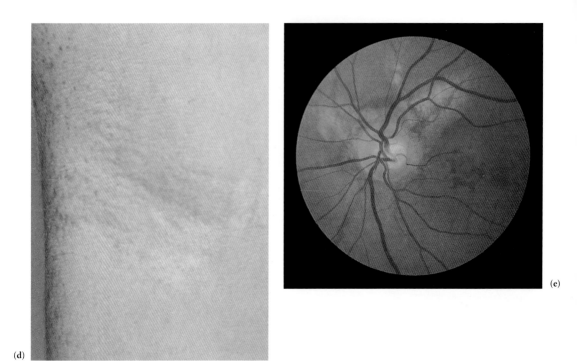

(d)

(e)

**Figure I5.8** (*Continued*) (d) Antecubital fossa. (e) Angioid streaks in the retina. There is a dark ring with irregular margins around the optic disc. Note a streak radiating outwards from it at 1 o'clock and another at 10 o'clock.

# Case 11 | Lichen planus

**Frequency in survey for 3rd edition**: main focus of a short case in 2% of attempts at PACES Station 5, Skin.

## *Record*

This young (or middle-aged) patient has *flat-topped, polygonal, shiny*, reflecting light, violaceous *papules* on the wrists (and other flexor surfaces usually, though it may affect any part of the skin). Fine white streaks (*Wickham's striae*) are seen on the surface of the lesions (better seen with a hand lens). The *Koebner phenomenon* is present (i.e. lesions appear in a linear pattern along a scratch mark or on a surgical scar). There are also asymptomatic lesions in the *buccal mucosa* (in 50% of cases – white, lacy pattern).

This patient has lichen planus (itching is usual and may be quite severe, though there are seldom any excoriations because the patients tend to rub rather than scratch).

---

Male to female ratio is 1:1.

Lichen planus is a cell-mediated immune response and there is an association with hepatitis C (16%). Lichen planus usually resolves in 6–24 months but it may recur. Steroids (systemic, local or intralesional) may be required if pruritus is severe and in the hypertrophic variety (see below). Certain drugs such as thiazides, angiotensin-converting enzyme (ACE) inhibitors, leflunomide, β-blockers, phenothiazines, gold, quinidine and antimalarials can cause lichen planus-like, generalized eruptions. Some patients with graft-versus-host disease develop a skin reaction that closely resembles lichen planus. There may be aetiological clues in this.

## Other sites for lichen planus

Scalp (scaly pruritic papules on the scalp leading to atrophy of the skin with patchy, permanent alopecia)

Nails (dystrophy of the nail plate with longitudinal streaking of the nail; if it is severe there may be complete loss of the nail plate)*

Palms and soles (yellowish rather than violaceous)

Genitals (annular papules in men, vulval involvement ranges from papules to erosive disease)

## Other forms

Hypertrophic lichen planus (plaque-like lesions with a thick, warty surface on the front of the legs). This form is more common in Afro-Caribbean races

Erosive lichen planus (oral and genital and may be chronic >5 years)

Bullous lichen planus (lower limbs and mouth)

## Treatment

Intralesional triamcinolone is helpful for symptomatic cutaneous or oral mucosal lesions. Steroid mouthwashes may be used in patients with erosive oral lesions. In resistant, generalized, erosive oral and hypertrophic varieties, systemic therapy with corticosteroids, cyclosporin, retinoids and PUVA photochemotherapy have all been tried with some success.

---

*A characteristic change of lichen planus of the nail is *pterygium* in which the cuticle invades the nailbed.

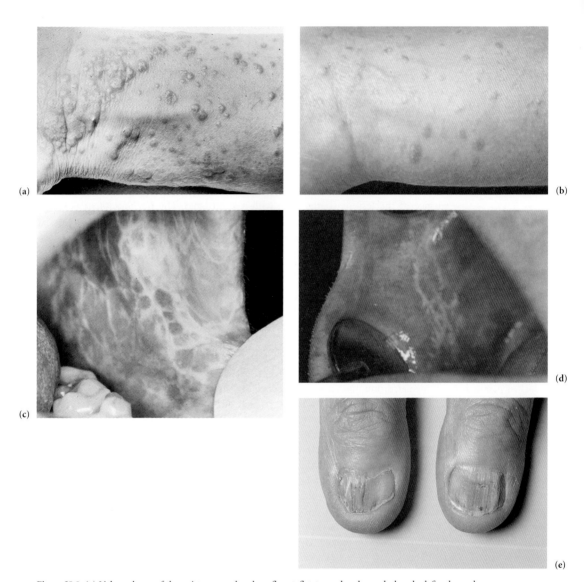

**Figure I5.9** (a) Lichen planus of the wrist: grouped and confluent, flat-topped, polygonal, sharply defined papules. (b) Flat-topped violaceous, polygonal papules on the wrist. Note Wickham's striae. (c,d) The buccal mucosa is exposed to show the characteristic lacy, white pattern. (e) Pterygium (left) and longitudinal ridging of the nails – lichen planus.

# Case 12 | **Yellow nail syndrome**

**Frequency in survey for 3rd edition:** main focus of a short case in 2% of attempts at PACES Station 5, Skin.

### *Record*

The *nails* are thick, *excessively curved* from side to side and slow growing, leaving *bulbous fingertips* uncovered and pale yellow (or greenish yellow). The *cuticles* are *lost*, the lunulae are absent and there is onycholysis (though the degree is variable).

This suggests the yellow nail syndrome (check for *lymphoedema* of the extremities which may also be present).

---

Yellow nail syndrome consists of the triad of yellow slow-growing nails, lymphoedema and pleural effusion. It is usually associated with lymphatic hypoplasia, ankle oedema and a number of *pulmonary conditions* may occur, such as bronchiectasis, pleural effusion, recurrent pneumonias and sinusitis.

Other associations include D-penicillamine therapy, nephrotic syndrome, hypothyroidism and AIDS.

(a)
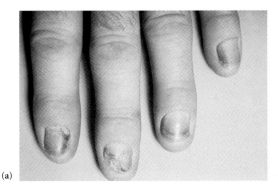

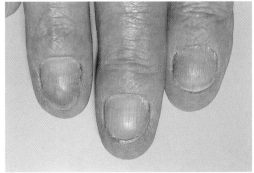
(b)

**Figure I5.10** Yellow nail syndrome. (a) Thickened nails and onycholysis. (b) No cuticles or lunulae. Bulbous uncovered fingertips are suggestive of stunted nail growth.

# Case 13 | **Gouty tophi**

**Frequency in survey for 3rd edition:** main focus of a short case in 2% of attempts at PACES Station 5, Skin.

Tophaceous gout is dealt with in Station 5, Locomotor, Case 5.

# Case 14 | Alopecia areata

**Frequency in survey for 3rd edition:** main focus of a short case in 2% of attempts at PACES Station 5, Skin.

## Record 1

There is a *discrete, well-circumscribed*, round (or oval) patch of *hair loss* over the back of the scalp (may involve the beard) of this patient. There is no evidence of inflammation or scarring. The empty hair follicles are easily seen and in the periphery there are tiny hairs, about 4 mm in length, with tapered ends, the so-called *exclamation mark hairs*.* The eyebrows and eyelashes are preserved.

This is alopecia areata.†

## Record 2

There is a complete *loss* of *hair* over the *scalp* and body. Both the *eyebrows* and *eyelashes* are *absent*.

This is alopecia universalis (nail pitting occurs in up to 50% of patients).

---

Alopecia areata has an autoimmune cause. It is sometimes associated with Hashimoto's thyroiditis but it can also occur with other thyroid disorders, pernicious anaemia, diabetes mellitus and vitiligo (see Station 5, Skin, Case 8). Most patients with alopecia areata localized to the scalp have a good prognosis. Alopecia universalis (also known as alopecia totalis) has a poor prognosis. Topical or intralesional triamcinolone leads to localized tufts of regrowth and may be used to establish eyebrows but does not affect the overall outcome. Diphencyprone immunotherapy and PUVA therapy may be used in patients with extensive hair loss but the results are often unsatisfactory.

### Other types of alopecia

Diffuse hair loss may occur during an acute febrile illness or after childbirth (telogen effluvium = hair follicles going into the resting phase), and in association with an endocrine disorder (hypopituitarism, hypo- and hyperthyroidism, hypoparathyroidism), drugs (antimitotics, anticoagulants, vitamin A excess, oral contraceptives), severe chronic illness, iron deficiency or malnutrition. Androgenetic alopecia may become diffuse and occurs in men and women.

Sparse hair with poor development of nails and teeth, with or without defective sweat glands, is characteristic of a group of rare inherited disorders, the ectodermal dysplasias (Station 5, Skin, Case 43).

### Some causes of localized alopecia

#### Non-scarring alopecia

Alopecia areata
Androgenetic (male-pattern baldness)
Self-induced (hair-pulling habit and traction alopecia caused by rollers)
Scalp ringworm from human source

#### Scarring alopecia

Burns, radiodermatitis
Tinea capitis (from animal source)
Aplasia cutis
Cicatricial basal cell carcinoma
Carbuncle
Lichen planus
Lupus erythematosus
Necrobiosis lipoidica diabeticorum
Sarcoidosis

---

*These are broken-off hairs about 4 mm from the scalp, and are narrower and less pigmented proximally. They may be seen around the edges of enlarging areas of alopecia and are pathognomonic of alopecia areata.

†Hair loss of the entire scalp is called alopecia totalis. Alopecia affecting the entire epidermis is called alopecia universalis.

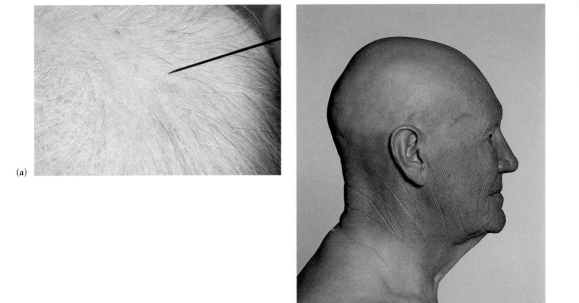

**Figure I5.11** (a) Alopecia areata. Note the empty hair follicles and short, tapering, exclamation mark hairs. (b) Alopecia universalis in a patient with diabetes mellitus.

# Case 15 | Eczema

**Frequency in survey for 3rd edition:** main focus of a short case in 2% of attempts at PACES Station 5, Skin.

## Record 1

There is a *papulovesicular* eruption on the *face* (may be on the trunk, hands or legs) with *excoriation, scratch marks* and *lichenification.** The *skin* is *dry*.

This is chronic atopic eczema.

## Record 2

There is an area of *lichenification** on the *arm* (usually in the flexural areas) with *dryness, scratch marks* and some *vesicular lesions*.

This is chronic atopic eczema.

## Record 3

There is a bilateral, *hyperpigmented, erythematous* eruption over the *face* with some *vesicular* and *crusted papules* and *fine scales*. There is *lichenification** with *prominent skin markings* secondary to repeated scratching and rubbing.

This is contact dermatitis probably secondary to the use of black hair dye (or other cosmetic agent).

---

## Some common forms of eczema (*syn.* dermatitis)

### Atopic dermatitis

Atopic dermatitis is a chronic condition often associated with a personal or family history of asthma, allergic rhinitis and/or atopic eczema. It often begins around the age of 6 months but the onset may be delayed to childhood or adult life. About 40% of affected babies will 'outgrow' their eczema but the others will manifest some features of atopic dermatitis as adults. In most cases, the condition starts as an acute or subacute, red, vesicular eruption affecting the face, upper chest and the antecubital and popliteal fossae (flexural dermatitis). Pruritus is a major symptom and the consequent rubbing and scratching lead to lichenification, most typically in the flexural areas of the arms and legs. Patients with chronic atopic dermatitis have a characteristic facies with diffuse erythema, perioral pallor and loose folds below the lower eyelids. The palms tend to be dry with an increased number of skin lines.

The incidence of atopic dermatitis is increasing in industrialized countries and the cause is thought to be due to inherited defective barrier function that leads to increased transepidermal penetrance of environmental allergens. Atopic patients demonstrate excessive T-cell activation, specifically with increased helper T-cell cytokines such as interleukin (IL)-4 and IL-10, usually with elevated serum IgE levels. These patients have depressed cell-mediated immunity, and a defective epithelial barrier function which probably accounts for their increased susceptibility to cutaneous infections by herpesvirus, vaccinia and molluscum contagiosum virus, and human papillomavirus. Abnormal neutrophil and monocyte chemotaxis may explain frequent staphylococcal infections, which often flare or complicate atopic dermatitis.

The treatment consists of education, emollients, topical calcineurin inhibitors, topical steroids and systemic antihistamines. Refractory cases may require immune modulators such as azathioprine, methotrexate, cyclosporin or tacrolimus.

*Lichenification is dry, leathery thickening of the skin with exaggerated skin markings. It is testimony to patients' bitter complaint of itching and is a characteristic sign of rubbing rather than scratching (which leads to excoriations).

## Contact dermatitis

Contact dermatitis may be due to a direct toxic or irritant effect of a substance (e.g. acids, solvents, detergents, etc.) or through an allergic, delayed (type IV) type of hypersensitivity. The original site of the eruption suggests a clue to the likely irritant or allergen, since both irritant and allergic contact eczemas are initially confined to sites of contact. In chronic cases, the eczema and the maculopapular or papulovesicular rash spread to other parts of the skin, as the skin reacts as an organ.

The most common allergens causing allergic contact dermatitis are pentadecylcatechol in poison oak, ivy, cashews and mangoes, paraphenylenediamine (a substance in hair dyes that cross-reacts with benzocaine and hydrochlorthiazide), nickel, mercaptobenzothiazole and thiuram (components in rubber), and ethylenediamine (a preservative found in many medications and also found in industrial dyes and insecticides).

## Photodermatitis

Areas of skin exposed to ultraviolet light become red and painful. Repeated exposure leads to pigmentation and desquamation. Photodermatitis has an immunological basis. A specific wavelength of ultraviolet light is absorbed by a topical substance or systemic drug, which is deposited in the skin from the circulation (amiodarone, chlorpropamide, nalidixic acid, oral contraceptives, phenothiazines, sulphonamides, tetracyclines and thiazides). The offending rays cause chemical conversion of the substance or drug to a hapten, that binds cutaneous proteins to become a complete antigen, capable of inducing a type IV delayed hypersensitivity reaction similar to that of allergic contact dermatitis.

## Stasis dermatitis

A chronic, patchy, ill-defined eczematous eruption occurs on the lower legs secondary to peripheral venous insufficiency, with a consequent increased hydrostatic pressure and extravasation of red blood cells and serum. These blood substances set up an inflammatory, brawny, oedematous, red, scaling or weeping reaction on the distal one-third of the lower legs, which in due course becomes hyperpigmented due to haemosiderin deposition.

## Nummular dermatitis (discoid eczema)

Nummular dermatitis often affects the legs and arms of middle-aged males with groups of vesicles on an erythematous base. These lesions may coalesce into rounded or coin-shaped (Latin *nummularis* – like a coin) plaques, 4–6 cm in diameter, and have an erythematous base with an indistinct border.

## Seborrhoeic dermatitis

Seborrhoeic dermatitis often affects those with a tendency to dandruff. It manifests as a red, exudative eruption with yellow, greasy scales localized to hairy regions of the skin, or areas with a high population of sebaceous glands (i.e. middle of the face, nasolabial folds, eyebrows, retroauricular folds, presternal and interscapular areas). Some lesions develop follicular papules or pustules (seborrhoeic folliculitis) and some manifest as intertriginous lesions of the armpits, groins and umbilicus or under spectacles or hearing aids.

It is sometimes difficult to distinguish seborrhoeic dermatitis from psoriasis when the latter is confined to the scalp, ears and face. The cause of seborrhoeic dermatitis is unknown but it is sometimes associated with emotional stress and neurological disease. Patients with Parkinson's disease or stroke may have a dramatic flare up of their seborrhoeic dermatitis. Extensive, intractable seborrhoeic dermatitis may also signal infection with HIV regardless of CD4 counts or viral load and may be one of the first cutaneous clues to the diagnosis.

Antiseborrhoeic shampoos containing tar, sulphur, salicylic acid, selenium sulphide, pyrithione zinc or ketoconazole provide the most effective treatment. Continual use of shampoo and topical steroids is sometimes required for control. This should be stressed to the patient.

## Lichen simplex chronicus

This occurs as a single, lichenified plaque on the nape of the neck in women, legs in men, and on genital areas in both sexes.

## Erythroderma/exfoliative dermatitis

The whole skin may become red and scaly (exfoliative dermatitis) or red with little or no scaling (erythroderma) in patients with a previous skin disease (psoriasis, pityriasis, pemphigus, contact dermatitis, Reiter's syndrome and cutaneous T-cell lymphoma). Most patients have lymphadenopathy with improper temperature regulation and fluid and electrolyte disturbance.

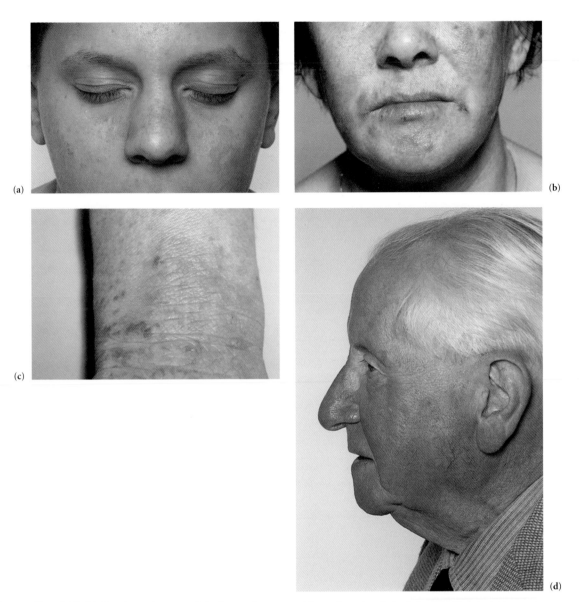

**Figure I5.12** (a) Chronic atopic eczema of the face: erythematous patches and papulovesicular lesions. (b) Chronic atopic eczema. Note perioral pallor, erythematous patches and papulovesicular lesions. (c) Chronic atopic eczema of the arm with marked lichenification. (d) Photodermatitis (amiodarone face).

# Case 16 | **Pretibial myxoedema**

**Frequency in survey for 3rd edition:** main focus of a short case in 2% of attempts at PACES Station 5, Skin.

Pretibial myxoedema is dealt with in Station 5, Endocrine, Case 9.

# Case 17 | Clubbing

**Frequency in survey for 3rd edition:** main focus of a short case in 2% of attempts at PACES Station 5, Skin. Additional feature in many cases in all stations.

## Record

There is finger clubbing*(*thickening of the nailbed†* with *loss of the obtuse angle* between the nail and the dorsum of the finger – becomes >180°‡; *increased curvature* of the nailbed, both side-to-side and lengthwise; increased *sponginess or fluctuation* of the nailbed; and sometimes, when there is marked swelling of the nailbed, the fingers may have a *drumstick appearance*).

## Causes of clubbing

**1** Carcinoma of the bronchus (the most common cause – ?nicotine staining, obvious weight loss with temporal dimples, lymph nodes, chest signs, evidence of secondaries, etc; see Vol. 1, Station 1, Respiratory, Case 13)

**2** Fibrosing alveolitis (?basal crackles; see Vol. 1, Station 1, Respiratory, Case 1)

**3** Cyanotic congenital heart disease (?cyanosis, thoracotomy scars, Fallot's; see Vol. 1, Station 3, Cardiovascular, Case 23, Eisenmenger's; see Vol. 1, Station 3, Cardiovascular, Case 27)

**4** Bronchiectasis (?productive cough, crepitations, etc; see Vol. 1, Station 1, Respiratory, Case 4)

**5** Cirrhosis (?icterus, spider naevi, palmar erythema, Dupuytren's, xanthelasma – especially in primary biliary cirrhosis, hepatosplenomegaly, etc; see Vol. 1, Station 1, Abdominal, Case 4)

---

## Other causes

Subacute bacterial endocarditis (heart murmur, fever, splenomegaly, petechiae, splinter haemorrhages, Osler's nodes, Janeway's lesions, Roth's spots, etc.)
Empyema
Lung abscess
Crohn's disease

Ulcerative colitis
Asbestosis (especially with mesothelioma)
Thyroid acropachy (?exophthalmos, pretibial myxoedema, goitre, thyroid status, etc; see Station 5, Endocrine, Case 3)
Hereditary (rare; dominant)

---

*Indisputable clubbing is one of the important fundamental clinical signs which, when present, has clear implications. Less clear-cut changes in the fingernails are susceptible to assessment which (even if dogmatic) may be very subjective. Such fingernails are best described as showing 'debatable clubbing' (in that physicians will disagree as to whether there are significant changes or not). Genuine 'debatable clubbing' occurring in the examination may cause trouble if you recognize it as such but you are not sure what your examiners' opinion is. The safest course in a case of doubt is to use nailbed thickening as your guide and quote the nail angle rule in a way that cannot be argued with. For example, 'The appearance of the nails (e.g.

increased curvature) is initially suggestive of clubbing, but the obtuse angle between the nail and the dorsum of the finger is preserved, and therefore by definition (loss of the angle being the "official" first sign) the diagnosis of definite clubbing cannot be accepted in this case.'

†Before palpating, always inspect the fingers in profile for a slightly bulbous appearance due to thickening of the nailbed.

‡*Shamroth's sign:* if you put the fingernails of the same fingers of each of your hands together, against each other, you will see a gap at their base between them. This gap may be lost when the angle is lost in finger clubbing.

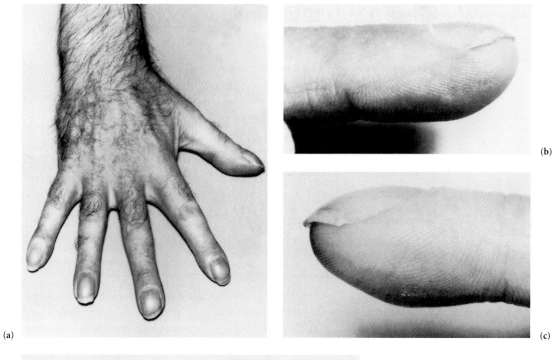

(a)

(b)

(c)

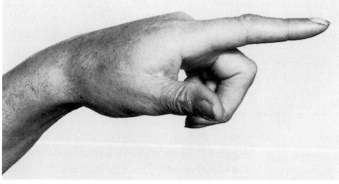

(d)

**Figure I5.13** (a) Clubbing (carcinoma of the bronchus). (b) Loss of the angle. (c) Thickening of the nailbed (early drumstick appearance – same patient as in (a)). (d) Clubbing and leuconychia (cirrhosis of the liver).

# Case 18 | Necrobiosis lipoidica diabeticorum

**Frequency in survey for 3rd edition:** main focus of a short case in 2% of attempts at PACES Station 5, Skin.

## *Record*

There are *sharply demarcated*, coalescing *oval plaques* on the *shins* (occasionally arms and elsewhere) of this lady (usually a female aged <40). The lesions have a *shiny atrophic surface,* with characteristic *waxy yellow centres* and *brownish-red edges.* There is (usually) telangiectasia over the surface.

The diagnosis is necrobiosis lipoidica diabeticorum.

---

It is uncommon, usually associated with diabetes, but can occur in the patient with prediabetes and on its own. It may have to be differentiated from granuloma annulare, from xanthomas when small, and from localized scleroderma or sarcoidosis when larger.

The lesions may ulcerate. Opinions vary as to whether good diabetic control can improve healing, but this should be tried. Gradual healing, with scarring, occurs over a period of years. Steroids (topical or local injection) can reduce inflammation in early plaques. Topical tacrolimus and PUVA have been used with success. Pulsed dye laser therapy can reduce redness. The histology varies, some containing large amounts of lipid, some not. There is necrosis of collagen, surrounded by pallisades of granulomatous epithelioid cells, and the aetiology is obscure.

**Granuloma annulare** (did not occur in original survey): pale or flesh-coloured, non-scaly (distinguishable from tinea/ringworm which has fine scales over the surface) papules coalescing in rings of usually 1–3 cm diameter, especially on the backs of the hands and fingers. Blanching by pressure reveals a characteristic beaded ring of white dermal patches. It is sometimes associated with diabetes, especially when the lesions are generalized and atypical. The histology is almost identical to necrobiosis lipoidica diabeticorum. The lesions regress spontaneously.

**Diabetic dermopathy** (did not occur in original survey): atrophic pigmented patches (start as dull red oval papules, sometimes with a small blister) occurring mostly on the shins of patients with diabetes. It has been suggested that they are precipitated by trauma in association with neuropathy. It tends to arise in long-standing diabetes or with multiple complications.

### Other skin lesions in patients with diabetes

Infective (bacterial – boils, etc.; fungal – candidiasis)

Foot/leg ulcers (ischaemic and neuropathic)

Vitiligo (?other associated organ-specific autoimmune disease; see Station 5, Skin, Case 8)

Fat atrophy (very rare with highly purified insulins)

Fat hypertrophy (recurrent injection of insulin into the same site)

Xanthomata (associated hyperlipidaemia – may disappear with control of diabetes as this causes improvement in the hyperlipidaemia; see Station 5, Skin, Case 7)

Sulphonylurea allergy (erythema multiforme, phototoxic and other eruptions)

Acanthosis nigricans (see Station 5, Skin, Case 48)

Peripheral anhidrosis (due to autonomic neuropathy)

Scleroderma diabeticorum – insidious onset of thickened skin on the back of a patient with long-standing diabetes. May cause restriction of movement. Rare

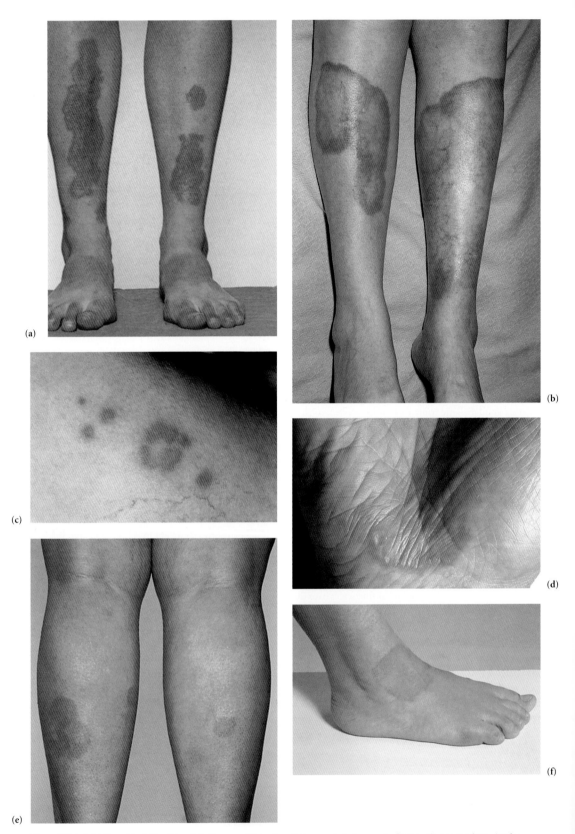

**Figure I5.14** (a,b) Necrobiosis lipoidica diabeticorum: bilateral, well-demarcated plaques. (c–f) Granuloma annulare: circular, well-demarcated plaques with central regression.

# Case 19 | Lupus pernio

**Frequency in survey for 3rd edition**: main focus of a short case in 2% of attempts at PACES Station 5, Skin.

**Survey note**: candidates often gave differential diagnoses such as systemic lupus erythematosus (SLE) and rosacea before being led to the correct diagnosis. We suggest that candidates try to see real-life cases of all three conditions affecting the face before the examination so that they can recognize the differences.

## Record

There is (in this female patient) a *diffuse*, livid, *purple-red infiltration* of the *nose* (and/or cheeks, ears, hands and feet).* The diagnosis is lupus pernio (usually associated with *chronic pulmonary sarcoidosis* which progresses to *fibrosis; chronic uveitis* and *bone cysts* in the phalanges are often present).

---

Lupus pernio usually affects the nose, cheeks, ears and lips but can occur on the dorsa of the hands, fingers, toes and forehead. When it affects the nose it has been associated with granulomatous involvement of the upper respiratory tract (50%) and lungs (75%).

## Other complications which may occur in chronic sarcoidosis

Facial palsy (may be bilateral; parotid enlargement not always present)

Peripheral neuropathy

Meningeal infiltrations and tumour-like deposits

Hypopituitarism and diabetes insipidus (granulomata extending from the meninges into the hypothalamus)

Hypercalcaemia and its nephropathy (probably hypersensitivity to vitamin D)

Mikulicz's syndrome (diffuse swelling of lachrymal and salivary glands with conditions such as sarcoidosis, lymphoma or leukaemia; see Station 5, Other, Case 1)

Cardiomyopathy (clinical evidence rare; there may be arrhythmias or heart block; cor pulmonale is more likely to be the cardiac consequence)

Chronic arthritis

Hypersplenism if sufficient splenomegaly

Infiltration of old scars by sarcoid tissue

Polymyositis (progressive muscle wasting)

Hepatic granulomata can be found in two-thirds of patients with sarcoidosis (symptoms rare). Sarcoidosis may affect most tissues.

*Other skin lesions*: multiple scattered maculopapular or papular lesions, 0.5–1 cm, yellowish brown or purple, that occur mainly on the face and extremities. Larger, brownish-purple plaques with annular, polycyclic or serpiginous margins and central atrophy also occur mainly on the extremities, buttocks and trunk. Sarcoid granulomata tend to infiltrate old scars, as translucent, purple or yellowish papules and nodules. On the scalp, sarcoidosis may cause scarring alopecia with brownish infiltration of the scarred tissue.

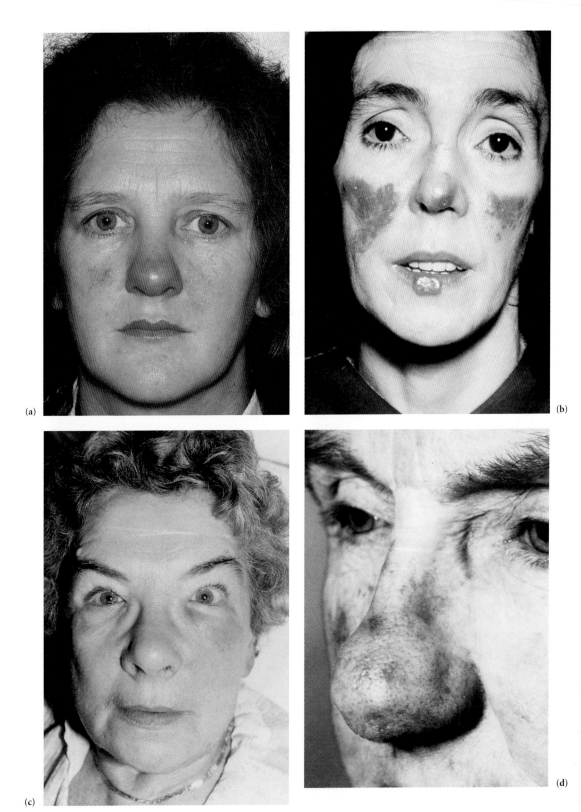

**Figure I5.15** (a,b) Lupus pernio on cheeks, nose and lip. (c) Lesions under the eyes, especially on the left. (d) A close-up of lupus pernio on the nose. The treated case may just show a faint purplish discolouration on the end of the nose or cheeks.

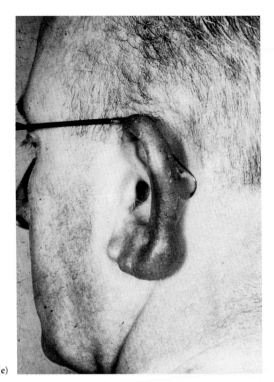

(e)

**Figure I5.15** (*Continued*) (e) Lupus pernio of the ear.

# Case 20 | Tinea

**Frequency in survey for 3rd edition:** main focus of a short case in 2% of attempts at PACES Station 5, Skin.

## Record 1

There is a well-defined, *annular, erythematous plaque* with *central clearing* on the *face* and *scalp* (can be on the trunk or limbs). The *erythema* and papular lesions with *fine scaling* are more *pronounced* at the *periphery of the plaque.*\* This is tinea capitis caused by a fungal (dermatophyte) infection of the keratin.

## Record 2

The *palms* of this patient are *erythematous* with *exaggerated creases* and *hyperkeratosis*. There is characteristic *powdery, dry scaling* in the creases. There may be similar changes on the soles (ask to examine the feet). The appearance is characteristic of chronic dermatophyte infection (tinea) of the hands.

## Record 3

There are widespread but *well-demarcated, erythematous plaques* in both *groins* spreading over the thighs (look over the abdomen for contiguous spread) with *scaling in the periphery*. There is some *clearing* in the *centre*. This is tinea of the groins (tinea cruris).

## Record 4

The skin between the fourth and fifth toes (most common site of infection) is *soggy* and *macerated* with *fine scaling*. This is tinea pedis, also known as athlete's foot.†

---

Dermatophyte infections (ringworm) are transmitted to humans by animals (zoophilic) or from person to person (anthropophilic fungi). Dermatophytes invade keratin only, live on dead tissue and cause inflammation by their metabolic products and/or by delayed hypersensitivity. The sites of predilection are the trunk (tinea corporis), scalp (tinea capitis), groins (tinea cruris), hands, feet, fingernails and toenails.

### Diagnosis

The appearances are sufficiently characteristic for a clinical diagnosis to be made, though the lesion may have to be distinguished from eczema, psoriasis, erythrasma, interdigital intertrigo and granuloma annulare. Microscopic examination of a skin scraping, nail clipping or a plucked hair can provide confirmatory evidence.

### Treatment

Local application of one of the imidazole preparations such as miconazole may be all that is necessary for tinea of the trunk, hands and feet. Systemic treatment with griseofulvin or terbinafine is often needed for tinea of the scalp and of the nails, and for widespread or chronic infection of the skin that has not responded to local measures.

---

\*The lesions expand slowly outwards and healing in the centre leaves a ring-like pattern, hence the name ringworm.

†This is the most common type of fungal infection in humans. The sharing of wash places and swimming pools predisposes to infection, which is often aggravated by occlusive footwear.

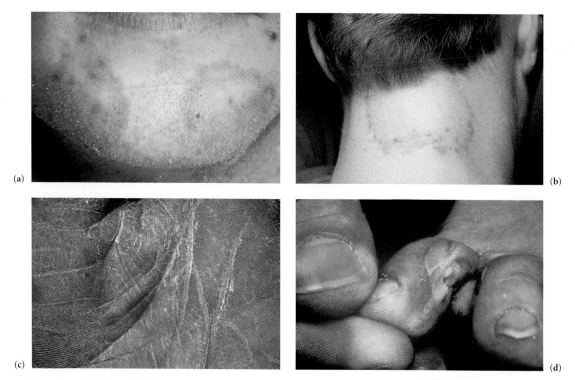

**Figure I5.16** (a) Tinea of the face: annular, erythematous border. (b) Tinea of the neck: note central clearing. (c) Tinea of the hand: prominent creases with powdery scales. (d) Tinea of the toes.

# Case 21 | Koilonychia

**Frequency in survey for 3rd edition:** main focus of a short case in 2% of attempts at PACES Station 5, Skin.

## *Record*
The nails are thin, concave and spoon-shaped with everted edges in this patient who also has pallor of the skin and conjunctivae (check for this). This is koilonychia associated with iron deficiency anaemia.

---

Koilonychia is common in infancy as a benign feature. In adults it has a familial pattern and is most commonly associated with iron deficiency anaemia and haemochromatosis. All fingers and toes may be affected, most prominently the thumb or great toe, which are sometimes the only nails that show the characteristic appearance.

### Causes of koilonychia
#### *Hereditary and congenital forms*
Ectodermal dysplasia
Adenoma sebaceum
Osteo-onychodysplasia (the nail–patella syndrome)

#### *Acquired forms*
Iron deficiency states (e.g. Plummer–Vinson syndrome, polycythaemia rubra vera)
Some haematological conditions (e.g. haemoglobinopathy, haemochromatosis)
Endocrine disorders (e.g. acromegaly, hypothyroidism)
Traumatic
Malnutrition
Dermatoses (e.g. lichen planus, psoriasis, acanthosis nigricans)
Connective tissue diseases

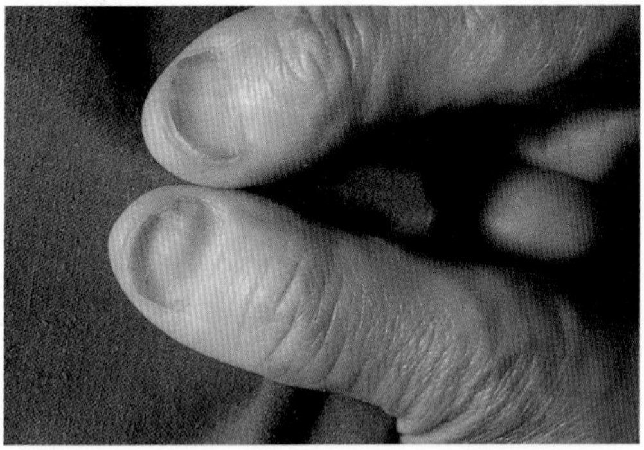

**Figure I5.17** Koilonychia.

# Case 22 | Raynaud's phenomenon

**Frequency in survey for 3rd edition:** main focus of a short case in 0.5% of attempts at PACES Station 5, Skin. Additional feature in a further 2% of Station 5, Locomotor.

## *Record*

The *fingers* are *cold* and *cyanosed*\* with (maybe) *atrophy* of the *finger pulps* (and in severe cases gangrene of the fingertips). The patient is likely to have Raynaud's phenomenon (now look for features of underlying connective tissue diseases, especially systemic sclerosis).

---

## Causes of Raynaud's phenomenon

**1** Idiopathic Raynaud's disease\* (common, especially in young women, thumbs often spared, starts in childhood, usually benign)

**2** Vibrating tools (e.g. pneumatic drills, polishing tools)

**3** Systemic sclerosis (Raynaud's may be the first symptom; ?smooth, tight, shiny skin on the hands and face, typical mask-like facies, telangiectasia, etc; see Station 5, Locomotor, Case 3)

**4** Other connective tissue disorders (especially mixed connective tissue disease but also SLE, polymyositis, Sjögren's syndrome and rheumatoid arthritis)

**5** Cervical rib (?supraclavicular bruit, ipsilateral diminished radial pulse especially during a Raynaud's attack, wasting of the small muscles of the hand and C8/T1 sensory impairment though neurological signs of cervical rib are often minimal if vascular signs are prominent)

## Other causes

Cold agglutinins

Cryoglobulinaemia

Hypothyroidism

Heavy metal poisoning

Women who develop toxaemia of pregnancy are more likely to have a history of Raynaud's disease (suggesting an abnormal vascular reactivity or unidentified humoral agent underlying both conditions)

## Treatment

Hand warmers, vasodilators both oral (calcium channel blockers, ACE inhibitors) and, if necessary, parenteral (prostacyclin analogues and calcitonin gene-related peptide). In severe cases, lumbar (feet) and digital sympathectomy may help.

---

\*In idiopathic Raynaud's disease, the arteries show an exaggerated physiological response to cold and go into intense spasm to produce numb, dead-white fingers. With rewarming, the classic colour sequence is white to blue (cyanosis) then blue to red (rebound hyperaemia which is painful). If taking a history from the patient, ask about precipitating events, frequency, severity, progression, ulcers and for features of associated connective tissue diseases. The patient (usually with systemic sclerosis) in whom Raynaud's is discussed in the MRCP examination may have chronically impaired arterial circulation leading to cyanosis even in the warm hospital environment.

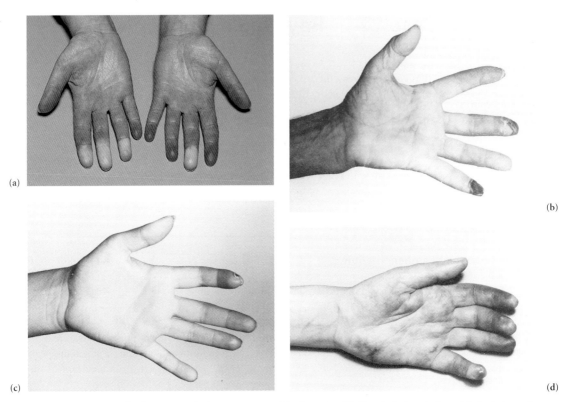

(a)

(b)

(c)

(d)

**Figure I5.18** (a) Raynaud's phenomenon. (b,c) Note gangrene of the fingertips. (d) Chronically impaired arterial circulation and atrophy of the finger pulps.

# Case 23 | Erythema nodosum

**Frequency in survey for 3rd edition:** did not occur in the initial small survey of PACES Station 5, Skin.

**Predicted frequency from older, more extensive MRCP short case surveys:** main focus of a short case in 5% of attempts at PACES Station 5, Skin.

**Survey note:** in the original, pre-PACES survey this usually occurred as a spot diagnosis followed by questions about the possible causes. Histology was asked for on one occasion.

## Record

There are in this (usually) female patient *raised* (become flat with healing) *red* (pass through the changes of a *bruise* with healing), *tender* plaques 2–6 cm in diameter on the *shins* (and occasionally thighs and upper limbs). The diagnosis is erythema nodosum (?fever, arthralgia).

## Possible causes

1 Acute sarcoidosis (bilateral hilar lymphadenopathy; fever, arthralgia, palpable cervical and axillary lymph nodes, mild iridocyclitis)
2 Bacterial infection (e.g. *Streptococcus*, *Mycoplasma*)
3 Ulcerative colitis and Crohn's disease
4 Rheumatic fever (tachycardia, murmur, nodules, etc.)
5 Primary tuberculosis (?ethnic origin, chest signs, etc.)
6 Drugs (sulphonamides, penicillin, oral contraceptives, codeine, salicylates, barbiturates)

## Other causes

Pregnancy
*Yersinia* enterocolitis
Malignancies (lymphoma and leukaemia)
Syphilis
Leprosy (important cause on a worldwide basis)
Coccidioidomycosis
Toxoplasmosis
Lymphogranuloma venereum
Behçet's disease (orogenital ulceration, iridocyclitis, etc.)
Idiopathic

## Histology

This is a classic example of septal panniculitis where the inflammation is mostly in the septa of fat, with little or no vasculitis.* These septa are thickened and infiltrated with inflammatory cells that extend to the periseptal areas of the fat lobules. The composition of the infiltrate varies with age of the lesion. In early stages, oedema, haemorrhage and neutrophils cause septal thickening, whereas fibrosis, periseptal granulation tissues, lymphocytes and giant cells are found in late-stage erythema nodosum.

*The idea that erythema nodosum is vasculitic in origin is a misleading one which has been passed from book to book for far too long!

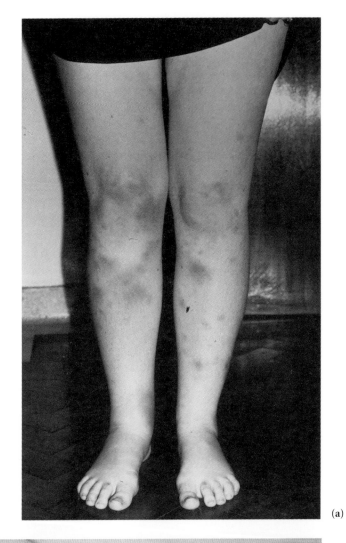

(a)

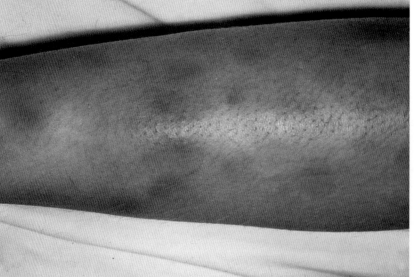

(b)

**Figure I5.19** Erythema nodosum: subcutaneous swellings with erythematous overlying skin.

## Treatment

The ideal treatment, though not always possible, is to identify and eliminate the cause (e.g. penicillin if a streptococcal infection is confirmed). Non-steroidal anti-inflammatory drugs (NSAIDs), elevation and bedrest are helpful. Systemic steroids are seldom necessary. Empirically, a short course of potassium iodide in a dose of 400–900 mg/day may be helpful.

# Case 24 | Sturge–Weber syndrome

**Frequency in survey for 3rd edition**: did not occur in the initial small survey of PACES Station 5, Skin.

**Predicted frequency from older, more extensive MRCP short case surveys**: main focus of a short case in 5% of attempts at PACES Station 5, Skin.

**Survey note**: patients with unilateral and bilateral lesions were seen. One case had buphthalmos. There was discussion on the skull X-ray appearance, including the site of calcification and, on one occasion, temporal lobe epilepsy.

## Record

There is a *port-wine stain* (capillary haemangioma) involving the area supplied by the first (and/or second) division of the trigeminal nerve on the R/L side (it does not cross the mid-line although the skin supplied by the opposite nerve may also be involved). There may be an associated ipsilateral intracranial capillary haemangioma* of the pia arachnoid with *tramline calcification* (which outlines the cortical mantle in an undulating manner) on skull X-ray and a history of *epilepsy*, in which case the diagnosis would be Sturge–Weber syndrome.†

---

There may be a genetic predisposition.

**Congenital abnormalities** may be found in the eye on the affected side:
Glaucoma (blindness frequent)
Strabismus
Buphthalmos or ox eye
Angiomata of the choroid
Optic atrophy

If the port-wine stain is in the area supplied by the first division of the trigeminal nerve, the intracranial lesion is often in the occipital lobe. A facial naevus is more commonly associated with involvement of parietal and frontal lobes. The calcification seen on skull X-ray is in the cortical capillaries. The capillary haemangioma does not contain large vessels and does not fill on arteriography. The underlying brain damage is a rare cause of infantile hemiplegia (?hemi-smallness) and mental retardation as well as epilepsy. Most lesions occur on the face or trunk in a dermatomal distribution. The lesion is present at birth and persists throughout life. In middle age it may darken and become studded with angiomatous nodules. Treatment is unsatisfactory but encouraging results have been obtained with careful, and time-consuming, laser therapy.

---

*Rare association with port-wine stain in real life but common in the examination!

†A phakomatosis; see Footnote, Station 5, Skin, Case 2.

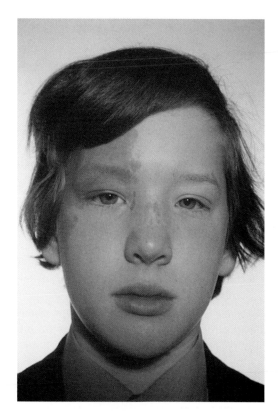

**Figure I5.20** Sturge–Weber syndrome (note strabismus).

# Case 25 | Purpura

**Frequency in survey for 3rd edition:** did not occur in the initial small survey of PACES Station 5, Skin.

**Predicted frequency from older, more extensive MRCP short case surveys:** main focus of a short case in 4% of attempts at PACES Station 5, Skin. Additional feature in some others in all stations (Cushingoid patients on therapeutic steroids).

## *Record*
There is purpura.*
   Now look at the patient and note:
?*Age* ('senile purpura')
?*Cushingoid features* with thin skin (if present, observe for features of underlying steroid-treated disease, e.g. asthma, rheumatoid arthritis, cryptogenic fibrosing alveolitis)
?*Rheumatoid arthritis* (phenylbutazone and gold as well as steroids)
?*Anaemia* (leukaemia, bone marrow aplasia or infiltration)
– as well as the distribution and type of purpura.

## Causes of purpura
Can be divided into:
**Thrombocytopenic purpura such as:**
*Idiopathic thrombocytopenic purpura* (purpuric rash in a young woman, ?spleen – may respond to steroids and/or splenectomy)
*Marrow replacement by leukaemia* (acute and chronic; ?spleen, nodes, liver, anaemia, oral and pharyngeal infection)
*Marrow replacement by secondary malignancy* (?cachexia, evidence of primary)
*Marrow aplasia* (idiopathic, secondary to drugs, hepatitis A or B).
**Capillary defect (vascular; platelet count normal) such as:**
*Senile and steroid-induced purpura* (purpura over loose skin areas); skin atrophy/ fragility
*Henoch–Schönlein purpura* (children > adults); purpuric rash (a leucocytoclastic vasculitis, with appearance ranging from papular to vesiculopustular) over the extensor surfaces of the limbs, particularly at the ankles and on the buttocks; associated with arthritis of medium-sized joints, colicky abdominal pains, occasionally gastrointestinal bleeding and acute nephritis; see Station 5, Skin, Case 33.
**Coagulation deficiency such as:†**
*Haemophilia A*
*Christmas disease (haemophilia B)*
*Anticoagulant therapy.*

*Purpura refers to a spontaneous extravasation of blood from the capillaries into the skin; petechiae = pin-head size, ecchymoses = large lesions. The lesions are non-blanching.

†These conditions may cause ecchymoses rather than purpura.

## Other causes of purpura

Other drugs (e.g. sulphonamides, chloramphenicol, thiazides)

Hypersplenism (large spleen)

Von Willebrand's disease

Infective endocarditis (?heart murmur, splenomegaly, splinters, clubbing, Osler's nodes, etc.)

Systemic lupus erythematosus (?typical rash)

Polyarteritis nodosa (?arteritic lesions)

Osler–Weber–Rendu syndrome (see Station 5, Skin, Case 3)

Venous stasis (ankle and lower legs; obesity or varicose veins; accompanied by progressive pigmentation due to deposition of haemosiderin)

Scurvy (NB: the neglected elderly patient with ecchymoses on the legs)

Paroxysmal nocturnal haemoglobinuria

Amyloidosis (periorbital purpura)

Uraemia (pale, brownish-yellow tinge to skin)

Disseminated intravascular coagulation

Thrombotic thrombocytopenic purpura

Haemolytic-uraemic syndrome

Paraproteinaemia

Meningitis (especially meningococcal)

Septicaemia (especially meningococcal)

Viral haemorrhagic fevers

Factitious purpura

Ehlers–Danlos syndrome (see Station 5, Skin, Case 28)

Scarlet fever

Measles

Rubella

Glandular fever

Typhoid

Cyanotic congenital heart disease

## Investigations

These will be dictated by the clinical circumstances. For example, it may be immediately clear that the patient is on steroids and that this is the cause and no further investigation is required. If it is not clear, in addition to a full blood count and biochemical screen, protein electrophoresis (to exclude paraproteinaemia and hypergammaglobulinaemia) and a full coagulation screen, including measurement of fibrin degradation products, should be carried out. A bone marrow biopsy will establish the diagnosis of idiopathic thrombocytopenic purpura. A trephine biopsy of the iliac crest may be necessary if marrow aplasia is suspected. Skin biopsy will confirm a small vessel vasculitis.

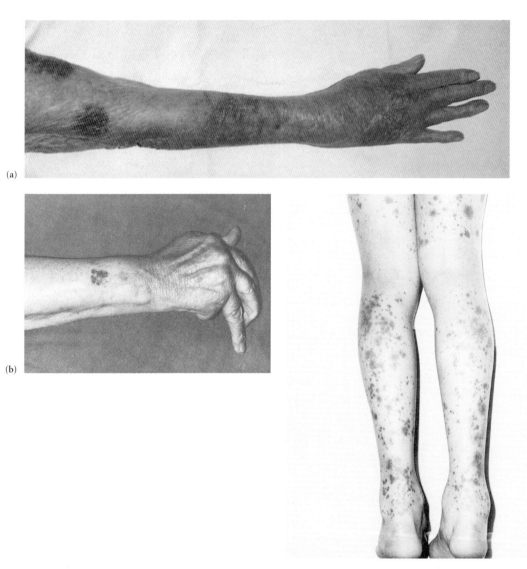

**Figure I5.21** (a) Purpura from steroid therapy for rheumatoid arthritis. (b) Purpura on forearm (note rheumatoid arthritis). (c) Henoch–Schönlein purpura.

# Case 26 | Peutz–Jeghers syndrome

**Frequency in survey for 3rd edition**: did not occur in the initial small survey of PACES Station 5, Skin.

**Predicted frequency from older, more extensive MRCP short case surveys**: main focus of a short case in 4% of attempts at PACES Station 5, Skin.

## *Record*

There are (sparse or profuse) small brownish-black *pigmented macules* (2–5 mm) (lentigines) on the lips, around the *mouth* (and/or eyes or nose) and *buccal mucosa* (but never on the tongue). They are also (may be) seen on the hands and fingers. This pigmentation (which tends to reduce in adult life\*) may be associated with *intestinal polyposis* (single or multiple polyps, which are *hamartomata*, and may occur in the small and large bowel) in which case the diagnosis would be Peutz–Jeghers syndrome.

---

Autosomal dominant.

### Complications
Recurrent colicky abdominal pain
Intestinal obstruction or intussusception
Iron deficiency anaemia
Frank gastrointestinal haemorrhage

Malignant transformation (rare)†
Increased incidence of breast, ovarian (approximately 10% of affected women) and pancreatic cancer

Multiple polypectomy may be required for disabling symptoms but excision of bowel is to be avoided, if possible, as polyps may recur.

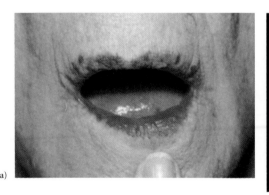
(a)

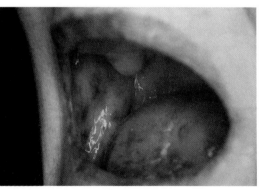
(b)

**Figure I5.22** (a) Peutz–Jeghers syndrome. (b) Pigmentation of the buccal mucosa.

---

\*Macules on the lips may disappear over time but mouth pigmentation persists, and is the *sine qua non* for the diagnosis.
†Cf. familial polyposis coli – adenomatous tumours in which malignant transformation is inevitable and for which premalig-

nant treatment is colectomy, ileorectal anastomosis and fulgarization of remaining rectal polyps. This is followed by careful life-long 6-monthly follow-up with sigmoidoscopy and polyp fulgarization.

# Case 27 | **Vasculitis**

**Frequency in survey for 3rd edition**: did not occur in the initial small survey of PACES Station 5, Skin.

**Predicted frequency from older, more extensive MRCP short case surveys**: main focus of a short case in 4% of attempts at PACES Station 5, Skin. Additional feature in some others in Station 5, Locomotor.

## *Record*

There are (may be) small *nailfold* and nail-edge *infarcts* (due to small vessel vasculitis affecting the terminal digital arteries – in severe cases there may be *digital gangrene*). There is (may be) a purpuric rash (macules, papules, nodules or pustules). There are (may be) chronic leg ulcers. There is (may be) a peripheral neuropathy (due to involvement of the vasa nervorum). This patient has vasculitis (look for obvious signs of a cause, e.g. rheumatoid arthritis, SLE).

---

The term 'vasculitis' refers to a broad grouping of disorders involving the small vessels and larger arteries of the skin, either alone or in association with other organs (there is chronic inflammation in and around the vessel wall). This is usually caused by deposition of immunoglobulin and is sustained by complement activation. The clinical hallmark is *palpable purpura*. The papules may coalesce to form plaques which may ulcerate.

### Conditions associated with vasculitis

Rheumatoid arthritis (?hands, nodules, etc; see Station 5, Locomotor, Case 1)

SLE (?rash, etc; see Station 5, Locomotor, Case 16)

Polyarteritis nodosa* (medium and small arteries and adjacent veins – fever, hypertension, abdominal pain, mononeuritis multiplex, peripheral neuropathy, proteinuria, haematuria, renal failure, myocardial infarction)

Churg–Strauss syndrome (eosinophilic granulomatous vasculitis – similar to polyarteritis nodosa but asthma, eosinophilia, IgE elevation and pulmonary infiltrates are prominent; it may present as asthma)

Australia antigenaemia and vasculitis (a variant of polyarteritis nodosa)

Infectious diseases – hepatitis B and C viruses, group A haemolytic streptococci, *Staphylococcus aureus*, *Mycobacterium leprae*

Wegener's granulomatosis* (granulomatous ulceration of the upper and lower respiratory tract associated with generalized arteritis and glomerulitis)

Antiphospholipid antibody syndrome (?livedo reticularis, history of recurrent deep vein thrombosis [DVT], recurrent spontaneous abortion; see Station 5, Skin, Case 29)

Other connective tissue diseases (systemic sclerosis, etc.)

Drug reactions – sulphonamides, penicillin, serum, etc.

Infective endocarditis

Mixed cryoglobulinaemia

Hypergammaglobulinaemia

Lymphoproliferative disorders

Henoch–Schönlein syndrome (leucocytoclastic vasculitis; children > adults; purpuric rash over the extensor surface of the limbs, particularly at the ankles and often on the buttocks; associated with arthritis of

---

*Antineutrophil cytoplasmic antibodies (ANCA) occur in two staining patterns: cytoplasmic (cANCA) and perinuclear (pANCA). High-titre cANCA strongly suggests necrotizing vasculitis of the Wegener's granulomatosis type. pANCA is particularly associated with microscopic polyarteritis nodosa.

medium-sized joints, colicky abdominal pains, occasionally GI bleeding and acute nephritis; see Station 5, Skin, Case 33)

Persistent (>24 h) urticaria (urticarial vasculitis)

Giant cell arteritis (large and medium-sized vessels; elderly patients – headache, temporal artery tenderness, polymyalgia rheumatica – danger of blindness)

Behçet's disease (oral ulcers, uveitis, phlebitis, photosensitivity, spontaneous pustules)

Thromboangiitis obliterans – Buerger's disease (young man, nicotine staining, peripheral ischaemia, gangrene, migratory superficial thrombophlebitis; see also Station 5, Other, Case 3)

## Rheumatoid patients with vasculitis often have

Nodules

Circulating immune complexes

Cryoglobulins

Low complement levels

Rheumatoid factor

Antinuclear factor

Immunoglobulins and complement in the cutaneous lesions.

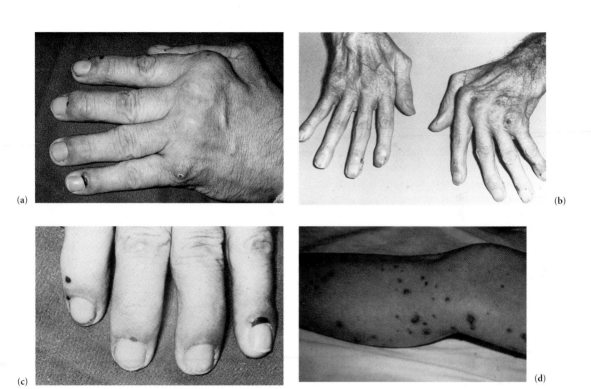

(a)

(b)

(c)

(d)

**Figure I5.23** (a,b) Vasculitis (rheumatoid arthritis). (c) Nailfold infarcts (rheumatoid arthritis). (d) Vasculitis with 'palpable purpura' (bright red, well-demarcated petechiae with a central, dot-like haemorrhage) on the lower limb.

# Case 28 | Ehlers–Danlos syndrome

**Frequency in survey for 3rd edition**: did not occur in the initial small survey of PACES Station 5, Skin.

**Predicted frequency from older, more extensive MRCP short case surveys**: main focus of a short case in 2% of attempts at PACES Station 5, Skin.

## Record

The patient (may be wearing glasses; myopia common) has *epicanthal folds*, a *flat nasal bridge* and prominent ears which point downwards. There is *hyperextensibility* of the skin which is *elastic* and *very thin*. There is evidence of *poor healing* with *thin*, *'cigarette-paper'* scars (the skin tears with minor injury, usually over the knees and elbows, producing *fish-mouth* wounds). *Purpura* is present and there are (commonly) *pseudotumours* over the knees and elbows (trauma → haematoma which organizes → fatty degeneration → calcification). The joints are (remarkably) *hyperextensible* and the patient has kyphoscoliosis, genu recurvatum and flat feet. The diagnosis is Ehlers–Danlos syndrome.

---

There are at least 10 distinct types which vary from mild to severe and show different patterns of inheritance (dominant, recessive, X-linked) of defects in connective tissue synthesis and structure.

### Complications

Bleeding (mostly from the gut)
Poor healing which makes surgery difficult
Recurrent dislocations of patellae, shoulders, hips, etc.
Recurrent hydrarthrosis
Repeated falls (poor control due to hypermobile joints), frequent skin lacerations and prominent scars – may suggest child abuse before the diagnosis is made
Diaphragmatic herniae
Diverticula of the GI and respiratory tracts
Spontaneous pneumothorax
Dissecting aneurysms
Spontaneous rupture of large arteries
Mitral valve prolapse (see Vol. 1, Station 3, Cardiovascular, Case 10).

### Other causes of hypermobile joints

Osteogenesis imperfecta\* (see Station 5, Other, Case 4)
Marfan's syndrome (tall, long bones, dislocated lens, etc; see Vol. 1, Station 3, Cardiovascular, Case 13)
Turner's syndrome (see Station 5, Endocrine, Case 11)
Noonan's syndrome (males and females; short stature, webbed neck, etc; see Station 5, Endocrine, Case 11)
Down's syndrome (see Station 5, Other, Case 5)
Pseudoxanthoma elasticum (see Station 5, Skin, Case 10)
Familial tendency in otherwise normal patients
**Cutis laxa**: in this condition the skin may also be hyperextensible but, in contrast to Ehlers–Danlos syndrome, it has decreased elasticity and hangs in loose folds. Late in Ehlers–Danlos, the skin in localized areas may resemble that seen in cutis laxa.

\*Blue sclerae often occur in Ehlers–Danlos also.

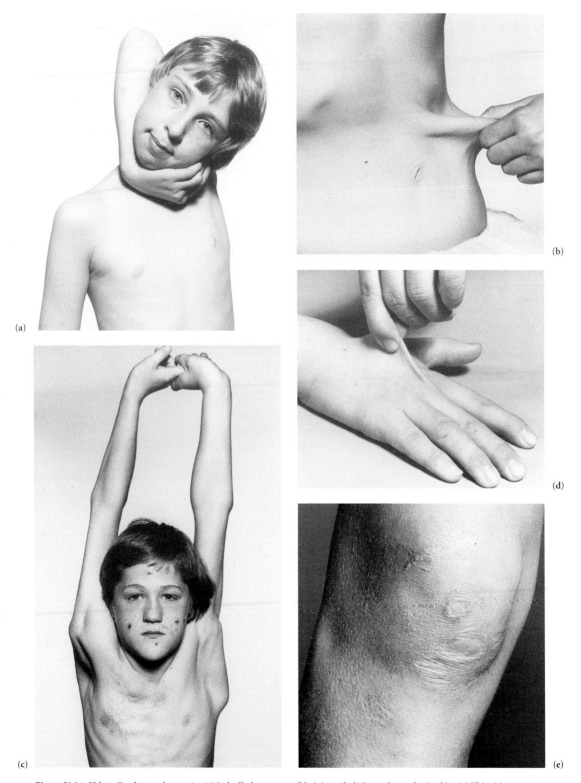

**Figure I5.24** Ehlers–Danlos syndrome. (a,c) Markedly hyperextensible joints. (b,d) Loose hyperelastic skin. (e) Thin, 'cigarette-paper' scars.

# Case 29 | Livedo reticularis

**Frequency in survey for 3rd edition**: did not occur in any of our MRCP surveys. Nevertheless, we suspect it has occurred in MRCP, in particular in the old Station 5 when a skin case was mandatory; and it is a skin marker of a systemic problem. (Erythema ab igne did not occur in the initial small survey of PACES Station 5, Skin. However, it did occur in our older, more extensive, MRCP short case surveys.)

## Record 1

There is (say where) an *arborescent pattern* of *reddish-blue* erythema (or pigmentary change). The changes are suggestive of livedo reticularis. (Now, if allowed, ask for any history of deep venous thrombosis, transient cerebral ischaemic attacks or cerebrovascular accidents, migraine, epilepsy or recurrent abortions.)

---

Livedo reticularis may be associated with antiphospholipid antibody syndrome (APAS), collagen vascular disease, especially polyarteritis nodosa, cryoglobulinaemia or a hyperviscosity syndrome. APAS is a hypercoagulable condition leading to both venous and arterial occlusions. Lupus anticoagulant and *anticardiolipin antibodies* are the serological markers. DVT, transient ischaemic attack, cerebrovascular accident, migraine, epilepsy and recurrent abortions may all be manifestations. Other arterial and venous thromboses may occur, as may heart valve disease. Sudden widespread organ failure may occur (catastrophic APAS). Sometimes, but not always, it may occur in the context of a connective tissue disease, particularly SLE (see Station 5, Locomotor, Case 16). APAS (or APS) is also recognized as occurring as a primary condition (PAPS). APAS now tends to be referred to as *Hughes' syndrome.*

Other conditions which show a reticuloid pattern in the skin are erythema ab igne (see below) and cutis marmorata (a physiological reaction to cold seen in 50% of normal children and many adults).

## Record 2

There is a *reticular pigmented* rash on the. . . (describe the site – usually lateral aspect of one *leg*).

It is characteristic of erythema ab igne.* (As it is due to long-term exposure to local heat, the patient obviously feels the cold. Look at the face and feel the pulse – ?hypothyroidism.)

*Erythema ab igne is due to repeated infrared heat injury. It can occur anywhere where heat is applied, e.g. on the back or abdomen where a hot water bottle is used over a prolonged period in an attempt to alleviate pain. The condition is common in northern Europe ('tinker's tartan') but rare in the USA where central heating is almost universal. In long-standing cases, premalignant keratosis and squamous cell carcinoma can develop.

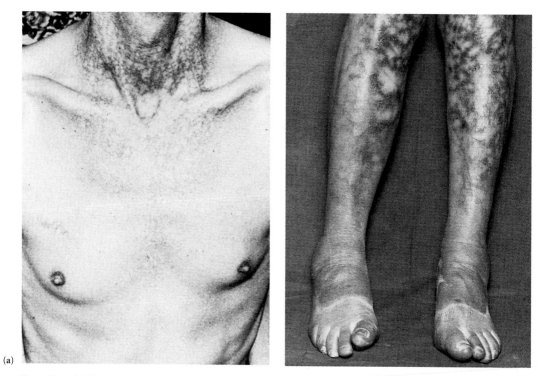

**Figure I5.25** (a) Livedo reticularis visible on the neck (SLE). (b) Erythema ab igne.

# Case 30 | Pemphigus/pemphigoid

**Frequency in survey for 3rd edition:** did not occur in the initial small survey of PACES Station 5, Skin.

**Predicted frequency from older, more extensive MRCP short case surveys:** main focus of a short case in 2% of attempts at PACES Station 5, Skin.

## Record 1

This middle-aged patient has flaccid, *thin-roofed blisters* containing serous fluid, and arising on normal skin (usually over the scalp, axillae and trunk), which vary in size (usually 1–2 cm in diameter). Most of the blisters have *burst*, leaving *red* and *exuding erosions* (which are extremely tender). There are also (not always) red denuded patches in the *mouth* (the first site involved in up to 50% and may precede by months the appearance of skin lesions), *pharynx* and *eyes*. The patient has pemphigus.

## Record 2

This elderly patient has *tense blisters* (containing serous/haemorrhagic fluid, arising on normal/erythematous skin) varying in size from a few millimetres to a few centimetres in diameter involving. . . (describe where – usually it is the limbs but it can be widespread). There are also *reddened* and *urticated* (sometimes eczematous) *plaques* surrounding and separate from the blisters. There are no lesions in the mouth (they do occur but are uncommon). The diagnosis is pemphigoid.

---

### Pemphigus vulgaris

This is an autoimmune blistering disease of skin and mucous membranes. It occurs most commonly in Jewish people. The site of the blister is in the epidermis. Occasionally lesions may occur without initial blister formation. The mucous membranes never have blisters, only denuded, painful patches. It is a progressive and fatal condition if not treated with corticosteroids in very high doses (initially 1–2 mg/kg/day of prednisolone). Azathioprine may reduce the maintenance dose of steroid. Drug-induced pemphigus can be caused by penicillamine, captopril, phenylbutazone and rifampicin. In most cases, the eruption resolves after withdrawal of the offending drug. There is an increased incidence in patients with thymoma and myasthenia gravis. *Acantholysis* (rounded keratinocytes floating free within the blister) is a characteristic histological feature. Nikolsky's sign* is invariably present. Immunofluorescence of a biopsy shows intercellular epidermal deposits of immunoglobulins (usually IgG) and/or complement factor C3.

### Pemphigoid

The site of the blisters is at the basement membrane between the epidermis and the dermis; therefore the blister is thicker and less likely to rupture than in pemphigus. Mucosal lesions are less common in pemphigoid. Though it is self-limiting (2 years) systemic steroids are usually given (initially 60–80 mg/day) and azathioprine may reduce the maintenance dose. It does not have a high mortality like pemphigus. It has been alleged that it is sometimes a manifestation of underlying malignancy but this point is not proven. Biopsy shows a band of IgG and complement at the basement membrane zone.

*Firm pressure on apparently normal skin causes it to slide off. Nikolsky's sign may also occur in other severe bullous eruptions, such as toxic epidermal necrolysis.

## Other bullous disorders

Dermatitis herpetiformis (groups of blisters on the elbows, knees and buttocks; associated with coeliac disease; see Station 5, Skin, Case 39)

Epidermolysis bullosa congenita (congenital blistering disorders usually of the hands and feet; genetically determined; range from simple blisters to severe scarring with contractures (e.g. epidermolysis bullosa dystrophica); teeth and nails abnormal in some forms)

Epidermolysis bullosa acquisita (associated with inflammatory bowel disease, amyloidosis and internal malignancy)

Pemphigoid gestationis – pregnancy-associated autoimmune disease previously called herpes gestationis (pregnancy or early puerperium, erythematous/urticated plaques with blistering; no relation to herpes virus; resolves a few weeks to months after the birth; may require steroids; recurs with increased severity in subsequent pregnancies); higher rate of premature and small-for-dates babies but no increased mortality

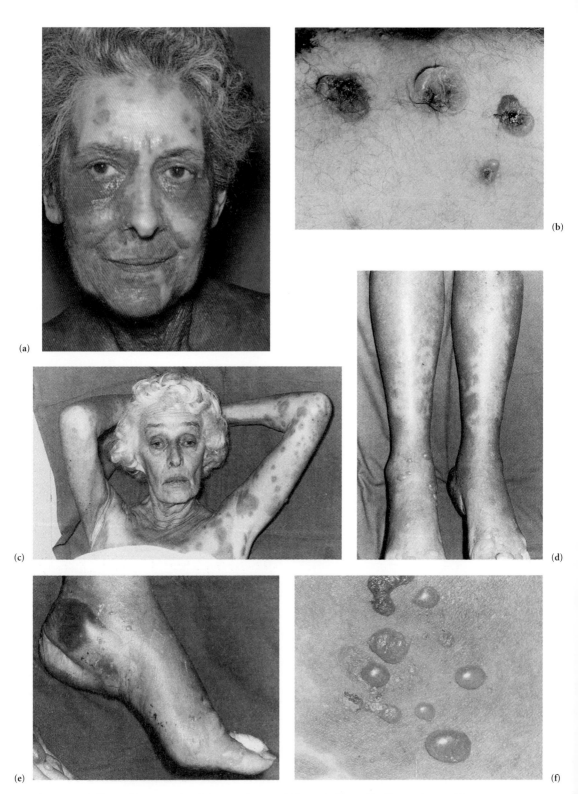

(a)

(b)

(c)

(d)

(e)

(f)

**Figure I5.26** (a,b) Pemphigus. Note denuded areas and ruptured blisters. (c–f) Pemphigoid. Note the tense blisters.

# Case 31 | Radiation burn on the chest

**Frequency in survey for 3rd edition:** did not occur in the initial small survey of PACES Station 5, Skin.

**Predicted frequency from older, more extensive MRCP short case surveys:** main focus of a short case in 1% of attempts at PACES Station 5, Skin. Additional feature in some others in Station 1, Respiratory.

**Survey note:** may be one of many physical signs in a patient with carcinoma of the bronchus (see Vol. 2, Section F, Experience 108), sometimes causing superior vena cava obstruction. Rarely other intrathoracic malignancy.

## Record

There is an area of *erythema* on the *chest* wall. The chest has been marked (radio-therapy *field markings* or 'Red Indian' marks*) for deep X-ray therapy and this (or the signs of *intrathoracic malignancy*) suggests that it is due to a radiotherapy burn (see Vol. 1, Station 1, Respiratory, Case 13).

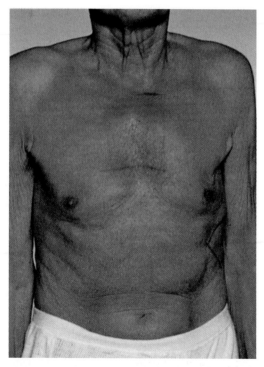

**Figure I5.27** Radiation burn between the two field marks over the chest, and marks over the left lower chest wall (carcinoma of the lung).

*Radiotherapy tattoo marks may be found in other cases of malignancy; see Vol. 2, Section F, Anecdote 100.

# Case 32 | Herpes zoster

**Frequency in survey for 3rd edition:** did not occur in the initial small survey of PACES Station 5, Skin.

**Predicted frequency from older, more extensive MRCP short case surveys:** main focus of a short case in 1% of attempts at PACES Station 5, Skin.

## Record

This elderly (or middle-aged) patient has *grouped and confluent papules, vesicles* and *crusted erosions* in the *area supplied by the . . . nerve* (say which/where).* The lesions are in *clusters* at different stages of development – papule → vesicle → (pustule, sometimes haemorrhagic) → crusting → scar. The regional lymph nodes are enlarged. The diagnosis is herpes zoster.

---

About two-thirds of patients are older than 50 years of age. Risk factors include diminishing immunity to varicella zoster virus with advancing age, malignancy and immunosuppression from lymphoproliferative disorders, chemotherapy, radiotherapy and HIV infection (eight times more susceptible than normal subjects).

### Complications

Cranial nerve palsy – especially facial nerve palsy which may occur not only with lesions of the external auditory meatus (Ramsay Hunt syndrome) but also with trigeminal zoster and zoster of the head, neck and mouth†

Peripheral motor palsy (lower motor neurone deficit from involvement of the motor root – sometimes permanent)

Postherpetic neuralgia (10%; more common in the elderly, approaching 40% in patients older than 60 years of age; can be very severe and difficult to treat)

Eye damage (ophthalmic zoster)

Zoster sine herpete (typical pain, etc., but no rash – serological evidence confirms)

**Other complications** include visceral nerve involvement (pain or dysfunction in an organ), myelitis (transverse or ascending – rare), disseminated encephalitis (rare), cerebellar ataxia (rare) and diffuse polyneuritis (rare).

**Generalized herpes zoster** is usually associated with an underlying reticulosis (especially Hodgkin's), leukaemia, HIV or carcinoma (especially bronchogenic).

---

*The most common is a thoracic dermatome (>50%). Cranial nerve involvement is next in frequency (10–20%). The ophthalmic division of the trigeminal nerve is the most common cranial nerve. With cranial nerve involvement there are often signs of meningeal irritation and sometimes mucous membranes are affected.

†In true Ramsay Hunt (see Vol. 1, Station 3, CNS, Case 35), the zoster is probably of the geniculate ganglion. In other cases there

may be multiple cranial ganglia involvement (see Vol. 2, Section F, Anecdote 278) and an associated localized encephalitis and neuronitis. Eighth nerve involvement (vertigo and deafness) is a particularly common association with facial palsy due to herpes zoster. Aciclovir given as soon as possible after the start of the infection is the treatment of choice.

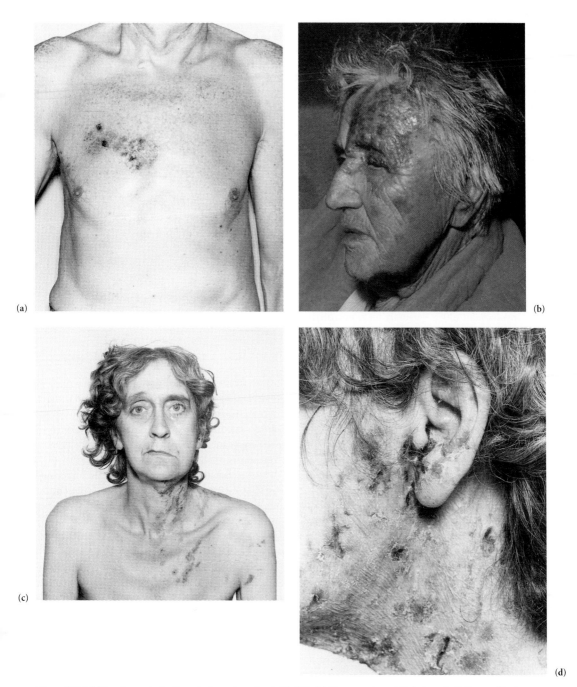

**Figure I5.28** (a) Involvement of a thoracic dermatome (probably T3). (b) Herpes zoster ophthalmicus. (c,d) Ramsay Hunt syndrome.

# Case 33 | Henoch–Schönlein purpura

**Frequency in survey for 3rd edition:** did not occur in the initial small survey of PACES Station 5, Skin.

**Predicted frequency from older, more extensive MRCP short case surveys:** main focus of a short case in 1% of attempts at PACES Station 5, Skin.

## Record

This patient (usually a male child or a young adult) has a *palpable purpuric rash* (initially macules which rapidly urticate and become purpuric and may go on to develop central necrosis with overlying crusts) over the *extensor* surfaces of his *limbs* (usually forearms and the back of the legs) and *buttocks*.

The rash is typical of Henoch–Schönlein purpura. The patient may have other features of the Henoch–Schönlein syndrome: *polyarthralgia* (70% – large joints, usually knees and ankles), *bowel involvement* (25% – colic and haemorrhage) and *renal involvement* (30% – usually focal necrotizing glomerulonephritis).

---

The Henoch–Schönlein syndrome is also called *anaphylactoid purpura* or leucocytoclastic vasculitis.

### Other features of Henoch–Schönlein syndrome

There may be a history of *recent infectious illness* (most commonly viral). Usually remits after 1 week but the cutaneous lesions may take several weeks to regress and the course is often punctuated by recurrent flare-ups of the symptoms and/or signs. There may be self-limiting hypertension.

Polyarthralgia is common but frank arthritis is rare. Colicky abdominal pain may mimic an acute surgical abdomen. Patients may experience nausea, vomiting, diarrhoea, constipation and occasionally the passage of blood and mucus per rectum. *Intussusception* may occur rarely.

Renal disease typically develops within 3 months of the onset of the other systemic manifestations of the Henoch–Schönlein syndrome. It is usually only a glomerulitis with microscopic haematuria and without any significant impairment of renal function. Renal failure is rare in children. Up to 25% of adults develop a severe crescentic lesion with rapidly progressive glomerulonephritis; nephrotic syndrome occurs in 50%.

Patients usually recover spontaneously and completely. Corticosteroids may lead to symptomatic improvement and should be considered in patients with renal involvement. In difficult cases colchicine or dapsone may be worth a trial, but such patients will require careful monitoring for side-effects.

Involved tissues, including the skin, demonstrate vasculitis with IgA and complement deposition. IgA nephropathy (*Berger's disease*) is now regarded as a monosymptomatic form of the Henoch–Schönlein syndrome with manifestations usually confined to the kidney. Histology of the biopsy shows leucocytoclastic vasculitis.

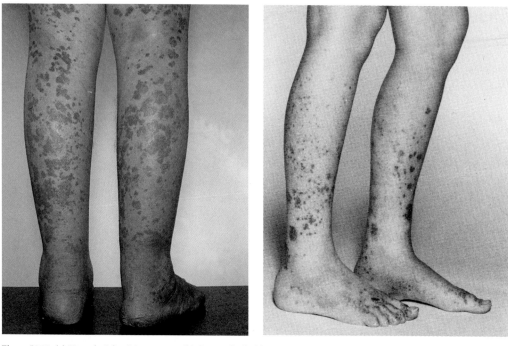

**Figure I5.29** (a) Henoch–Schönlein purpura. (b) Crops of palpable purpura, some lesions with central, haemorrhagic necrosis.

# Case 34 | Mycosis fungoides

**Frequency in survey for 3rd edition:** did not occur in the initial small survey of PACES Station 5, Skin.

**Predicted frequency from older, more extensive MRCP short case surveys:** main focus of a short case in 0.9% of attempts at PACES Station 5, Skin.

## Record

There are (in this middle-aged or elderly patient) erythematous, *well-defined, thick-ened, indurated, scaly plaques* (which itch) over. . . (describe the site; can be on any part of the body though in the early stages exposed areas are often spared). There are also (may be) raised ulcerated nodules. The appearances are suggestive of mycosis fungoides (cutaneous lymphoma*).

---

Male to female ratio is 2:1.

Mycosis fungoides is the most common type of cuta-neous T-cell lymphoma (CTCL). It is a T-cell (CD4+) tumour of the skin* which usually shows no evidence of visceral involvement for several years. The initial lesions may be confused with psoriasis or eczema.† They usually progress very slowly to nodules which may ulcerate.

Diffuse exfoliative erythroderma may develop in 5% (Sezary's syndrome). Extensive nodular infiltra-tion of the face can cause characteristic *leonine facies*. Extracutaneous involvement (especially lung, liver and spleen) does not usually become manifest for many years (though it can be found in two-thirds of patients at autopsy). Lymph node involvement suggests the like-lihood of further extracutaneous spread.

Other reticuloses, for example Hodgkin's disease and leukaemia, may present as infiltrative papules or plaques in the skin diagnosed by skin biopsy.

### Treatment

Treatment depends on staging and previous treatment history. It includes steroids, cytotoxic agents, PUVA and radiotherapy. Topical steroids, topical retinoids, topical chemotherapy (e.g. nitrogen mustard), UVB or PUVA photochemotherapy is used for patch and plaque stage disease. Electron beam therapy and local radiotherapy may be used with systemic treatment (retinoids, inter-feron, extracorporeal photopheresis) for more advanced disease.

---

*Cutaneous T-cell lymphomata are lymphoproliferative disor-ders of helper T-lymphocytes with an affinity for the skin in which atypical lymphocytes accumulate in clusters in the epider-mis. They represent at least three types of lymphoma: mycosis fungoides, Sézary's syndrome and adult T-cell lymphoma (HTLV-1 antibodies, hepatosplenomegaly, osteolytic bone lesions, *hypercalcaemia*).

†In fact, a high index of suspicion should be maintained in patients with atypical or refractory 'eczema' or 'psoriasis'.

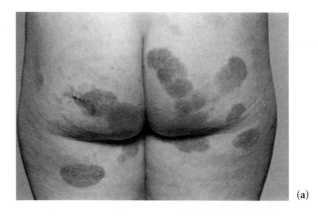

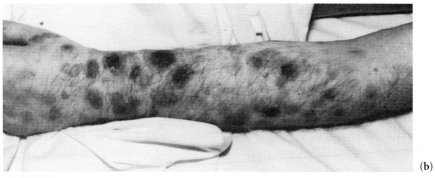

**Figure I5.30** (a) Early lesions of mycosis fungoides showing well-demarcated, scaly, atrophic, erythematous patches. (b) Mycosis fungoides showing early ulceration of plaques.

# Case 35 | Morphoea

**Frequency in survey for 3rd edition:** did not occur in the initial small survey of PACES Station 5, Skin.

**Predicted frequency from older, more extensive MRCP short case surveys:** main focus of a short case in 0.9% of attempts at PACES Station 5, Skin.

## Record 1

There is an *indurated, poorly defined plaque* under the breast (may be anywhere on the trunk, face, axillae or perineum). The lesion is multicoloured (initially violaceous, later ivory coloured) with a central yellowish area, 2–5 cm in diameter (say how big), the surface is (may be) *smooth* and *shiny* with *no hair follicles* and *no sweat ducts*. There is (may be) a *lilac border* (diagnostic, if present). There is *hypoaesthesia* over the plaque which is adherent to deeper tissues. The plaque looks like a depressed area due to *atrophy* of the *underlying tissue*.\* The appearances are suggestive of localized scleroderma (morphoea).

## Record 2

There is a solitary indistinct induration over the trunk (say where). The area looks *discoloured* and *depressed* and there is (may be) telangiectasis. This is probably a small patch of solitary, localized scleroderma.

---

Morphoea is also known as *localized* or *circumscribed scleroderma*. The aetiology is unknown but some patients (predominantly in Europe) with classic morphoea have sclerotic skin changes due to *Borrelia burgdorferi* infection. Occasionally, morphoea develops after X-ray irradiation for breast cancer.

Lichen sclerosus is a chronic atrophic disorder characterized by a *white*, angular, *well-defined indurated* plaque or plaques, which can usually be distinguished from morphoea by its characteristic clinical and histological features.

## Treatment

Treatment of localized morphoea with superpotent topical steroids may prevent progression. Morphoea-like lesions associated with borreliosis may be treated successfully in the early stages with parenteral penicillin or cefotaxime. The course is slowly progressive, but spontaneous remission may occur in some cases. Generalized, linear or deep morphoea requires early treatment with systemic steroids and/or methotrexate to prevent progression.

---

\*Deep involvement may be associated with *atrophy* of *muscles* and *bone*. There may be *scarring alopecia* on the scalp. A variant of morphoea, involving the frontoparietal scalp and face usually in a linear distribution, with or without hemiatrophy of the face, is rarely seen (*en coup de sabre*).

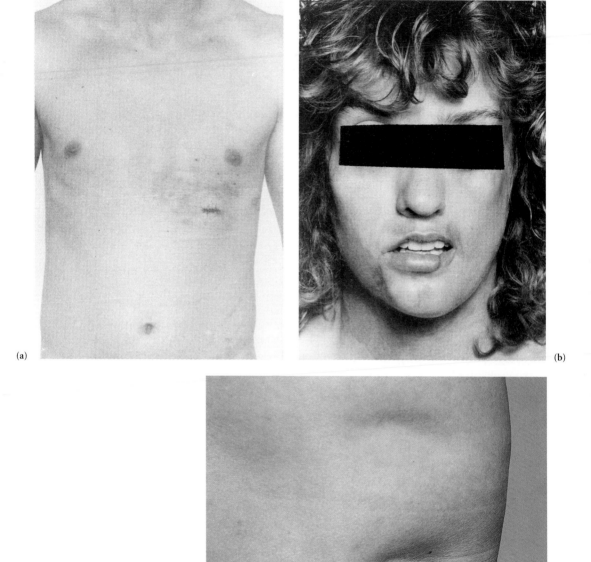

(a)

(b)

(c)

**Figure I5.31** (a) Morphoea – central pale area from which a biopsy has been taken. (b) Localized scleroderma of the lower lip. (c) Depression caused by the atrophy of underlying tissues.

# Case 36 | Kaposi's sarcoma (AIDS)

**Frequency in survey for 3rd edition:** did not occur in the initial small survey of PACES Station 5, Skin.

**Predicted frequency from older, more extensive MRCP short case surveys:** main focus of a short case in 0.9% of attempts at PACES Station 5, Skin.

## Record

There are (may be numerous or solitary; may be firm; are palpable even at the macular stage) well-demarcated, reddish-purple and bluish-brown macules, plaques and nodules (may appear initially as a dusky stain, especially about the toes). The lesions are suggestive of Kaposi's sarcoma.

---

Kaposi's sarcoma classically occurs in four major clinical settings:

1 African – endemic Kaposi's (extremities; 9–12.8% of all malignancies in Zaïre)

2 Elderly Jewish or Mediterranean males (purplish on distal extremities; indolent course)

3 Immunodeficiency conditions (widespread, reddish-purple papules; rapidly progressive; may regress if immunosuppression discontinued)

4 AIDS* (reddish-brown; wide distribution).

### Features of Kaposi's sarcoma

Herpesvirus type 8 is thought to be involved in the pathogenesis of all variants of Kaposi's sarcoma

May also occur in the viscera

May infiltrate the lymphatics of the leg leading to chronic oedema

Associated with cytomegalovirus on electron microscopy

May complicate treatment with immunosuppression for SLE or renal transplant

Especially affects homosexual men (most commonly fourth decade): smaller lesions than non-AIDS Kaposi's. May affect viscera first

### Human immunodeficiency virus

Human immunodeficiency virus (HIV) is an RNA retrovirus that infects human cells that express CD4 and one type of chemokine receptor (CCR5 or CXCR4) on their surface. Agents that prevent HIV attachment to its host (target) cells are called entry inhibitors.

Once inside the cytoplasm, HIV undergoes reverse transcription, the viral RNA acting as a template for a complementary DNA molecule. Synthetic nucleotides and non-nucleotide inhibitors can be used to interfere with this process.

In the absence of antiretroviral agents, the completed HIV DNA chain migrates inside the host cell's nucleus and becomes integrated into the cell's DNA. The process involves viral integrase. Agents that block viral integrase are called integrase inhibitors.

In the absence of HIV drugs, viral DNA is transcribed into chains of RNA that enter a host cell's cytoplasm where building of new viral particles takes place. The new viral particles need to undergo a 'maturation' process before being infective. This process relies on HIV protease. Protease inhibitors prevent maturation of new viral particles, making them incapable of infecting new cells.

### Epidemiology

In the UK, it has been estimated that 83,000 individuals had HIV and 27% were unaware of their diagnosis in 2009.

### Routes of HIV transmission

Human immunodeficiency virus is a blood-borne virus that can be transmitted sexually. Sexual transmission of

---

*In HIV-infected individuals, the risk for Kaposi's sarcoma is 20 000 times that of the general population.

the virus is responsible for the majority of HIV epidemics globally. In the beginning of the epidemics, sexual transmission of HIV was mostly reported amongst men who have sex with men (MSM) in developed nations whereas heterosexual transmission of HIV has been the main route of transmission in developing nations. In the UK, this distinction has disappeared and heterosexual transmission of HIV has been the main route of transmission since 2000.

Human immunodeficiency virus can also be transmitted during pregnancy and delivery from an infected mother to the child. Implementation of antenatal screening programmes has significantly reduced the rate of HIV mother-to-child transmission.

Sharing of injection equipment between intravenous drug users (IVDU) is another identified route of HIV transmission. Transmission via infected blood products can also lead to HIV transmission.

### Clinical features

Acute infection with HIV may present with non-specific flu-like symptoms (maculopapular rash, pharyngitis, myalgia, lymphadenopathy, headache or rarely aseptic meningitis) and lasts for 12 weeks. After that period, patients remain asymptomatic for an average of 8 years (latency period of HIV infection). At the end of this period, HIV viral load starts to increase, whilst patients' CD4 count starts to decline. Unless treated with antiretroviral agents, patients become immuno-compromised and at risk of developing acquired

immunodeficiency syndrome (AIDS)-defining illnesses. AIDS-defining illnesses are infections and malignancies strongly associated with immunocompromised HIV-infected patients. It is important to ensure that patients with any AIDS-defining illness are tested for HIV.

### Laboratory diagnosis

Serology including immunoassays for HIV antigen and antibody. There is an interval between infection and development of detectable amounts of anti-HIV antibodies during which HIV-infected patients may test antibody negative (window period). The duration of the window period is 3–4 weeks with the new HIV assays.

### Treatment

Antiretroviral therapy is the most effective treatment for medium- and long-term survival for patients with any of the AIDS defining illnesses.

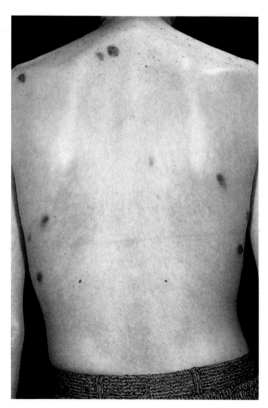

**Figure I5.32** Kaposi's sarcoma: multiple, well-demarcated, purplish macules, papules and plaques.

**Table I5.2** AIDS-defining illnesses

| | |
|---|---|
| Bacterial infections | *Mycobacterium avium* complex |
| | Disseminated tuberculosis |
| | Disseminated or extrapulmonary mycobacterial infection |
| | Recurrent *Salmonella* septicaemia |
| | *Notes* |
| | • Any person with any form of mycobacterial infection must be tested for HIV. Not everyone with mycobacterial infection will be HIV infected |
| | • Mycobacterial (tuberculosis or non-tuberculosis) infections commonly cause long-standing fever, weight loss, lymphadenopathy. Patients may also present with cough, anaemia and hepatosplenomegaly |
| | • Treatment of non-tuberculosis mycobacterial infections is complex and depends on the antibiotic sensitivity of the species. All mycobacterial infections require combined anti-TB therapy for several months |
| Fungal infections | *Pneumocystis jiroveci* pneumonia (formerly *Pneumocystis carinii* |
| | • Most often presenting with shortness of breath, fever and dry cough. |
| | • Treatment is with high-dose co-trimoxazole. Patients with severe hypoxia should also receive short-term steroids |
| | Candidiasis of bronchi, trachea or lungs |
| | Oesophageal candidiasis |
| | Disseminated or extrapulmonary coccidioidomycosis |
| | Extrapulmonary cryptococcosis, cryptococcal meningitis |
| Protozoal infections | Chronic intestinal cryptosporidiosis (for longer than 1 month) |
| | Disseminated or extrapulmonary histoplasmosis |
| | Toxoplasmosis of the brain |
| | Chronic intestinal isosporiasis (for more than 1 month) |
| Viral infections | Cytomegalovirus disease (other than liver, spleen or lymph nodes) |
| | • Most commonly involving retina and gastrointestinal tract |
| | • Is mostly associated with severe immunosuppression (CD4 count <50 cells/mm$^3$) |
| | Chronic ulcer(s) (for more than 1 month); bronchitis, pneumonitis or oesophagitis caused by herpes simplex virus |
| | Progressive multifocal leucoencephalopathy |
| | • Caused by JC virus, is associated with severe immunosuppression |
| | • Presents with visual field defects, gait instability, and disrupted co-ordination |
| Malignancy | Invasive cervical cancer |
| | Kaposi's sarcoma (KS) |
| | • Caused by human herpes virus 8 |
| | • Can develop on skin and mucosa involving internal organs. Internal KS can affect lungs or gastrointestinal tract |
| | • Antiretroviral therapy is the most effective treatment of local KS. Internal KS often requires chemotherapy as well |
| | Non-Hodgkin's lymphoma |
| | • Mostly presenting as anaemia, hepatosplenomegaly, lymphadenopathy and fever |
| | • Strong association with Epstein–Barr virus and HIV infections; hence the need for testing patients for HIV |
| | • Prognosis has significantly improved with antiretroviral therapy and combined chemotherapy regimes |
| Others/general | HIV-related encephalopathy |
| | Recurrent pneumonia |
| | • Patients with two episodes of pneumonia in 12 months must be tested for HIV infection |
| | Wasting syndrome due to HIV |

# Case 37 | Porphyria

**Frequency in survey for 3rd edition:** did not occur in the initial small survey of PACES station 5, Skin.

**Predicted frequency from older, more extensive MRCP short case surveys:** main focus of a short case in 0.9% of attempts at PACES Station 5, Skin.

**Survey note:** only variegate porphyria and porphyria cutanea tarda were reported as short cases in the original, pre-PACES surveys.

## Record 1

There is *muscular weakness* in the upper and lower limbs, particularly in the *proximal* groups. The *tendon reflexes* are *absent* (or diminished) and the plantars are flexor (or unresponsive). There are no sensory changes. The backs of the hands show *crusts*, *scarring*, areas of *fragility of the skin* and *blisters*. These features suggest a diagnosis of variegate porphyria.*

## Record 2

The skin on the backs of the hands shows *thin* and *traumatized areas*, *vesicles* and *bullae*, *crusts* and *scarring* and a few (say how many) *pearly white* to *yellow, subepidermal papules* or *milia*, 1–5 mm in diameter, particularly over the knuckles. There are areas of hyperpigmentation with some patches of hypopigmentation, periorbital suffusion and *hypertrichosis* over the temples and cheeks. There is one crusted lesion on the pinna of the ear, presumably a remnant of a bulla.

The features of *cutaneous fragility*, *photosensitivity* and *bullous lesions* suggest a diagnosis of porphyria (possibly porphyria cutanea tarda†), though one has also to consider the possibility of a pseudoporphyria.‡ A complete clinical assessment and laboratory investigations are necessary for a more specific diagnosis.

---

*Variegate porphyria has both the cutaneous changes of porphyria cutanea tarda and the systemic features of acute intermittent porphyria. The latter does not show photosensitivity or have any cutaneous changes.

†Patients with porphyria cutanea tarda excrete increased amounts of porphyrin into the urine, which can be demonstrated with a Wood's lamp as pinkish-red fluorescence. Freshly voided urine may look orange-red. A quick way to demonstrate orange-red fluorescence is by adding a few drops of 10% hydrochloric acid or acetic acid to the urine sample. A rapid screening test demonstrating excess porphobilinogen (PBG) in the urine can be done to diagnose acute intermittent porphyria. Freshly voided urine should be *exposed to sunlight* for several hours after which time a *deep red colour develops* which suggests that there is some excess PBG. Alternatively, a *few drops* of freshly voided

urine are added to 2 mL of *Ehrlich's reagent* and the urine forms a *cherry-red* colour, suggesting the presence of PBG. A markedly elevated faecal protoporphyrin level is diagnostic of variegate porphyria.

‡The term 'pseudoporphyria' is applied when patients clinically exhibit cutaneous manifestations of porphyria cutanea tarda without the characteristic abnormal porphyrin profile. The disorder may develop in association with certain drugs (frusemide [furosemide], tetracycline, naproxen and pyridoxine), diabetes mellitus and chronic renal failure on maintenance haemodialysis. In the initial stages the porphyrin levels in the urine, faeces and plasma may be normal in the last condition, but some studies have reported true porphyria cutanea tarda with excess porphyrins in dialysed patients.

*Acute intermittent porphyria* (the skin is not affected), *variegate porphyria*\* and *hereditary coproporphyria* (very rare) all exhibit acute episodes, the clinical features of which may be abdominal pain, vomiting and constipation, peripheral neuropathy with weakness or paralysis, confusion and psychosis, tachycardia and hypertension. Drugs and chemicals associated with the clinical expression of acute hepatic porphyria include ethyl alcohol, oestrogen hormones, hexachlorobenzene, chlorinated phenols, iron, etc. There is a long list of potentially hazardous drugs including barbiturates, carbamazepine, amphetamines, chloroquine, danazol, ethosuximide, frusemide (furosemide), methyldopa, sulphonamides, rifampicin, hydralazine and valproic acid.

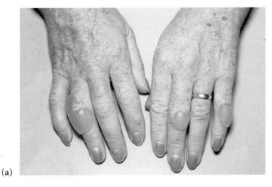

(a)

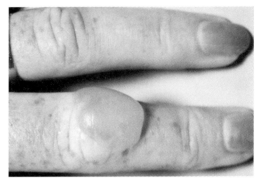

(b)

**Figure I5.33** (a,b) Porphyria cutanea tarda.

# Case 38 | Lupus vulgaris

**Frequency in survey for 3rd edition:** did not occur in the initial small survey of PACES Station 5, Skin.

**Predicted frequency from older, more extensive MRCP short case surveys:** main focus of a short case in 0.9% of attempts at PACES Station 5, Skin.

## Record

There is a *reddish-brown flat plaque* with irregular edges of about $5 \times 7$ cm on the R/L side of the face.\* The appearance is smooth (may be hyperkeratotic in later stages) and glistening but there is *fine scaling* over the middle (look for this). The *consistency* is *soft*† and there is some *scarring* (say where). The characteristic appearance of this plaque, with scarring and its soft consistency, supports the diagnosis of lupus vulgaris.‡

---

Lupus vulgaris is a progressive form of cutaneous tuberculosis occurring in a person with a moderate or high degree of immunity. A cool, moist, dull climate (as in northern Europe) seems to favour its development but nowadays it is rare in Europe and the USA. Lupus vulgaris is disproportionately uncommon in Eastern countries where other forms of TB are frequently seen. Its clinical presentation falls into five general patterns.

1 Plaque form – starts as a tiny reddish-brown, flat plaque and extends gradually with little or no scarring. There may be excessive scaling which gives it a psoriasiform appearance. The edges often become thickened and hyperkeratotic

2 Ulcerative form – scarring and ulceration with crusts over the areas of necrosis are the major features of this type. The lesion erodes into deep tissues and cartilages, producing deformities and contractures

3 Vegetating forms – ulcerates, sometimes quite rapidly, producing necrosis but there is minimal scarring. Mucous membranes may be invaded. Response to chemotherapy is excellent

4 Tumour-like forms – these lesions are deeply infiltrating and stand out over the surface of the skin as a group of soft, smooth nodules. Scaling and scarring are absent. In the 'myxomatous' form, large soft tumours occur, mostly on the ear lobes which become enlarged. The response to treatment may be poor

5 Papular and nodular forms – this is often the disseminated variety and multiple papular and nodular lesions may occur on the body ('miliary lupus'). The papulonodular lesions may be confined to the face and resemble acne

## Treatment

Standard antituberculous therapy should be given. Despite long periods of indolence, the natural course of an untreated lesion is inexorably progressive. The older the patient, the more rapid is the spread of the lesion. Spontaneous resolution may occur but leaves contractures, scars and mutilation.

---

\*The lesion commonly appears on normal skin of the head and neck in about 80% of the cases in Europe. The face, particularly around the nose, is the area of predilection. The arms and legs are sometimes involved but the trunk is often spared. In India, the face is affected less frequently than the buttocks and trunk.
†The lesions of lupus vulgaris are soft and this, together with the associated scarring, is the main feature that distinguishes it from the lupus pernio of sarcoidosis. If the lesion is probed, the instrument breaks through the overlying epidermis. Diascopy (i.e. looking at a glass slide pressed against the lesion) reveals an 'apple-jelly' (yellowish-brown) colour of the infiltrate.

‡In the early stage (i.e. a small plaque/nodule on the face), lupus vulgaris may be confused with lymphocytoma, lupus pernio, lupus erythematosus and a 'port-wine' stain. Of these, lupus pernio and lymphocytoma are the two conditions which may have solitary lesions on the face without any other manifestations and may present a diagnostic problem. Lymphocytoma cutis is often a red, even violaceous, nodule with an indurated centre. Lupus pernio (see Station 5, Skin, Case 19) is usually a purple-red induration of the skin. On diascopy these lesions look pale, brownish-red.

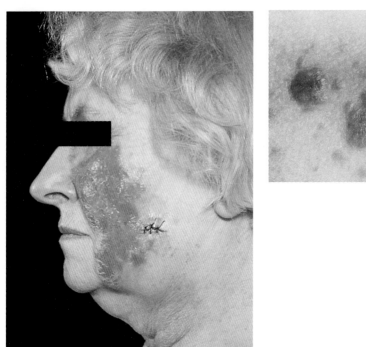

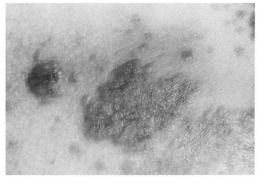

(b)

(a)

**Figure I5.34** (a) Lupus vulgaris: note the glistening, transparent surface of the lesion. (b) Plaques with scaling and irregular edges.

# Case 39 | Dermatitis herpetiformis

**Frequency in survey for 3rd edition:** did not occur in the initial small survey of PACES Station 5, Skin.

**Predicted frequency from older, more extensive MRCP short case surveys:** main focus of a short case in 0.5% of attempts at PACES Station 5, Skin.

## *Record*

This middle-aged (or elderly) patient has *groups* of *erythematous papules* and *excoriations* on the *elbows, knees, buttocks, scalp, upper back* and at *pressure points* (very occasionally it is generalized). There are (may be) *vesicles* which have (usually) a raised, reddened background (vesicles may be present but have usually been ruptured by scratching – the lesions are intensely *pruritic*). The diagnosis is dermatitis herpetiformis and this is nearly always associated with a gluten-sensitive enteropathy* (*coeliac disease*).

---

Male to female ratio is 2:1.

About 85% of patients are HLA-B8/DRw3.

Ingestion of iodides and gluten overload may bring on an attack.

Dermatitis herpetiformis can occur at any stage of adult life (rare in childhood). Once developed, it is persistent. It is treated with a gluten-free diet and/or dapsone (has a dramatic response, often within hours of starting dapsone, but side-effects include rashes, haemolysis and agranulocytosis). The G6PD level should be checked before starting sulfones, methaemoglobin levels should be determined during the initial 10 weeks, and blood counts should be monitored for the first few months. The differential diagnosis is from pemphigus, pemphigoid and other bullous disorders (see Station 5, Skin, Case 30) and from scabies. Involvement of the oral mucosa is uncommon. There may be a higher incidence of developing malignancies than in the general population.

Histology – subepidermal blister with microabscesses at dermal papillae. Direct immunofluorescence (diagnostic) – IgA deposit at basement membrane (dermal papillae).

*There may not be overt symptoms of malabsorption, which occurs in 10–20% of patients, though an abnormal D-xylose absorption may be found in up to 70% of patients.

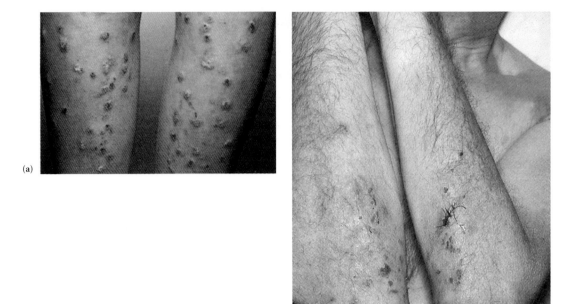

(a)

(b)

**Figure I5.35** (a) Dermatitis herpetiformis. (b) Grouped lesions.

# Case 40 | Urticaria pigmentosa (mastocytosis)

**Frequency in survey for 3rd edition:** did not occur in the initial small survey of PACES Station 5, Skin.

**Predicted frequency from older, more extensive MRCP short case surveys:** main focus of a short case in 0.5% of attempts at PACES Station 5, Skin.

## Record

There are *multiple*, small, discrete, round (or oval), reddish-brown (or yellowish-brown) *pigmented macules* (and/or papules). After *friction, rubbing* or *stroking, itching, urticarial weals* develop (due to histamine release from the mast cells – *Darier's sign*). The diagnosis is urticaria pigmentosa.

---

Urticaria pigmentosa, the most common skin manifestation, is seen in more than 90% of patients with indolent mastocytosis, and in less than 50% of patients with mastocytosis and an associated haematological disorder or those with aggressive mastocytosis.

If involvement is extensive, a hot bath followed by vigorous drying and certain drugs (alcohol, dextran, polymyxin B, morphine, codeine and NSAIDs) may lead to flushing, hypotension, bronchospasm and diarrhoea. In a minority, systemic involvement may occur with involvement of the liver, spleen and bone marrow. Bowel involvement may lead to malabsorption. A small percentage of patients develop leukaemia which can be, but is not usually, mast cell leukaemia.

## Treatment

Drugs that may cause mast cell degranulation should be avoided (see above). Both H1 and H2 antihistamines and disodium cromoglycate can ameliorate itching, flushing, diarrhoea and abdominal pains.

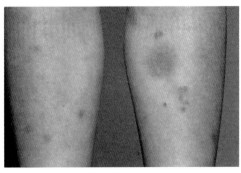

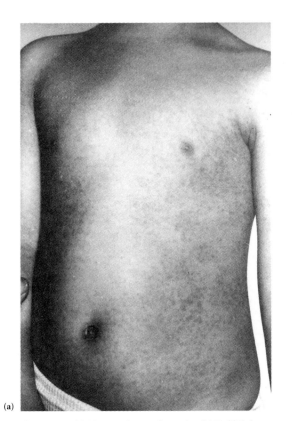

**Figure I5.36** (a) Discrete pigmented macules. (b) Reddish-brown macules.

# Case 41 | Palmoplantar keratoderma (tylosis)

**Frequency in survey for 3rd edition:** did not occur in the initial small survey of PACES Station 5, Skin.

**Predicted frequency from older, more extensive MRCP short case surveys:** main focus of a short case in 0.5% of attempts at PACES Station 5, Skin.

## *Record*

There is *diffuse, thick, yellowish hyperkeratosis* of the *palms* and (ask to see the feet) of the *soles* with painful fissuring. The margins are delineated by a reddish line at the lateral border of the feet and at the wrist, beyond which there is no hyperkeratosis (does not involve the extensor surfaces). The areas are *moist* (*hyperhidrosis*) and there is (may be) evidence of dermatophyte infection. The diagnosis is diffuse palmoplantar keratoderma (PPK) or tylosis.

---

Palmoplantar keratodermas can be inherited or acquired.

### Inherited palmoplantar keratodermas

*Diffuse* – affects palms and soles uniformly. Usually evident in infancy

*Focal* – affects localized areas, particularly friction and pressure points. This is autosomal dominant and may be associated with oesophageal cancer in the fifth decade of life

*Punctate* – features small hyperkeratotic papules that may include the whole palm or sole or just affect the creases

In addition there may also be other skin signs and other organs involved.

### Acquired palmoplantar keratodermas

Keratoderma climactericum seen in menopausal women

Keratoderma associated with internal malignancy (oesophagus, stomach, breast, lung)

Due to inflammatory dermatoses, e.g. pityriasis rubra pilaris, keratoderma blennorrhagicum

Due to infections, e.g. dermatophytes, syphilis

Drug-related, e.g. arsenic, lithium, venlafaxine

Systemic disease associated, e.g. hypothyroidism

Regular paring emollients and keratolytic ointments may be helpful.

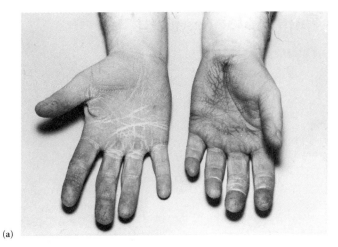

(a)

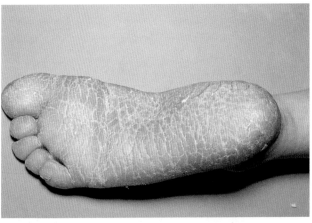

(b)

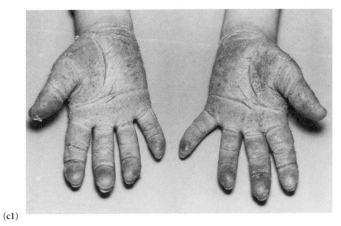

(c1)

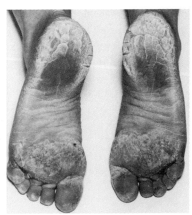

(c2)

**Figure I5.37** Palmoplantar keratoderma. (a) Palms. (b) Sole. Note the diffuse hyperkeratotic areas. (c) Hyperkeratosis with secondary fungal infection in (1) palms and (2) soles.

# Case 42 | Secondary syphilis

**Frequency in survey for 3rd edition**: did not occur in the initial small survey of PACES Station 5, Skin.

**Predicted frequency from older, more extensive MRCP short case surveys**: main focus of a short case in 0.5% of attempts at PACES Station 5, Skin.

## *Record*

There are *firm, well-demarcated* round to oval *papules*, 0.5–1 mm in diameter, on the *palms* and (ask to see the feet) the *soles* of this patient. There are (may be) similar lesions on the *trunk*, *face* and *legs*. Scattered among the papules are some *macules*. Both of these lesions are *pinkish-brown*, and many of the papules have some *fine scaling* in the centre.

The differential diagnosis lies between secondary syphilis, pityriasis rosea, a drug eruption (especially captopril), tinea versicolor, lichen planus and infectious mono-nucleosis.* The characteristic maculopapular (sometimes pustular, papulosquamous or acneiform) lesions with scaling and their predilection for the palms and soles favour the diagnosis of secondary syphilis.

---

## Mucosal and other associated findings

Small, asymptomatic, flat-topped, round or oval, some-what elevated macules and papules, covered with a hyperkeratotic greyish membrane, occur on the oral or genital mucosa. There may be mucocutaneous papules (*split papules*) at the angles of the mouth. About 80% of patients with secondary syphilis have cutaneous or mucocutaneous lesions. The patient may have lymph-adenopathy (cervical, suboccipital, epitrochlear and axillary), splenomegaly or hepatosplenomegaly, perios-titis of the long bones, diffuse pharyngitis and acute iritis. The diagnosis can be confirmed by dark-field examination and serology.

---

*In *pityriasis rosea* there is often (about 80%) a bright red, oval, 2–5 cm, *herald plaque*, with *delicate scaling, adherent peripherally* (a collarette), and a fine scaling maculopapular rash is usually scattered on the trunk in a 'Christmas tree' distribution. A *drug eruption* will mimic any rash but generally tends to be distributed symmetrically over the trunk. *Tinea versicolor* is a chronic, asymptomatic fungal infection of the *trunk* characterized by sharply marginated scaly macules which often take on a colour in contrast with the normal colour of the patient's skin. The flat-topped maculopapules of *lichen planus* (see Station 5, Skin, Case 11) may be mistaken for secondary syphilis but their pre-dilection for the wrist and the presence of characteristic mucosal lesions should help make the diagnosis.

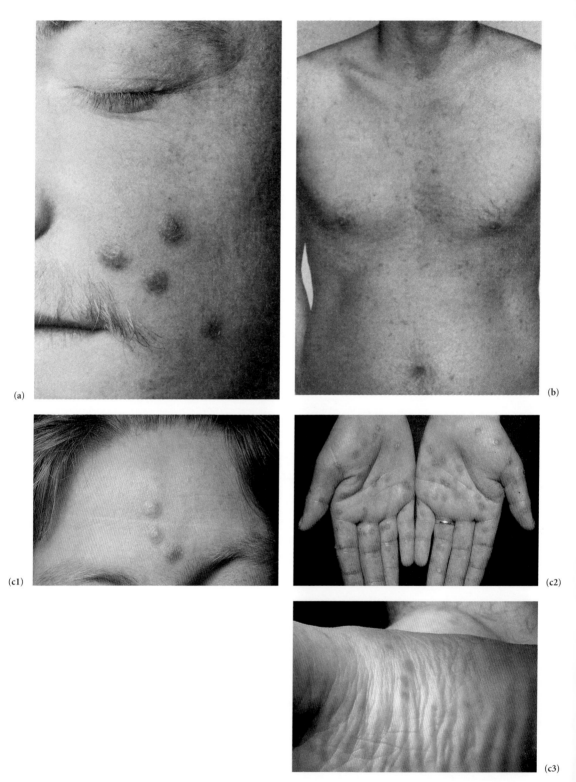

(a)

(b)

(c1)

(c2)

(c3)

**Figure I5.38** (a) Round papules with a keratotic top of secondary syphilis. (b) Scattered papules and macules (c) on the forehead (1), palms (2) and sole (3).

# Case 43 | Ectodermal dysplasia

**Frequency in survey for 3rd edition:** did not occur in the initial small survey of PACES Station 5, Skin.

**Predicted frequency from older, more extensive MRCP short case surveys:** main focus of a short case in 0.5% of attempts at PACES Station 5, Skin.

## Record 1

The striking feature in this patient is *alopecia* with *sparse, dry, thin, spindly*, short hair. The *skin is dry* and finely wrinkled around the eyes. The nails are short, thin, ridged and brittle (ask the patient to show his teeth). The *incisors* and *canine teeth* are *underdeveloped, conical* and *pointed*. These features suggest that this patient has hypohidrotic ectodermal dysplasia.

## Record 2

The *scalp hair* is *sparse, fine* and *brittle*. The eyebrows are (may be) absent. The *teeth* are *normal*. The *palms* and *soles* show diffuse *hyperkeratosis*. The *nails* are *short, thickened* and *discoloured*. The *skin feels moist*. The nail dystrophy and sparse hair with normal teeth and facial appearance suggest that this patient has hidrotic ectodermal dysplasia.

---

Ectodermal dysplasia is a congenital condition with one or more defects of hair, teeth, nails and sweating. Two main groups are identified. Hypohidrotic (or anhidrotic) ectodermal dysplasia is X-linked (over 90% of patients are male but female carriers may show dental defects, sparse hair and reduced sweating) and characterized by partial or complete *absence of sweat glands*, *hypotrichosis* and *hypodontia*. In the complete form, the facial features are distinctive with prominent frontal ridges and chin, saddle nose, sunken cheeks, thick lips, large ears and sparse hair. Absent or reduced sweating causes heat intolerance and affected individuals may present with unexplained fevers.

The *sweat glands* are *normal* in the other main group (hidrotic ectodermal dysplasia) which is transmitted as an autosomal dominant trait. This variety is characterized by *nail dystrophy, defects of the hair* and *keratoderma of the palms and soles*.

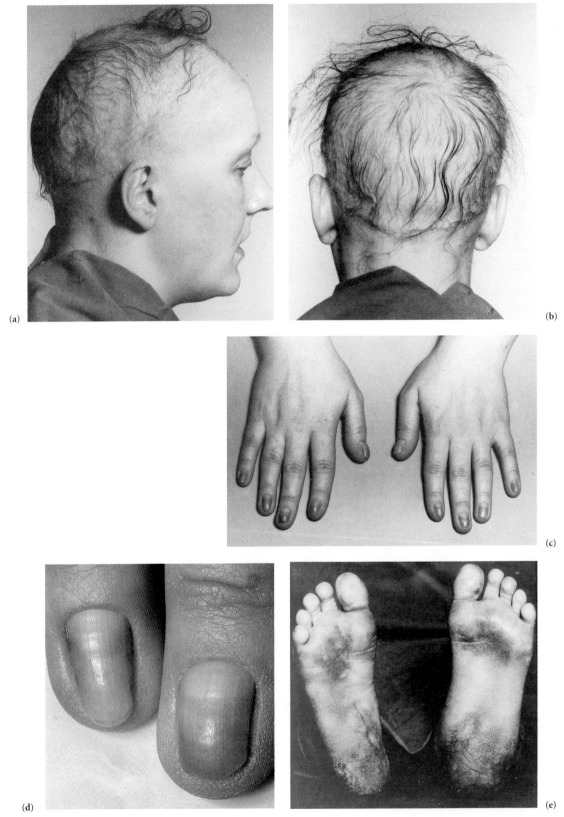

**Figure I5.39** (a,b) Hydrotic ectodermal dysplasia showing alopecia with sparse, thin, spindly hair. (c,d) Thin, ridged, discoloured and excessively curved nails. (e) Diffuse hyperkeratosis.

# Case 44 | **Partial lipodystrophy**

**Frequency in survey for 3rd edition:** did not occur in the initial small survey of PACES Station 5, Skin.

**Predicted frequency from older, more extensive MRCP short case surveys:** main focus of a short case in 0.5% of attempts at PACES Station 5, Skin.

## Record

There is *loss of fat* in the *face* and *upper half* of the body.* The prominent muscles and inframaxillary dimples give the face a characteristic masculine appearance. There is (may be) hypertrophy of fat† on the lower half of the body. This suggests the diagnosis of partial lipodystrophy, a condition which may be associated with *renal disease*.

---

Male to female ratio is 1:5.

Usually begins in children or young adults. A history of infection, frequently measles, has often been noted prior to onset.

*Retinitis pigmentosa* has been reported to occur in patients with partial lipodystrophy. Sometimes there is deterioration in vision. Eye examinations, including dark adaptation, electroretinography and electro-oculography, should be performed upon first presentation and periodically thereafter. Retinal angiogram may reveal dense deposits in the ciliary epithelial membrane.

## Association with renal disease

Patients with partial lipodystrophy often develop progressive mesangiocapillary glomerulonephritis and hypocomplementaemia. The prognosis depends on the severity of the renal disease.

## HIV-associated lipodystrophy syndrome

A curious combination of *lipohypertrophy* (buffalo hump and axial adiposity involving the neck, breast and abdomen) and *lipoatrophy* (face and proximal extremities) occurs in HIV-infected patients treated with a protease inhibitor. The pathogenesis is not clear though it is thought that it is not a drug toxicity effect and probably results from the substantial suppression of HIV in advanced patients. Carbohydrate tolerance is impaired in 16% and type 2 diabetes mellitus develops in 7% of these patients.

## Total lipoatrophy

Complete loss of subcutaneous fat* may occur in children or young adults with associated diabetes, which may be difficult to treat because of extreme insulin resistance. Severe hepatic dysfunction may occur, sometimes with terminal liver failure.

---

*The lack of fat may give the appearance of emaciation but closer inspection reveals that the muscles are not wasted, being well developed with clearly visible outlines beneath the skin. The whole appearance may give a false suggestion of virilization in females.

†The legs may be grossly fat and may give chronic discomfort.

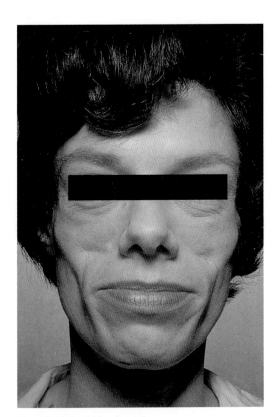

**Figure I5.40** Partial lipodystrophy.

# Case 45 | Fabry's disease

**Frequency in survey for 3rd edition:** did not occur in the initial small survey of PACES Station 5, Skin.

**Predicted frequency from older, more extensive MRCP short case surveys:** main focus of a short case in 0.5% of attempts at PACES Station 5, Skin.

### *Record*

The *skin* is *dry* and *lax*, and there is (may be) *arthropathy* of the *terminal interphalangeal joints*. There is conjunctival injection with dilated and tortuous vessels. There are groups of *darkish-red* and *black telangiectatic macules* and *papules* (*angiokeratomata*), about 2–4 mm in diameter, over the thigh and around the umbilicus in this young man. The skin is somewhat roughened because of *hyperkeratosis*, and the *papules do not fade on pressure*.

These lesions are characteristic of Anderson–Fabry disease. The patient also has *superficial corneal dystrophy* (cornea verticillata) which is almost specific to this condition.*

---

Most cases of Fabry's disease occur in males and the female carriers are mostly symptomless. The cutaneous eruption first appears at, or soon after, puberty. The prognosis is usually grave, with death occurring in the third or fourth decade from a *vascular accident* or *uraemia*. Patients are often mildly *hypertensive*, and there may be *varicose veins* and *stasis oedema*. *Albuminuria, haematuria* and *specific lipophages* may be seen in the urine resulting from lipid infiltration of the glomerular vessels. The homozygous males have attacks of excruciating unexplained pain in their hands, transient ischaemic attacks (TIAs) and myocardial infarction.

Fabry's disease is also called *Anderson–Fabry disease* and *angiokeratoma corporis diffusum*. It is a rare hereditary disorder (X-linked recessive) characterized by a *deficiency* of the *lysosomal hydrolase α-galactosidase A*, resulting in the progressive deposition of uncleaved, neutral glycosphingolipids in the small blood vessels of the skin and viscera. The characteristic cutaneous eruption (*angiokeratomata*) may be seen on the limbs, buttocks, around the umbilicus (periumbilical rosette), lower trunk and on the shaft of the penis.

---

*Superficial corneal dystrophy is frequently present both in affected patients and in female carriers. It is asymptomatic but of great diagnostic importance since the only other condition resembling it is *chloroquine keratopathy*.

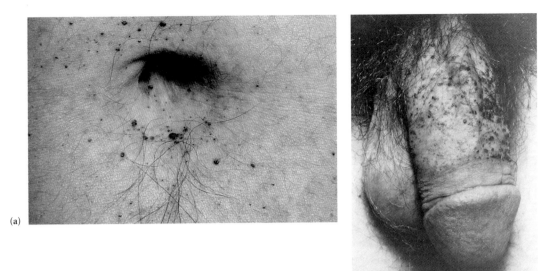

(a)

(b)

**Figure I5.41** Fabry's disease. (a) Groups of fleshy macules and papules (angiokeratomata) around the umbilicus (periumbilical rosette). (b) Macules and papules with fine, keratotic crusts.

# Case 46 | Reiter's syndrome/reactive arthritis/keratoderma blennorrhagica

**Frequency in survey for 3rd edition:** did not occur in the initial small survey of PACES Station 5, Skin.

**Predicted frequency from older, more extensive MRCP short case surveys:** main focus of a short case in 0.5% of attempts at PACES Station 5, Skin.

## *Record*

On the *soles* of this patient's feet* and on the *palms* of his hands* there are *brownish-red macules* (early lesions), some *vesicopustules* (further developed lesions) and some crusted limpet-like masses of yellowish-brown scales (late lesions). The appearances are those of keratoderma blennorrhagica.* If the patient has a history of *urethritis, conjunctivitis, arthritis, buccal ulceration* or *balanitis*, the combination would suggest the diagnosis of Reiter's syndrome (reactive arthritis).

---

The classic triad of Reiter's syndrome is urethritis, conjunctivitis and arthritis. However, this triad is only present in one-third of cases. It may manifest as a tetrad with the addition of buccal ulceration or balanitis; alternatively, only two of the cardinal features may be present. Classically, arthropathy develops within 1 month of urethritis or *cervicitis*. However, it may follow either a dysenteric (e.g. *Shigella*) or venereal infection. Its prevalence is higher in patients with AIDS, especially men who are HLA-B27 positive.

## Other features which may occur

Uveitis
Balanitis may progress to *balanitis circinata* (scaling red patches evolve encircling the glans penis and within the groin)
Plantar fasciitis

Sausage-shaped digit is a typical manifestation of the arthropathy
Sacroiliitis†
Ascending spinal disease†
Nail involvement with subungual pustules that progress to onycholysis and extensive subungual hyperkeratosis with erythema surrounding the nail
Plantar spurs on X-ray
Periosteal new bone formation on X-ray
Cardiac complications similar to ankylosing spondylitis as a late manifestation
HLA-B27 may predispose
Appears much less common in women but the sex distribution is difficult to define as the syndrome is diagnosed in women with difficulty because the urethritis and cervicitis are often clinically unapparent

---

*At times Reiter's syndrome may be confused with psoriasis as pustular psoriasis on the palms and soles looks like keratoderma blennorrhagica. Psoriatic arthropathy is also a seronegative arthropathy with an HLA-B27 association. In severely affected Reiter's disease, the skin lesions may occur anywhere on the body. The toes and fingernails in Reiter's may be affected with thickening, ridging and opacity of the nails. The skin lesions of psoriasis and Reiter's are often indistinguishable clinically or histologically. In Reiter's the lesions are typically confined to the palms and soles and the presence of urethritis, iritis or conjunctivitis, balanitis, asymptomatic lesions on the tongue and buccal mucosa, and occasionally diarrhoea should suggest the diagnosis.

†Occasionally the diagnosis of ankylosing spondylitis and Reiter's syndrome may be difficult to disentangle. The original urethritis of Reiter's may be forgotten or the patient with ankylosing spondylitis may happen to have an unrelated episode of urethritis.

*Formes frustes* of the syndrome (e.g. a woman with an inflammatory arthropathy of the knee, in association with HLA-B27, with or without uveitis, may have Reiter's syndrome)

High level of complement in synovial fluid (low level in rheumatoid arthritis)‡

About 80% of patients still have evidence of disease activity after 5 years

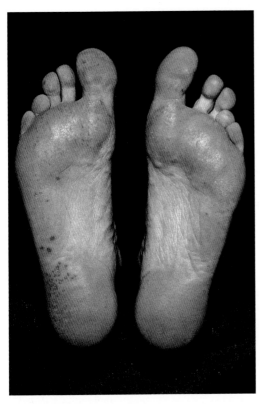

**Figure I5.42** Keratoderma blennorrhagica.

‡The high level in Reiter's reflects a non-specific inflammatory reaction whereas the low level in rheumatoid reflects immune complex disease.

# Case 47 | Malignant melanoma

**Frequency in survey for 3rd edition:** did not occur in the initial small survey of PACES Station 5, Skin.

**Predicted frequency from older, more extensive MRCP short case surveys:** main focus of a short case in 0.5% of attempts at PACES Station 5, Skin.

## Record

There is a *violaceous* (or darkish-brown, reddish-brown or black)* nodule with *variegated* appearance and *irregular edges* on this patient's leg (it may also be present on the trunk or face). It is about 8 mm in diameter (measure). The shape is asymmetrical (i.e. *one half is unlike the other half*), it is unevenly pigmented* and it is elevated above the level of the skin.† These features suggest the diagnosis of a malignant melanoma.

## Diagnosis

A seven-point check list is used when taking a history. It consists of three major (the first three) and four minor criteria: (i) change in size; (ii) change in shape; (iii) change in colour; (iv) diameter more than 7 mm; (v) the presence of inflammation; (vi) oozing or bleeding; and (vii) mild itch. When examining, the ABCDE mnemonic is used:

A = *asymmetry*
B = *irregular border*
C = *colour variation*, mottled, haphazard shades of brown, black, grey and white
D = *diameter > 6 mm*
E = *elevated* above the skin.

## Types of cutaneous malignant melanomata

*Superficial spreading melanoma*: this variety appears mostly in the fourth or fifth decade on the trunk (mostly males) or legs (mostly females). Starts as a brown macule with well-defined but irregular margins. It may be present for years before it becomes invasive. The majority of invasive melanomata are preceded by a superficial and radial growth phase, seen as an expanding, irregularly pigmented macule. It is then fol-

lowed by a horizontal growth phase. As it expands and becomes palpable, it is entering a vertical growth phase. Partial regression may cause central pigment loss while extension continues peripherally.

*Nodular melanoma*: this usually occurs in the fifth or sixth decade and the male : female ratio is 2:1. It presents as an elevated, dome-shaped or pedunculated nodule with reddish-brown colour. There may be a varied red central area, with only a faint brown ring of melanin peripherally. Ulceration and bleeding occur frequently. This variety of malignant melanoma is frequently confused with a vascular lesion because of its rapid growth and paucity of melanin pigment. It is a tumour in the vertical growth phase and carries a poor prognosis.

*Lentigo maligna melanoma*: this occurs equally in males and females on sun-exposed areas, and tends to occur in the elderly. Most lesions occur on the face, commonly on the upper cheek or forehead. Initially, it is a flat, brown, stain-like lesion. This flatness with loss of skin markings is useful in distinguishing it from such lesions as actinic or seborrhoeic keratoses.

*Acral lentiginous melanoma (palmoplantar malignant melanoma)*: this represents 10% of all melanomata on white skin but almost 50% of all melanomata in Japan.

---

*There is usually an array of colours in a gradation of red, grey or blue and mixed with brown or black. The colour may vary from one part to the other, and from the centre to the periphery, of the tumour.

†The prognosis of malignant melanoma depends on the thickness of the tumour (Breslow thickness).

The lesions are found mainly on the sole of the foot or the palm of the hand, and are characterized by a large, macular, lentiginous pigmented area around an invasive raised tumour.

*Desmoplastic melanoma*: a rare variant of melanoma which may complicate any of the above, but is most commonly seen in lentigo maligna.

A *pigmented naevus* without any inflammation or granulation is unlikely to be mistaken for a malignant melanoma. The most common errors occur with *benign pigmented lesions, seborrhoeic keratosis, haemangiomas* and pigmented *basal cell carcinoma*. In general, *any change* in a *pigmented lesion* in an adult between 20 and 40 years of age should be regarded with suspicion, and any *unusual pigmented lesion* on the lower leg of a female should be examined carefully. The correct diagnosis can be made on excision biopsy.

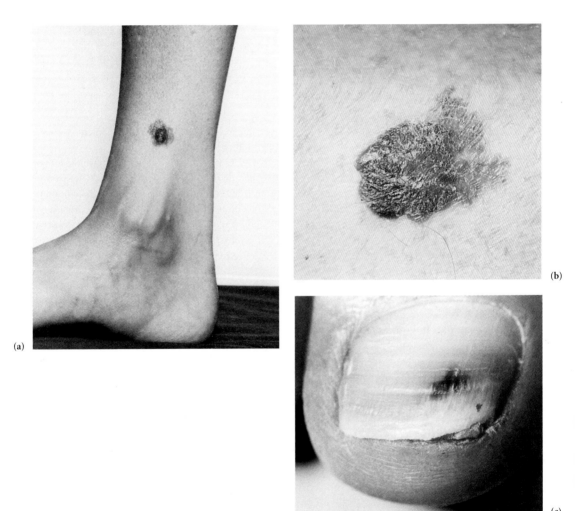

(a)

(b)

(c)

**Figure I5.43** Malignant melanoma. (a) Note the variegated appearance and irregular edge. (b) Irregular edge with variegated surface. (c) Subungual melanoma.

# Case 48 | Acanthosis nigricans

**Frequency in survey for 3rd edition**: did not occur in the initial small survey of PACES Station 5, Skin.

**Predicted frequency from older, more extensive MRCP short case surveys**: main focus of a short case in 0.5% of attempts at PACES Station 5, Skin.

## Record

There is a soft, *velvety*, verrucous, *brown* hyperpigmentation of the body folds, especially those of the *neck*, *axillae* and groin. The diagnosis is acanthosis nigricans.

### Patient aged under 40 years (most common)

Associated with:

*Obesity** and *insulin resistance* (high insulin levels; there may be glucose intolerance or frank diabetes, though glucose tolerance may be normal, depending on the severity of the insulin resistance; rarely insulin receptor antibodies are found)

*Endocrinopathies* (it is said that it may also be associated with a variety of endocrinopathies such as Cushing's disease, acromegaly, polycystic ovaries, hypothyroidism and hyperthyroidism)

May be familial.

### Patient aged over 40 years

May indicate *underlying malignancy* (usually adenocarcinoma, especially of the *stomach*, gastrointestinal tract and uterus; less commonly, ovary, prostate, breast and lung; rarely lymphomata. Involvement of the tongue and oral mucosa highly suggestive of malignancy. Acanthosis nigricans may appear before the malignant neoplasm becomes manifest in 20% of cases. May regress with response to therapy for the tumour and worsen again with reactivation of the tumour, raising the possibility of a humoral secretion from the tumour as the cause of the skin lesion).

---

## Other cutaneous manifestations of malignancy

### Non-genetic

*Paget's disease of the breast* (underlying intraductal mammary carcinoma)

*Stewart–Treves syndrome* (angiomatous, livid or dusky-red blebs and nodules exuding fluid, indicating lymphangiosarcoma as a complication of chronic lymphoedema, especially after radical mastectomy)

*Dermatomyositis* (heliotrope rash around eyes and backs of hands, proximal muscle weakness, but see

Footnote, Vol. 1, Station 3, CNS, Case 45). Neoplasm should be suspected if the dermatomyositis is unresponsive to conventional treatment, if there are atypical symptoms or the patient has a history of previous malignant disease.

*The Leser–Trélat sign* (sudden appearance and growth of multiple seborrhoeic keratoses in the elderly may be a sign of underlying malignancy; however, there is increasing doubt about this nowadays. Multiple seborrhoeic keratoses are very common in the elderly and one needs to exercise caution in

---

*Particular concern should be raised over the appearance of acanthosis nigricans in non-obese adults.

chasing internal malignancy in everyone with multiple seborrhoeic keratoses)

*Necrolytic migratory erythema* (associated with glucagonomata of the pancreas; gradually enlarging erythematous patches with central superficial blister formation, progressing to central crusting and healing; annular and figurate lesions result, with exudative, erosive and crusting areas, especially in the perineum, groin and perioral areas; similar lesions are seen in severe zinc deficiency)

*Bazex's syndrome* or *acrokeratosis paraneoplasia* (red to violaceous scaling, psoriatic-like patches confined to the bridge of the nose, fingers, toes and margins of the ear helices; nailfolds may be red, scaling and tender with nail grooving and onycholysis; associated with asymptomatic squamous cell carcinomata of the oral, pharyngeal, laryngeal and bronchial areas primarily in men; as the tumour progresses, the rash may spread and develop, and can become very widespread)

*Clubbing of the fingers* (see Station 5, Skin, Case 17)

*Hypertrophic pulmonary osteoarthropathy* (clubbing in association with subperiosteal new bone formation, shafts of long bones of extremities and digits; ankles, knees, wrists and hands may be painful and swollen†)

*Carcinoid* erythema (eventually the flush becomes permanent and telangiectasis and tortuous veins evolve in the flushed areas; see Vol. 1, Station 1, Abdominal, Case 18)

*Urticaria pigmentosa* (multiple reddish-brown or yellowish-brown macules showing Darier's sign, see Station 5, Skin, Case 40; may rarely be associated with myeloproliferative disorders: mast cell leukaemia, myelofibrosis, myeloid metaplasia, polycythaemia, granulocytic leukaemia)

*Bowen's disease* of the skin (multiple, discrete, red, scaling, flat to slightly raised patches that mimic eczematous or psoriatic patches, occurring in non-sun-exposed areas; each represents a squamous cell cancer [*in situ*]; may progress to invasive squamous carcinoma if not excised; relationship to internal malignancy controversial; particularly associated with long-term exposure to arsenicals – well water, insecticides, industrial chemicals)

## Genetic

*Gardner's syndrome* (multiple epidermoid and sebaceous cysts of the face and scalp, fibrous tissue tumours of the skin, osteomata of the membranous bones of the face and head, and polyps of the colon and rectum; all patients develop adenocarcinoma of the bowel before the seventh decade)

*Cowden's disease* (numerous hamartomata of the skin, mucous membranes and internal organs; present as keratotic, warty papules and nodules on the hands, arms and central face; may be papular, cobblestone lesions on the gingiva, palate, tongue and larynx; associated with malignant neoplasms of the breast and thyroid in a high percentage of cases)

*Torre's syndrome* (dominant; multiple sebaceous gland tumours, sebaceous adenomata, sebaceous hyperplasia, and basal cell cancers with sebaceous differentiation; present as yellowish or red papules and nodules; associated with cancers of the colon, duodenum, ampulla of Vater, uterus and genitourinary tract)

*MEN type IIb* (multiple whitish to pink papular mucosal neuromata studding the lips, tip of tongue and, less often, the buccal mucosa, gingivae, palate and pharynx; neuromata on the conjunctivae and corneas; associated with medullary carcinoma of the thyroid and phaeochromocytoma; see Footnote, Station 5, Endocrine, Case 4)

*Ataxia telangiectasia* (recessive; telangiectasia over the ears, eyelids, nose, butterfly facial area and conjunctivae in association with progressive cerebellar ataxia, profound immunological deficiency and sinopulmonary infections; lymphoma develops in 10%; other malignancies may occur less frequently)

*Wiscot–Aldrich syndrome* (skin changes similar to atopic dermatitis; there may be petechiae due to thrombocytopenia; widespread humoral and cell-mediated immunological abnormalities; 80% have lymphoma and 15% leukaemia by the age of 10 years)

*Neurofibromatosis* (dominant; *café-au-lait* spots, axillary freckles, multiple neurofibromata; 10% develop phaeochromocytoma by the age of 60; acoustic neuromata and neurofibrosarcomata are also associated; see Station 5, Skin, Case 2)

---

†Occasionally in hypertrophic pulmonary osteoarthropathy, cutaneous thickening of the forearms and legs leads to cylindrical enlargement of the limbs. Facial features may become coarse with deep facial furrows reminiscent of acromegaly. Deep confluent skin wrinkles may evolve over the forehead and scalp, these latter in association with the acromegalic features being termed *pachydermoperiostosis*.

*Peutz–Jeghers syndrome* (dominant; numerous brown-black macules on the lips, perioral regions and hands and feet; associated with hamartomatous polyps of the small bowel, stomach and, less commonly, colon; see Station 5, Skin, Case 26)

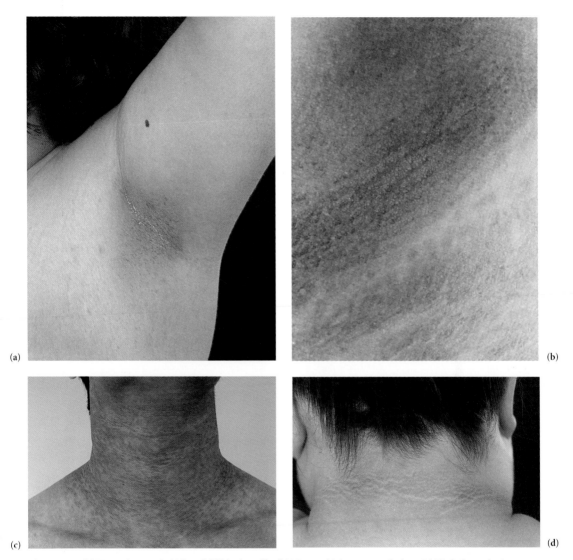

(a)     (b)

(c)     (d)

**Figure I5.44** (a) Hyperpigmented, thickened fold in the axilla. (b) Note multiple verrucous lesions. (c) Marked acanthosis nigricans of the neck, and (d) less marked acanthosis nigricans at the back of the neck in an overweight female.

# Case 49 | **Keratoacanthoma**

**Frequency in survey for 3rd edition**: did not occur in the initial small survey of PACES Station 5, Skin.

**Predicted frequency from older, more extensive MRCP short case surveys**: main focus of a short case in 0.5% of attempts at PACES Station 5, Skin.

## *Record*

There is (say where – usually *sun-exposed areas*, face, backs of hands and forearms) a *round*, firm, cherry-sized, *flesh-coloured, shouldered nodule* with a *central crater containing horny material*. It is well demarcated and seems to be stuck on the skin. The likely diagnosis is keratoacanthoma.

---

More common in males (3:1); also called *molluscum sebaceum*.

Microscopic appearance is so like a low-grade squamous cell carcinoma that differentiation is often impossible. In keratoacanthoma (self-healing epithelioma), however, the edge is regular, the surrounding skin is undamaged and the age of onset is younger (middle age) than in squamous cell carcinoma.

They begin as flesh-coloured papules that *rapidly grow* to full size (1–2.5 cm diameter) over a period of about 6 weeks, evolving a central keratin-filled crater. The lesions remain for about 6 or 8 weeks and then undergo spontaneous involution, leaving a depressed scar.

Although spontaneous regression occurs within a few months, lesions are best excised because the scars are unsightly and because of the difficulty of differentiation from squamous cell carcinoma.

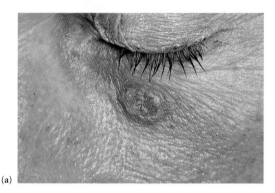

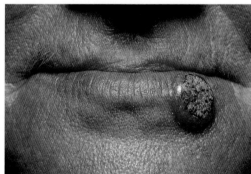

(a)

(b)

**Figure I5.45** (a,b) Keratoacanthoma.

# Case 50 | Pyoderma gangrenosum

**Frequency in survey for 3rd edition**: did not occur in the initial small survey of PACES Station 5, Skin.

**Predicted frequency from older, more extensive MRCP short case surveys**: main focus of a short case in 0.2% of attempts at PACES Station 5, Skin.

## *Record*

There are large *necrotic ulcers* with *ragged* bluish-red *overhanging edges* together with areas containing erythematous plaques with pustules. They are situated... (describe site – usually legs but can occur anywhere on the body).* The appearances are suggestive of pyoderma gangrenosum. The patient may have *ulcerative colitis* or Crohn's disease.

---

It may also be associated with *rheumatoid arthritis* and myeloproliferative disorders. Fifty per cent of patients with pyoderma gangrenosum have ulcerative colitis.† It is frequently an indicator of the severity of the disease. Healing often parallels that of the colitis and colectomy may allow this to be rapid. Systemic corticosteroids often help. The adjunctive use of minocycline may reduce corticosteroid requirements. The histopathological findings are non-specific.

## Other skin manifestations of inflammatory bowel disease

Aphthous ulcers
Angular stomatitis
Erythema nodosum
Perianal fistulae and abscess formation
Abdominal fistulae
Cutaneous vasculitis

Sweet's syndrome‡
Erythema multiforme

## Other causes of leg ulcers

Venous ulceration (only 50% have superficial varices)
Ischaemic arterial ulceration (usually anterior or lateral lower leg, pain, cold pulseless cyanotic feet, shiny hairless lower legs; see Station 5, Other, Case 3)
Diabetes mellitus (see Station 5, Locomotor, Case 4)
Vasculitis (rheumatoid arthritis or other connective tissue disorder)
Infection (acute pyogenic, tuberculous, syphilitic, cutaneous leishmaniasis)
Tumour (squamous cell, basal cell, melanoma)
Haematological (sickle cell, thalassaemia, acholuric jaundice, paroxysmal nocturnal haemoglobinuria)
Neurological (diabetes, tabes dorsalis, leprosy, syringomyelia)

---

*Pyoderma gangrenosum may occur as an example of *Koebner's phenomenon* in which skin diseases occur in scars or sites of trauma. It may rarely complicate surgical wounds and needs to be recognized and distinguished from infection as it responds to corticosteroids.
†Pyoderma gangrenosum can precede the onset of chronic inflammatory bowel disease.

‡Sweet's syndrome, also known as acute febrile neutrophilic dermatosis, is a skin disease characterized by the sudden onset of fever, leucocytosis, and tender, erythematous, well-demarcated papules and plaques that show dense infiltrates by neutrophil granulocytes on histological examination.

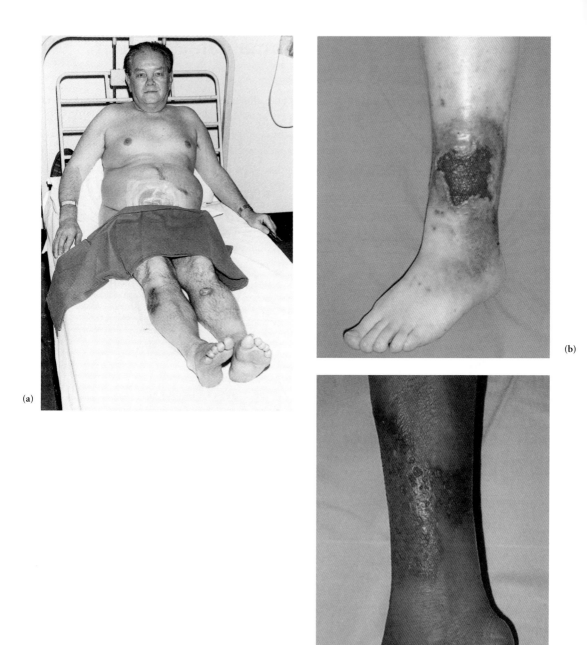

**Figure I5.46** (a) Note scarred abdomen and ileostomy bag of this patient with inflammatory bowel disease. Note pyoderma gangrenosum on the legs. (b,c) Pyoderma gangrenosum. Note ragged, bluish-red edge to the ulcer.

# Case 51 | Psychogenic/factitious

Psychogenic and factitious illnesses occur in everyday clinical practice and it would seem from the following anecdote and from those in Vol. 1, Station 3, Central Nervous System, Case 47, from our original, pre-PACES surveys, that it is possible that they have also occasionally appeared in the Membership!

## *Anecdote*

A candidate was shown a rash on a female patient. The rash was only in accessible areas and there were some bullae. He asked the patient a few questions and then gave a differential diagnosis of bullous lesions. The examiners asked if there were any other causes. There was a period of silence. One examiner said 'Yes, it seems to be in accessible areas'. The candidate asked the invigilating registrar later about the case and was told that 'Apparently no one yet knows the cause!'. In retrospect, the candidate feels it may have been a case of dermatitis artefacta.

For discussion, see Vol. 1, Station 3, Central Nervous System, Case 47.

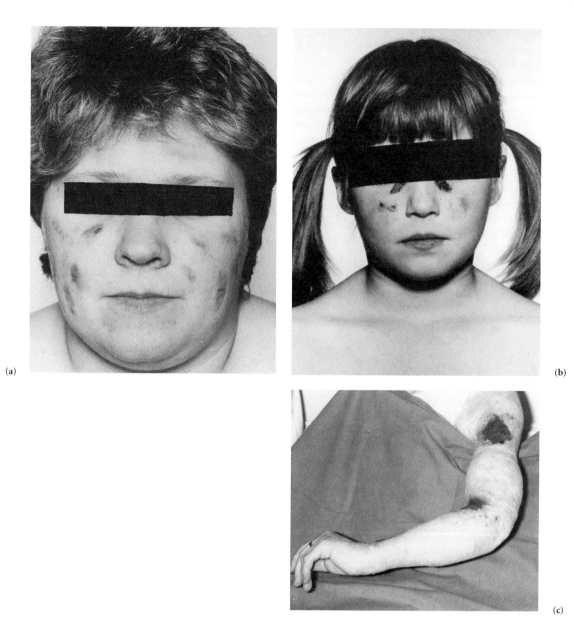

(a)

(b)

(c)

**Figure I5.47** (a,b) Dermatitis artefacta – self-inflicted lesions. (c) Self-inflicted ulcers.

# Station 5
# Locomotor

| Short case | Checked and updated as necessary for this edition by |
|---|---|
| **1** Rheumatoid arthritis | Dr David Carruthers* |
| **2** Psoriatic arthropathy | Dr David Carruthers* |
| **3** Systemic sclerosis/CREST syndrome | Dr David Carruthers* |
| **4** Diabetic foot/Charcot's joint | Dr Fran Game* |
| **5** Tophaceous gout | Dr David Carruthers* |
| **6** Ankylosing spondylitis | Dr David Carruthers* |
| **7** Paget's disease | Dr David Carruthers* |
| **8** Osteoarthritis | Dr David Carruthers* |
| **9** Marfan's syndrome | Dr David Carruthers* |
| **10** Vasculitis | Dr David Carruthers* |
| **11** Proximal myopathy | Dr Saiju Jacob* |
| **12** One leg shorter and smaller than the other | Dr David Carruthers* |
| **13** Radial nerve palsy | Dr Steve Sturman* |
| **14** Arthropathy associated with inflammatory bowel disease | Dr David Carruthers* and Dr Brian Cooper* |
| **15** Polymyositis | Dr David Carruthers* |
| **16** Systemic lupus erythematosus | Dr David Carruthers* |
| **17** Old rickets | Dr David Carruthers* |
| **18** Juvenile idiopathic arthritis | Dr David Carruthers* |
| **19** Swollen knee | Dr David Carruthers* |

*All suggested changes by these specialty advisors were considered by Dr Bob Ryder and were either accepted, edited, added to or rejected with Dr Ryder making the final editorial decision in every case.

Dr David Carruthers, Consultant Rheumatologist, City Hospital, Birmingham, UK
Dr Fran Game, Consultant Physician/Diabetologist, Royal Derby Hospital, Derby, UK
Dr Saiju Jacob, Consultant Neurologist, Queen Elizabeth Neurosciences Centre, Birmingham, UK
Dr Steve Sturman, Consultant Neurologist, City Hospital, Birmingham, UK
Dr Brian Cooper, Consultant Gastroenterologist, City Hospital, Birmingham, UK

# Case 1 | Rheumatoid arthritis

**Frequency in survey for 3rd edition:** main focus of a short case in 31% of attempts at PACES Station 5, Locomotor. Additional feature in some others, especially Station 1, Respiratory.

## *Record*

There is a symmetrical deforming polyarthropathy. There is spindling of the fingers due to soft tissue swelling at the proximal interphalangeal joints and metacarpophalangeal joints. The distal interphalangeal joints are spared. There is generalized wasting of the small muscles of the hand and use is restricted by weakness, deformity and pain. There are nodules at the elbow, over the extensor tendons and in the palm. There is ulnar deviation of the fingers (consequent upon subluxation and dislocation at the metacarpophalangeal [MCP] joints). There are arteritic lesions* in the nailfolds. (The presence of erythema, warmth, pain and swelling suggests that there is active inflammation at present.) The patient has rheumatoid arthritis.

---

The ratio of males to females is 1:3.

## Other features which may occur

'Swan neck' deformity (*hyperextension of proximal interphalangeal* joint with fixed flexion of MCP and distal interphalangeal joints)

Boutonnière's deformity (flexion deformity of proximal interphalangeal joint with *extension contracture of distal interphalangeal* and MCP joints)

Z deformity of the thumb

Triggering of the finger (flexor tendon nodule)

Palmar erythema

Iatrogenic Cushing's (?facies, thin atrophic skin, purpura)

Swollen or deformed knees (see Station 5, Locomotor, Case 19)

Elbow and shoulder disease

Cervical spine disease (upper cervical spine, especially atlantoaxial joint – subluxation can occur with *spinal cord compression*; a lateral X-ray centred on the odontoid peg with the neck in full flexion shows the distance from the odontoid to the anterior arch of the atlas as abnormal at more than 3 mm – general anaesthesia is dangerous and requires extreme care in neck handling)

Anaemia (five causes†)

Chest signs (?pleural effusions; fibrosing alveolitis‡)

Neurological signs (?peripheral neuropathy, mononeuritis multiplex, carpal tunnel syndrome, cervical myelopathy)

Eye signs (episcleritis, painful scleritis, scleromalacia perforans, cataracts due to chloroquine or steroids)

---

*As well as causing nailfold infarcts and chronic leg ulceration, the vasculitis (see Station 5, Skin, Case 27), which is immune complex induced and may affect small, medium or large vessels, may also lead to digital gangrene. A purpuric rash may occur due to capillaritis. Raynaud's phenomenon (see Station 5, Skin, Case 22) may occur. Pyoderma gangrenosum (see Station 5, Skin, Case 50) is a rare cause of ulceration.

†Five causes of anaemia in rheumatoid arthritis are:

1 Anaemia of chronic disease (normochromic normocytic)

2 Gastrointestinal bleeding related to non-steroidal anti-inflammatory drugs (NSAIDs)

3 Bone marrow suppression (indomethacin, methotrexate, sulphasalazine, gold)

4 Megaloblastic anaemia (folic acid deficiency or associated pernicious anaemia; see organ-specific autoimmune disease, Station 5, Skin, Case 8 and Footnote)

5 Felty's syndrome (see Vol. 1, Station 1, Abdominal, Case 23).

‡The lungs may also be affected in other ways. Rheumatoid nodules may occur in the lung fields on chest X-ray and in patients exposed to certain dusts, especially coal miners, nodules may be accompanied by massive fibrotic reactions (Caplan's syndrome). Obliterative bronchiolitis is a severe but rare complication which may be associated with penicillamine therapy.

Sjögren's syndrome (?dry eyes, dry mouth)

Felty's syndrome (?spleen; see Vol. 1, Station 1, Abdominal, Case 23)

Leg ulceration (vasculitic)*

Cardiac signs (pericarditis is present in up to 40% of patients at autopsy but is rarely apparent clinically; myocarditis, conduction defects and valvular incompetence are rare consequences of granulomatous infiltration)

Secondary amyloidosis (?proteinuria, hepatosplenomegaly, etc; see Footnote, Vol. 1, Station 1, Abdominal, Case 4)

Other autoimmune disorders (see Vol. 1, Station 3, CNS, Case 27; Station 5, Skin, Case 8 and Station 5, Endocrine, Case 5)

## Treatment

### General measures

Education (patient, carer)

Exercise (affected joints, general)

Physiotherapy (heat, cold or specific exercise techniques; joint protection in the form of splinting to prevent deformity during episodes of acute pain; advice regarding transference of load or alternative ways of performing)

Dietary advice (weight reduction, fish oil, fish supplements or evening primrose oil§)

### NSAIDs

These have no effect on long-term disability but provide symptom relief. Pure analgesic agents such as paracetamol can provide pain relief and reduce the dose requirements for NSAIDs. NSAIDs reduce prostaglandin synthesis. Prostaglandins have a major role in maintaining normal body function, particularly in the gastric and renal tracts and interference with these processes leads to a variety of adverse reactions (see below).¶ Patients need to try these drugs for up to 10 days before it can be decided whether they are likely to respond.

### Potential adverse effects of NSAIDs

Gastrointestinal (common; indigestion, ulceration, haemorrhage, perforation, small bowel ulceration, stomatitis)

Renal (common; increased serum creatinine, renal failure, oedema, worsening of heart failure, interstitial nephritis, papillary necrosis)

Neurological (uncommon; headache, dizziness, nausea)

Pulmonary (rare; asthma)

Dermatological (rare; erythema multiforme or variants [Stevens–Johnson syndrome, toxic epidermal necrolysis], bullous eruptions, fixed drug eruption, urticaria)

Haematological (rare; aplastic anaemia, haemolytic anaemia [mefenamic acid only])

Hepatic (rare; hepatitis)

Systemic (rare; anaphylactoid reactions)

### Disease-modifying antirheumatic drugs (DMARDs)

Early introduction of DMARD therapy significantly improves response rates. Early referral of patients from primary care is essential

Adverse events (require monitoring – Table I5.3) are relatively common, though the incidence of toxicity is probably similar to that with NSAIDs

Onset of effect is usually delayed (4 weeks to 3 months)

Various mechanisms of action

Can alter laboratory markers of inflammation such as C-reactive protein and erythrocyte sedimentation rate (ESR)

Meta-analyses of randomized controlled trials of DMARDs show a favourable benefit-to-toxicity ratio with low-dose methotrexate and antimalarial drugs. Hydroxychloroquine is significantly less effective than other DMARDs but is still better than placebo

Despite this efficacy, most patients commenced on a DMARD will not be taking that particular drug 3–4 years later because of adverse drug reactions or lack of efficacy. Some patients respond initially to these drugs but their disease subsequently reactivates

Most patients are given combinations of DMARDs

### DMARDs include:

Methotrexate (the most widely used and effective; given weekly – oral or intramuscular; associated with pulmonary disease in up to 10% of patients, including opportunistic infections and pneumonitis)

---

§Fish oil substitutes have enabled reduction or discontinuation of NSAIDs in some patients with rheumatoid arthritis.

¶The cyclo-oxygenase (COX) enzyme system involved in producing prostaglandins comprises two enzymes: (i) COX-1, which produces prostaglandins for normal body functions, and

(ii) an inducible enzyme, COX-2, which produces prostaglandins found at sites of tissue inflammation. NSAIDs selective for COX-2 seem to be associated with a lower incidence of gastric and renal side-effects.

**Table I5.3** Major adverse effects of antirheumatic drugs

| Drug | Recommended monitoring* |
|------|-------------------------|
| *Methotrexate*<br>Hepatic fibrosis, nausea, cytopenia, pneumonitis | Full blood count and liver function tests every 2 weeks, then 1–3 monthly; liver biopsy in at-risk patients |
| *Antimalarials*<br>Visual disturbances, retinopathy (occasionally)<br>Rash | Baseline check of visual acuity and annually thereafter using a reading chart. Ophthalmology review if patient develops visual symptoms |
| *Sulphasalazine*<br>Hepatic reactions, nausea, dizziness, rash, discoloration of urine and sweat, oligospermia | Full blood count and liver function tests fortnightly for 3 months, then 3 monthly |
| *Leflunomide*<br>Hepatitis, myelosuppression, rash, diarrhoea | Full blood count and liver function tests every 2 weeks initially, then 2 monthly |
| *Gold*<br>Rash, eosinophilia, cytopenia, proteinuria, diarrhoea (oral gold) | Intramuscular: full blood count and urinalysis before each injection<br>Beware coadministration of ACE inhibitors<br>Oral: full blood count and urinalysis every 2 weeks to monthly |
| *D-penicillamine*<br>Rash, proteinuria, thrombocytopenia<br>Taste disturbances | Full blood count and urinalysis every 2 weeks on initiating or changing dose, then monthly full blood count and urinalysis |
| *Corticosteroids*<br>Weight gain, bruising, fluid retention, susceptibility to infection, diabetes<br>Osteoporosis | Consider bone density measurement in line with national guidelines |
| *Azathioprine*<br>Oncogenicity<br>Cytopenia | Full blood count and liver function tests every 1–2 weeks initially, then 3 monthly |
| *Cyclosporin*<br>Renal impairment<br>Hypertension | Full blood count, serum creatinine level and blood pressure measurement weekly, then every 2–4 weeks with maintenance dose |
| *Cyclophosphamide*<br>Interstitial nephritis, haemorrhagic cystitis<br>Oncogenicity | Full blood count and urinalysis monthly after initial weekly tests |

*None of these monitoring strategies has been tested for cost-effectiveness.
ACE, angiotensin-converting enzyme.

Sulphasalazine (has been shown to slow joint erosions)

Leflunomide (similar efficacy to sulphasalazine but more rapid onset of action)

Chloroquine and hydroxychloroquine (3–4 months before steady-state concentrations and maximal efficacy are achieved)

Gold complexes (suppresses disease activity in many patients; intramuscular gold is more effective than oral; can be used over long periods of time)

Penicillamine (now seldom used but effective in some patients; has multiple mechanisms of action)

Other DMARDs (such as azathioprine, cyclophosphamide, chlorambucil and cyclosporin) can be tried in refractory patients

Combinations of DMARDs (may prove beneficial in some patients; leflunomide and methotrexate or methotrexate and sulphasalazine have been shown to be superior to methotrexate alone)

### Corticosteroids
**Features of corticosteroid therapy in rheumatoid arthritis include:**

Still commonly used

Dose of 7.5 mg/day effective in slowing the rate of erosion

May be used as:

Continuous oral background therapy (up to 7.5 mg daily)

Short courses of a rapidly decreasing dose for disease flares

Intra-articular injections into inflamed joints

Intravenous pulse therapy during a flare-up or as induction treatment at the time of commencement of DMARDs

Intramuscular injection during a flare-up

High doses should be given only to patients who demonstrate severe systemic features and/or vasculitis

Low-dose background therapy may be beneficial in maintaining mobility in patients with active disease on other DMARDs

Variety of long-term side-effects (see Station 5, Endocrine, Case 6)

Antiosteoporotic therapies (calcium supplements, 1,25-dihydrocholecalciferol or bisphosphonates) should be considered in all patients on long-term (>3 months) therapy

A slow dose reduction (1 mg every month) should be tried in patients in whom disease is relatively quiescent or in whom the side-effects are becoming a problem

### Biological agents (Table I5.4)

**Include molecules targeted at:**

Proinflammatory cytokines (e.g. tumour necrosis factor [TNF]-α, interleukin [IL]-6, IL-1)

Cells involved in inflammation (e.g. B-cells)

Clinical trials of these agents show a dramatic improvement in symptoms and apparent halting of disease progression, especially when used in combination with methotrexate

**Table I5.4** Biological agents

| Biological agent | Notes |
|---|---|
| *TNF-α inhibition* | |
| Infliximab | Chimeric molecule (mouse-human monoclonal antibody) |
| | 8-weekly infusion |
| Etanercept | Recombinant TNF receptor:Fc fusion protein |
| | Weekly subcutaneous injection |
| Adalimumab | Recombinant human TNF-α inhibitor |
| | 2-weekly subcutaneous injection |
| *IL-6 inhibition* | |
| Tocilizumab | Humanized monoclonal antibody against IL-6R |
| | 4-weekly infusion |
| *IL-1 inhibition* | |
| Anakinra | Recombinant IL-1 receptor antagonist |
| | Daily subcutaneous injection (less effective than TNF-α inhibition) |
| *B-cell depletion* | |
| Rituximab | Anti-CD20 chimeric monoclonal antibody |
| | 2 infusions 2 weeks apart then re-treat when disease flares (9–12 months on average) |

IL, interleukin; TNF, tumour necrosis factor.

TNF-α inhibitors are NICE approved after failure of two DMARDs, including methotrexate, over a 6-month period. Those intolerant of or who fail TNF-α inhibition can receive rituximab

Nevertheless there is caution because of the potential for long-term side-effects, possibly associated with immunosuppression, and the cost of therapy. TB reactivation has been reported with TNF inhibitors

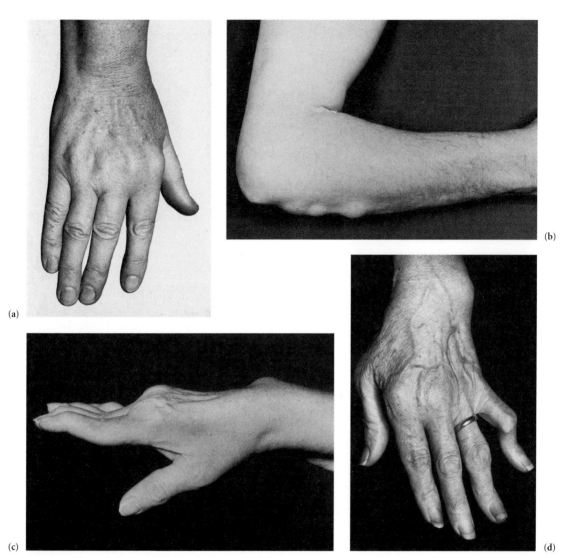

**Figure I5.48** (a) Early changes: swelling of the MCP joints, slight ulnar deviation. (b) Rheumatoid nodules. (c) 'Swan neck' deformity. (d) Boutonnière deformity.

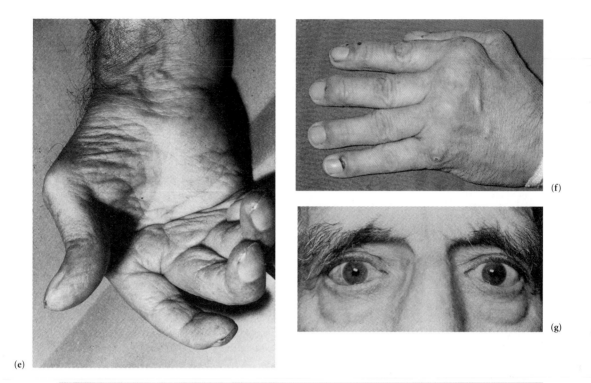

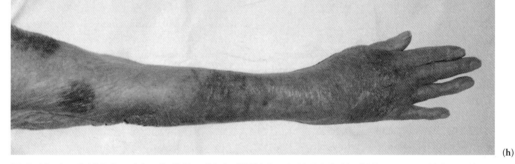

**Figure I5.48** (*Continued*) (e) Z-shaped thumb. (f) Vasculitis (nailfold infarcts). (g) Episcleritis. (h) Purpura: steroid therapy for rheumatoid arthritis.

# Case 2 | Psoriatic arthropathy

**Frequency in survey for 3rd edition:** main focus of a short case in 12% of attempts at PACES Station 5, Locomotor. Additional feature in a further 1%.

**Survey note:** patients had arthropathy and/or skin lesions. Questions such as treatment were only occasionally asked.

## Record

There is an *asymmetrical arthropathy* involving mainly the *distal interphalangeal joints*. There is *pitting* of the fingernails and *onycholysis*. Some of the nail plates (say which) are thickened and there is a thick scale (*hyperkeratosis*) under them. There are patches of psoriasis at the *elbows*. The plaques are circular with well-defined edges and they are *red* with a *silvery scaly* surface. The patient has psoriatic arthropathy.

---

Psoriatic arthropathy (even if severe) can occur with minimal skin involvement.* If there is no obvious psoriasis at the elbows, the following areas should particularly be checked for skin lesions.

1 Extensor aspects
2 Scalp
3 Behind the ears
4 In the navel

### Other forms of psoriatic arthropathy

Arthritis mutilans
Arthritis clinically indistinguishable from rheumatoid arthritis but consistently seronegative
Asymmetrical oligo- or monoarthropathy
Ankylosing spondylitis occurring alone or in conjunction with any of the other forms

### Treatment

Treatments of the skin lesions include sunlight, ultraviolet (UV) light, coal tar, dithranol, local steroids, calcipotriol and psoralen and UVA light (PUVA). Systemic treatment with acitretin (a retinoid) or antimetabolites (methotrexate, azathioprine, hydroxyurea), because of their side-effects, should be reserved for severe widespread disease unresponsive to topical measures. Analgesic anti-inflammatory agents are used for the pain of the arthropathy. Sulphasalazine and methotrexate are becoming established as effective agents for the treatment of psoriatic arthropathy. Gold and penicillamine may be useful but few controlled studies have been done. Cyclosporin may also have a place in refractory disease. Choroquine is contraindicated as it may exacerbate the skin lesions (exfoliative dermatitis). Intra-articular steroids are useful for a single inflamed troublesome joint. TNF-α inhibitors can be used for more severe skin and/or joint disease.

### Incidence

One to 5% of Caucasians in north western Europe and USA. Uncommon among Japanese, North American Indians and Afro-Americans.

---

*There is no evidence of a link between the activity of the skin lesions and the arthropathy.

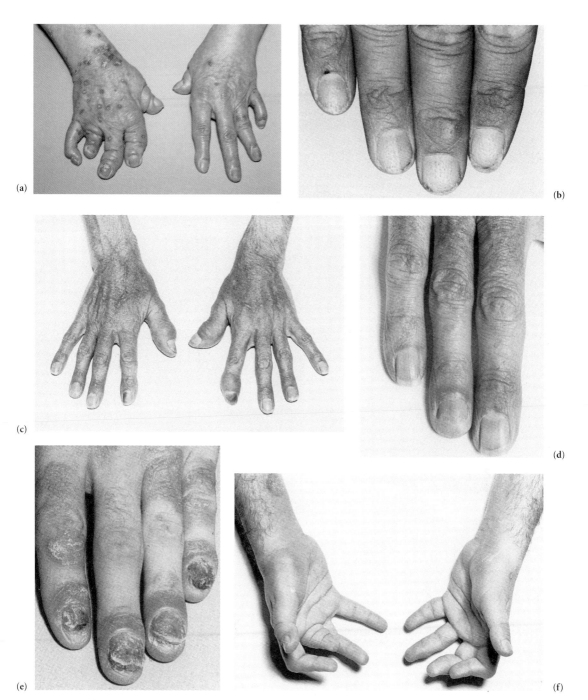

**Figure I5.49** (a) Psoriasis and arthritis mutilans. Note the telescoping of the thumbs and the fingers on the right. (b) Nail pitting. (c) Distal interphalangeal arthropathy and nail changes. (d) Onycholysis. (e) Advanced nail changes (note the psoriatic plaques and hyperkeratosis of the nail beds). (f) Note the typical plaque on the forearm and telescopic middle finger. (*Continued*)

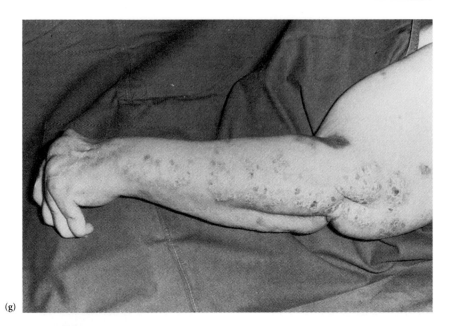

(g)

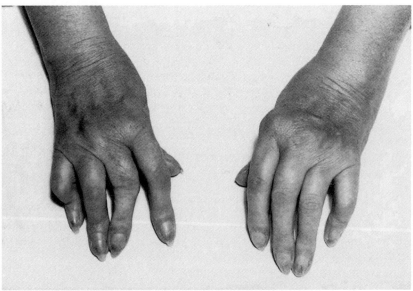

(h)

**Figure I5.49** (*Continued*) (g,h) Indistinguishable from rheumatoid arthritis. Note plaques in (g) and nails in (h).

# Case 3 | Systemic sclerosis/CREST syndrome

**Frequency in survey for 3rd edition:** main focus of a short case in 12% of attempts at PACES Station 5, Locomotor. Additional feature in a further 1%.

## *Record*

The *skin* over the *fingers* and *face* (of this middle-aged female) is *smooth, shiny* and *tight*. There is *sclerodactyly*, the *nails* are *atrophic* and there is evidence of *Raynaud's phenomenon* (see Station 5, Skin, Case 22). There is atrophy of the soft tissues at the ends of the fingers. There is *telangiectasia* of the face and pigmentation. There are nodules of *calcinosis*\* palpable in some of the fingers. The diagnosis is systemic sclerosis or CREST† syndrome.

---

## Other signs which may be present

Skin ulcers

Vitiligo (see Station 5, Skin, Case 8)

Dry eyes and dry mouth (Sjögren's syndrome; see Station 5, Other, Case 1)

Dyspnoea or inspiratory crackles (diffuse interstitial fibrosis‡ – decreased pulmonary diffusion capacity is the first sign; overspill pneumonitis may also occur)

## Other systems which may be involved

Oesophagus (dysphagia or other oesophageal symptoms are present in 45–60%; oesophageal manometry is abnormal and shows diminished peristalsis in 90%)

Kidney (renal failure occurs in 20% – it is late but often fatal; it may be associated with malignant hypertension which tends to be responsive to ACE inhibitors but is otherwise resistant to therapy)

Heart (pericardial effusion is not an uncommon finding if careful echocardiography is performed; cardiomyopathy may occur but is rare)

Musculoskeletal (inflammatory arthritis or myositis – their presence raises the possibility of mixed connective tissue disease§ and therefore increased likelihood of improvement with steroid therapy)

Intestine (rarely hypomotility with a dilated second part of the duodenum leads to bacterial overgrowth, which in turn leads to steatorrhoea and malabsorption; wide-mouthed colonic diverticuli and the rare pneumatosis cystoides are other abnormalities which may occur)

Liver (may be associated with primary biliary cirrhosis; see Vol. 1, Station 1, Abdominal, Case 17)

## Treatment

No drug or treatment has proved safe and effective in altering the underlying disease process in scleroderma.

Management includes:

General – education, counselling and family support

Contractures – exercises and lubricants may limit

---

\*If there is diffuse deposition of calcium in subcutaneous tissue in the presence of acrosclerosis, this is termed the Thibierge–Weissenbach syndrome.

†CREST is the association of calcinosis, Raynaud's, oesophageal involvement, sclerodactyly and telangiectasia. It may be a variant of systemic sclerosis associated with a more benign prognosis.

‡Pulmonary hypertension may develop independent of parenchymal changes, suggesting primary pulmonary vessel disease. Renal failure has now been replaced by pulmonary complications as the major cause of death in systemic sclerosis. Pleural effusions, pulmonary hypertension, interstitial lung disease, progressive

pulmonary fibrosis and obstructive airways disease all contribute to respiratory failure. Pulmonary hypertension can develop suddenly; all patients should be followed closely for the changes in $P_2$. The appearance of tricuspid regurgitation is evidence of established pulmonary hypertension. Endothelin receptor antagonists can now be used to treat pulmonary hypertension.

§Mixed connective tissue disease is a clinical overlap between systemic sclerosis, systemic lupus erythematosus (SLE) and polymyositis. The serum has a high titre of antiribonuclear protein antibody. The fluorescent antinuclear antibodies are typically distributed in a speckled pattern.

Raynaud's – hand warmers, vasodilators both oral (calcium channel blockers, ACE inhibitors) and parenteral (prostacyclin analogues and calcitonin gene-related peptide). In severe cases lumbar and digital sympathectomy may help

Oesophageal symptoms – proton pump inhibitors and prokinetic drugs (cisapride)

Malabsorption – low-residue diets, nutritional supplements, rotational antibiotics

Renal – intensive hypertensive control (with either ACE inhibitors or calcium antagonists). High-dose corticosteroids should be avoided and may precipitate renal crisis

Pulmonary vascular disease – vasodilators

Fibrotic process – D-penicillamine and interferon-γ are suggested therapies. The treatment of lung fibrosis has paralleled that of cryptogenic fibrosing alveolitis and has been a mixture of corticosteroids and cyclophosphamide or azathioprine

The efficacy of these treatments remains to be proven in placebo-controlled trials.

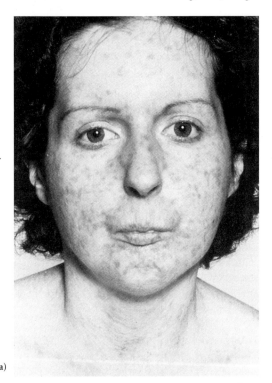

(a)

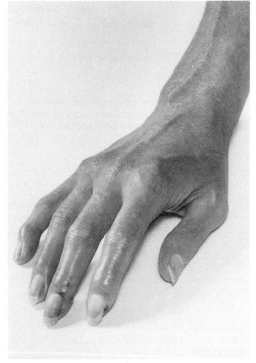

(b)

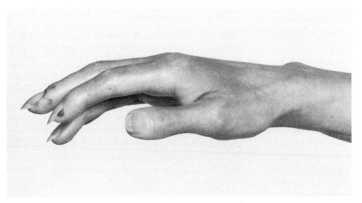

(c)

**Figure I5.50** (a) Perioral tethering with pseudorhagades. (b) Tight, shiny, adherent skin and vasculitis. (c) Atrophy of the finger pulps.

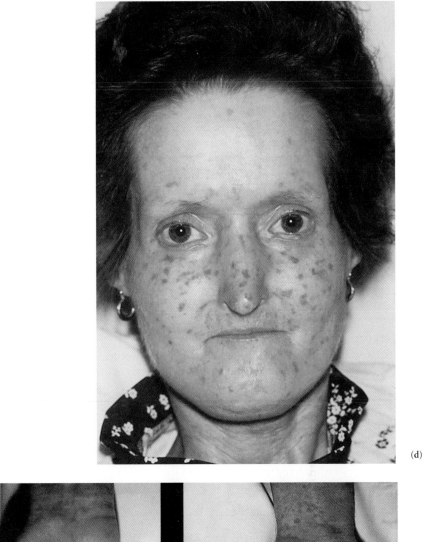

(d)

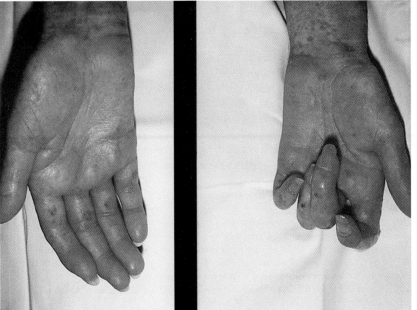

(e)

**Figure I5.50** (*Continued*) (d,e) The face and hands of the same patient, note the tight, shiny skin, pinched nose and telangiectasia.

# Case 4 | Diabetic foot/Charcot's joint

**Frequency in survey for 3rd edition:** main focus of a short case in 7% of attempts at PACES Station 5, Locomotor. Additional feature in a further 2%, especially Station 3, CNS.

## Record 1

There is an *ulcer* on the sole of the R/L foot (most commonly at the site of the pressure point under the head of the first metatarsal) and two of the toes have previously been amputated. There is thick *callous\** formation over the pressure points of the feet, and the normal concavity of the transverse arch at the head of the metatarsals is lost. There is *loss of sensation* to light touch, vibration and pinprick in a *stocking distribution*. The foot pulses are not palpable\* and there is *loss of hair* on the lower legs which are *shiny*.

   This patient has *peripheral neuropathy*, a *neuropathic ulcer* on the sole of his foot and evidence of *peripheral vascular disease*. It is likely that he has underlying diabetes mellitus (?fundi).

## Record 2

As relevant from *record* 1, plus the ankle joint† is greatly *deformed* and (may be) *swollen*.‡ If the foot were examined there would be loud *crepitus* accompanying *movement,* which would be of *abnormal range*. (**However, in the exam, the swollen Charcot foot should *not* be manipulated as the crepitus would be the sound of you breaking bones!**)

   This is a Charcot's joint (neuropathic arthropathy – gross osteoarthrosis and new bone formation from repeated minor trauma without the normal protective responses which accompany pain sensation; the joint is painlessly destroyed).

---

**Factors which may contribute to the production of diabetic foot lesions**

Injury – always a provocative factor

Neuropathy – trivial injury is not noticed

Consequent formation of callosities at repeatedly traumatized pressure points

Small vessel disease

Large vessel disease producing ischaemia and gangrene of the foot

Increased susceptibility to infection

Maldistributed pressure and foot deformity leading to increased likelihood of friction and trauma

   From the list of the other causes of peripheral neuropathy (see Vol. 1, Station 3, CNS, Case 1), **neuropathic ulcers** are particularly associated with:

1 Tabes dorsalis (?facies, pupils, etc; see Vol. 1, Station 5, CNS, Case 50)

2 Leprosy

---

\*NB: in the predominantly neuropathic foot the pulses may be present or even bounding, and the veins may be prominent (Ward's sign). Autonomic denervation opens up arteriovenous shunts; as a consequence, blood passes down the arteries, through the shunts and back up the veins, missing out the nutrient capillaries on the way – this contributes to the poor healing. The above short case combines features of neuropathic and

ischaemic aetiologies. In practice, cases are often predominantly one or the other. In severe arterial disease thick callous is unlikely, the feet are cold, pulseless and the skin is usually thin.

†Another area that can be affected is the mid-foot – typical rocker bottom foot.

‡Not swollen in chronic Charcot.

3 Porphyria (?vesicles, crusts; see Station 5, Skin, Case 37)

4 Amyloidosis

5 Progressive sensory neuropathy (both familial and cryptogenic) and rarely as a late manifestation of

6 Charcot–Marie–Tooth disease (distal muscle wasting, pes cavus, etc; see Vol. 1, Station 5, CNS, Case 4).

## Main causes of a Charcot's joint

Diabetes mellitus (toes – common; mid-foot – more common; ankles – rare)

Tabes dorsalis (especially hip and knee; ?facies, pupils, etc.)

Syringomyelia (elbow and shoulder; ?Horner's, wasted hand muscles, dissociated sensory loss, etc; see Vol. 1, Station 5, CNS, Case 29)

Leprosy (important on a worldwide basis)

Other rare causes include yaws, progressive sensory neuropathy (familial and cryptogenic), other hereditary neuropathies (e.g. Charcot–Marie–Tooth) and neurofibromatosis (pressure on sensory nerve roots), though any cause of loss of sensation in a joint may render it susceptible to the development of a neuropathic arthropathy.

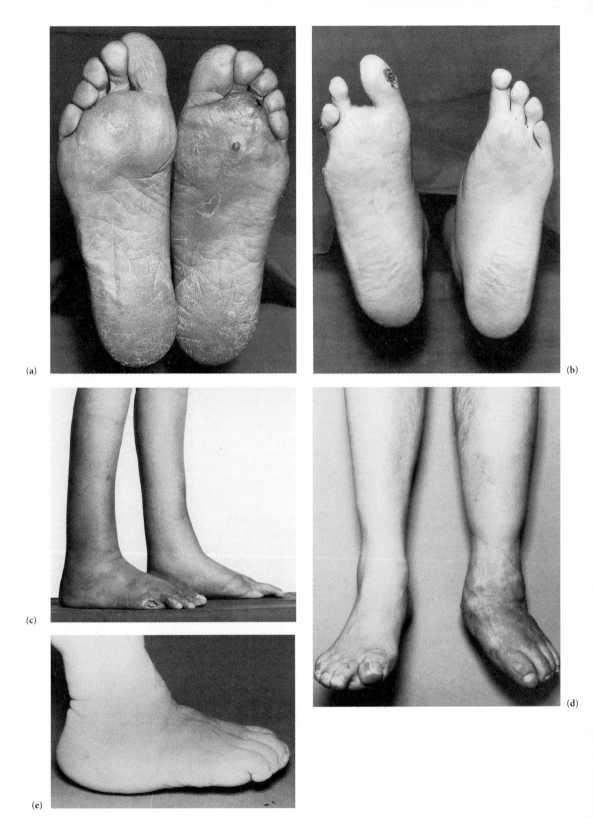

**Figure I5.51** (a–c) Note ulcers, missing digits, hyperkeratinization over pressure areas and loss of arches. (d,e) Charcot's ankle.

# Case 5 | Tophaceous gout

**Frequency in survey for 3rd edition:** main focus of a short case in 6% of attempts at PACES Station 5, Locomotor.

## Record

There is *asymmetrical swelling* affecting the *small joints* of the *hands* and feet with *tophi* formation (in the periarticular tissues). These joints are (occasionally) severely *deformed*. There are tophi on the *helix* of the *ear* and in some of the tendon sheaths (especially the ulnar surface of the forearm, olecranon bursa, Achilles tendon and other pressure points). This patient has chronic tophaceous gout.

---

Chronic tophaceous gout results from recurrent acute attacks. Tophus formation is proportional to the severity and duration of the disease. However, patients with severe tophaceous disease appear to have milder and less frequent acute attacks than non-tophaceous patients. Large tophi may have areas of necrotic skin overlying them and may exude chalky or pasty material containing monosodium urate crystals. Sinuses may form. Tophi may resolve slowly with effective treatment of hyperuricaemia. Effective antihyperuricaemic therapy has reduced the incidence and severity of the tophaceous disease. A major complication is renal disease (urolithiasis, urate nephropathy). Carpal tunnel syndrome may occur.

**Associations** include obesity, type IV hyperlipidaemia and hypertension. These may be the cause of an association which has also been recognized between gout and two other conditions – diabetes mellitus and ischaemic heart disease.

**Secondary hyperuricaemia** may occur in many situations including:
Drugs – diuretics (especially thiazides), ethambutol, nicotinic acid, cyclosporin
Myeloproliferative and lymphoproliferative disorders (and other conditions with increased turnover of preformed purines)
Chronic renal failure
Alcoholism
Obesity.

## Treatment

### Acute attack

Non-steroidal anti-inflammatory drugs* (oral or suppository) or oral colchicine (effective but can cause nausea, diarrhoea or abdominal pain) are the first-line treatments. Intra-articular injection of a corticosteroid or a short course of systemic corticosteroids may be used if necessary. NSAIDs should be avoided in patients with renal insufficiency, recent gastrointestinal (GI) ulceration/bleeding or severe heart failure.

Allopurinol or uricosuric (probenecid, sulphinpyrazone) drugs should not be started until the acute attack has settled for 2–3 weeks because they can prolong the acute attack or trigger further episodes.

### Long-term treatment

Prolonged administration of drugs that lower the serum urate level should be considered following complete resolution of the acute attack when:
there is associated renal disease
there have been recurrent attacks (>3/year)
there is evidence of tophi or chronic gouty arthritis
the patient is young with a high serum uric acid and a family history of renal or heart disease
normal levels of serum uric acid cannot be achieved by lifestyle modifications (gradual weight loss and restriction of intake of alcohol and food with a high purine content).

*Avoid aspirin as it causes uric acid retention unless given in very high doses.

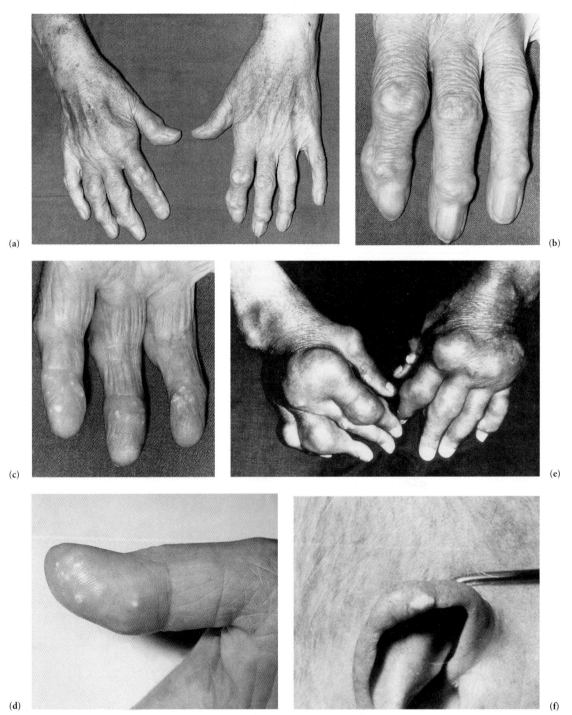

**Figure I5.52** (a–d) Gouty tophi and arthropathy. (e) An extreme case of tophaceous gout. (f) A tophus on the helix of the ear.

# Case 6 | Ankylosing spondylitis

**Frequency in survey for 3rd edition:** main focus of a short case in 4% of attempts at PACES Station 5, Locomotor.

**Survey note:** in the original, pre-PACES, survey, candidates were asked to examine the chest, the back, the neck, to watch the patient walk or to watch the patient 'look at the ceiling'. One-third of candidates made the point that the diagnosis was not apparent with the patient lying down.

## Record

There is (in this male patient) *loss of lumbar lordosis* and *fixed kyphosis* which is compensated for by extension of the cervical spine (to attempt to keep the visual axis horizontal) producing a *stooped*, 'question mark' posture. When I ask the patient to turn his head to look to the side his whole body turns as a block (the spine being rigid with little movement). *Chest expansion* is *reduced*; the patient breathes by increased diaphragmatic excursion which is the cause of the *prominent abdomen*.

The diagnosis is ankylosing spondylitis. (If allowed, look at the *eyes* – iritis; listen to the *heart* – aortic incompetence; and examine the *chest* – apical fibrosis).

---

Ratio of males to females is 8:1.

## Complications and extra-articular manifestations

Iritis – 30% (acute, deep aching pain, redness, photophobia, miosis, sluggish pupillary reflex, circumcorneal conjunctival injection; may result in synechiae or cataracts)

Aortitis – 4% (?collapsing pulse and early diastolic murmur of aortic incompetence; ascending aortic aneurysm)

Apical fibrosis – rare (?apical inspiratory crackles; probably secondary to diminished apical ventilation; there may be calcification and cavitation; may get secondary aspergillus infection)

Cardiac conduction defects – 10% (usually atrioventricular [AV] block; other cardiac abnormalities may occur – pericarditis and cardiomyopathy)

Neurological (atlantoaxial dislocation or traumatic fracture of a rigid spine may injure the spinal cord – tetra/paraplegia; involvement of the sacral nerves at the sacroiliac joints may cause sciatica; rarely cauda equina involvement can cause urinary or rectal sphincter incompetence)

Secondary amyloidosis (kidneys, adrenals, liver – ?hepatomegaly)

## Other features

There is a strong (87%) association with HLA-B27. There is a familial tendency; 50% of relatives are HLA-B27 and 9% have sacroiliitis, which may be symptomless.* Ankylosing spondylitis usually starts before the age of 45.† It may present as an asymmetrical peripheral arthritis usually of large, weight-bearing joints; the small joints of the hands and feet are only rarely involved.‡ It commonly presents with low back pain:

*Ankylosing spondylitis* – pain worse on waking, eases with exercise

Compared with

*Mechanical back pain* – no pain on waking; pain brought on by exercise.

---

*The disease is more severe in sporadic cases (about 80%) than in the familial form (20%). Sibling pairs concordant for the disease tend to have disease of comparable severity.

†In the early stages, loss of lateral flexion of the lumbar spine is usually the first sign of spinal involvement, followed by loss of lumbar lordosis.

‡Enthesitis may occur (plantar fasciitis, Achilles tendinitis).

In the 'heels, hips, occiput' test the patient is asked to demonstrate that he can put all three against a wall at once. (The patient with ankylosing spondylitis fails this test.) *Schober's test* examines lumbar mobility. While the patient stands upright with heels together, a mark is made in the mid-line at the level of the sacral dimples. Two additional marks are made 10 cm above and 5 cm below this first mark. On full forward flexion, the distance between the upper and lower mark should increase by >5 cm. Movement of <5 cm indicates decreased lumbar spine movement.

## Treatment

Physiotherapy with regular exercise regime
NSAIDs
Methotrexate for peripheral not axial disease
TNF-α inhibitors for severe disease – improve stiffness and pain

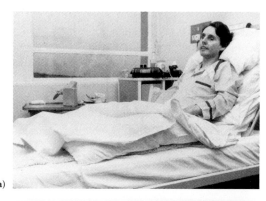

(a)

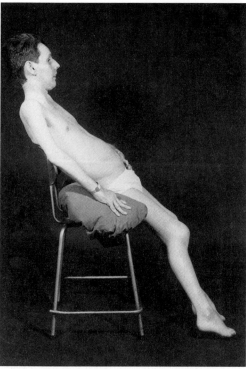

(b)

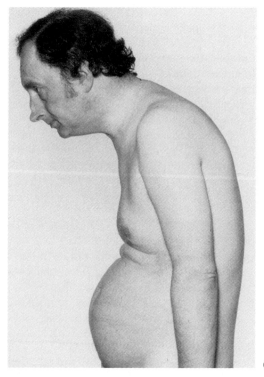

(c)

**Figure I5.53** (a) The ankylosing spondylitis is less obvious when reclining in bed. (b) In the same patient as (a), a rigid and immobile spine was revealed by his attempt at sitting up (note the generalized involvement of the joints in this severe case). (c) Patient attempting to look straight ahead (note the kyphosis, loss of lumbar lordosis and protuberant abdomen).

# Case 7 | Paget's disease

**Frequency in survey for 3rd edition:** did not occur in the initial small survey of PACES Station 5, Locomotor.

**Predicted frequency from older, more extensive MRCP short case surveys:** main focus of a short case in 23% of attempts at PACES Station 5, Locomotor.

## *Record*

There is (in this elderly patient) *enlargement* of the *skull*. There is also *bowing* of the R/L *tibia* (or femur) which is *warmer* (due to increased vascularity) than the other and the patient is (may be) *kyphotic* (vertebral involvement may lead to *loss of height* and kyphosis from disc degeneration and vertebral collapse).

The diagnosis is Paget's disease. (There may be evidence of complications, e.g. a *hearing aid* – see below.)

---

Paget's disease occurs in 3% (autopsy series) of the population over the age of 40, rising to 10% over the age of 70, though it is not clinically important in the vast majority of these. Though it is often asymptomatic, patients may have symptoms such as bone pain, headaches, tinnitus and vertigo. Serum *alkaline phosphatase* and *urinary hydroxyproline* are elevated except sometimes in very early disease. Serum calcium and phosphate concentrations are usually normal in mobilized patients but may be increased or decreased. Urinary calcium and hydroxyproline rise in immobilized patients. High serum uric acid and ESR may also occur. Genetic factors play an important role in pathogenesis of Paget's, with mutated genes identified. Environmental factors such as viruses (e.g. paramyxoviruses) may also play a role, but none has been identified yet. Specific therapies which can be considered if indicated* include bisphosphonates and α-calcitonin.

### Complications

Progressive closure of skull foramina may lead to:
1 Deafness (also results from pagetic involvement of the ossicles†)

2 Optic atrophy‡
3 Basilar invagination (platybasia causing brainstem signs).

Other complications include:
1 High-output cardiac failure (?bounding pulse – occurs when more than 30–40% of the skeleton is involved)
2 Pathological fractures
3 Urolithiasis
4 Sarcoma (incidence is probably <1%; increase in pain and swelling may occur; 'explosive rise' in alkaline phosphatase occurs only occasionally).

### Causes of 'bowed tibia'

*True bowing* due to soft bone:
    Paget's disease (asymmetrical)
    Rickets (bilateral, symmetrical; see Station 5, Locomotor, Case 17).
*Apparent bowing* due to thickening of the anterior surface of the tibia secondary to periostitis:
    Congenital syphilis (?saddle nose, bulldog jaw, rhagades, Hutchinson's teeth, Moon's molars, etc; see Vol. 1, Station 5, CNS, Case 39)
    Yaws.

---

*Bisphosphonates (e.g. pamidronate, zoledronic acid) are now the first-line treatment with short courses leading to long-term suppression of disease activity and improvement in bone pain, etc. Indications for specific therapy in Paget's disease are: bone pain; osteolytic lesions in weight-bearing bones; neurological complications (except deafness); delayed or non-union of fractures; immobilization hypercalcaemia; before and after orthopaedic surgery.

†Although hearing loss is frequently attributed to compression of the VIIIth cranial nerve in the canal in the temporal bone, this is unlikely to be the major cause because the facial nerve, which follows the same course, is rarely affected.

‡The other ophthalmological finding which may occur in Paget's disease is angioid streaks in the retina (see Section I, Figure I5.8d, Station 5, Skin, Case 10).

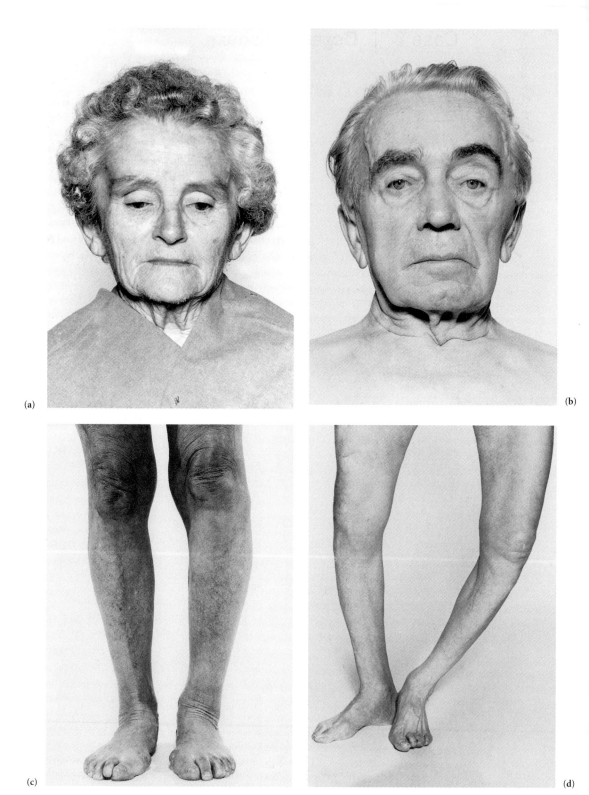

**Figure I5.54** (a,b) Note the hearing aids. (c) Bowing of tibiae. (d) Gross deformity.

# Case 8 | **Osteoarthritis**

**Frequency in survey for 3rd edition:** main focus of a short case in 2% of attempts at PACES Station 5, Locomotor.

## *Record*

There are *Heberden's nodes* present at the bases of the distal phalanges (and less commonly Bouchard's nodes at the proximal interphalangeal joints). There is a 'square hand' deformity due to subluxation of the base of the first metacarpal. Signs of joint inflammation are (generally) absent. There is swelling and deformity of the knee joints with development of varus (or valgus) deformity. There is crepitus in these joints. There is wasting and weakness of the quadriceps and glutei, and there is downward tilting of the pelvis when the patient stands on the affected leg (Trendelenburg's sign).

This patient has osteoarthritis.*

---

**Complications**

Pain

Deformity

Ankylosis

Entrapment of nerves (e.g. ulnar nerve palsy or carpal tunnel syndrome)

Cervical spondylosis

---

*Osteoarthrosis is probably a better term as the 'itis' suggests an inflammatory disease. However, regardless of this, osteoarthritis is the term in common parlance.

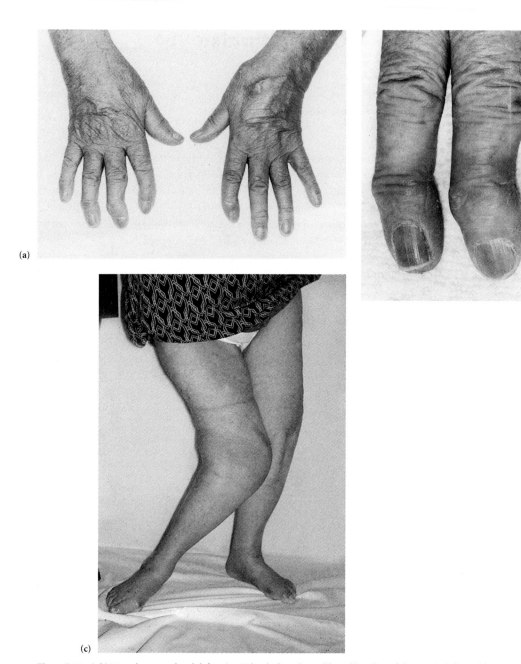

(a)

(b)

(c)

**Figure I5.55** (a,b) Note the square hand deformity, Heberden's nodes and lateral bending of the terminal digits. (c) Osteoarthritis of the knee joint with valgus deformity.

# Case 9 | Marfan's syndrome

**Frequency in survey:** main focus of a short case in 2% of attempts at PACES Station 5, Locomotor.

## *Record*

The patient is *tall* with disproportionately *long extremities* (pubis–sole > pubis–vertex) and elongated fingers and toes (*arachnodactyly*). He has a *high-arched palate* (gothic), a long, narrow face and his span is greater than his height. His musculature is underdeveloped and hypotonic (and he may have a funnel or pigeon chest, pectus excavatum, kyphoscoliosis, flat feet, genu recurvatum, hyperextensibility of joints and recurrent dislocations). The tremor of the iris (*iridodonesis*) is evidence of *lens dislocation* (50–70% of patients; a slit lamp may be needed for detection in minor cases). He has (may have) a collapsing pulse (auscultate if allowed) suggestive of *aortic incompetence* (cystic necrosis of the aortic media leading to steadily progressive* dilation of the aorta; aortic dissection can occur).

The diagnosis is Marfan's syndrome.

---

Autosomal dominant.
Defects in fibrillin (gene responsible is on the long arm of chromosome 15).

### Other features which may occur in Marfan's syndrome
Heterochromia of the iris
Blue sclerae
Myopia
Undue liability to retinal detachment
Cystic disease of the lungs (tendency to spontaneous pneumothorax which is often recurrent and may be bilateral; other pulmonary manifestations are bullae, apical fibrosis, aspergilloma and bronchiectasis)
Mitral valve prolapse (common, see Vol. 1, Station 3, Cardiovascular, Case 10; severe mitral incompetence may occur)

Coarctation of the aorta
Bacterial endocarditis even on valves with only minor abnormalities
Inguinal or femoral herniae
Decreased subcutaneous fat
Miescher's elastoma (small nodules or papules in the skin of the neck)
Death due to cardiovascular component (average age is mid-forties)

NB: *Homocystinuria* (autosomal recessive) may produce a similar clinical picture to Marfan's except in addition mental retardation, a malar flush and osteoporosis are common and ocular lens dislocation is downwards (in Marfan's it is upwards). Homocystine can be detected in the urine by the cyanide–nitroprusside test.

---

*Prophylactic β-blockade may slow the rate of aortic dilation and reduce the development of aortic complications in some patients with Marfan's.

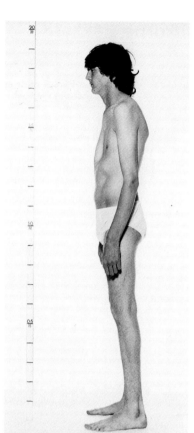

(a)

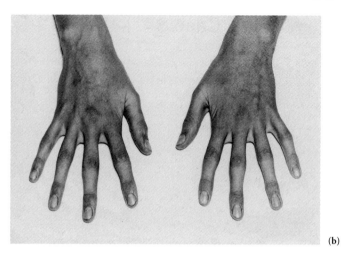

(b)

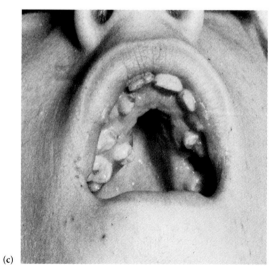

(c)

**Figure I5.56** (a–c) Marfan's syndrome.

# Case 10 | **Vasculitis**

**Frequency in survey for 3rd edition:** main focus of a short case in 2% of attempts at PACES Station 5, Locomotor.

Vasculitis is dealt with in Station 5, Skin, Case 27.

# Case 11 | **Proximal myopathy**

**Frequency in survey for 3rd edition:** main focus of a short case in 2% of attempts at PACES Station 5, Locomotor.

Proximal myopathy is dealt with in Vol. 1, Station 3, CNS, Case 23.

# Case 12 | One leg shorter and smaller than the other

**Frequency in survey for 3rd edition:** main focus of a short case in 2% of attempts at PACES Station 5, Locomotor.

This case appearing in Station 5, Locomotor was presumably either old polio (see Vol. 1, Station 3, CNS, Case 15) or infantile hemiplegia (see Vol. 1, Station 3, CNS, Case 42).

# Case 13 | **Radial nerve palsy**

**Frequency in survey for 3rd edition:** main focus of a short case in 1% of attempts at PACES Station 5, Locomotor.

**Survey note:** see Vol. 2, Section F, Experience 18.

Radial nerve palsy is dealt with in Vol. 1, Station 3, CNS, Case 48.

# Case 14 | Arthropathy associated with inflammatory bowel disease

**Frequency in survey for 3rd edition:** main focus of a short case in 1% of attempts at PACES Station 5, Locomotor.

## Record

There is *symmetrical* (may be asymmetrical) *arthropathy* of the *hands* with *swelling* of the *metacarpophalangeal* and *proximal interphalangeal joints*. There is *wasting* of the *small muscles* of the *hand* with *guttering* in between the metacarpals. There are no nodules or arteritic lesions (check for these). The patient cannot make a complete fist but can pick up a paperclip, suggesting a reasonable retention of function. I also noticed an *operation scar* on the *abdomen* (check for extraintestinal signs; see Table I5.5), possibly from a hemicolectomy in the past.

The appearances suggest rheumatoid arthritis but I would also have to consider peripheral arthropathy associated with inflammatory bowel disease.

---

## Enteropathic arthropathies

Two distinct forms of arthritis have been recognized in association with inflammatory bowel disease (IBD): peripheral and axial arthropathies.

### Peripheral arthropathy

About 15% of patients with Crohn's disease and 10% with ulcerative colitis develop peripheral arthritis. It is commonly non-erosive, reversible and migratory, affecting the large joints (i.e. knees, ankles and elbows) but, in chronic cases, it may be indistinguishable from seronegative rheumatoid arthritis (but joint deformity is rare). Peripheral arthritis frequently occurs in those who have other extraintestinal manifestations such as uveitis and erythema nodosum in Crohn's disease. It affects all age groups and both sexes equally. In adults the arthritis usually develops in cases with well-established intestinal inflammation but the converse is true in children. Peripheral arthritis usually, but not always,

parallels gut inflammation and measures to control the bowel disease may ameliorate the articular activity. Total colectomy is associated with remission of arthritis in half of the patients with ulcerative colitis though sometimes the arthritis may begin after surgery. Septic arthritis in the hip joint has been reported in Crohn's disease.

### Axial arthropathy

Spinal involvement, which occurs in 3–6% of IBD patients, may be symptomatic or silent sacroiliitis/spondylitis and it may precede or coincide with the onset of bowel symptoms. Spondylitis is more common in males and it is clinically and radiologically indistinguishable from ankylosing spondylitis. The course of sacroiliitis and spondylitis may be independent of active bowel inflammation. HLA-B27 is found in 50% of patients with IBD-associated spondylitic colitis.

**Table I5.5** Extraintestinal signs of inflammatory bowel disease

| Area | Sign/manifestation |
| --- | --- |
| Joints | Peripheral and axial–sacroiliac arthritides, septic arthritis rarely in Crohn's disease and not reported in ulcerative colitis |
| Eyes | Uveitis, iritis and scleritis* – all occur in both conditions but are more common in Crohn's disease |
| Mouth | Aphthous ulcers and swollen lips in Crohn's disease but never in ulcerative colitis |
| Hands | Finger clubbing – more common in Crohn's disease |
| Skin | Erythema nodosum – up to 9% in Crohn's disease, up to 20% in ulcerative colitis |
| | Pyoderma gangrenosum† – 0.5% in Crohn's disease, occurs more often and mostly on the limbs in ulcerative colitis, usually with a bout of acute colitis |
| | Pallor – resulting from anaemia in either condition |
| | Erythema multiforme – occurs but is rare in either condition, has some association with erythema nodosum |
| Abdomen | Fistulae and laparotomy scars in Crohn's disease, operation scar of a colectomy, with or without ileostomy, in ulcerative colitis |
| Vasculitis | Cutaneous polyarteritis nodosa (painful skin nodules) reported in both conditions. Digital ischaemia and gangrene are rare complications |
| Nutritional status | Weight loss in both conditions |

* These changes also occur in rheumatoid arthritis without inflammatory bowel disease.

† Ulcerative colitis should be considered in any patient presenting with diarrhoea and pyoderma gangrenosum. Unfortunately, the latter is often misdiagnosed as a simple ulcer, unrelated to the bowel problem, in such patients.

# Case 15 | Polymyositis

**Frequency in survey for 3rd edition:** main focus of a short case in 1% of attempts at PACES Station 5, Locomotor.

Polymyositis is dealt with in Vol. 1, Station 3, CNS, Case 45.

# Case 16 | Systemic lupus erythematosus

**Frequency in survey for 3rd edition:** did not occur in the initial small survey of PACES Station 5, Locomotor.

**Predicted frequency from older, more extensive MRCP short case surveys:** main focus of a short case in 4% of attempts at PACES Station 5, Locomotor.

## *Record*

There is (in this *young female* patient) a *red, papular butterfly rash* on the face (and elsewhere, especially light-exposed areas) with *scaling, follicular plugging\** and *scarring.* These features suggest lupus erythematosus (chronic discoid lupus erythematosus if only the skin is affected; SLE if there is evidence of multisystem involvement).

---

Discoid LE: ratio of males to females is 1:2.
SLE: ratio of males to females is 1:9.

### Look for other features

Buccal mucosa (sharply defined whitish patches with red borders)

Scalp (scarring alopecia)

Hands and joints (arthritis; deformity may occur but is usually mild and non-erosive; Raynaud's in 20%)

Skin (vasculitis – see below)

Lungs† (pleural effusions, or rarely crepitations from interstitial involvement)

Ankles (oedema – SLE is an important cause of nephrotic syndrome)

Heart (for pericardial friction rub, rarely pericardial effusion; cardiac enlargement or failure – myocarditis; or murmurs – Libman–Sachs endocarditis)

Proximal muscles (myalgia is common; polymyositis may occur)

Eyes (Sjögren's syndrome; fundal haemorrhages or white exudates called cytoid bodies; papilloedema)

Reticuloendothelial system (lymph nodes; splenomegaly)

Mucous membranes for pallor – anaemia is normochromic normocytic and/or haemolytic (Coombs' positive or negative); thrombocytopenia often occurs; haematological changes may antedate other features of the disease by years

Hepatomegaly (chronic passive congestion – usually transient‡)

Urine (proteinuria and haematuria)

NB: in SLE vasculitic rashes can occur in addition to the classic butterfly rash. They characteristically affect

---

\*Very close examination of the butterfly rash reveals that the scales in many areas appear as dots. These dots indicate where the follicle has been plugged by a scale. When the scales are removed (very unlikely to be required in the examination) and the undersurface is inspected, they clearly appear as tiny spicules projecting from the scaly mass. No other scaly condition produces this phenomenon. Healing of the discoid lesions occurs with atrophy, scarring (telangiectasia), hyperpigmentation or hypopigmentation (vitiligo).

†Drug-induced SLE involves the lungs more commonly and kidneys less commonly than classic SLE. The most common (90%) drugs are hydralazine (slow acetylators), isoniazid, pheny-

toin and procainamide (rapid acetylators). Other drugs include hydrochlorothiazide, oral contraceptives, penicillin, reserpine, streptomycin, sulphonamides, minocycline and tetracycline.

‡Liver biopsy may be normal or show fatty infiltration and/or fibrosis. These manifestations in SLE should not be confused with the form of chronic active hepatitis, which often has a positive antinuclear factor, called 'lupoid hepatitis'. The liver biopsy in the latter shows an inflammatory infiltrate extending into the liver lobule, causing erosion of the limiting plate and piecemeal necrosis. Fibrous septa isolate rosettes of cells. Cirrhosis is usually present and eventually hepatic failure may develop.

the elbows, knees, hands and feet. The rash may be a punctate erythematous rash, palmar erythema, periungual erythema or livedo reticularis (see Station 5, Skin, Case 29). Subcutaneous nodules may occur (5%), somewhat resembling those encountered in rheumatoid arthritis.

Table I5.6 Autoantibodies and their antigens in systemic lupus erythematosus

| Antigen | Autoantibody |
| --- | --- |
| Nucleosome | Anti-dsDNA |
| | Antihistone antibody |
| Small nuclear | Anti-RNP |
| ribonucleoprotein | Anti-Sm |
| Small cytoplasmic | Anti-Ro |
| ribonucleoprotein | Anti-La |
| Ribosome | Antiribosomal RNA |
| | Antiribosomal P protein |

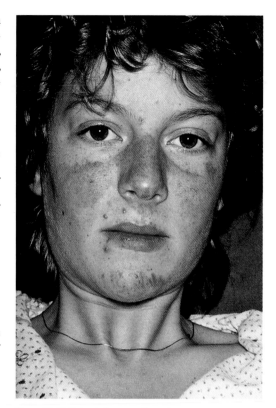

Figure I5.57 Systemic lupus erythematosus.

# Case 17 | Old rickets

**Frequency in survey for 3rd edition:** did not occur in the initial small survey of PACES Station 5, Locomotor.

**Predicted frequency from older, more extensive MRCP short case surveys:** focus of a short case in 0.6% of attempts at PACES Station 5, Locomotor.

## Record

The legs are *bilaterally* and *symmetrically curved laterally* in this *short-statured* patient. The bowing involves both the thighs (femurs) and the lower legs (tibiae). The curved areas are not warmer than the neighbouring areas, joints and feet.

The deformity is probably of long standing* and the symmetrical appearance* suggests the diagnosis of old rickets. Although there are many causes of rickets and osteomalacia, the old age (may be 80 years or older) of this patient suggests that he/she may have suffered nutritional deprivation during childhood.†

---

### Main causes of rickets and osteomalacia‡

Decreased availability of vitamin D:
  insufficient sunlight exposure
  low dietary intake
Malabsorption:
  Billroth type II gastrectomy
  coeliac disease
  jejunoileal bypass
  regional enteritis
  pancreatic insufficiency
  biliary cirrhosis
Abnormal metabolism:
  chronic renal failure
  liver disease

X-linked hypophosphataemia
renal tubular disorders
anticonvulsants
vitamin D-resistant rickets
Miscellaneous:
  aluminium toxicity
  etidronate
  hypophosphatasia
  nephrotic syndrome (urinary loss)
  total parenteral nutrition

---

*Unlike Paget's disease (see Station 5, Locomotor, Case 7), the deformity of old rickets is present from childhood. The bilateral involvement of the tibiae and the symmetrical appearance of the bowing are highly suggestive of old rickets. Bilateral Paget's disease of the legs is very rare and the deformity is very unlikely to be symmetrical.

†Bowing of the long bones results when poor exposure to sunlight and a low dietary intake of vitamin D occur during active skeletal growth, e.g. child refugees of the First and Second World Wars. Rickets with gross bony deformities is also seen in patients with *familial hypophosphataemia*, renal tubular disorders and in Asian immigrants of all ages.

‡After closure of the epiphyses, vitamin D deficiency manifests as *osteomalacia*. Severe osteomalacia may present with bone pain, proximal muscle weakness, difficulty in climbing stairs and rising from chairs, and waddling gait. Pseudofractures (also known as Looser's zones or Milkman's fractures) on X-ray of pelvis, ribs, clavicles or lateral scapulae are pathognomonic of osteomalacia and rickets. However, osteomalacia is often diagnosed in relatively asymptomatic individuals. A raised alkaline phosphatase with low or low normal calcium should arouse suspicion. The level of vitamin D in the blood may be low, though elevation of serum parathyroid hormone level (secondary rise) is a more sensitive indicator.

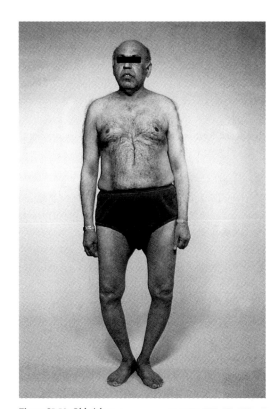

**Figure I5.58** Old rickets.

# Case 18 | Juvenile idiopathic arthritis

**Frequency in survey for 3rd edition:** did not occur in the initial small survey of PACES Station 5, Locomotor.

**Predicted frequency from older, more extensive MRCP short case surveys:** main focus of a short case in 0.6% of attempts at PACES Station 5, Locomotor.

## Record

This (febrile) *teenager* with painful joints (*polyserositis*) has an evanescent salmon-coloured *rash*, lymphadenopathy and hepatosplenomegaly.

These features are suggestive of Still's disease (juvenile idiopathic arthritis* [JIA] of *systemic onset*).

---

### Other features of Still's disease

Twenty per cent of patients with JIA
Rheumatoid factor and antinuclear antibodies not found
Usually a childhood disease but can begin at any age
Anaemia, leucocytosis and thrombocytosis common (can be confused with leukaemia or infection)

### Other forms of JIA

#### *Polyarticular onset*

Forty per cent of patients with JIA
Female predominance
Usually seronegative† (if seropositive, HLA-DR4 common and follows a course similar to adult rheumatoid arthritis)

#### *Pauciarticular onset*

Forty per cent of patients with JIA.

#### *Early age of onset and female preponderance*

Antinuclear antibodies positive, rheumatoid factor negative
Risk of chronic iridocyclitis (prophylactic ophthalmological surveillance mandatory)
Arthritis usually resolves without deformity
HLA-DR5 and HLA-DRw8 associated

#### *Strong male predominance and later age of onset*

Mostly HLA-DR27
Follows a course consistent with spondyloarthropathy‡

---

*Also called *juvenile chronic arthritis* (JCA). Has been termed in the past juvenile rheumatoid arthritis, though the majority of cases do not resemble adult rheumatoid arthritis.

†No HLA association except a small subset with HLA-B27 who develop cervical spine fusion and less often sacroiliitis or ankylosing spondylitis.

‡The seronegative spondyloarthritides are characterized by sacroiliac joint involvement, peripheral inflammatory arthropathy and the absence of rheumatoid factor. Pathological changes are concentrated around the *enthesis* – at sites of ligamentous inser-tions into bones (rather than the synovium). Changes may also develop in the eye, aortic valve, lung parenchyma and skin. Types include ankylosing spondylitis (see Station 5, Locomotor, Case 6), Reiter's syndrome (see Station 5, Skin, Case 46), psoriatic arthropathy (see Station 5, Locomotor, Case 2) enteropathic sacroiliitis (ulcerative colitis and Crohn's disease, see Vol.1, Station 1, Abdominal, Case 9), reactive arthritides (infections such as with *Yersinia, Salmonella, Helicobacter, Campylobacter*), certain subsets of JIA, and perhaps a group of rarer disorders (Whipple's disorders, Behçet's syndrome and pustular arthro-osteitis).

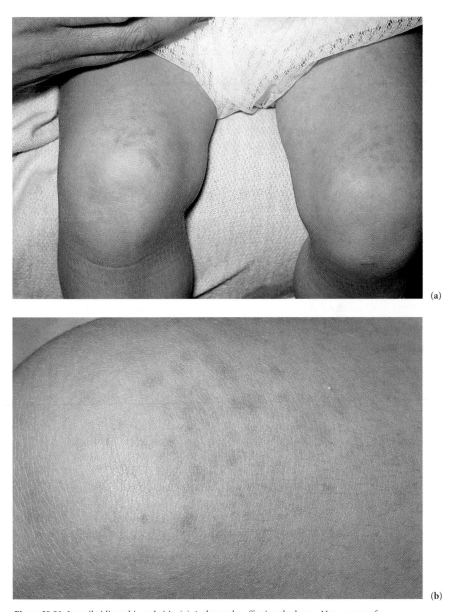

(a)

(b)

**Figure I5.59** Juvenile idiopathic arthritis. (a) Arthropathy affecting the knees. Note a crop of characteristic macular lesions. (b) Close-up view of the rash.

# Case 19 | Swollen knee

**Frequency in survey for 3rd edition:** did not occur in the initial small survey of PACES Station 5, Locomotor.

**Predicted frequency from older, more extensive MRCP short case surveys:** main focus of a short case in 2% of attempts at PACES Station 5, Locomotor. Additional feature in a further 3%.

**Survey note:** half of the cases were due to rheumatoid arthritis.

## *Record*

There is generalized *swelling* of the R/L *knee joint* obscuring the medial and lateral dimples. The *patellar tap sign*\* is *positive*, suggesting the presence of fluid in the synovial cavity. The swelling does not extend to the back in the popliteal fossa (always check).† The joint is *painful* to move and it is *warm*.

There is an *effusion* in the knee joint. (Now look at the hands for evidence of rheumatoid arthritis; see Station 5, Locomotor, Case 1.)

---

### Causes of a swollen knee

Rheumatoid arthritis (the swelling may be due to synovial thickening – synovium is palpable as boggy tissue around the joint margin)

Osteoarthritis (osteophytes on X-ray)

Rupture of a Baker's cyst (?rheumatoid arthritis; see Station 5, Other, Case 2)

Pseudogout (calcified menisci; birefringent calcium pyrophosphate crystals; associated with a large variety of conditions including hyperparathyroidism, haemochromatosis, acromegaly, diabetes mellitus,

Wilson's disease, hypothyroidism, alkaptonuria and gout; there are also idiopathic and hereditary varieties)

Septic arthritis (purulent fluid, organisms in a smear)

Gout (urate crystals)

Trauma

Charcot's knee (painless, ?tabes dorsalis; see Vol. 1, Station 3, CNS, Case 50)

Haemarthrosis of haemophilia

Oedematous states (congestive cardiac failure, nephrotic syndrome)

---

\*With one hand above the knee joint, exert pressure to drive fluid from the suprapatellar pouch into the knee joint proper. With the index finger of the other hand, depress the patella with a sharp jerky movement. If the patella rebounds this is definite evidence of fluid in the knee joint. The sign may not be positive if there is too much or too little fluid. To test for a small amount of fluid in the knee joint, displace fluid by sweeping fluid from the medial aspect of the patella laterally, and then back again. The medial hollow will slowly refill.

†Swelling in the popliteal fossa extending down to the upper third of the calf in cases of ruptured Baker's cyst; see Station 5, Other, Case 2.

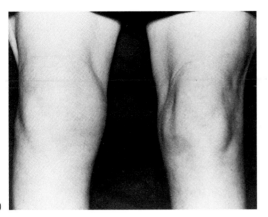 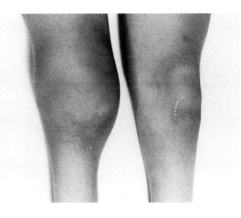

(a)                                                                                          (b)

**Figure I5.60** (a) Osteoarthritis with effusion of the knee joint. (b) Charcot's knee (spina bifida).

# Station 5
# Endocrine

| Short case | Checked and updated as necessary for this edition by |
|---|---|
| **1** Exophthalmos | Professor Hugh Jones* |
| **2** Acromegaly | Professor Hugh Jones* |
| **3** Graves' disease | Professor Hugh Jones* |
| **4** Goitre | Professor Hugh Jones* |
| **5** Hypothyroidism | Professor Hugh Jones* |
| **6** Cushing's syndrome | Professor Hugh Jones* |
| **7** Addison's disease | Professor Hugh Jones* |
| **8** Hypopituitarism | Professor Hugh Jones* |
| **9** Pretibial myxoedema | Professor Hugh Jones* |
| **10** Gynaecomastia | Professor Hugh Jones* |
| **11** Turner's syndrome | Professor Hugh Jones* |
| **12** Klinefelter's syndrome/hypogonadism | Professor Hugh Jones* |
| **13** Bitemporal hemianopia | Professor Hugh Jones* |
| **14** Diabetic foot/Charcot's joint | Dr Fran Game* |
| **15** Necrobiosis lipoidica diabeticorum | Dr Shireen Velangi* |
| **16** Short stature | Professor Hugh Jones* |
| **17** Pseudohypoparathyroidism | Professor Hugh Jones* |
| **18** Pendred's syndrome | Professor Hugh Jones* |

*All suggested changes by these specialty advisors were considered by Dr Bob Ryder and were either accepted, edited, added to or rejected with Dr Ryder making the final editorial decision in every case.

Professor T Hugh Jones, Consultant Physician and Endocrinologist and Honorary Professor of Andrology, Barnsley Hospital and University of Sheffield, UK
Dr Fran Game, Consultant Physician/Diabetologist, Royal Derby Hospital, Derby, UK
Dr Shireen Velangi, Consultant Dermatologist, City Hospital, Birmingham, UK

# Case 1 | Exophthalmos

**Frequency in survey for 3rd edition**: main focus of a short case in 26% of attempts at PACES Station 5, Endocrine. Additional feature in a further 19%.

## Record 1

There is (may be) bilateral *swelling* of the *medial caruncle* and *vascular congestion* of the *lateral canthus* with exophthalmos (protrusion of the eye revealing the *sclera above the lower lid* in the position of forward gaze) which is greater on the R/L side.*

Likely causes include:

1 Hyperthyroid Graves' disease† (?lid retraction or lag, tachycardia, bruit over the goitre; exophthalmos usually symmetrical)
2 Euthyroid Graves' disease (?no lid lag, *normal* pulse rate, no sweating or tremor, etc.)
3 Hypothyroid Graves' disease (?facies, scar of thyroidectomy, hoarse voice, slow pulse, ankle jerks, etc.).

## Record 2

There is severe exophthalmos, *chemosis, exposure keratitis, corneal ulceration* and *ophthalmoplegia*‡ which is reducing the upward and lateral gaze most and which is responsible for the *diplopia*. Convergence (check for this) is also impaired. Testing the eye movements caused the patient discomfort (or pain). The diagnosis is Graves' malignant exophthalmos (patient may be hyper-, eu- or hypothyroid).

---

Graves' malignant exophthalmos (congestive ophthalmopathy) can cause severe pain and the patient is at risk of blindness due to pressure on the optic nerve, if not treated. The condition may require large doses of systemic steroids and sometimes *tarsorrhaphy* (which may be in evidence in the examination patient) or orbital decompression may even be necessary. Radiotherapy has also been successfully used. Mild exophthalmos is associated with an increased risk of optic neuropathy. Ophthalmopathy may precede onset of hyperthyroidism.

### Protective measures for the eye with exophthalmos

Eyedrops/lubrication
Stop smoking/avoid smoky atmospheres

'Cataract glasses', i.e. wrap-around glasses
Optimize thyroid status (improves lid lag and retraction but will have little effect on exophthalmos itself)

Eye disease may deteriorate with radioiodine therapy (if possible, avoid radioiodine therapy in moderate-to-severe disease. Use glucocorticoid prophylaxis in mild-to-moderate disease).

### Other causes of exophthalmos
**Bilateral (though asymmetrical) with conjunctival oedema**

Cavernous sinus thrombosis (follows infection of the orbit, nose and face; eyeball is painful and there is extreme venous congestion)
Caroticocavernous fistula (pulsating exophthalmos)

---

*Look for pretibial myxoedema (see Station 5, Skin, Case 16) if the legs are exposed and for thyroid acropachy (see Station 5, Endocrine, Case 3) if pretibial myxoedema is present.
†There are some studies that suggest that radioactive iodine therapy for Graves' disease may worsen exophthalmos, though this is a controversial area.

‡The ophthalmoplegia is due to infiltration, oedema and subsequent fibrosis of the external ocular muscles. It may occur with oedema of the lids and conjunctivae and precede the exophthalmos. For this reason the term 'congestive ophthalmopathy' may be preferable to 'malignant exophthalmos'.

### Unilateral

Retro-orbital tumour (the protrusion measured with the Hertel exophthalmometer is usually >5 mm more than the unaffected eye by the time of presentation, whereas Graves' eyes rarely achieve a difference of 5 mm§)

Orbital cellulitis

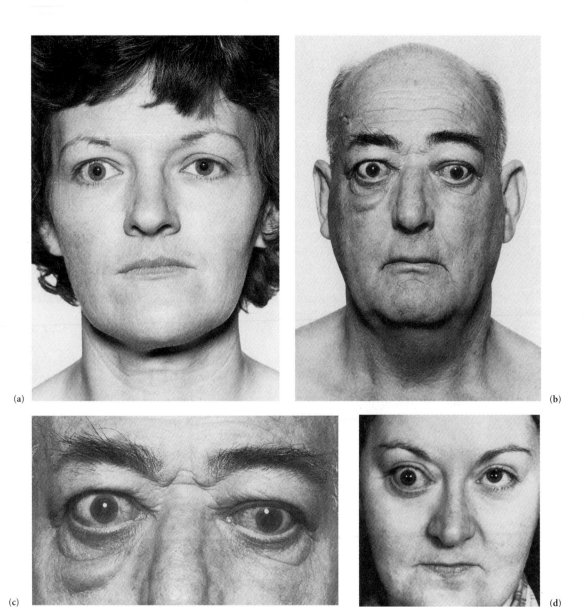

**Figure I5.61** (a) Unilateral exophthalmos. (b,c) Bilateral exophthalmos (note proptosis, ophthalmoplegia, conjunctival congestion, swelling of the medial caruncle and periorbital swelling). (d) Ophthalmoplegia of the right eye. (*Continued*)

§Unless the diagnosis is unquestionably Graves' disease, the possibility of a retro-orbital tumour should always be investigated with computed tomography (CT) scan, etc., regardless of the Hertel exophthalmometer measurement.

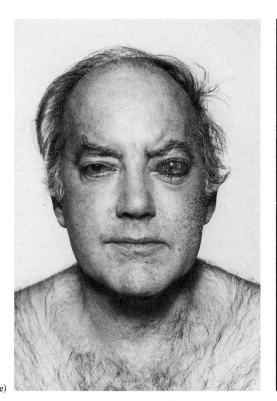

(e)

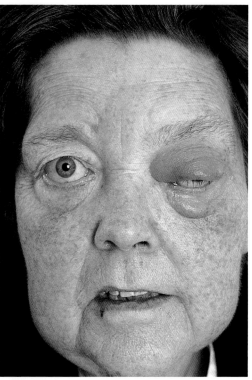

(f)

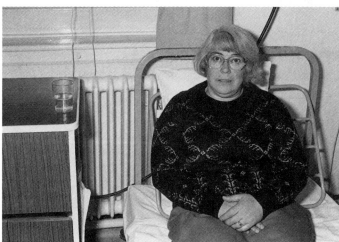

(g)

**Figure I5.61** (*Continued*) (e) Severe congestive ophthalmopathy, chemosis and corneal ulceration. (f) Severe congestive ophthalmopathy on the left. (g) Tell-tale glass of water (for examination of the goitre) in a patient with exophthalmos.

# Case 2 | Acromegaly

**Frequency in survey for 3rd edition:** main focus of a short case in 24% of attempts at PACES Station 5, Endocrine. Additional feature in a further 3%.

**Survey note:** candidates were sometimes asked questions on subjects such as presentation, investigation and complications.

## *Record*

The patient has prominent *supraorbital ridges* and a *large lower jaw*. The facial wrinkles are exaggerated and the lips are full. There is *malocclusion* of the teeth, the *lower teeth overbiting* in front of the upper (prognathism), and there is an increase in the *interdental spaces*. The *nose, tongue* and *ears* are enlarged and the patient is *kyphotic*. The *hands* are *large*, doughy and spade-shaped,* and the *skin* over the back of them is *thickened* (shake hands and examine the dorsum). There is (may be) loss of the thenar eminence bilaterally with impaired sensation in the median nerve distribution (*carpal tunnel syndrome*). The patient is *sweating* excessively and is mildly *hirsute* (one-third of cases). The *voice* is husky and cavernous.† There is a *bitemporal peripheral visual field defect*. The diagnosis is acromegaly.

---

## Other physical signs which may be present

Increased foot (shoe) size
Increased head (hat) size
Bowed legs
Rolling gait
Goitre
Gynaecomastia
Galactorrhoea
Large testes
Small testes (if hypogonadal)
Greasy skin
Acne
Multiple skin tags (correlate with the occurrence of colonic polyps)
Skin thickening and skinfolds on scalp (cutis verticis gyrata)

Acanthosis nigricans
Osteoarthrosis
Prominent superficial veins of extremities
Proximal muscle weakness
Cardiomegaly (hypertension and cardiomyopathy)
Third nerve palsy

## Other features

Diabetes mellitus (glycosuria, glucose intolerance or frank diabetes (10–20%) may occur; it is usually mild and ketoacidosis is rare; it is somewhat resistant to insulin)
Hypertension (20–50%)
Hypercalciuria (common)
Hypercalcaemia‡ (occasionally)
Urolithiasis (5–10%)

---

*Shaking hands with the patient may give the impression of losing one's hands in a mass of dough.
†Thick vocal cords in conjunction with sinus enlargement results in the characteristic deep, resonant voice.
‡Most likely to be due to associated hyperparathyroidism as part of *multiple endocrine neoplasia (MEN) type I* (Werner's syndrome) which is two or more of:
1  Pituitary tumour (prolactinoma, acromegaly, Cushing's)
2  Islet cell tumour (gastrin, insulin, glucagon and pancreatic polypeptide)

3  Primary hyperparathyroidism (adenoma or hyperplasia)
4  Adrenocortical adenoma (see Station 5, Endocrine, Case 6 and Footnote).
MEN type 1 should probably be regarded as a complex of separate genetic abnormalities rather than as a consequence of a single primary disease. It should not be confused with MEN type 2 which is usually an autosomal dominant trait with a high degree of penetrance (see Footnote, Station 5, Endocrine, Case 4).

Hypertriglyceridaemia (20–40%)

Diabetes insipidus (normally due to hypothalamic pressure effect; if there is impaired cortisol secretion symptoms may be masked)

Hypopituitarism (see Station 5, Endocrine, Case 8).

## Symptoms before presentation§

Excessive sweating

Increasing size of shoes, gloves, hats, dentures and rings

Paraesthesiae of hands and feet

Digital pain and stiffness (of slowly expanding fingers and toes)

Arthralgia

Hypogonadism (amenorrhoea, loss of libido)

Headache (may be severe; may occur without clinically detectable enlargement of the pituitary tumour; the mechanism is not clear)

Visual field or acuity disturbance

## Investigations

Insulin-like growth factor (IGF)-I (not diagnostic but good initial screening test)

Glucose tolerance test with growth hormone (GH) response (lack of suppression; sometimes a paradoxical rise)

Magnetic resonance imaging (MRI) scan of pituitary fossa (CT scan if MRI scan cannot be done)

Visual fields

Comparative study of old photographs of the patient can be useful to date onset

Tests of anterior pituitary function (*adrenocorticotroph:* short Synacthen test,¶ insulin tolerance test; *thyro-*

*troph:* thyroid-stimulating hormone [TSH] plus total or free T4; *gonadotroph:* menstrual history plus oestradiol, luteinizing hormone [LH] and follicle-stimulating hormone [FSH] (female), potency plus testosterone (male); *lactotroph:* prolactin\*\*).

## Treatment
### Surgery

Trans-sphenoidal hypophysectomy – GH falls to <5 µg/L in >60% (more successful in those with smaller tumours)

Transfrontal hypophysectomy in some cases with large extensive adenomata (rarely used)

### Medical

Long-acting somatostatin analogues – octreotide/lanreotide (require parenteral administration); effective in lowering GH before and (if necessary) after surgery/radiotherapy; tumour may shrink in some cases

Dopamine agonists – cabergoline/bromocriptine (70% respond by reducing GH levels but few suppress to <5 µg/L; the size of the tumour is not reduced; useful for GH hypersecretion after surgery)

GH receptor antagonist – pegvisamont (for somatostatin analogue-resistant tumours)

### Radiotherapy

Stereotactic radiosurgery (gamma-knife)

Conventional radiotherapy – external irradiation (especially if surgery fails or patient is unfit for surgery; takes 1–10 years to take effect)

§The mean age of onset has been estimated at about 27 years whereas the mean age of presentation is over 40 years, i.e. there is an average pre-presentation lapse of 13–14 years. The prevalence is 40–70 per million; the incidence is 3 per million. Males = females. Ninety-nine per cent are due to pituitary adenomata; <1% due to excess growth hormone-releasing hormone (GHRH) production from gangliocytomata of the hypothalamus or pituitary or from peripheral tumours (ectopic), especially carcinoid (see Vol. 1, Station 1, Abdominal, Case 18).

¶In hypopituitarism, the adrenal cortex does not respond sufficiently in the short Synacthen test. It needs to be primed con-

tinually by adrenocorticotrophic hormone (ACTH) from a functioning pituitary in order to be responsive.

\*\*The prolactin may be low in hypopituitarism. However, production may also be elevated because (i) some GH-secreting pituitary tumours co-secrete prolactin, and (ii) any pituitary macroadenoma that presses on the pituitary stalk will interfere with dopamine suppression of prolactin production and lead to hyperprolactinaemia.

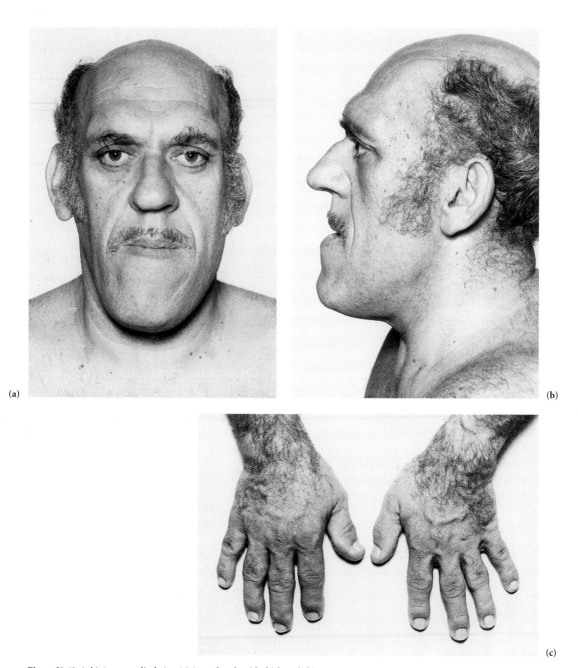

**Figure I5.62** (a,b) Acromegalic facies. (c) Large hands with thickened skin.

# Case 3 | Graves' disease

**Frequency in survey for 3rd edition:** main focus of a short case in 9% of attempts at PACES Station 5, Endocrine. Additional feature in a further 9%.

## Record 1

The patient (usually female) is *thin*, has *sweaty palms*, a *fine tremor* of the outstretched hands, a *tachycardia*,* and she is *fidgety* and nervous. There is a small diffuse *goitre* with a *bruit*, and she has *exophthalmos* (see Station 5, Eyes, Case 12) with *lid lag*.† This patient is *thyrotoxic* and has Graves' disease.

## Record 2

There is *exophthalmos* (?chemosis, ophthalmoplegia, diplopia, lateral tarsorrhaphy), *thyroid acropachy*,‡ and the lesions on the front of the shins are *pretibial myxoedema* (see Station 5, Skin, Case 16). The pulse is regular* and the *pulse rate* is *normal* (give rate), the palms are *not sweaty*, and there is *no hand tremor* or *lid lag*. There is a *thyroidectomy scar*. The diagnosis is *euthyroid* Graves' disease,§ the patient having been treated by thyroidectomy in the past.

---

Male to female ratio is 1:5.

## Record 3

This patient with *exophthalmos* (?chemosis, ophthalmoplegia, diplopia, lateral tarsorrhaphy, goitre, thyroidectomy scar, pretibial myxoedema, thyroid acropachy) has *hypothyroid facies*, a *hoarse voice, slow pulse** and *slowly relaxing reflexes*.

The patient has Graves' disease and is clinically *hypothyroid*. It is likely that she had hyperthyroidism treated in the past (?thyroidectomy or radioactive iodine) and is probably now on inadequate thyroxine replacement. (Because of the close links between the autoimmune thyroid diseases – see below – patients with Graves' disease occasionally go on to develop hypothyroidism spontaneously.)

### Other signs which may occur

Fever (rarely hyperpyrexia)
Systolic hypertension with wide pulse pressure
Cutaneous vasodilation
Systolic murmur due to increased blood flow
Proximal muscle weakness (thyrotoxic myopathy)
Hyperactive reflexes

---

*The pulse may be regular or irregular – the patient may have sinus rhythm or atrial fibrillation whatever the thyroid status (hyperthyroid; eu- or hypothyroid due to treatment).

†Graves' disease may be present in the absence of the eye signs and in an elderly male patient. There may be evidence of humoral autoimmunity, more specifically a circulating antibody to the thyrotrophin receptor. The thyroid gland may even have a nodular enlargement but its radioactive iodine uptake is uniformly increased throughout the gland between the nodules in autoimmune disease (Graves' disease). The patient with nodular goitre and thyrotoxicosis due to autonomous hypersecretion of nodule(s) that does not have an autoimmune (thyrotoxicosis) basis will have some nodules with increased uptake (hot nodules) on the isotope scan. Such patients are more likely to relapse after antithyroid drug therapy than patients with Graves' disease.

‡Thyroid acropachy may resemble finger clubbing in hypertrophic pulmonary osteoarthropathy (HPOA). However, in thyroid acropachy new bone formation seen on X-ray has the appearance of soap bubbles on the bone surface with coarse spicules. In HPOA new bone is formed in a linear distribution. Sometimes the new bone formation in acropachy is both visible and palpable along the phalanges.

§Graves' exophthalmos is due to increased retro-orbital fat and enlarged intraorbital muscles infiltrated with lymphocytes and containing increased water and mucopolysaccharide. It may develop in the absence of hyperthyroidism and remit, persist or develop further despite successful treatment of hyperthyroidism. Though there are no hard and fast rules, pretibial myxoedema tends to develop after the hyperthyroidism has been treated, especially with radioactive iodine.

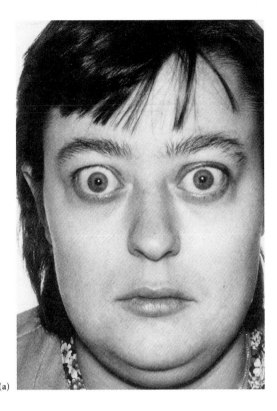

(a)

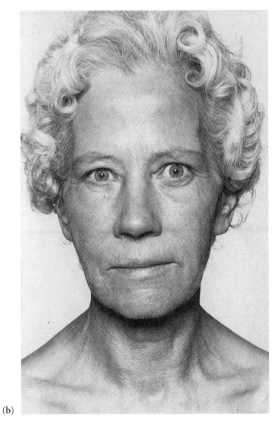

(b)

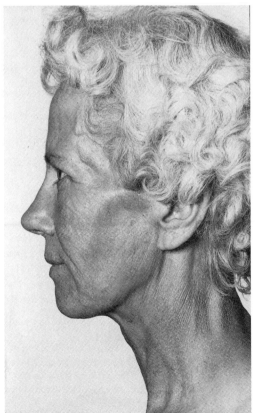

(c)

**Figure I5.63** (a) Graves' disease. (b,c) Hyperthyroidism in a patient who presented with the complaint that she had noticed a staring appearance of her left eye (note thinning of the hair in the temporal region). (*Continued*)

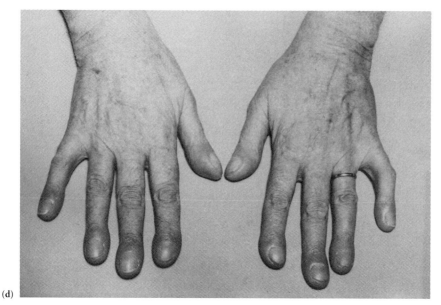

**(d)**

**Figure I5.63** (*Continued*) (d) Thyroid acropachy.

Thrill over goitre in addition to a bruit

Choreoathetoid movements (in children)

Fine thin hair (females may show temporal recession of the hairline)

Onycholysis (Plummer's nails, typically found bilaterally on the fourth finger)

Palmar erythema

Spider naevi

Splenomegaly (minimal)

Hepatomegaly (minimal)

Palpable lymph nodes (especially axillae)

Thyrotoxic osteoporosis (only rarely causes kyphosis or loss of height)

**Important symptoms** of hyperthyroidism (if asked to ask the patient some questions) are heat intolerance, weight loss, increased appetite, diarrhoea, exertional dyspnoea, undue fatiguability, 'can't keep still', irritability, nervousness and menstrual problems in females.

**Other organ-specific autoimmune diseases** (see also Station 5, Skin, Case 8) of which autoimmune thyroid disease¶ is an example include:

1 Pernicious anaemia
2 Atrophic gastritis with iron deficiency anaemia
3 Diabetes mellitus
4 Addison's disease
5 Idiopathic hypoparathyroidism
6 Premature ovarian failure
7 Renal tubular acidosis
8 Fibrosing alveolitis
9 Chronic active hepatitis
10 Primary biliary cirrhosis.

All of these diseases show a *marked female preponderance*. Premature greying of the hair, alopecia areata and vitiligo (see also Station 5, Skin, Case 8) are all associated with this group of diseases. Autoimmune thyroiditis is also associated with:

1 Sjögren's syndrome
2 Myasthenia gravis
3 Systemic sclerosis
4 Mixed connective tissue disease
5 Cranial arteritis
6 Polymyalgia rheumatica.

¶Graves' disease is one of the three closely related autoimmune thyroid diseases, the others being Hashimoto's thyroiditis and its atrophic variant, myxoedema. Among patients with one of these three, it is typical to find relatives with one of the other two. Some patients appear to have a combination which has been termed 'hashitoxicosis'.

# Case 4 | Goitre

**Frequency in survey for 3rd edition**: main focus of a short case in 7% of attempts at PACES Station 5, Endocrine. Additional feature in a further 6%.

## Record 1

There is a *multinodular* goitre, the R/L lobe being enlarged more than the L/R. There are *no lymph nodes* palpable, there is *no retrosternal* extension, there is *no bruit* and the patient is clinically *euthyroid* (having checked pulse, palms, tremor, lid lag, tendon reflexes). The diagnosis (in this middle-aged or elderly patient) is likely to be a simple multinodular goitre.

---

*Simple multinodular goitre* is due to relative iodine deficiency in a susceptible person. The multinodular nature suggests that it is of long standing. If there has been no recent rapid increase in size and if the gland is not causing symptoms or worrying the patient then no further investigation or treatment is required. The patient should be observed in 6 months or a year to confirm that there is still no change. Fine-needle aspiration should be undertaken if there is any doubt.

## Record 2

There is a *firm, diffusely enlarged* goitre without retrosternal extension (check for bruit and, if allowed, feel the pulse and assess thyroid status).

### Possible causes

Simple goitre (euthyroid, no bruit, relative iodine deficiency, especially females, ?puberty, ?pregnancy)

Treated Graves' disease* (?exophthalmos ± bruit, patient is euthyroid – normal pulse, no tremor or sweatiness – or even hypothyroid – slow pulse, facies, ankle jerks)

Hyperthyroid Graves' disease* (?bruit, tachycardia, exophthalmos, tremor, sweatiness, etc.)

Hashimoto's disease* (goitre usually, but not always, finely micronodular, firm and symmetrical; ?hypothyroid facies, pulse, ankle jerks, etc.)

De Quervain's (viral) thyroiditis (thyroid tender ± constitutional upset; absent radioactive iodine uptake on scan though the serum thyroxine may be elevated with TSH suppressed†)

Goitrogens (e.g. lithium, iodide in large doses, phenylbutazone, para-aminosalicylic acid and others are all rare causes)

Dyshormonogenesis (six different types of congenital enzyme defect, all rare)

## Record 3

There is a *solitary nodule* in the thyroid (check for lymphadenopathy).

### Possible causes

Only one palpable nodule in a multinodular goitre

Thyroid adenoma (if a scan were done it may show decreased, normal or increased [subclinical toxic nodule] uptake)

Toxic adenoma (hot nodule on scan, tachycardia, sweaty palms, lid lag, etc.)

Thyroid cyst

Thyroid carcinoma (?hard, lymph nodes, recent change, cold on scan)

As well as assessment of thyroid function, fine-needle aspiration to attempt to establish histological diagnosis

---

*Note the possibility of associated autoimmune disease adding extra interest to the case of goitre in the Membership (see Vol. 2, Section F, Experience 127), e.g. diabetes mellitus, rheumatoid arthritis, Addison's disease or pernicious anaemia. About 7% of patients with Graves' disease have vitiligo. About 5% of patients with myasthenia gravis have thyrotoxicosis at some time. (See

also Station 5, Skin, Case 8 and Station 5, Endocrine, Case 3 and Case 5)

†By contrast, when the goitre and raised serum thyroxine are due to Graves' disease, there is high radioactive iodine uptake on scan.

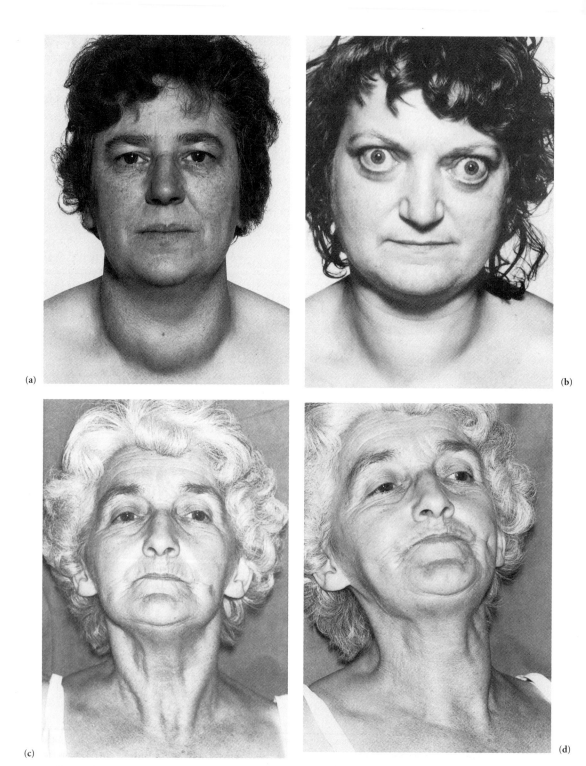

**Figure I5.64** (a) Multinodular goitre. (b) Diffusely enlarged thyroid (Graves' disease). (c,d) A solitary nodule only made obvious by swallowing (right).

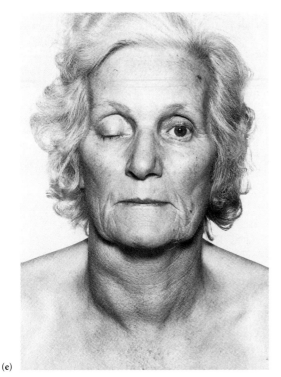

**(e)**

**Figure I5.64** (*Continued*) (e) Follicular carcinoma of the thyroid with secondaries in the cavernous sinus (total ophthalmoplegia and absent corneal reflex on the right).

should be undertaken in most cases of solitary thyroid nodule. As an adjunct, the nodule may be scanned radioisotopically though this is not usually necessary. If the nodule is hot it is not malignant but if it is cold it may be. In an older patient in whom the nodule has been present without changing for a long time, observation only (perhaps with full-dose thyroxine therapy which will reduce some nodules) may sometimes be justified initially. In any case of doubt, exploration of the neck and biopsy of the nodule are indicated, proceeding to subtotal lobectomy if the nodule is benign.

### Types of thyroid carcinoma

Papillary carcinoma is the most common form. It occurs in children and the middle-aged. It spreads to regional lymph nodes but is often resectable and has a good prognosis. It is often TSH dependent and may respond to thyroxine

Follicular carcinoma is the next most common and tends to arise later in life. Blood-borne metastases may occur but following surgery and suppressive thyroxine treatment, the prognosis is fair. It and its secondaries often take up and respond to radioactive iodine

Anaplastic carcinoma tends to arise in the elderly and is highly malignant

Medullary carcinoma‡ is rare, tends to arise in young adults, secretes calcitonin and sometimes ACTH, but usually carries a good prognosis

Lymphoma (B-cell) generally arises in a gland affected by Hashimoto's thyroiditis. A rapidly enlarging mass in the thyroid of a patient with Hashimoto's should arouse suspicion

‡Multiple endocrine neoplasia (MEN) type 2a (Sipple's syndrome, also known as multiple endocrine adenopathy [MEA] syndrome) describes the association of:
1 Medullary cell carcinoma of the thyroid
2 Phaeochromocytoma (may be bilateral)
3 Parathyroid hyperplasia (50%).
In MEN type 2b, medullary cell carcinoma of the thyroid and sometimes phaeochromocytoma are associated with a variety of neurological abnormalities including mucosal neuromata (lumpy, bumpy lips and eyelids), marfanoid habitus, hyperplastic corneal nerves, skin pigmentation, proximal myopathy and intestinal disorders such as megacolon and ganglioneuromatosis.

Parathyroid hyperplasia is less common. In MEN type 2a medullary carcinoma may occasionally secrete other substances such as ACTH, histaminase, vasoactive intestinal peptide, prostaglandins and serotonin, whereas in MEN type 2b production of hormones other than calcitonin is rare. Both are autosomal dominant. MEN type 2 is associated with *RET gene mutation*. Family members can be screened for this mutation. Those who are RET positive can be offered prophylactic thyroidectomy (or annual calcitonin measurement) and can undertake annual screening of urinary catecholamines and serum calcium. Type 2b is sometimes called type 3.

# Case 5 | Hypothyroidism

**Frequency in survey for 3rd edition**: main focus of a short case in 6% of attempts at PACES Station 5, Endocrine. Additional feature in a further 1%.

## Record 1

The patient is *overweight* with myxoedematous facies (*thickened* and *coarse facial features, periorbital puffiness* and pallor). The *skin* is rough, *dry, cold* and inelastic with a distinct yellowish tint (due to carotenaemia), and there is generalized *non-pitting swelling* of the subcutaneous tissues. The patient's voice is *hoarse* and *croaking*, she is somewhat hard of hearing and her movements are *slow*. There is *thinning* of the *hair* which is *dry* and *brittle* and there is (may be) loss of the outer third of the eyebrows (not a reliable sign). The pulse is *slow* (give rate). There is no palpable goitre. The relaxation phase of the *ankle jerks* (and other reflexes) is delayed and *slow*. This patient has *myxoedema\** (?evidence of associated autoimmune disease – see below).

## Record 2

As appropriate from the above, plus: in view of the symmetrical, firm, finely micro-nodular (typical features of a Hashimoto's goitre though there are many exceptions) *goitre* the likely diagnosis is hypothyroidism due to *Hashimoto's thyroiditis\** (?associated autoimmune disease – see below).

## Record 3

As appropriate from the above, plus: in view of the *exophthalmos* it is likely that this patient was treated in the past for *Graves' disease* by radioactive iodine (or thyroidectomy if there is a scar) and is now hypothyroid (occasionally Graves' disease progresses spontaneously to hypothyroidism; see Station 5, Eyes, Case 12).

---

**Associated autoimmune diseases†**

Pernicious anaemia (?spleen, subacute combined degeneration of the cord [SACD])
Addison's disease (?buccal + scar pigmentation)
Vitiligo
Alopecia (areata, totalis, universalis)
Rheumatoid arthritis (?hands, nodules)
Sjögren's syndrome (?dry eyes and mouth)
Ulcerative colitis
Idiopathic (presumed to be autoimmune) chronic active hepatitis (?icterus, etc.)

Systemic lupus erythematosus (?rash)
Haemolytic anaemia
Diabetes mellitus (?fundi)
Graves' disease
Hypoparathyroidism
Premature ovarian failure

**Important symptoms** (if asked to ask the patient some questions; NB: deafness and hoarse voice):
Cold intolerance
Tiredness and depression

*In hypothyroidism, accumulation of hyaluronic acid in the dermis as well as other tissues alters the composition of the ground substance. This material binds water, producing the mucinous oedema that is responsible for the thickened features and puffy appearance of full-blown hypothyroidism which is termed myxoedema. Hypothyroidism due to autoimmune thyroiditis may present as primary thyroid atrophy (*record* 1) or Hashimoto's disease (*record* 2).
†See also Station 5, Skin, Case 8.

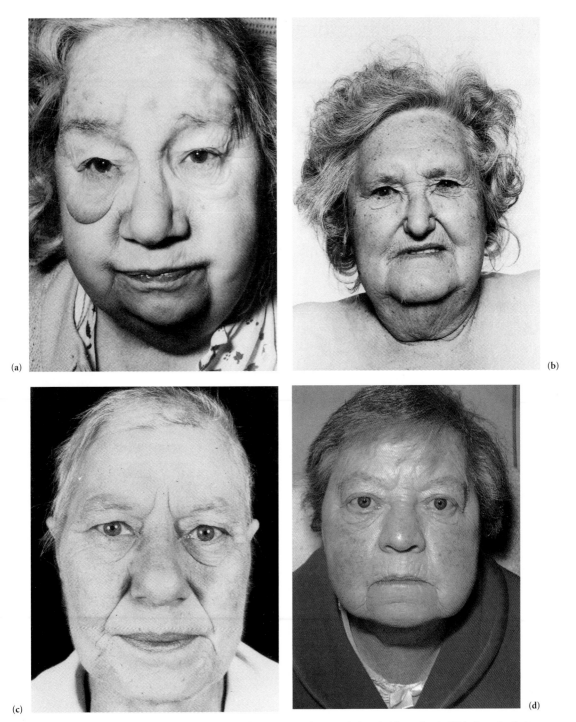

(a)

(b)

(c)

(d)

**Figure I5.65** (a–d) Note thickened skin, periorbital swelling, sparse eyebrows and alopecia. The patient in (d) had a malar flush.

Mental sluggishness

Constipation (may occasionally present to the surgeons with faecal impaction)

Angina (treatment may unmask, therefore start with low doses if age >50 or if patient has angina)

Menorrhagia (middle-aged women)

Primary or secondary amenorrhoea (younger patients)

**Other features**

Anaemia (normochromic, iron deficient – atrophic gastritis, or megaloblastic – frank pernicious anaemia; slight macrocytosis may occur in hypothyroidism without a megaloblastic change in the marrow)

Carpal tunnel syndrome (see Vol. 1, Station 3, CNS, Case 33)

Peripheral cyanosis (there may be a malar flush)

Raynaud's phenomenon

Hypertension

Accident proneness (may present to the emergency department)

Hypothermia (especially the elderly living alone)

Hoffman's syndrome (pain, aching and swelling in muscles after exertion together with signs of myotonia)

Psychosis (myxoedematous madness)

Hypothyroid coma

Associated with Down's syndrome

A variety of other central nervous system (CNS) disorders may occur,‡ such as peripheral neuropathy, cerebellar ataxia, pseudodementia, drop attacks and epilepsy.

---

‡Always exclude concomitant vitamin B12 deficiency as the association with pernicious anaemia is strong. If you find peripheral neuropathy, think also of concomitant diabetes mellitus before putting it down to the hypothyroidism.

# Case 6 | Cushing's syndrome

**Frequency in survey for 3rd edition:** main focus of a short case in 5% of attempts at PACES Station 5, Endocrine. Additional feature in many others in all stations (steroid treatment).

**Survey note:** almost all cases were secondary to therapeutic steroids, especially for asthma and rheumatoid arthritis but also for cryptogenic fibrosing alveolitis and chronic active hepatitis, amongst others.

## *Record*

The patient has a *moon face* with *acne* and *truncal obesity* with a *buffalo hump*. The skin is thin (demonstrate by raising a skinfold at the back of the patient's hand) and shows excessive bruising (*purpuric patches*, often at venesection sites), and there are purple *striae* on the abdomen (must be differentiated from the pale pink striae of obese adolescents and the stretch marks of pregnancy [striae gravidarum] and simple obesity) and she is *hirsute*. There is *proximal muscle weakness* and wasting (few patients with Cushing's syndrome can rise normally from the squatting position; as a simple clinic test, ask the patient to stand up from sitting without using her hands). The diagnosis is Cushing's syndrome (?evidence of underlying steroid-responsive inflammatory or immunological disorder).

---

## Other features of Cushing's syndrome

Hypertension and peripheral oedema (salt retention)

Irregular menstruation

Impotence

Back pain (osteoporosis and vertebral collapse leading to kyphosis and loss of height)

Diabetes mellitus

Pigmentation (especially ectopic or exogenous ACTH or Nelson's syndrome)

Psychiatric disorder (commonly depressive illness)

## Causes of Cushing's syndrome*

Therapeutic corticosteroids

Therapeutic ACTH

Cushing's disease – pituitary (basophilic or chromophobe pituitary adenoma) or hypothalamic lesion leading to excessive ACTH†

Adrenocortical adenoma (occasionally part of *MEN type 1* with one or more of primary hyperparathyroidism, islet cell tumour, pituitary tumour; see Station 5, Endocrine, Case 2‡)

Adrenocortical carcinoma

Ectopic ACTH-secreting non-endocrine tumours:

  **(a)** oat cell carcinoma of bronchus (weight loss, pigmentation, hypokalaemic alkalosis and oedema)

  **(b)** bronchial adenoma

  **(c)** carcinoid tumour (usually bronchial)

  **(d)** carcinoma of the pancreas

  **(e)** non-teratomatous ovarian tumour

*When the syndrome is not iatrogenic, then in about 80% of affected adults the cause is Cushing's disease whereas adrenal adenoma, carcinoma and ectopic ACTH syndrome contribute equally to the remaining 20%.

†ACTH-secreting pituitary adenoma is also associated with MEN 1.

‡In MEN type 1, the islet cell tumour may secrete gastrin (Zollinger–Ellison syndrome) or insulin (insulinoma). The pituitary tumour may be eosinophilic (acromegaly) or a chromophobe adenoma which is non-secreting (bitemporal hemianopia, headaches, blindness, hypopituitarism and other pressure symptoms – tumour may become very large). Pituitary tumours may also secrete prolactin (impotence, amenorrhoea, galactorrhoea) or ACTH (Cushing's disease).

**Table I5.7** Tests for Cushing's syndrome

1 *Classic low-dose dexamethasone suppression test*
   Dexamethasone, 2 mg/day administered orally for 2 days in eight divided doses. Normal individuals almost totally suppress cortisol production (24-h urinary cortisol excretion <10 μg or 100 mmol). Used for the positive diagnosis of Cushing's syndrome

2 *Overnight dexamethasone suppression test*
   Dexamethasone 1 mg administered orally between 2300 and 2400 h. Plasma cortisol is measured the next morning at 0800 h. Normal individuals almost totally suppress cortisol production (plasma cortisol <20 ng/mL, 60 mmol/L). Used for the positive diagnosis of Cushing's syndrome

3 *Classic high-dose dexamethasone suppression test*
   Dexamethasone 8 mg/day administered orally for 2 days in eight divided doses. Patients with Cushing's disease show partial suppression of cortisol production (a significant decrease in 24-h urinary 17-OH steroids or cortisol excretion, usually more than 50%). Patients with other causes of Cushing's syndrome (ectopic ACTH syndrome, adrenal tumours) typically show no significant variation of cortisol production

4 *Corticotrophin-releasing hormone (CRH) test*
   Synthetic ovine (or less often human) CRH is administered IV 100 μg or 1 μg/kg body weight, and plasma ACTH and cortisol are measured during the next 60 min. Patients with Cushing's disease are typically responsive (ACTH and/or cortisol plasma levels increase by more than 50%) and/or 20% of patients with ectopic ACTH syndrome or adrenal tumour are typically unresponsive

## Diagnosis of Cushing's syndrome

The best clinical discriminating signs are easy bruising and proximal muscle weakness. There are two stages to diagnosis: (1) establish diagnosis of Cushing's, and (2) establish the cause.

1 Establishing the diagnosis
Screening:
Overnight dexamethasone suppression test (Table I5.7)
24-h urinary free cortisol (false positives in obesity, depression, oral contraceptive pill and alcohol abuse).

If screening test positive, proceed to low-dose dexamethasone suppression with measurement of 9.00am ACTH.

Loss of circadian rhythm (measure midnight cortisol – usually done as inpatient)
2 Establishing the cause: see Figure I5.66.

## Treatment of Cushing's disease

Trans-sphenoidal hypophysectomy (usually small microadenoma) is the first-line treatment (80% cure). If surgery fails, hypercortisolism can be controlled with antiadrenocortical drugs such as metyrapone or ketoconazole. Simultaneous radiotherapy may allow antiadrenocortical therapy to be discontinued later. In some cases, total bilateral adrenalectomy (laparoscopic or laparotomy) may eventually become necessary, though it has a low and unpredictable risk of Nelson's syndrome (further development of a pituitary tumour).

## Nelson's syndrome

This is due to an ACTH-secreting pituitary tumour in 20% of patients with Cushing's disease who have undergone bilateral adrenalectomy. Untreated, the tumour may enlarge and cause mass effects, in particular visual field defects. May be prevented by external pituitary irradiation at the time of (or prior to) adrenalectomy. The patient is pigmented because of the excess ACTH. The syndrome is rare now that adrenalectomy is no longer a primary treatment for Cushing's disease. Patients with Nelson's syndrome become pigmented due to ACTH causing increased melanin in the skin.

## Prophylaxis and treatment of corticosteroid-induced osteoporosis

The therapeutic options for prophylaxis and treatment of corticosteroid-induced osteoporosis are the same: hormone replacement therapy (HRT) in women, testosterone in men; bisphosphonates; calcitriol. Consider

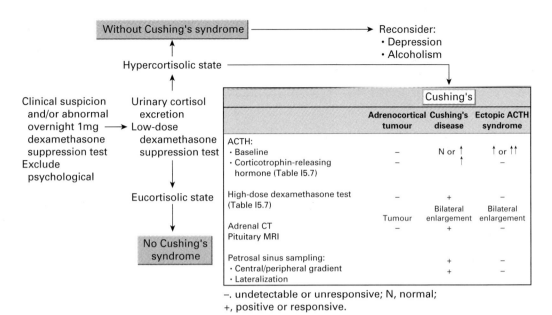

Figure I5.66 Diagnosis of Cushing's syndrome.

The diagram above contains the following text elements:

Without Cushing's syndrome → Reconsider:
• Depression
• Alcoholism

Hypercortisolic state

Clinical suspicion and/or abnormal overnight 1mg dexamethasone suppression test
Exclude psychological

Urinary cortisol excretion → Low-dose dexamethasone suppression test

Eucortisolic state

No Cushing's syndrome

Cushing's

| | Adrenocortical tumour | Cushing's disease | Ectopic ACTH syndrome |
|---|---|---|---|
| **ACTH:** | | | |
| • Baseline | – | N or ↑ | ↑ or ↑↑ |
| • Corticotrophin-releasing hormone (Table I5.7) | – | ↑ | – |
| High-dose dexamethasone test (Table I5.7) | – | + | – |
| Adrenal CT | Tumour | Bilateral enlargement | Bilateral enlargement |
| Pituitary MRI | – | + | – |
| Petrosal sinus sampling: | | | |
| • Central/peripheral gradient | | + | – |
| • Lateralization | | + | – |

–. undetectable or unresponsive; N, normal;
+, positive or responsive.

prophylaxis in all patients taking (or about to commence) prednisolone >7.5 mg/day (or equivalent) for a period of 3 months or more:

1 Prednisolone dose 7.5–15 mg – offer prophylaxis if there are one or more other risk factors§ (in absence of risk factors consider dual-energy X-ray absorptiometry (DEXA) scan to assess bone mineral density and offer prophylaxis if reduced)

2 Prednisolone dose >15 mg – offer prophylaxis at onset.

§Risk factors for osteoporosis:
• long-term steroid treatment
• age greater than 65 years
• premature menopause at less than 45 years
• family history of low trauma fracture
• previous low trauma fracture
• history of amenorrhoea
• slender build
• immobility
• endocrine disorders including Cushing's disease and thyrotoxicosis
• male hypogonadism.

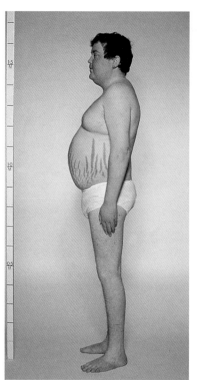

(a)

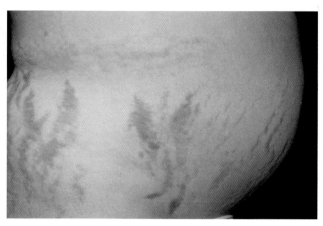

(b)

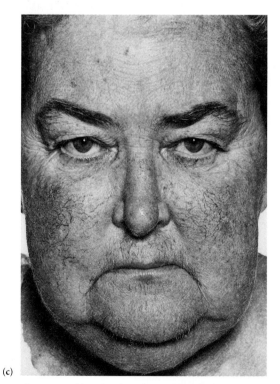

(c)

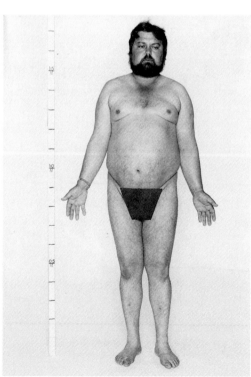

(d)

**Figure I5.67** (a) Cushing's syndrome. (b) Abdominal striae. (c) Cushingoid facies (steroid therapy for cerebral lupus erythematosus). (d) Truncal obesity (Cushing's disease).

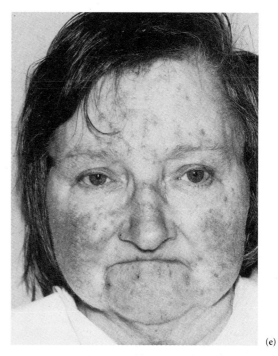

(e)

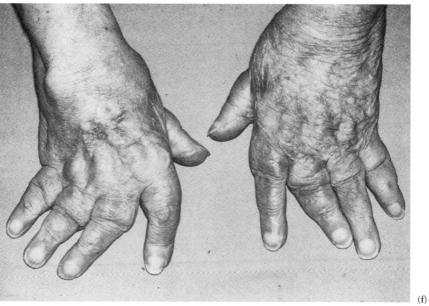

(f)

**Figure I5.67** (*Continued*) (e,f) Corticosteroid therapy in a patient with rheumatoid arthritis.

# Case 7 | Addison's disease

**Frequency in survey for 3rd edition:** main focus of a short case in 3% of attempts at PACES Station 5, Endocrine.

## *Record*

There is *generalized pigmentation* (due to the direct action of ACTH causing increased melanin in the skin), which is more marked in the *skin creases* (e.g. palmar), in *scars* (especially more recent ones), in the *buccal mucosa* (look in the mouth), in the *nipples, axilla* and at *pressure points*. This suggests Addison's disease or Nelson's syndrome (?temporal field defect, ?abdominal scar of bilateral adrenalectomy; see Station 5, Endocrine, Case 6).

---

Patchy, almost symmetrical areas of skin depigmentation surrounded by areas of increased pigmentation may occur due to vitiligo (15% of patients with idiopathic Addison's) which is one of the associated organ-specific autoimmune diseases. (For the others, which include autoimmune thyroiditis, diabetes mellitus, pernicious anaemia and hypoparathyroidism, see Station 5, Skin, Case 8. Premature ovarian failure is particularly associated with Addison's disease.)

### Common causes of primary hypoadrenalism

Autoimmune adrenalitis

Tuberculosis (in endemic areas – ?lung signs)

### Other causes of primary hypoadrenalism

Bilateral adrenalectomy (malignant disease, e.g. breast cancer, Cushing's syndrome)

Secondary deposits

Amyloidosis (hypoadrenalism preceded by nephrotic syndrome; see Footnote, Vol. 1, Station 1, Abdominal, Case 4)

Haemochromatosis

Granulomatous disease (rarely sarcoidosis)

Fungal diseases (e.g. histoplasmosis)

Congenital adrenal hyperplasia*

Meningococcal and pseudomonal septicaemia

AIDS

Adrenal haemorrhage (newborn, especially breech delivery; patients on anticoagulants)

Adrenal vein thrombosis after trauma or adrenal venography

**Skin pigmentation** is usually racial (including buccal pigmentation) or due to sun-tanning. Other causes of abnormal generalized pigmentation include the following:

Endocrine

ACTH therapy (e.g. asthma)

Cushing's disease (?facies, truncal obesity, striae, etc; see Station 5, Endocrine, Case 6)

Thyrotoxicosis (?exophthalmos, goitre, etc; see Station 5, Endocrine, Case 3)

Ectopic ACTH (especially oat cell carcinoma)

Uncontrolled congenital adrenal hyperplasia.

*Chronic debilitating disorders* (also, like Addison's, associated with lassitude and weight loss)

Malignancy (including reticuloses and leukaemias)

Malabsorption syndromes

Chronic infections (especially TB)

Cirrhosis (?icterus, spider naevi, etc; see Vol. 1, Station 1, Abdominal, Case 1 and Case 17)

Uraemia (pale, brownish-yellow tinge to skin)

---

*Series of inherited defects in adrenocortical steroidogenesis (e.g. 21-hydroxylase deficiency). Homozygotes present neonatally with salt wasting, hypotension and ambiguous genitalia in females.

*Pigments other than melanin* such as:

Haemochromatosis (slate-grey pigmentation, hepato-splenomegaly, etc; see Vol. 1, Station 1, Abdominal, Case 16)

Argyria

Chronic arsenic poisoning.

*Drugs*

Phenothiazines (blue-grey pigmentation)

Antimalarials (blue-grey pigmentation)

Amiodarone (grey pigmentation)

Cytotoxics

Minocycline (purple-blue pigmentation; may get blue oral discoloration due to blue-black discoloration of alveolar bone and hard palate – 'black-bone disease')

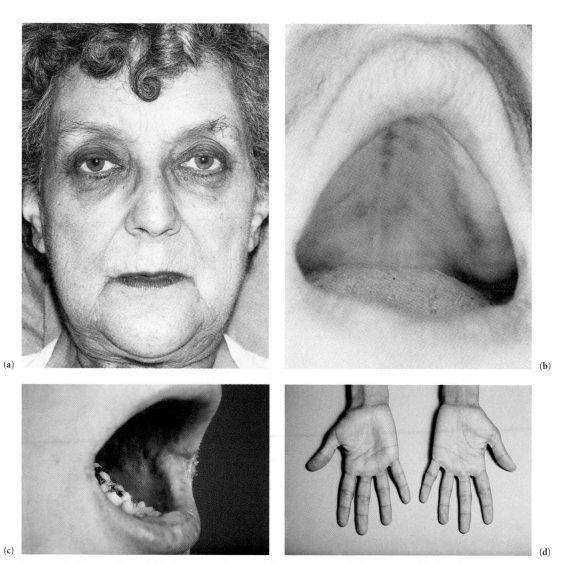

(a)

(b)

(c)

(d)

**Figure I5.68** Addison's disease. (a) Facial pigmentation, especially periorbitally. (b,c) Pigmentation of the buccal mucosa. (d) Palmar crease pigmentation. (*Continued*)

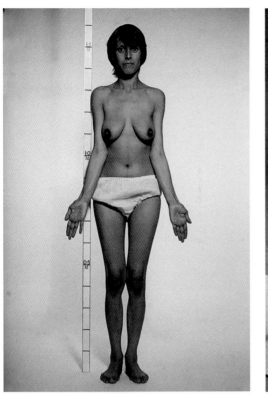

(e)

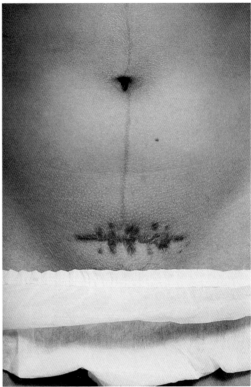

(f)

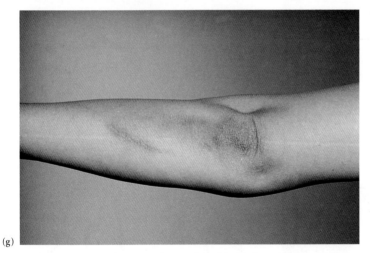

(g)

**Figure I5.68** (*Continued*) (e) Note pigmentation of the nipples and areolae. (f) Pigmentation of the scar and linea alba. (g) Pigmentation of the elbow (a pressure point).

# Case 8 | **Hypopituitarism**

**Frequency in survey for 3rd edition:** main focus of a short case in 2% of attempts at PACES Station 5, Endocrine. Additional feature in a further 1%.

## *Record*

The patient's *skin* is *soft, wrinkled* and *pale* with a *yellow tint* (the pallor is due to a combination of lack of melanocyte-stimulating hormone and anaemia – marrow hypofunction). The areolae of the breasts are (may be) depigmented. *Pubic, axillary, facial* and *body hair* is *reduced* (and the *genitals* and *breasts* are *atrophied*).

These features suggest hypopituitarism (now check for a bitemporal visual field defect).

---

With progressing hypopituitarism, gonadotrophin secretion is usually impaired first, followed by growth hormone, TSH, ACTH* and antidiuretic hormone, in that order. Hypogonadism causes loss of libido, erectile dysfunction, fatigue and loss of physical strength in the male, and fine facial wrinkling and amenorrhoea/oligomenorrhoea in the premenstrual female. Growth hormone deficiency may lead to weight gain and mood changes associated with a reduced quality of life. With the onset of thyroid failure, the features of hypothyroidism (see Station 5, Endocrine, Case 5) are superimposed on those in the above *record*. Lassitude, cold intolerance, dryness of skin and prolongation of the relaxation phase of the tendon reflexes occur, though swelling of the subcutaneous tissues is usually less prominent. The insidious onset of asthenia, nausea, vomiting, postural hypotension, hypoglycaemia, collapse and coma mark progressive ACTH lack. Diabetes insipidus (most commonly occurs post pituitary surgery) develops with lack of antidiuretic hormone, though impaired glomerular filtration caused by cortisol deficiency may mask the symptoms.

**The main causes of adult panhypopituitarism** (male-to-female ratio is 1:2) are:
Pituitary tumour† (especially chromophobe adenoma)
Head injury
Idiopathic
Meningioma or parasellar tumour
Craniopharyngioma
Iatrogenic (hypophysectomy, radiotherapy to sella or nasopharynx)
Pituitary granulomatous lesion (tuberculoma, sarcoidosis, Hand–Schüller–Christian disease, syphilitic gumma)
Sheehan's syndrome (following severe obstetric haemorrhage or shock – much less common nowadays with good obstetric practice).

**The factors that lead to coma** in hypopituitarism include hypoglycaemia, sodium depletion, water intoxication, cerebral anoxia, hypothyroidism, hypothermia and pressure on the midbrain or hypothalamus.

---

*Pituitary hypothyroidism may protect the patient from the effects of failing ACTH secretion. In this situation, misdiagnosing the cause of hypothyroidism and waking the patient from hibernation with thyroxine alone may precipitate Addisonian crisis.

†Suprasellar extension may cause compression of the optic chiasm (visual field defect); lateral extension may cause mononeuropathies (IIIrd, IVth, Vth [Va and Vb], VIth cranial nerves).

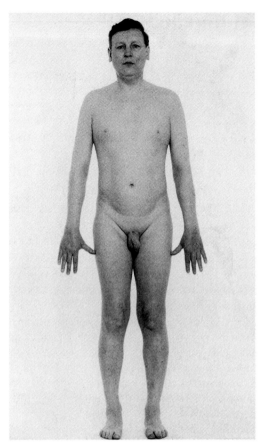

**Figure I5.69** Hypopituitarism (8 years after removal of pituitary adenoma).

# Case 9 | Pretibial myxoedema

**Frequency in survey for 3rd edition:** main focus of a short case in 2% of attempts at PACES Station 5, Endocrine. Additional feature in a further 5%.

## *Record*

There are *elevated symmetrical* skin lesions over the anterolateral aspects of the *shins* (may spread onto the feet; may affect other parts of the body, e.g. the face or the dorsa of the hands). The lesions are coarse, *purplish-red* (may be skin colour, pink or, rarely, brown) in colour and raised with *well-defined* serpiginous *margins*. The skin is *shiny* and has an *orange peel appearance*. The hairs in the affected areas are coarse and the lesions are *tender* (and itch). The patient has *exophthalmos** (*?thyroid acropachy**) and is likely to have been rendered *euthyroid* (?pulse, etc.) by surgery (*?thyroidectomy scar*) or, more particularly, with *radioactive iodine*. The diagnosis is pretibial myxoedema (occurs in about 5% of patients with Graves' disease).

---

The superficial layer of the skin is infiltrated with the mucopolysaccharide hyaluronic acid. Biopsy scars of the area almost invariably develop keloid.

The latent interval between the treatment for hyper-thyroidism and the clinical onset of pretibial myxo-edema varies from 4 to 32 months with a mean time of 1 year.

Pretibial myxoedema in its most extreme form clini-cally resembles lymphoedema. It may be that mucin deposition in the dermis causes compression of the dermal lymphatics which results in dermal oedema and the clinical features of lymphoedema.

Early treatment with topical, strong glucocorticoid preparations can clear or improve the lesions. Larger and long-standing disease is more resistant.

---

*Pretibial myxoedema is almost always accompanied by exoph-thalmos. Thyroid acropachy (see Station 5, Endocrine, Case 5) is occasionally associated – diffuse thickening of distal extremities, subperiosteal new bone formation simulating clubbing of the digits. Exophthalmos has also been termed *infiltrative ophthal-mopathy* and pretibial myxoedema, *infiltrative dermopathy*.

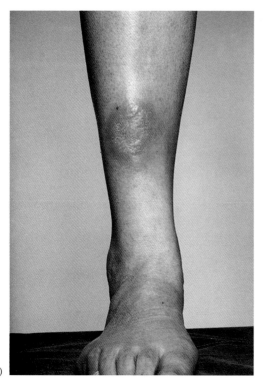 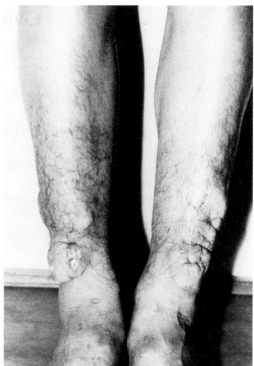

(a)                                                                                    (b)

**Figure I5.70**  (a,b) Pretibial myxoedema.

# Case 10 | Gynaecomastia

**Frequency in survey for 3rd edition:** main focus of a short case in 2% of attempts at PACES Station 5, Endocrine. Additional feature in a further 5%, especially Station 3, Cardiac and Station 1, Abdominal.

**Survey note:** all cases were due to either drugs or cirrhosis.

## *Record*

There is gynaecomastia (it may be unilateral). This is confirmed on palpation by the presence of *increased glandular tissue*.\* (Now look for signs of *cirrhosis, heart failure* [spironolactone], *atrial fibrillation* [digoxin], *clubbing and cachexia* [carcinoma of the lung], *absence of body hair* [hypogonadism, oestrogen therapy] or evidence of an *endocrine disorder* – see below. The *testes* are small and firm in Klinefelter's and asymmetrical with a tumour. If tall stature, most likely to have Klinefelter's syndrome.)

---

There may be feminization of the nipples and tenderness of the breasts. Gynaecomastia must be differentiated from tumours of the breast and simple adiposity. Gynaecomastia is due to an imbalance in the free androgen to free oestrogen ratio – an imbalance in production or drug effects on metabolism.

## Causes of gynaecomastia

### *Physiological*

Pubertal (very common,† often unilateral – due to transient dominance of circulating oestradiol over testosterone)

Senile (normal rise in oestrogens and fall in androgens with age)

### *Pathological*

Cirrhosis of the liver (?stigmata; see Vol. 1, Station 1, Abdominal, Case 1)

Thyrotoxicosis (?exophthalmos, goitre, etc; see Station 5, Endocrine, Case 3)

Carcinoma of the lung (5% of patients; sometimes with hypertrophic pulmonary osteoarthropathy; human chorionic gonadotrophin [HCG] secreted by the tumour)

Carcinoma of the liver (HCG secreting)

Klinefelter's syndrome (47,XXY, small testes, mental deficiency, incomplete virilization, raised LH and FSH and can have tall stature)

Pituitary disease,‡ i.e. acromegaly, hypopituitarism (?visual field defect)

Isolated gonadotrophin deficiency (e.g. Kallman's syndrome – hypogonadotrophic hypogonadism and anosmia, often with harelip or cleft palate)

Testicular tumours (due to HCG secretion, oestrogen secretion or excess aromatase activity in the tumour tissue)

Testicular failure

Addison's disease (?pigmentation – buccal and scar; see Station 5, Endocrine, Case 7)

Adrenal carcinoma

Testicular feminization (androgen insensitivity)

Drug induced (Table I5.8)§

---

\*A disc of tissue arising from beneath the nipple and areola – concentric, firm and mobile.

†Thirty-nine per cent of 1855 adolescent boys of different ages at one boy scout camp, though other surveys have found it less common.

‡NB: prolactin excess in the absence of oestrogens produces galactorrhoea rather than gynaecomastia.

§The letters of the word MADRAS form a useful mnemonic: methyldopa, aldactone, digoxin, reserpine, alkylating agents and stilboestrol. These were the drugs of this mnemonic in the 20th century; today they could be marijuana, angiotensin-converting enzyme (ACE) inhibitors, digoxin, ranitidine, amiodarone and spironolactone.

**Table I5.8** Drugs that may cause gynaecomastia

| | |
|---|---|
| Hormonal | Oestrogens |
| | Aromatizable androgens (e.g. testosterone enanthate, testosterone propionate) |
| | Antiandrogens (cyproterone acetate) |
| Cardiac | Calcium-channel blockers |
| | Angiotensin-converting enzyme inhibitors |
| | Digoxin |
| | Amiodarone |
| | Spironolactone |
| | Methyldopa |
| CNS | Dopamine receptor antagonists (phenothiazines, metoclopramide) |
| | Tricyclic antidepressants |
| | Benzodiazepines |
| | Opiates |
| | Marijuana |
| Gastrointestinal | Omeprazole |
| | Cimetidine |
| | Ranitidine |
| Anti-infective | Isoniazid |
| | Metronidazole |
| | Ketoconazole |
| Cytotoxic | Alkylating agents (cause testicular damage) such as busulphan and nitrosureas |
| Alcohol | |

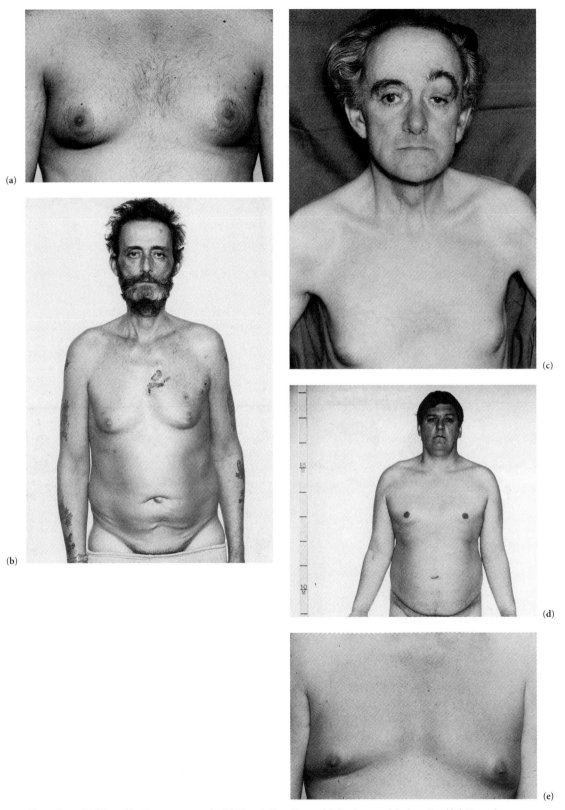

**Figure I5.71** (a) Bilateral benign gynaecomastia. (b) Chronic liver disease. (c) Carcinoma of the lung (note left Horner's syndrome). (d,e) Hypogonadism. (e) Close-up view of the same patient as (d).

# Case 11 | Turner's syndrome

**Frequency in survey for 3rd edition:** main focus of a short case in 2% of attempts at PACES Station 5, Endocrine.

## Record

The patient (who probably presented with primary amenorrhoea) is *short* (usually less than 1.5 m) with a *short webbed neck*\* (only found in 54%) and shows *cubitus valgus* deformity. She has a *shield-like chest* (and may have widely separated nipples). The *nails* are *hypoplastic* and she has *short fourth metacarpals* (other metacarpals may also be short). The *hairline* is *low*, she has a *high-arched palate* and there are *numerous naevi*. The secondary sexual characteristics are underdeveloped (unless the patient has been treated with oestrogens).

The diagnosis is Turner's syndrome. (If allowed, examine the cardiovascular system – abnormal in 20%, especially coarctation of the aorta (see Vol. 1, Station 3, Cardiovascular, Case 26) but also atrial septal defect (see Vol. 1, Station 3, Cardiovascular, Case 28), ventricular septal defect (see Vol. 1, Station 3, Cardiovascular, Case 12) and aortic stenosis (see Vol. 1, Station 3, Cardiovascular, Case 5).

---

One in 2500–3500 female births.

The patient with Turner's syndrome is likely to have streak gonads and a chromosome constitution which is mostly 45,XO,† though mosaicism (XO,XX) does occur. Red-green colour blindness (an X-linked recessive character) occurs as frequently in Turner's as it does in normal males, and other X-linked conditions may occur.

**Other features which sometimes occur**

Lymphoedema
Genitourinary abnormality (e.g. horseshoe kidney)
Hypertelorism
Epicanthal fold
Mental retardation is rare

Strabismus
Ptosis
Intestinal telangiectasia
Premature osteoporosis
Premature ageing in appearance
Higher incidence of diabetes mellitus and Hashimoto's thyroiditis

**Noonan's syndrome**

May affect both sexes. Females have Turner's phenotype but normal 46,XX, normal ovarian function and normal fertility. Noonan's are more likely to have right-sided cardiac lesions (especially pulmonary stenosis) whereas Turner's are more likely to have left-sided lesions. Mental retardation is frequent.

---

\*A feature especially associated with cardiovascular abnormalities in this condition.

†Most 45,XO pregnancies end in spontaneous abortion.

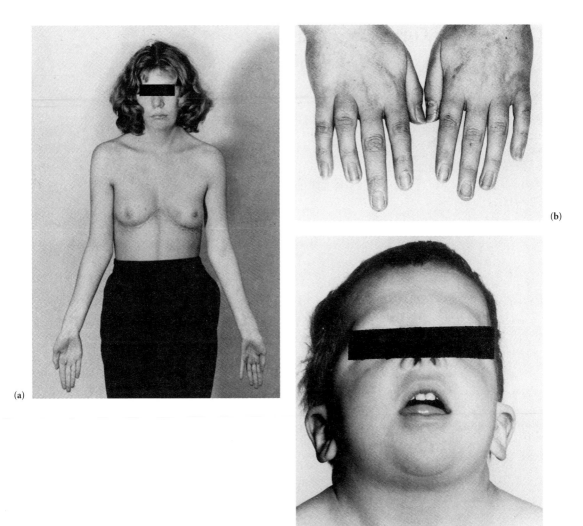

**Figure I5.72** (a) XO,XX mosaic. Note the webbed neck, increased carrying angle and scar under the breasts (special incision for atrial septal defect repair). (b) The hands of another patient showing a short fourth metacarpal. (c) Noonan's syndrome.

# Case 12 | Klinefelter's syndrome/ hypogonadism

**Frequency in survey for 3rd edition:** main focus of a short case in 2% of attempts at PACES Station 5, Endocrine.

**Survey note:** it does not often happen but occasionally candidates are allowed to examine the testes (see Vol. 2, Section F, Experience 216 and Vol. 2, Section F, Anecdote 291).

## Record

The patient is *tall*, has *gynaecomastia* (may be asymmetrical), sparse body hair and has a *eunuchoid habitus.** He has very small testes (<2 cm length, often termed *pea-sized*; lower limit of normal for adults is 3.5 cm length). The features suggest Klinefelter's syndrome.

---

See Vol. 2, Section F, Anecdote 291.

## Other features of Klinefelter's syndrome

Affects 1 in 400–500 men (1/20 if maternal age >45)

Classically 47,XXY but also XXYY, more than two X (poly X) plus Y and mosaics

Azoospermia and raised gonadotrophins

Though the majority have normal intelligence there is a higher than normal incidence of mental retardation (especially if more than two X chromosomes)

Higher incidence of somatic abnormalities (especially if more than two X chromosomes) such as hypospadias, cryptorchidism and bony abnormalities of the radius and ulna

If there is an additional Y chromosome, patients tend to be tall with very aggressive antisocial behavioural abnormalities

Less severe manifestations in mosaics (fertility has been recorded in XXY, XY)

Character and personality disorders common (may be in part related to the psychosocial consequences of androgen deficiency)

Slightly increased incidence of certain systemic diseases (diabetes, chronic obstructive airways disease, autoimmune disorders such as systemic lupus erythematosus (SLE) and Hashimoto's thyroiditis, malignancy such as breast, lymphoma and germ cell neoplasms, and varicose veins)

## Features of eunuchoid appearance

Average height or above (growth until mid-twenties)

Span > height†

Pubis–heel > pubis–crown

Body fat tends to be in feminine contours; broad hips, musculature poor

Sparse body hair/beard

Poorly developed genitalia

Gynaecomastia

Timid behaviour

---

*The degree of eunuchoidism is variable depending on the degree of androgen deficiency which is seldom complete; indeed, the occasional Klinefelter's patient may have normal testosterone levels and virilization, the only abnormality being the pea-sized testes and azoospermia. The patient treated with exogenous testosterone may also be well virilized.

†In contrast to other conditions which result in prepubertal androgen deficiency, Klinefelter's patients often have a disproportionate increase in lower extremity compared to upper extremity long bone growth (i.e. span may not be > height).

## Causes of primary hypogonadism (with deficiency of both sperm and androgen production)

### Congenital or developmental disorders

Klinefelter's syndrome and variants

Functional prepubertal castrate syndrome (congenital anorchia – no testicular tissue from birth; testes must have been active in fetal life because the phenotype is male; hence sometimes referred to as 'vanishing testis syndrome')

Noonan's syndrome (?short stature, triangular micrognathic facial appearance and posteriorly angulated low-set ears with a thick helix, webbed neck, shield-like chest, pectus excavatum, cubitus valgus, mental retardation, right-sided cardiovascular abnormalities; often cryptorchidism as well as primary testicular dysfunction; see also Station 5, Endocrine, Case 11)

Myotonic dystrophy – see Vol. 1, Station 3, CNS, Case 2 (though most cases develop testicular atrophy with maintained androgen production but impaired spermatogenesis in middle age, 20% have manifestations of androgen deficiency as a result of primary testicular failure – testosterone in these patients may help maintain or improve muscle function)

Polyglandular autoimmune disease – see Station 5, Skin, Case 8 (though much less common than autoimmune primary ovarian failure, primary testicular failure associated with antitesticular antibodies and androgen deficiency may also occur)

Complex genetic disorders (Alström, ataxia telangiectasia, Sohval–Soffer, Weinstein's and Wermer's syndromes)

Cryptorchidism (failure of testicular descent)

NB: normal ageing (in healthy men is associated with a relative fall in testosterone with associated elevation of gonadotrophins)

### Acquired disorders

Orchitis (viral, especially mumps; also gonorrhoea, leprosy, tuberculosis [TB], brucellosis, glanders, syphilis, filariasis, bilharziasis)

Surgical and traumatic castration

Drugs (which may produce antiandrogen effects include spironolactone, ketoconazole, H2-blockers such as cimetidine, alcohol, marijuana, digitalis, cytotoxics)

Irradiation

### Systemic disorders

Chronic liver disease – see Vol. 1, Station 1, Abdominal, Case 1 (total testosterone low or normal, LH usually elevated, high circulating oestrogens due to impaired hepatic clearance of adrenal androgens leading to increased substrate for peripheral aromatization to oestrogens; treatment with aromatizable androgens may worsen the gynaecomastia)

Chronic renal failure (?uraemic pallor; testosterone replacement may improve the anaemia)

Malignancy (Hodgkin's disease, testicular cancer)

Sickle cell disease

Paraplegia (transient reduction in testosterone initially)

Vasculitis (may involve the testes)

Infiltrative disease (amyloidosis, leukaemia)

HIV

## Causes of secondary hypogonadism (with deficiency of both sperm and androgen production)

### Congenital and developmental disorders

Isolated hypogonadotrophic hypogonadism‡ (?associated anosmia or hyposmia due to developmental failure of the olfactory lobes in which case *Kallman's syndrome* – may also exhibit other mid-line defects [e.g. cleft lip or cleft palate, colour blindness, renal agenesis, nerve deafness], cryptorchidism and skeletal abnormalities [e.g. syndactyly, short fourth metacarpals, craniofacial asymmetry])

Isolated LH deficiency ('*fertile' eunuch syndrome*; variant of Kallman's syndrome in which FSH secretion is preserved, resulting in near normal-sized testes and well-advanced, though not normal, spermatogenesis; despite the name, patients are not fertile without HCG therapy)

Haemochromatosis – see Vol. 1, Station 1, Abdominal, Case 16 (iron deposition in the pituitary selectively inhibits gonadotrophins whilst other anterior pituitary hormone secretion remains unaffected)

‡Differentiation from the much more common constitutional delayed puberty is difficult. Withdrawal of androgen therapy can eventually be achieved in constitutional delayed puberty but not in hypogonadotrophic hypogonadism. Fertility can be facilitated in hypogonadotrophic hypogonadism by treatment with gonadotrophins or gonadotrophin-releasing hormone instead of androgens.

Complex genetic syndromes (e.g. Prader–Willi;§ Laurence–Moon–Bardet–Biedl – see Station 5, Eyes, Case 19; familial cerebellar ataxia; familial icthyosis)

### Acquired disorders

Hypopituitarism – see Station 5, Endocrine, Case 8

Hyperprolactinaemia (either *microprolactinoma, macroprolactinoma* or other large pituitary tumour causing stalk compression;¶ prolactin inhibits gonadotrophin secretion; macroadenomata may destroy pituitary gonadotrophs)

Oestrogen excess (therapy for prostatic cancer; oestrogen-producing neoplasms)

Opiate-like drugs (such as morphine, methadone and heroin) inhibit gonadotrophin production

### Systemic disorders

Cushing's – see Station 5, Endocrine, Case 6 (high levels of glucocorticoids suppress gonadotrophin secretion)

Acute stress or illness (high glucocorticoids)

Nutritional deficiency (protein–calorie malnutrition or anorexia nervosa; gonadotrophin production inhibited)

Chronic illness (malnutrition may contribute)

Massive obesity§

§*Prader–Labhart–Willi syndrome.* Our survey has raised the possibility that this has occurred rarely as an MRCP short case. The syndrome consists of poor fetal activity, infantile hypotonia and neonatal failure to thrive. Compulsive hyperphagia with *massive obesity* in later childhood. May be *cryptorchidism*. Thin turned-down upper lips and up-slanting palpebral fissures often seen (*almond-shaped eyes*). Poor dentition is often present. Fair skin and hair darkens with age. Hands and feet characteristically small (*acromicria*). Pickwickian syndrome (see Vol. 1, Station 1, Respiratory, Case 18) may occur. Diabetes mellitus is common. Mild-to-severe *mental retardation* with behaviour and personality problems is usual. Hypothalamic dysfunction and *hypogona-*dotrophic hypogonadism are often present. *It should be remembered that low testosterone and gonadotrophins may be found in association with any case of massive obesity.*

¶Microprolactinomata are <1 cm in diameter and macroprolactinomata >1 cm. Any pituitary macroadenoma which compresses the pituitary stalk and interferes with the prolactin-inhibiting dopaminergic neurones there may lead to hyperprolactinaemia. Serum prolactin levels >5000 mIU/L are not usually associated with stalk compression alone and usually reflect a true prolactinoma. Other causes of hyperprolactinaemia include CNS-active drugs such as phenothiazines and other antipsychotic drugs, opiates, sedatives, antidepressants and stimulants.

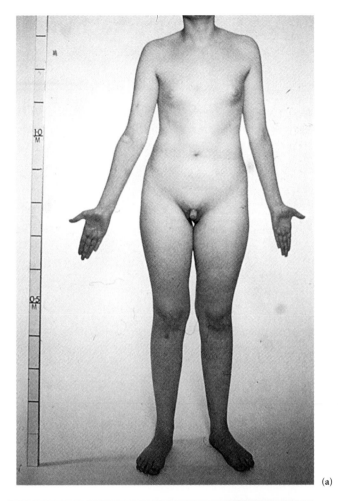

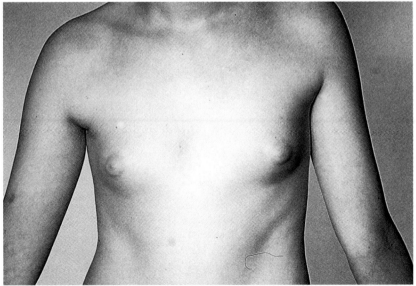

**Figure 15.73** Klinefelter's syndrome. (a) Note the disproportionately long lower limbs in relation to the upper torso, the underdeveloped genitalia and the absent axillary and pubic hair. (b) Gynaecomastia.

# Case 13 | Bitemporal hemianopia

**Frequency in survey for 3rd edition:** main focus of a short case in 2% of attempts at PACES Station 5, Endocrine.

Bitemporal hemianopia is dealt with in Vol. 1, Station 3, CNS, Case 13.

# Case 14 | Diabetic foot/Charcot's joint

**Frequency in survey for 3rd edition:** main focus of a short case in 2% of attempts at PACES Station 5, Endocrine.

Diabetic foot/Charcot's joint is dealt with in Station 5, Locomotor, Case 4.

# Case 15 | Necrobiosis lipoidica diabeticorum

**Frequency in survey for 3rd edition:** main focus of a short case in 1% of attempts at PACES Station 5, Endocrine.

Necrobiosis lipoidica diabeticorum is dealt with in Station 5, Skin, Case 18.

# Case 16 | **Short stature**

**Frequency in survey for 3rd edition:** main focus of a short case in 0.8% of attempts at PACES Station 5, Endocrine.

## *Record*

The patient is abnormally short (?features of a major systemic disease or of one of the classic syndromes).

## Causes of a short adult* include

### *Genetic*

Familial (correlation between a patient's height and the mid-parental height)

Achondroplasia (?short limbs, relatively normal trunk, large head with bulging forehead and scooped nose)

*Turner's syndrome* (?webbed neck, cubitus valgus, short metacarpals, female phenotype, left-sided heart lesions; see Station 5, Endocrine, Case 11)

Noonan's syndrome (?triangular micrognathic facial appearance and posteriorly angulated low-set ears with a thick helix, webbed neck, shield-like chest, pectus excavatum, cubitus valgus, mental retardation, right-sided cardiovascular abnormalities; see Figure I5.72c)

Growth hormone deficiency†

### *Nutritional or general diseases during childhood*

Low birth weight and subsequent slow growth (some cases end up as short adults)

Congenital heart disease (?cyanosis, young adult)

---

*The diagnoses in italics represent causes of short stature in adults that our surveys have shown have occurred in the MRCP with the short stature highlighted as a prominent feature. Short stature is a subject more commonly considered in childhood. Shortness which is out of keeping with parental height (familial) can usefully be considered as follows.

1 **Child looks normal**

  (a) *Normal growth velocity:* constitutional delay in growth and adolescence (common; short throughout childhood; pubertal growth spurt delayed; bone age lags behind chronological age; patients usually attain normal height)

  (b) *Low growth velocity:*

  • *Thin child* (mostly due to a disease of a major system):

    Central nervous system (mental retardation)

    Cardiovascular system (congenital heart disease)

    Respiratory system (cystic fibrosis, asthma, TB)

    Gastrointestinal system (malabsorption, e.g. coeliac disease, Crohn's)

    Renal system (chronic renal failure, renal tubular acidosis)

    Psychosocial problems (emotional deprivation, anorexia nervosa)

  • *Fat child* (endocrine causes):

    Hypopituitarism

    Growth hormone deficiency†

    Laron's syndrome (same phenotype as growth hormone deficiency but cause is somatomedin deficiency – resting growth hormone levels are high; no response to growth hormone therapy)

    Hypothyroidism

    Cushing's

    Pseudohypoparathyroidism

2 **Child looks abnormal**

  (a) *Dysmorphic features:* recognizable syndrome (e.g. low birth weight, chromosomal abnormality)

  (b) *Disproportionate short stature:*

    Short limbs (e.g. achondroplasia, hypochondroplasia, dyschondrosteosis, metaphyseal chondroplasia, multiple epiphyseal dysplasia)

    Short back and limbs (e.g. metatrophic dwarf, spondyloepiphyseal dysplasia, mucopolysaccharidosis)

†Most short and tall people are normal, just at the extremes of the normal range. To make a diagnosis of GH deficiency, GH secretion must be measured during a standard stimulation test (e.g. insulin, glucagon). Children with GH deficiency, if diagnosed early and treated with adequate doses of GH, achieve adult heights in keeping with their parents. The untreated adult height in severe GH deficiency is approximately 137 cm. This group gains the most height for the smallest doses.

Renal disease

*Cystic fibrosis*\* (?clubbing, cyanosis, basal crackles, sputum pot, young person; see
  Vol. 1, Station 1, Respiratory, Case 17)

Chronic infection

Collagenosis

Mental retardation

Coeliac disease

*Rickets*\* (?lateral bowing of legs that is symmetrical; see Station 5, Locomotor,
  Case 17)

Diabetes

Craniospinal irradiation

### Social

Severe emotional deprivation suppresses growth hormone release.

### Endocrine problems during childhood

Isolated growth hormone deficiency

Panhypopituitarism

Hypothyroidism

Cushing's disease

Precocious puberty

*Pseudohypoparathyroidism*\* (?round face, short neck, short metacarpals, decreased
  intelligence, subcutaneous calcification; see also Station 5, Endocrine, Case 17)

# Case 17 | Pseudohypoparathyroidism

**Frequency in survey for 3rd edition:** main focus of a short case in 0.4% of attempts at PACES Station 5, Endocrine.

## Record

The patient is *short* and *obese* with a *round* face (with frontal bossing of the skull) and a short neck. There is *shortening* of the (most often) fourth and fifth *metacarpals* (ask the patient to make a fist to demonstrate this) and, maybe, metatarsals, as well as shortening and broadening of the distal phalanges. There are *subcutaneous calcifications*.*

These features suggest the diagnosis of type 1a pseudohypoparathyroidism (Albright's† hereditary osteodystrophy).

### Other features which may occur in Albright's hereditary osteodystrophy

Mental retardation (usually slight)
Hypothyroidism (without goitre)
Hypogonadism
Pseudopseudohypoparathyroidism‡ in first-degree relatives
Females affected twice as commonly as males
Parathyroid glands normal or hyperplastic
Usually presents early in life (mental deficiency, epilepsy or tetany)
Treatment is with vitamin D

---

In pseudohypoparathyroidism there is target organ resistance to the action of parathyroid hormone. The defect occurs proximal to the formation of the second messenger cAMP.§

### Types of pseudohypoparathyroidism

*Type 1a* – appearance as described in the above *record*. Deficiency in the Gs protein that couples parathyroid hormone receptors to adenylcyclase limits the normal cAMP production in response to parathyroid hormone as well as to other hormones such as TSH. As a result, patients with type 1a pseudohypoparathyroidism have many abnormalities (e.g. *hypothyroidism, hypogonadism*) as well as hypocalcaemia.

The causative mutations in the gene encoding the Gs protein are inherited as *autosomal dominant*

*Type 1b* – appearance is normal. Gs protein normal – resistance is limited to parathyroid hormone. A defective parathyroid hormone receptor is the postulated cause. Osteitis fibrosa cystica can occur in some subjects, suggesting selective renal (but not skeletal) resistance to parathyroid hormone action; this rare combination has been called *pseudohypohyperparathyroidism*.

### Other causes of hypoparathyroidism

Autoimmune (there may be an associated endocrine deficiency, most frequently Addison's disease, as well

---

*Ectopic deposits of bone may develop in muscles, tendons, connective tissue and skin.

†Albright described pseudohypoparathyroidism as the first example of a hormone-resistance disorder.

‡Physical features of Albright's osteodystrophy without evidence of hormone resistance.

§The diagnosis is suggested by the finding of an *elevated* parathyroid hormone in a patient with hypocalcaemia, hyperphosphataemia and normal renal function. Lack of urinary cAMP excretion in response to parathyroid hormone (commercially available 1–34 peptide) infusion confirms the parathyroid hormone resistance.

as a T-cell defect predisposing to mucocutaneous candidiasis [see Station 5, Skin, Case 8]; alopecia and vitiligo may also be seen)

Surgical (incidence varies widely as a function of the skill of the surgeon)

Iron deposition in parathyroids (e.g. repeated transfusions in thalassaemia)

Copper deposition in parathyroids (Wilson's disease)

Failure of development of parathyroids (Di George's syndrome)

Idiopathic (inherited mutations in the parathyroid hormone gene that prevent synthesis and secretion of parathyroid hormone)

Transient (hypomagnesaemia; transient suppression of normal parathyroids by a hyperparathyroid-adenoma;¶ surgical injury to the parathyroids is another postulated cause of transient postoperative hypoparathyroidism)

---

¶Though within a week the suppressed parathyroids should be functioning again, the major cause of hypocalcaemia following parathyroidectomy for hyperparathyroidism is 'bone hunger' – with removal of the high parathyroid hormone levels, the skeleton rapidly takes in calcium. It may take months for the skeleton to recover fully.

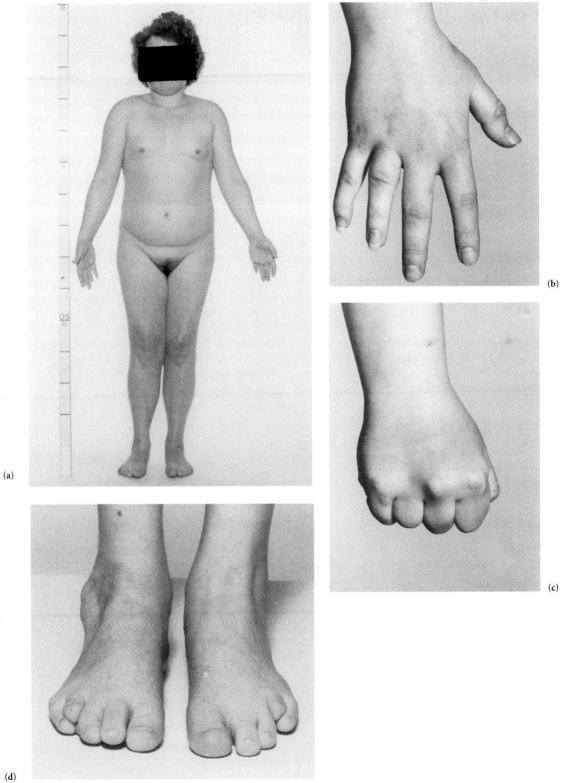

**Figure I5.74** Pseudohypoparathyroidism. (a) Note the short neck and short fourth finger. (b) Shortening of the fourth finger due to the short metacarpal. (c) Demonstrating the shorter fourth metacarpal. (d) Short fourth toes due to the shorter metatarsals.

# Case 18 | Pendred's syndrome

**Frequency in survey for 3rd edition:** did not occur in the initial small survey at PACES Station 5, Endocrine.

**Predicted frequency from older, more extensive MRCP short case survseys:** main focus of a short case in 0.6% of attempts at PACES Station 5, Endocrine.

## Record

This *deaf* patient has a smooth, firm, symmetrical *goitre*. In view of the combination of goitre and deafness, one would have to consider the possibility of Pendred's syndrome.*

---

### Congenital goitre (sporadic cretinism)

Goitrous infantile hypothyroidism is due to a defect in any of the steps of thyroid hormone synthesis (see Figure I5.75). Abnormalities that have been identified include defects in: (i) iodide transport; (ii) organification of iodide (defect in the enzyme peroxidase); (iii) synthesis of thyroglobulin; (iv) thyroglobulin proteolysis; or (v) iodotyrosine deiodination. All the defects are rare. The most common is the *inability to organify iodine* due to a defect in the enzyme peroxidase or to the synthesis of an abnormal thyroglobulin molecule. Large amounts of iodide accumulate in the thyroid and this can be demonstrated by the perchlorate discharge test. In some patients this defect is associated with an VIIIth nerve deafness and has the eponym *Pendred's syndrome*.

---

*Hearing impairment may be a manifestation of hypothyroidism *per se*, particularly in the elderly. In the adult with goitre and hypothyroidism, the hypothyroidism would be a much more common cause of hearing impairment than Pendred's syndrome.

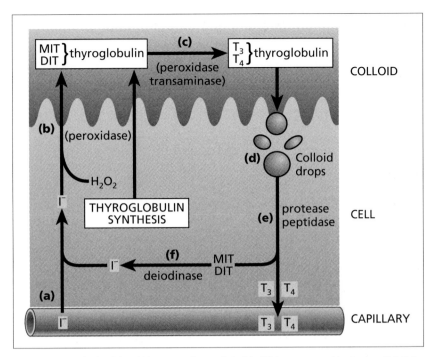

**Figure I5.75** Synthesis of thyroid hormones: inorganic iodide (I⁻) is concentrated in the thyroid follicles by active transport across the cell membrane (a) and then rapidly transferred across the cell into the colloid lumen. During this process, iodide is oxidized by peroxidase (b) and linked to tyrosine molecules to form monoiodotyrosines (MIT) and di-iodotyrosines (DIT) within a large protein, thyroglobulin. These are then coupled by further enzyme action (c) to form thyroxine (T4) and tri-iodothyronine (T3) and, still linked to thyroglobulin, are reabsorbed into the follicular cells in colloid drops by endocytosis (d). T4 and T3 are then separated from the thyroglobulin by proteases (e) contained within lysosomes. Any uncoupled MIT and DIT are further deiodinated (f) to release tyrosine and iodide which may be available for recycling. T4 and T3 are then secreted into the circulation.

# Station 5
# Eyes

| Short case | Checked and updated as necessary for this edition by |
|---|---|
| **1** Diabetic retinopathy | Professor Paul Dodson* |
| **2** Retinitis pigmentosa | Professor Paul Dodson* |
| **3** Optic atrophy | Professor Paul Dodson* |
| **4** Ocular palsy | Dr Saiju Jacob* |
| **5** Visual field defect | Dr Steve Sturman* |
| **6** Retinal vein occlusion | Professor Paul Dodson* |
| **7** Old choroiditis | Professor Paul Dodson* |
| **8** Papilloedema | Professor Paul Dodson* |
| **9** Cataracts | Professor Paul Dodson* |
| **10** Myasthenia gravis | Dr Steve Sturman* |
| **11** Albinism | Professor Paul Dodson* |
| **12** Exophthalmos | Professor Hugh Jones* |
| **13** Myelinated nerve fibres | Professor Paul Dodson* |
| **14** Hypertensive retinopathy | Professor Paul Dodson* |
| **15** Glaucoma/peripheral field loss | Professor Paul Dodson* |
| **16** Retinal artery occlusion | Professor Paul Dodson* |
| **17** Asteroid hyalosis | Professor Paul Dodson* |
| **18** Drusen | Professor Paul Dodson* |
| **19** Laurence–Moon–Bardet–Biedl syndrome | Professor Paul Dodson* |
| **20** Cytomegalovirus choroidoretinitis (AIDS) | Professor Paul Dodson and Dr Kaveh Manavi* |
| **21** Normal fundus | Professor Paul Dodson* |

*All suggested changes by these specialty advisors were considered by Dr Bob Ryder and were either accepted, edited, added to or rejected with Dr Ryder making the final editorial decision in every case.

Professor Paul Dodson, Consultant Medical Ophthalmologist and Diabetologist, Birmingham Heartlands Hospital, Birmingham, UK
Dr Saiju Jacob, Consultant Neurologist, Queen Elizabeth Neurosciences Centre, Birmingham, UK
Dr Steve Sturman, Consultant Neurologist, City Hospital, Birmingham, UK
Professor T Hugh Jones, Consultant Physician and Endocrinologist and Honorary Professor of Andrology, Barnsley Hospital and University of Sheffield, UK
Dr Kaveh Manavi, Consultant in GU/HIV Medicine, University Hospitals Birmingham NHS Foundation Trust, Birmingham, UK

# Case 1 | Diabetic retinopathy

**Frequency in survey for 3rd edition:** main focus of a short case in 41% of attempts at PACES Station 5, Eyes.

**Survey note:** historically, this has been one of the most common short cases; it will be less so with the new Station 5. It is one of the easiest short cases to fail. Some candidates who saw haemorrhages failed to note whether there were also micro-aneurysms. The uninitiated failed to recognize photocoagulation scars. The most common forms reported in the survey were background diabetic retinopathy (40%) and proliferative retinopathy treated with photocoagulation (40%). Most of the rest were fundi with untreated pre-proliferative and proliferative retinopathy. Advanced diabetic eye disease was only rarely reported.

## Record 1

There are *microaneurysms, blot haemorrhages* and *exudates* (due to lipid deposition in the retina).* The patient has background diabetic retinopathy.

## Record 2

The above, plus: in the R/L eye there is a *circinate formation* of *exudates* (indicating oedema) near† the R/L *macula* suggesting that macular oedema may be present or imminent. It would be important to assess the patient's visual acuity.

## Record 3

Any of the above, plus: there are *cotton-wool spots* (CWS), *flame-shaped haemorrhages* (both indicating ischaemia) and leashes of *new vessels* (say where). *Photocoagulation scars* are seen (say where). The patient has proliferative diabetic retinopathy treated by photocoagulation.

## Record 4

Any of the above, plus: *vitreous haemorrhage/vitreous scar/retinal detachment* (widespread and impairing vision) indicate advanced diabetic eye disease.

NB: with diabetic retinopathy there may also be:

1 Cataracts (see Station 5, Eyes, Case 9).
2 Arterioventricular (AV) nipping (indicating either coexistent hypertension or arteriosclerosis).

---

**Indications for photocoagulation** are the sight-threatening forms of retinopathy.

1 *Maculopathy* (especially type II = non-insulin-dependent diabetes): warning signs are hard exudates often in rings (indicating oedema) encroaching on the macula, sometimes with multiple haemorrhages (indicating ischaemia). Macular oedema itself is recognized by stereo biomicroscopy and not by direct ophthalmos-

*Say where the lesions are, particularly in relation to the macula – see criteria for referral to an ophthalmologist (Table I5.9).

†If you use the tiny spotlight of the ophthalmoscope and ask the patient to *look at* the light while you look in, you will be looking at the macula and this may help you assess whether there are hard exudates or haemorrhages involving the macula.

copy. Even slight visual deterioration is highly significant if there is any suspicion of maculopathy.

**2** *Pre-proliferative and proliferative retinopathy* (commonly type I = insulin-dependent diabetes). Pre-proliferative lesions suggesting that neovascularization is imminent are:

Multiple cotton-wool spots
Multiple large blot haemorrhages
Venous beading
Venous loops
Arterial sheathing
Atrophic-looking retina.

**Table I5.9** English National Screening Programme for Diabetic Retinopathy Grading standards

| | | |
|---|---|---|
| **Retinopathy (R)** | | |
| Level 0 | None | |
| Level 1 | Background | Microaneurysm(s) |
| | | Retinal haemorrhage(s) ± any exudates not within the definition of maculopathy |
| Level 2* | Pre-proliferative | Venous beading |
| | | Venous loop or reduplication |
| | | Intraretinal microvascular abnormality (IRMA) |
| | | Multiple deep, round or blot haemorrhages |
| | | (CWS† – make a careful search for above features) |
| Level 3* | Proliferative | New vessels on disc (NVD) |
| | | New vessels elsewhere (NVE) |
| | | Pre-retinal or vitreous haemorrhage |
| | | Pre-retinal fibrosis ± tractional retinal detachment |
| **Maculopathy (M)*** | | Exudate within 1 disc diameter (DD) of the centre of the fovea |
| | | Circinate or group of exudates within the macula |
| | | Retinal thickening within 1 DD of the centre of the fovea (if stereo available) |
| | | Any microaneurysm or haemorrhage within 1 DD of the centre of the fovea only if associated with a best visual acuity (VA) of ≤6/12 (if no stereo) |
| **Photocoagulation (P)** | | Evidence of focal/grid laser to macula |
| | | Evidence of peripheral scatter laser |
| **Unclassifiable (U)** | | Unobtainable/ungradable |

*Patients with retinopathy levels 2 and 3 or maculopathy should be referred to an ophthalmologist.
†Cotton-wool spots are indicators of retinal ischaemia.

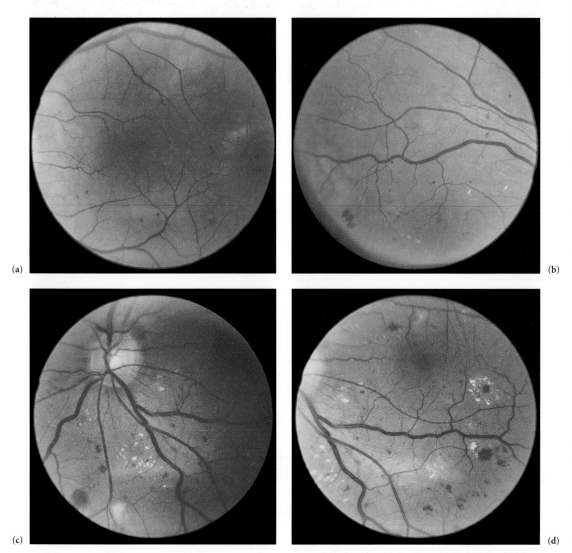

**Figure I5.76** Diabetic retinopathy. (a) Early background changes of microaneurysms and blot haemorrhages. (b) Background retinopathy (note microaneurysms, blot haemorrhages and punctate hard exudates). (c) Extensive background changes and cotton-wool spot 2.5 disc diameters inferior to the disc. (d) More extensive background changes (note small circinate temporal to the macula).

*Historical note. This is the actual photograph of the extreme case from the study that first exposed the potential value of photography in diabetic retinopathy screening – the circinate was missed by routine clinic ophthalmoscopy (see Ryder, REJ et al. BMJ 1985; 291: 1256–57). This photograph, and what it portended (that it was not safe to use direct ophthalmoscopy to screen for diabetic retinopathy), started a ball rolling which finally led, 20 years later, to the NHS national screening programme for diabetic retinopathy which is based on digital retinal photography.

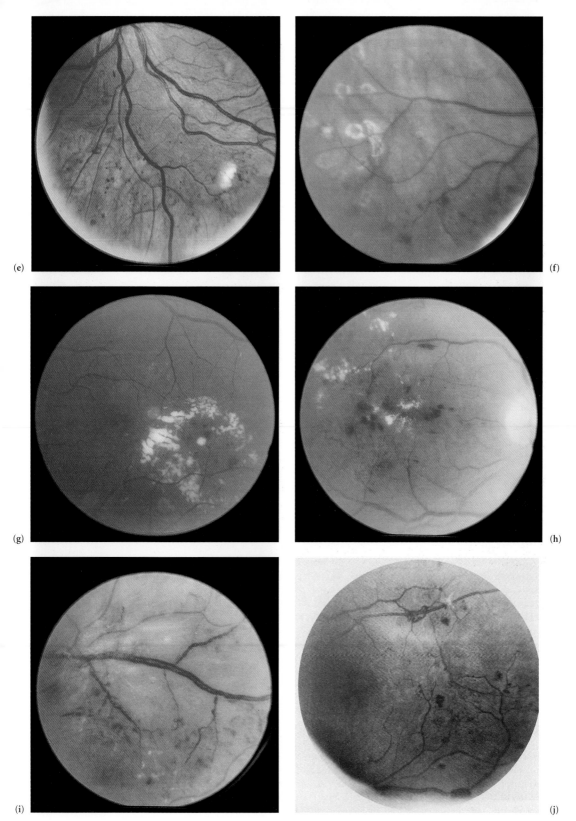

(e)

(f)

(g)

(h)

(i)

(j)

**Figure I5.76** (*Continued*) (e) The cotton-wool spot in the lower right of the picture indicates ischaemia which is the stimulus to new vessel formation. (f) Note photocoagulation scars. (g) The large circinate exudation temporal to the macula indicates oedema in that area.* (h) Haemorrhages and exudates at the macula (maculopathy). (i) Venous irregularity and beading (pre-proliferative sign). (j) Venous reduplication is seen in the upper part of this picture (a pre-proliferative sign). (*Continued*)

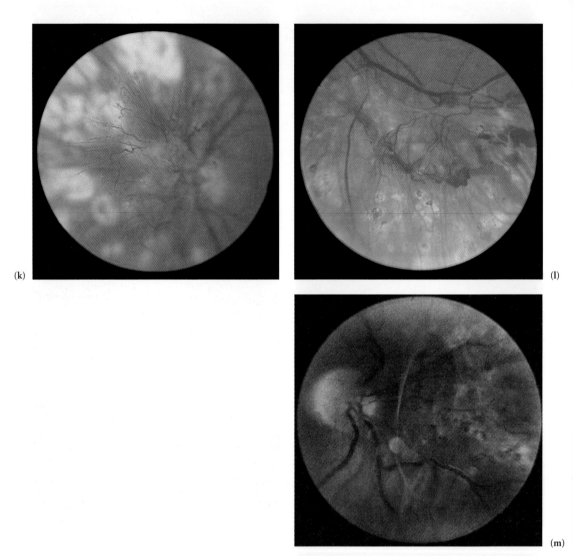

(k)

(l)

(m)

**Figure I5.76** (*Continued*) (k) The leash of new vessels protruding into the vitreous is in focus, whereas the retina with its photocoagulation scars is further away and therefore slightly out of focus. Note the leash of fibrous tissue accompanying the new vessels (previous haemorrhage).* (l) Peripheral new vessels which are haemorrhaging (note photocoagulation scars; same patient as [k]). (m) Advanced diabetic eye disease (note vitreous scar).

*Historical note. The plan of the authors of the first edition of this book, published in 1986, was to have this photograph on the front cover of the book. Our surveys had shown that in those days diabetic retinopathy was the commonest short case because an attempt was made to get everybody to have a fundus case. We thought that the photograph showing the important bit in focus was relevant to the concept of the good candidate focusing in the important bits. . . . We envisaged a black book with white writing and this fundus staring out at the reader. The publisher, however, came up with an entirely different idea – see http://www.ryder-mrcp.org.uk/first_edtion.htm. All these years later, the covers of the fourth edition are based on the original choice of the publisher.

# Case 2 | Retinitis pigmentosa

**Frequency in survey for 3rd edition:** main focus of a short case in 16% of attempts at PACES Station 5, Eyes.

## *Record*

There is *widespread* scattering of *black pigment* in a pattern resembling *bone corpuscles*. The macula is spared. There is *tunnel vision*. The diagnosis is retinitis pigmentosa.

---

The patient may well have presented with night blindness. The condition progresses remorselessly with increasing retinal pigmentation, deepening disc pallor of consecutive optic atrophy as the ganglion cells die, and increasing constriction of visual field. It may occur on its own although it is often associated with other abnormalities such as cataracts,* deaf-mutism and mental deficiency. Pigmentary degeneration of the retina may also occur in many conditions such as:

Laurence–Moon–Bardet–Biedl syndrome (autosomal recessive; ?obesity, hypogonadism, dwarfism, mental retardation and polydactyly; Station 5, Eyes, Case 19)

Refsum's disease (autosomal recessive; ?pupillary abnormalities, cerebellar ataxia, deafness, peripheral neuropathy, cardiomyopathy and icthyosis)

as well as some of the

Hereditary ataxias

Familial neuropathies

Neuronal lipidoses (ceroid lipofuscinosis).

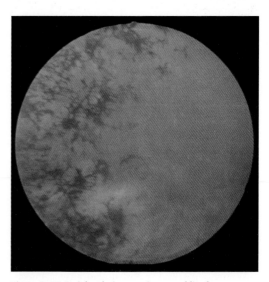

**Figure I5.77** Peripheral pigmentation resembling bone corpuscles.

*Visual acuity may sometimes be considerably improved by cataract removal.

# Case 3 | Optic atrophy

**Frequency in survey for 3rd edition:** main focus of a short case in 6% of attempts at PACES Station 5, Eyes. Additional feature in a further 2%, especially Station 3, CNS.

## *Record*

The disc is *pale* and *clearly delineated* and (in the severe case) the *pupil reacts consensually* to light but *not directly.** Field testing with the head of a hat pin (may reveal) reveals a *central scotoma*. The diagnosis is optic atrophy. The well-defined disc edge suggests that it is not secondary to papilloedema† (yellow/grey disc with blurred margins).

Common causes of primary optic atrophy are:

1 Multiple sclerosis† (may be temporal pallor only; ?nystagmus, scanning speech, cerebellar ataxia, etc; see Vol. 1, Station 3, CNS, Case 10)
2 Compression of the optic nerve by:
  **(a)** tumour (e.g. pituitary – ?bitemporal hemianopia)
  **(b)** aneurysm
3 Glaucoma (?pathological cupping).

---

### Other causes

Ischaemic optic neuropathy (abrupt onset of visual loss in an elderly patient; may be painful; thrombosis or embolus of posterior ciliary artery; temporal arteritis is sometimes the cause)
Leber's optic atrophy (males:females 6:1)
Retinal artery occlusion (see Station 5, Eyes, Case 16)
Toxic amblyopia (lead, methyl alcohol, arsenic, insecticides, quinine)
Nutritional amblyopia (famine, etc., tobacco-alcohol amblyopia, vitamin B12 deficiency, diabetes mellitus‡)

Friedreich's ataxia (?cerebellar signs, pes cavus, scoliosis, etc; see Vol. 1, Station 3, CNS, Case 12)
Tabes dorsalis (?Argyll Robertson pupils, etc; see Vol. 1, Station 3, CNS, Case 38)
Paget's disease (?large skull, bowed tibia, etc; see Station 5, Locomotor, Case 7)
Consecutive optic atrophy§

*In early unilateral optic neuritis before the direct reflex is lost, it may simply become more sluggish than the consensual reflex. In this situation it may be possible to demonstrate the *Marcus Gunn* phenomenon (relative afferent pupillary defect). In this, the direct reflex may at first appear to be brisk. However, when the light is alternated from one side to the other, the pupil on the affected side may be seen to dilate slowly when exposed to the light. The mechanism is as follows: when the light shines in the healthy eye a rapid constriction occurs in both eyes. As the light then moves to the affected eye, this fails to transmit the message to continue constriction as quickly as normal. As a result the pupils have time to recover and dilate, despite the light shining on the abnormal eye.

†Papillitis is often an early sign of multiple sclerosis. Papillitis is optic neuritis of the optic nerve head. In papillitis, the optic nerve head is hyperaemic with blurred margins and slightly oedematous. Haemorrhages and exudates may also appear. There is loss of visual acuity along with a central scotoma and impairment of colour vision. As well as multiple sclerosis, papillitis may also be associated with severe inflammation of the retina or choroid, vitamin B deficiency, diabetes mellitus, thyroid disease, lactation, toxicity or syphilis.

‡Optic atrophy in diabetes mellitus may also occur in the DIDMOAD syndrome, with diabetes insipidus, diabetes mellitus and deafness. It is a rare, recessively inherited disorder.

§Optic atrophy can be divided into primary, secondary and consecutive. Consecutive optic atrophy follows damage to the parent ganglion cells of the retina as in widespread choroidoretinitis, retinitis pigmentosa and retinal artery occlusion.

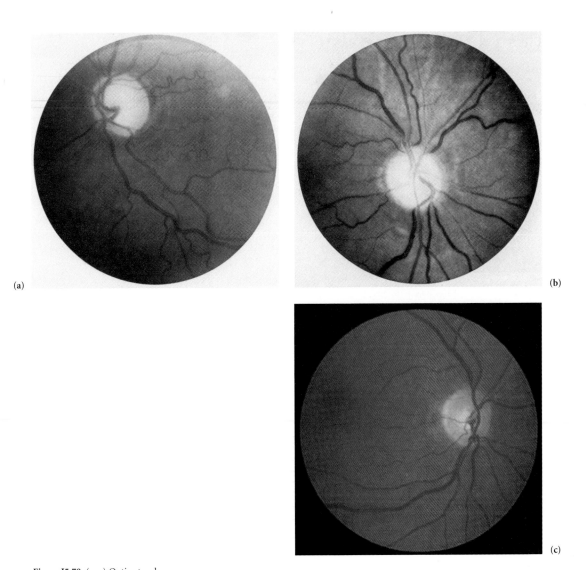

(a)

(b)

(c)

**Figure I5.78** (a–c) Optic atrophy.

# Case 4 | Ocular palsy

**Frequency in survey for 3rd edition:** main focus of a short case in 6% of attempts at PACES Station 5, Eyes.

Ocular palsy is dealt with in Vol. 1, Station 3, CNS, Case 16.

# Case 5 | **Visual field defect**

**Frequency in survey for 3rd edition:** main focus of a short case in 4% of attempts at PACES Station 5, Eyes.

Visual field defect is dealt with in Vol. 1, Station 3, CNS, Case 13.

# Case 6 | Retinal vein occlusion

**Frequency in survey for 3rd edition:** main focus of a short case in 2% of attempts at PACES Station 5, Eyes.

## Record

The veins are *tortuous* and *engorged*. *Haemorrhages* are *scattered riotously* over the whole retina, irregular and superficial, like bundles of straw alongside the veins (*papilloedema* and *soft exudates* may also be seen).

The diagnosis is central retinal vein occlusion (CRVO). There may be *hypertension, hyperlipidaemia* or *diabetes mellitus* or there may be an underlying *hyperviscosity syndrome,*\* especially *Waldenström's macroglobulinaemia* (?lymphadenopathy, hepatosplenomegaly, bruising and purpura), but also occasionally *myeloma* (?urinary Bence-Jones protein) and *connective tissue disorders.*

---

The condition is more common in eyes prone to simple glaucoma (which should, therefore, be excluded in the other eye), in the elderly arteriosclerotic, and the hypertensive and hyperlipidaemic, but may also arise in young adults (especially women – the contraceptive pill is a risk factor). It causes incomplete loss of vision and improvement may be scant. About 3 months after acute CRVO, 20% of cases lose the remaining sight in the affected eye because of an acute secondary glaucoma. This is due to new vessels on the iris root developing as a result of retinal hypoxia. Panretinal photocoagulation may decrease the risk of subsequent neovascular glaucoma. A less severe ophthalmoscopic appearance is encountered in younger patients when the terms *partial retinal vein occlusion* and *venous stasis retinopathy* are used; visual acuity in this situation is only slightly reduced and visual prognosis is good.

**In occlusion of a branch of the retinal vein** (also occurred in our survey), the occlusion usually occurs at an AV crossing with the changes confined to the sector beyond this – haemorrhages and cotton-wool spots spread out in a wedge from the AV crossing. Macula oedema and decreased visual acuity may occur or it may be asymptomatic. Neovascularization is a rare complication. Any loss of sight† mostly recovers and there is no secondary glaucoma, though sometimes the visual outcome is poor. Branch retinal vein occlusion must be distinguished from *viral retinitis* which it resembles ophthalmoscopically (see Station 5, Eyes, Case 20). In view of the association with hypertension, hypertensive changes may be visible in the rest of the fundus (thin arterioles, AV nipping, etc.).

---

\*The symptoms and signs of a hyperviscosity syndrome are principally neurological due to sluggish cerebral circulation. Cardiac failure may occur in the elderly. Waldenström's macroglobulinaemia is the cause in 90% of hyperviscosity syndromes.

†Think of this diagnosis if you find a quadrantic field defect in one eye only.

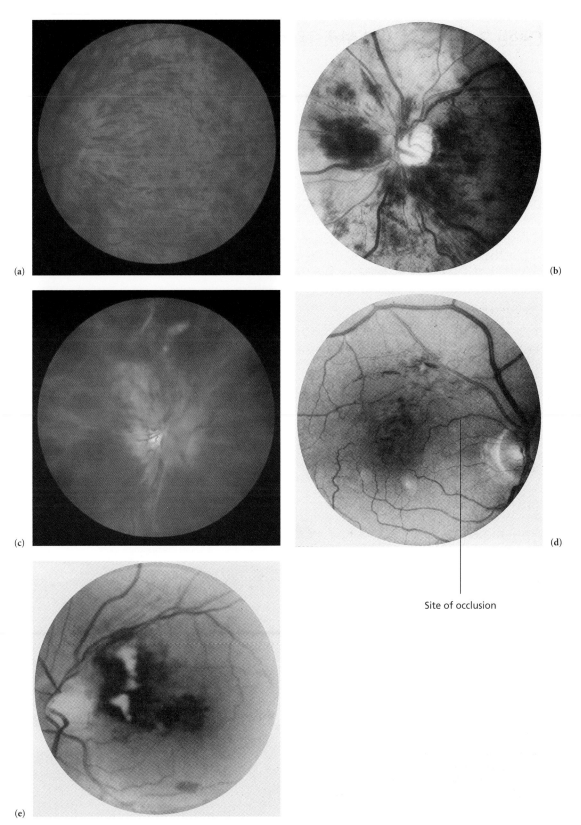

(a)

(b)

(c)

(d)

Site of occlusion

(e)

**Figure I5.79** (a–c) Three different cases of central retinal vein occlusion. (d) Branch retinal vein occlusion. (e) Macular branch retinal vein occlusion.

# Case 7 | Old choroiditis

**Frequency in survey for 3rd edition:** main focus of a short case in 2% of attempts at PACES Station 5, Eyes.

**Invigilator's observation:** easily confused with laser burn scars in the diabetic fundus.*

## *Record*
There is evidence of old choroiditis in the . . . region of the R/L fundus.

*or*

In the . . . region of the R/L fundus there is a *patch of white*\* (or yellow or grey). It suggests exposed sclera due to atrophy of the choroidoretina secondary to old choroiditis. Together with this, there are also scattered *pigmented patches* due to proliferation of the retinal pigment epithelium. In most cases the cause of the choroiditis is unknown but *toxoplasmosis* is commonly implicated.

---

## Other causes
Sarcoidosis (?lupus pernio, chest signs, etc.)

Tuberculosis (often inactive; ?ethnic origin, chest signs)

Syphilis (?tabetic facies and pupils, posterior column signs, extensor plantars, etc.)

Toxocara

Trauma

---

*Candidates sometimes call laser burns on the diabetic fundus (see Station 5, Eyes, Case 1) old choroiditis, and old choroiditis laser burns, thus diagnosing old choroiditis as diabetic retinopathy. The confusion can be understood when one realizes that laser burn scars are, in a way, a form of old choroiditis. The matter is made worse because the patient with diabetic retinopathy may also happen to have old choroiditis (as diabetics are the main group of people having their fundi carefully examined on a large scale, patients with old choroiditis among them are readily detected). Laser burns can usually be distinguished by their more regular uniform appearance as in Figure I5.76f.

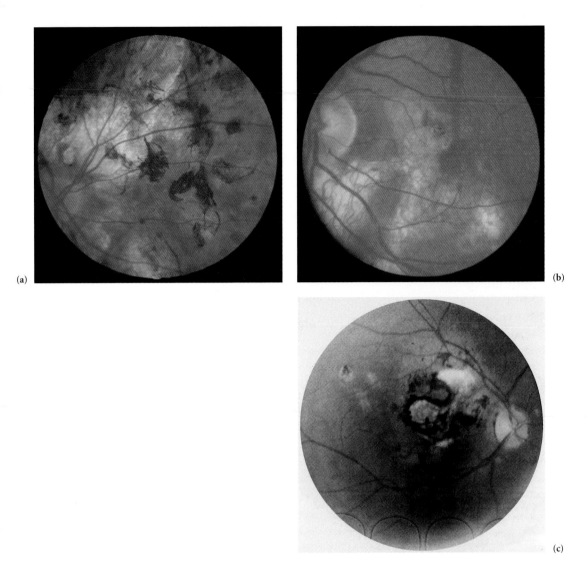

(a)

(b)

(c)

**Figure I5.80** (a–c) Three different cases of choroidoretinitis. The artefact on (b) is the shadow cast by the internal fixation device of the fundus camera.

# Case 8 | Papilloedema

**Frequency in survey for 3rd edition:** did not occur in the initial small survey at PACES Station 5, Eyes.

**Predicted frequency from older, more extensive MRCP short case surveys:** main focus of a short case in 4% of attempts at PACES Station 5, Eyes. Additional feature in a further 2%, especially Station 3, CNS.

## *Record*

There is bilateral papilloedema* (search carefully for haemorrhages, exudates and AV nipping).

## Possible causes

1 These include:
  (a) *an intracranial space-occupying lesion* (?localizing neurological signs†)
  (b) tumour (infratentorial more often than supratentorial)
  (c) abscess (fever not always present; ?underlying middle ear infection, underlying suppuration elsewhere – e.g. bronchiectasis or empyema)
  (d) haematoma.
2 *Accelerated (malignant) hypertension* (check blood pressure – haemorrhages and exudates are not always present; ?narrow tortuous arterioles that vary in calibre, AV nipping: see Station 5, Eyes, Case 14).
3 *Benign intracranial hypertension‡* (?obese female aged 15–45, no localizing neurological signs).

---

*The disc oedema of papillitis (disc usually pink due to hyperaemia) must be differentiated from developing papilloedema due to raised intracranial pressure. Papilloedema causes enlargement of the blind spot and constriction of the peripheral field, but visual acuity is unaffected. Papillitis (optic neuritis affecting the intraorbital portion of the optic nerve) causes central scotoma, diminished visual acuity, and sometimes tenderness and pain on eye movement during the acute attack. Furthermore, in papillitis there may be a pupillary reflex defect, loss of the central cup and cells may be present in the vitreous over the disc.
†Sixth nerve palsy in the presence of papilloedema may be a false localizing sign due to raised intracranial pressure stretching the nerve during its long intracranial course. A localizing sign may occasionally be rapidly apparent in the case of contralateral optic atrophy – the Foster–Kennedy syndrome (a frontal tumour pressing on the optic nerve to cause atrophy and at the same time raising intracranial pressure to cause papilloedema in the other eye). It must be remembered that tumours in and around the frontal lobes can present simply with dementia in the absence of signs and symptoms of raised intracranial pressure (i.e. without papilloedema). A classic lesion presenting in this manner is a subfrontal olfactory groove meningioma. These may grow to considerable size, initially causing only memory impairment and marked apathy. On examination and upon closer questioning, there is usually a history of diminished or absent sense of smell. Loss of urinary control associated with dementia should be regarded as indicating organic pathology until proven otherwise. A much shorter history of dementia and urinary incontinence together with increasingly severe headache may indicate an underlying malignant glioma of the corpus callosum or of one or other frontal lobe.
‡This syndrome (also called pseudotumour cerebri, serous meningitis or otitic hydrocephalus) is known to have occurred following middle ear infection which caused lateral sinus thrombosis. It may be that thrombosis of the venous sinuses is the aetiological factor in many other cases. The condition has been associated with the contraceptive pill, long-term tetracycline treatment for acne, corticosteroids (often reduction in dose during long-term therapy), head injury and times of female physiological hormone disturbance such as menarche, pregnancy and puerperium. The CSF pressure is high, frequently above 300 mm, but the composition of the fluid is normal; the protein content is usually low normal, below 20 mg/dL.

The first sign of raised intracranial pressure is loss of venous pulsation, but recognition of this sign requires much practice and experience (see Section G, Examination *routine* 12). If there is doubt about the normality of the disc, the presence of venous pulsation makes papilloedema and raised intracranial pressure unlikely.

## Other causes of papilloedema

Meningitis (especially TB)

Hypercapnoea (cyanosis, flapping tremor of the hands)

Central retinal vein thrombosis (sight affected, usually unilateral, dilated veins, widespread haemorrhages)

(Graves') congestive ophthalmopathy (= malignant exophthalmos though exophthalmos is not always present; prominent eyes, eyelids and conjunctivae swollen and inflamed, marked ophthalmoplegia, often pain)

Cavernous sinus thrombosis (usually becomes bilateral, follows infection of orbit, nose and face; eyeball(s) protrudes, is painful, immobile and there is extreme venous congestion)

Hypoparathyroidism (tetany, epilepsy, cataracts, etc.)

Severe anaemia especially due to massive blood loss and leukaemia (there may be haemorrhages and cotton-wool spots as well)

Guillain–Barré syndrome (papilloedema possibly due to impaired cerebrospinal fluid [CSF] resorption because of the elevated protein content)

Paget's disease (large head, bowed tibiae)

Hurler's syndrome (dwarf, large head, coarse features, hepatosplenomegaly, heart murmurs)

Poisoning with vitamin A, lead, tetracyclines or nalidixic acid

Ocular toxoplasmosis

(a)
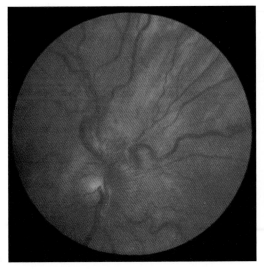
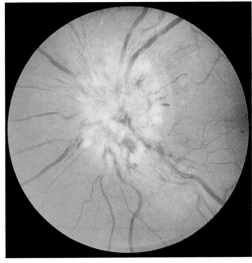
(b)

**Figure I5.81** (a,b) Papilloedema.

# Case 9 | **Cataracts**

**Frequency in survey for 3rd edition:** main focus of a short case in 2% of attempts at PACES Station 5, Eyes. Additional feature in a further 8%.

## *Record*

There are partial cataracts* in both eyes (may be localized to the lens nucleus or seen as flakes, dots or sector-shaped opacities within the lens periphery).

### Most common causes of cataract

**1** Old age (usually nuclear, with a brownish discoloration, or of the cortical spoke variety).
**2** Diabetic patients develop senile cataracts at younger ages than non-diabetics and this is the most common type of cataract in diabetes. Rarely,† a 'snowflake' (dot cortical opacities) cataract can develop in a young, poorly controlled diabetic, and may progress rapidly to a mature cataract in months or even days (good control may halt and even reverse development).

---

### Other causes of cataract in adults

Trauma

Chronic anterior uveitis

Hypoparathyroidism (Chvostek's and Trousseau's signs, tetany, paraesthesiae and cramps, ectodermal changes, moniliasis, mental retardation and psychiatric disturbances, papilloedema, epilepsy, bradykinetic-rigid syndrome)

Radiation (infrared, ultraviolet, X-rays and possibly microwaves)

Myotonic dystrophy (?frontal balding, ptosis, sternomastoid wasting, myopathic facies, myotonia, etc; See Vol. 1, Station 3, CNS, Case 2)

Retinitis pigmentosa (including Refsum's, Laurence–Moon–Bardet–Biedl; see Station 5, Eyes, Case 2 and Case 19)

Steroid therapy (10 mg prednisolone daily for more than 1 year)

Chlorpromazine (500 mg daily for 3 years or more)

Chloroquine

### Causes of cataracts in children

These include perinatal hypoglycaemia, perinatal hypocalcaemia, maternal rubella, galactosaemia, galactokinase deficiency, genetically inherited, Down's syndrome (trisomy 21), Patau's syndrome (trisomy 13), Edward's syndrome (trisomy 18), Alport's syndrome, Lowe's syndrome.

---

*Examine with direct ophthalmoscope focused to study the red reflex (see Section G, Examination *routine* 12).

†Rare in the era of modern insulin therapy. A case was seen in this era, however, in a type 1 patient who did not take insulin for prolonged periods for personal religious reasons.

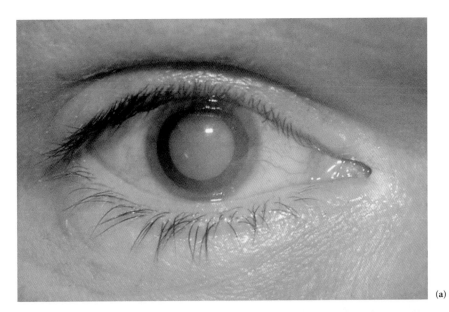

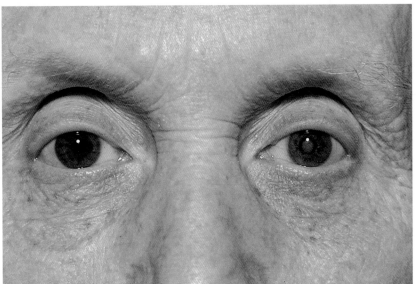

**Figure I5.82** (a) Cataract. (b) A cataract is seen in the left eye.

# Case 10 | Myasthenia gravis

**Frequency in survey for 3rd edition:** main focus of a short case in 2% of attempts at PACES Station 5, Eyes.

**Survey note:** the following anecdote was reported in our original PACES survey. A candidate in the Eyes section of Station 5 was asked to examine a patient's eye movements. He found unilateral partial ptosis and weakness of abduction of both eyes. When asked the causes, he said that cranial nerve lesions could not easily explain the findings and that the likely diagnosis was myasthenia gravis. There then took place a discussion on the other signs of myasthenia.

The old Station 5, Eyes, was supposed to be a fundal case. However, it was clear from our initial small PACES survey that myasthenia gravis has occasionally been used as a case in the Eyes section. It could turn up more easily in the new Station 5. Myasthenia gravis is dealt with in Vol. 1, Station 3, CNS, Case 27.

# Case 11 | Albinism

**Frequency in survey for 3rd edition:** main focus of a short case in 2% of attempts at PACES Station 5, Eyes.

### *Record*

The (?blind) patient is *very pale* skinned (marked hypomelanosis) and has *very white hair* (or faintly yellow blond). On examination of the eyes, there is *nystagmus* and the *irides* are *translucent*. The *fundus* is *pale*.

    The diagnosis is oculocutaneous albinism. (Now look for and comment on the presence [indicate the tyrosinase-positive type] or absence [indicate the tyrosinase-negative type] of *freckles.\**)

---

Oculocutaneous albinism is a group of autosomal recessive traits recognized by generalized hypomelanosis of the skin, hair and eyes. Albinism can be classified according to the presence or absence of tyrosinase, the enzyme crucial in the synthesis of eumelanin and phaeomelanin. Normal plucked hair bulbs darken when incubated *in vitro* with tyrosine. Tyrosinase-positive albinos display some minimal darkening (but not normal) of the hair bulb when incubated with tyrosinase, whereas tyrosinase-negative albinos show no darkening of the hair bulb. These two types of albinism have separate gene loci. Although melanogenesis is deficient in both forms, persons with the tyrosinase-positive form develop some pigmented naevi and have less eye damage than tyrosinase-negative albinos. Patients with phenylketonuria† have diffuse hypopigmentation, with light hair and blue eyes.

---

\*Another feature which distinguishes the two types of albinism is the colour of the eyes. The eyes are grey-blue in tyrosinase-negative individuals. In tyrosinase-positive individuals the eye colour may be brown or blue-yellow.

†*Phenylketonuria* is an autosomal recessive disorder in which the enzyme that converts phenylalanine to tyrosine is deficient. Consequently, melanin synthesis is deficient.

# Case 12 | Exophthalmos

**Frequency in survey for 3rd edition:** main focus of a short case in 2% of attempts at PACES Station 5, Eyes.

The old Station 5, Eyes, was supposed to be a fundal case. However, it was clear from our initial small PACES survey that exophthalmos has occasionally been used as a case in the Eyes section. Exophthalmos could readily turn up in the new Station 5, being connected to both eyes and endocrine. Exophthalmos is dealt with in Station 5, Endocrine, Case 1.

# Case 13 | Myelinated nerve fibres

**Frequency in survey for 3rd edition:** main focus of a short case in 1% of attempts at PACES Station 5, Eyes.

### *Record*

There are *bright white*, streaky, irregular patches with frayed margins at the edge of the disc. These are due to myelinated nerve fibres. They do not affect vision.

---

Normally the fibres of the optic nerve lose their myelin sheath as they enter the eye. Occasionally the sheath persists for some distance after the fibres leave the optic disc. If this phenomenon is extensive, the disc and emerging vessels can be obscured. This appearance may be mistaken for papilloedema and has been termed 'pseudopapilloedema'.

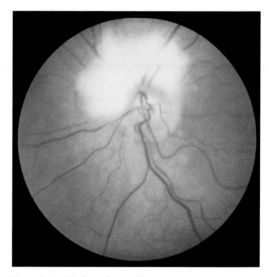

**Figure I5.83** Myelinated nerve fibres.

# Case 14 | Hypertensive retinopathy

**Frequency in survey for 3rd edition:** main focus of a short case in 1% of attempts at PACES Station 5, Eyes.

## *Record*

The retinal arterioles are *narrow* (normal ratio of vein to artery is 1.1:1), they are (may be) tortuous and (may) vary in calibre (localized constriction followed by segments of arteriolar dilation) with increased light reflex (copper or *silver wiring*) and *AV nipping* (these changes all occurring with ageing and arteriosclerosis as well as with hypertension). There are *flame-shaped* and (less frequently) *blot haemorrhages*, and *cotton-wool exudates* (all indicating grade 3 retinopathy and a diagnosis of malignant [accelerated] hypertension *even without* papilloedema), and there is *papilloedema* (indicating cerebral oedema; papilloedema may occur in malignant hypertension even without haemorrhages and exudates). This is grade 4 hypertensive retinopathy.

---

### Causes of hypertension

Essential – 94% (cause unknown)

Renal – 4% (renal artery stenosis – ?*bruit*, acute nephritis, pyelonephritis, glomerulonephritis, polycystic disease, systemic sclerosis, systemic lupus erythematosus [SLE], hydronephrosis, renin-secreting tumour and renoprival – after bilateral nephrectomy)

Endocrine – 1%* (Cushing's, Conn's, phaeochromocytoma,† acromegaly, hyperparathyroidism, hypothyroidism and oral contraceptive use)

Miscellaneous – <1% (coarctation of the aorta – ?*radiofemoral delay*, polycythaemia, acute porphyria, pre-eclampsia)

NB: cerebral tumour or raised intracranial pressure from any cause may lead to secondary hypertension (Cushing's reflex).

---

*The figure 1% does not include hypertension due to oral contraceptive use.

†All patients with phaeochromocytomata should be screened for multiple endocrine neoplasia (MEN) type 2 (see Station 5, Endocrine, Case 4) and von Hippel–Lindau disease (see Vol. 1, Station 1, Abdominal, Case 2) to avert further morbidity and mortality in the patients and their families. All patients in families with MEN 2 or von Hippel–Lindau disease should be screened for phaeochromocytoma even if they are asymptomatic.

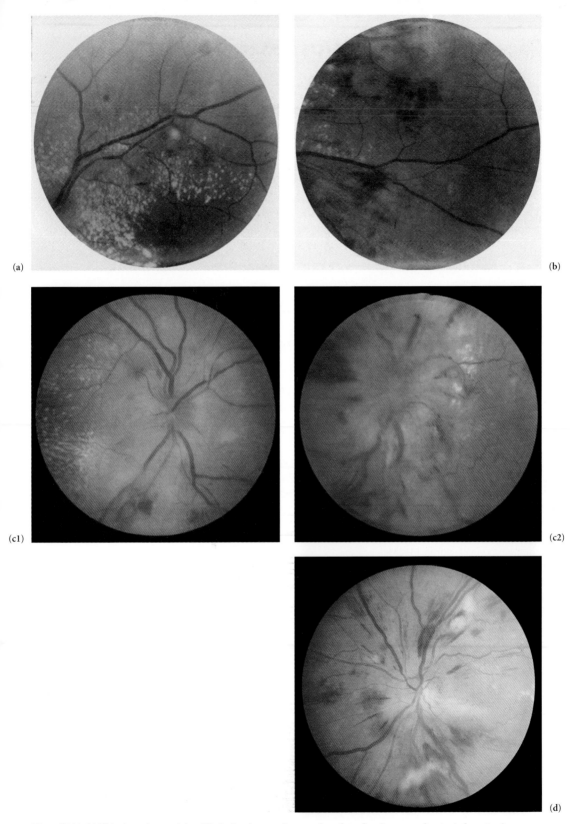

**Figure I5.84** (a) Thin, irregular arterioles, AV nipping, haemorrhages and exudates forming a macular star in hypertension. (b) Flame-shaped haemorrhages in hypertension. (c1) Hypertensive retinopathy grade 4; part of a macular star can be seen. (c2) Papilloedema–hypertension. (d) Hypertensive retinopathy grade 4; note papilloedema, flame-shaped haemorrhages and cotton-wool spots.

# Case 15 | Glaucoma/peripheral field loss

**Frequency in survey:** main focus of a short case in 1% of attempts at PACES Station 5, Eyes.

**Survey note:** in the original, pre-PACES, surveys the candidates were usually told that the patient had some difficulty with his vision, and they were asked to examine the visual fields. One candidate reported that he had found unilateral loss of the peripheral field and gave retinitis pigmentosa, extensive choroidoretinitis and diabetes mellitus with laser therapy as the possible causes; the examiner told him that the patient had chronic glaucoma.

## Record 1
There is a unilateral R/L nasal visual field defect. This could be due to a space-occupying lesion compressing the lateral part of the optic chiasma* or it could be due to chronic simple glaucoma.* (Ask to examine the fundi.†)

## Record 2
The visual fields are grossly constricted and the patient only has central vision (*tunnel vision*). The most likely causes are retinitis pigmentosa, advanced chronic glaucoma or diffuse choroidoretinitis.

---

Several mass screening studies have shown a prevalence of 1–2% for glaucoma in the age group of more than 40 years, the greatest incidence of simple glaucoma being between 60 and 70 years. Heredity is an important predisposing factor in 13–25% of cases.

In the early stages a sickle-shaped extension of the blind spot may be demonstrated and some impairment of the nasal field may be apparent on the Bjerrum screen. As the condition progresses, there is a contraction of the peripheral field, leaving only the central vision intact.

The problem is often one of when to start treatment in a patient suspected of having chronic open angle glaucoma. In general, patients who have a raised intraocular pressure of 24 mmHg or more, especially when it is persistent, those who have a family history of the disease and those who are in their seventh decade should all be considered. Medical treatment consists of the instillation of miotics (e.g. pilocarpine, neostigmine, carbachol, etc.) in the eyes, aiming to reduce the intraocular pressure to a normal level and thereby to slow the progression of visual failure.

---

*The nasal field loss can be bilateral in chronic glaucoma but would not be bilateral with lateral chiasmal compression. The condition is insidious and asymptomatic in its early stages. It may be discovered accidentally when the vision of one eye is almost lost and that of the other seriously impaired. The patient may need to change his/her presbyopic glasses frequently. There is usually accommodative failure. The patient finds it difficult to see in a less illuminated room. Dark and light adaptation are slower than in normal subjects. Periodic eye examinations by an expert are advisable *for those who have a family history of glaucoma.*

†*Cupping of the disc* is an essential feature of chronic glaucoma. The sides of the disc are steep and the retinal vessels have the appearance of *being broken* off at the margin of the disc. The edges of the disc overhang and the course of the vessels, as they climb the sides of the cup, is hidden.

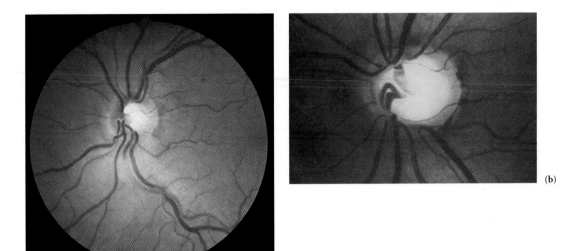

**Figure I5.85** (a) Early glaucoma with a cup:disc ratio of >0.6. (b) Advanced glaucoma. Note large optic disc with sharply angulated vessels (cupping).

# Case 16 | Retinal artery occlusion

**Frequency in survey for 3rd edition:** main focus of a short case in 0.5% of attempts at PACES Station 5, Eyes.

**Survey note:** in the original, pre-PACES, surveys, it was reported to have occurred as the underlying cause of optic atrophy with attenuated retinal arteries, and as a retinal artery branch occlusion causing a quadrantic field defect. No cherry-red spots were reported!

## Record

The eye is blind, the *fundus* is *pale*, the *arterioles* are *thin* and *scanty* and there is a *cherry-red spot* at the macula (because the underlying choroidal circulation is intact). The diagnosis is central retinal artery occlusion.

---

Retinal artery occlusion may occur in a central (CRAO) or branch (BRAO) form.

CRAO: in the acute phase the whole fundus (except for the cherry-red spot) is milky white due to retinal oedema. By the time the retinal oedema has faded, optic atrophy is generally apparent. The cherry-red spot is usually only seen for about 5–10 days.

BRAO: in retinal artery branch occlusion the fundoscopic appearances of thin arterioles and pale retina are limited to one area and there is a corresponding field defect (e.g. an inferior temporal field defect due to infarction of the superior nasal fundus).

The condition occurs most commonly in the elderly arteriosclerotic patient. It may be due to thrombosis, embolus (?carotid bruits, atrial fibrillation, heart murmurs) or spasm. Transient retinal artery occlusions associated with contralateral hemiparesis may occur from recurrent carotid emboli. Occlusion of the central retinal artery may also follow giant cell arteritis involving the arterioles around the optic disc (?headaches and temporal artery tenderness).

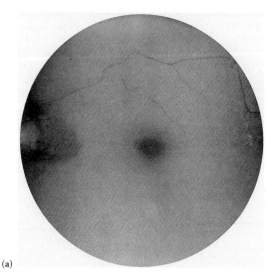
(a)

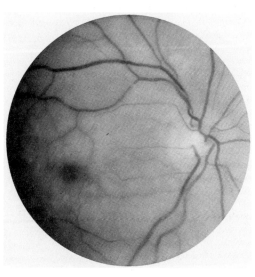
(b)

**Figure I5.86** (a,b) Acute CRAO. Note the macular cherry-red spots. The milky-white fundus due to retinal oedema is very pronounced in (a).

# Case 17 | Asteroid hyalosis

**Frequency in survey for 3rd edition:** did not occur in the initial small survey at PACES Station 5, Eyes.

**Predicted frequency from older, more extensive MRCP short case surveys:** main focus of a short case in 0.6% of attempts at PACES Station 5, Eyes.

## *Record*

With the ophthalmoscope focused in front of the retina, the vitreous is seen to be filled with *myriad tiny*, *white*, discrete, shiny *opacities*, like a galaxy of stars. The diagnosis is asteroid hyalosis.

---

*Asteroid hyalosis* is usually diagnosed in patients aged between 60 and 65 years. It may be more common in males. It is *unilateral* in the majority of patients. Biomicroscopically, there are *white* bodies of *oval* shape and varying size that are adherent to the framework of the vitreous gel. The opacities consist mainly of *calcium soaps*. Visual function is not disturbed and patients are unaware of the bodies which may be scattered throughout the entire vitreous cavity or may be accumulated in one part of it. Although it has been suggested by some authors that this condition is related to diabetes (approximately 30% of patients with asteroid hyalosis have diabetes), it is now generally agreed that the two are probably not connected. It probably reflects the fact that diabetic patients have their eyes examined more than others. It has also been suggested that the inci-dence of hypercholesterolaemia is higher and that of posterior vitreous detachment lower than expected for the age group concerned.

*Synchysis scintillans* appears to be rarer than asteroid hyalosis. Most descriptions relate it to injury or inflammation involving the vitreous cavity. In contrast to asteroid hyalosis, it is usually *bilateral* and the opacities, which are *cholesterol crystals*, appear more *golden*. The opacities do not appear to be attached to the collagen fibrils and float freely in the vitreous fluid with ocular motion; they settle together at the bottom of the vitreous when the eye ceases to move. They have a *flat, angular, crystalline* appearance in contrast to the white spheres of asteroid hyalosis.

# Case 18 | Drusen

**Frequency in survey for 3rd edition:** did not occur in the initial small survey at PACES Station 5, Eyes.

**Predicted frequency from older, more extensive MRCP short case surveys:** main focus of a short case in 0.4% of attempts at PACES Station 5, Eyes.

## *Record*

Multiple, discrete, round, yellow-white dots of variable size scattered around the macula and posterior pole of the eye. These are retinal drusen.

---

Retinal drusen represent abnormal accumulations in the retinal pigment epithelium basement (Bruch's) membrane in subjects usually over the age of 40 years. Drusen in the macular region are often precursors to visual loss from *senile macular degeneration*. The latter may lead to impairment of central vision early in its course – non-congruent central scotoma.

Once drusen have been discovered, the patient needs to be told to screen one eye at a time regularly for possible signs of neovascular macular degeneration. Such screening involves checking lines on a piece of graph paper or between tiles in a bathroom. Blank spots or distortion may be a sign of neovascularization. Photodynamic therapy using the drug verteporfin reduces the risk of vision loss.

Retinal drusen need to be distinguished from optic disc drusen (also called hyaline bodies) which are bright excrescences at the optic disc which may be-calcified. These are sometimes obvious but may be difficult to see in young persons, in whom the disc elevation they produce can be mistaken for papilloedema (*pseudopapilloedema*). Occasionally, these may be associated with tuberous sclerosis.

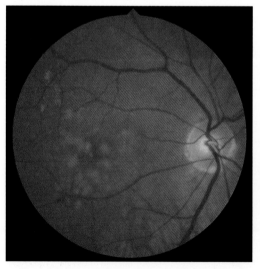 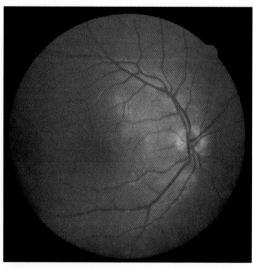

(a)  (b)

**Figure I5.87** (a) Retinal drusen in the macular area. (b) Optic disc drusen in a young person leading to pseudopapilloedema (when he presented to casualty with headache, the optic disc changes were noted and an urgent CT scan was ordered; this was normal and ultrasonography of the optic disc showed up the drusen as the only abnormality).

# Case 19 | Laurence–Moon–Bardet–Biedl syndrome

**Frequency in survey for 3rd edition:** did not occur in the initial small survey at PACES Station 5, Eyes.

**Predicted frequency from older, more extensive MRCP short case surveys:** main focus of a short case in 0.7% of attempts at PACES Station 5, Eyes. Additional feature in some others.

## Record

On examination of the fundi of this *blind** patient, there is a pigmentary retinopathy suggestive of *retinitis pigmentosa.** There is truncal *obesity*, *short stature* (not always) and *polydactyly*.† These features suggest the diagnosis of the Laurence–Moon–Bardet–Biedl syndrome. (There is likely to be *mental retardation*† of variable severity, and *hypogonadism*.†)

---

Autosomal recessive.

Renal structural and functional abnormalities are very common. Interstitial nephritis may lead to renal failure.

### The 'splitters' and the 'lumpers'

Some investigators (the 'splitters') consider the Bardet–Biedl syndrome and the Laurence–Moon syndrome to be distinct, the Laurence–Moon syndrome being characterized by the absence of polydactyly and obesity and the presence of spastic paraparesis. Other investigators (the 'lumpers') believe these distinctions relate to variable expression of a single disorder.

### Related disorders

*Alström's syndrome*: autosomal recessive; retinal dystrophy and obesity; blindness in early childhood; moderate deafness before the age of 10; diabetes mellitus and slowly progressive chronic nephropathy in early adulthood; *mental retardation and digital abnormalities do not occur*.

*Carpenter's syndrome* (acrocephalopolysyndactyly): autosomal recessive; acrocephaly; syndactyly; characteristic facial appearance associated with obesity, mental retardation, hypogonadism and polydactyly of the feet. In view of the characteristic skeletal findings, there should not be diagnostic difficulty.

---

*The retinal dystrophy of the Laurence–Moon–Bardet–Biedl syndrome is usually pigmentary. Though retinitis pigmentosa is commonly cited in this syndrome, the preferred term is *rod-cone dystrophy*, because it more accurately describes the pathological process and in the early stages no pigmentary changes may be seen despite significant visual disturbance. In one study mean age of night blindness was 9 years and of blindness registration was 15 years.

†Hypogonadism, mental retardation and polydactyly are less frequently found in females.

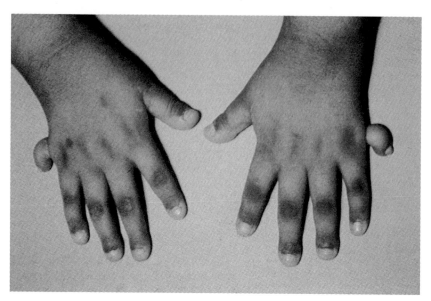

**Figure I5.88** Polydactyly.

# Case 20 | Cytomegalovirus choroidoretinitis (AIDS)

**Frequency in survey for 3rd edition:** did not occur in the initial small survey at PACES Station 5, Eyes.

**Predicted frequency from older, more extensive MRCP short case surveys:** main focus of a short case in 0.1% of attempts at PACES Station 5, Eyes.

## *Record*

The fundi show discrete areas of *white or yellow retinal opacification* with associated *haemorrhage* and *vascular sheathing* (the appearance resembles branch retinal vein occlusion (see Station 5, Eyes, Case 6), but is distinguished because one eye often has multiple foci, and there is a tendency for both eyes to be affected). The appearance (*'scrambled egg and tomato sauce'* and *'cottage cheese and jam'* are both terms that have been used to describe the typical appearance) is suggestive of cytomegalovirus choroidoretinitis in an *immunosuppressed patient*. The diagnosis could be substantiated by culture of throat and urine.

---

## Human immunodeficiency virus

The human immunodeficiency virus is an RNA retrovirus that infects human cells that express CD4 and one type of chemokine receptor (CCR5 or CXCR4) on their surface. Agents that prevent HIV attachment to its host (target) cells are called entry inhibitors.

Once inside the cytoplasm, HIV undergoes reverse transcription, the viral RNA acting as a template for a complementary DNA molecule. Synthetic nucleotides and non-nucleotide inhibitors can be used to interfere with this process.

In the absence of antiretroviral agents, the completed HIV DNA chain migrates inside the host cell's nucleus and becomes integrated into the cell's DNA. The process involves viral integrase. Agents that block viral integrase are called integrase inhibitors.

In the absence of HIV drugs, viral DNA is transcribed into chains of RNA that enter a host cell's cytoplasm where building of new viral particles takes place. The new viral particles need to undergo a 'maturation' process before being infective. This process relies on HIV protease. Protease inhibitors prevent maturation of new viral particles, making them incapable of infecting new cells.

## *Epidemiology*

In the UK, it has been estimated that 83,000 individuals had HIV and 27% were unaware of their diagnosis in 2009.

## *Routes of HIV transmission*

The human immunodeficiency virus is a blood-borne virus that can be transmitted sexually. Sexual transmission of the virus is responsible for the majority of HIV epidemics globally. In the beginning of the epidemics, sexual transmission of HIV was mostly reported amongst men who have sex with men (MSM) in developed nations whereas heterosexual transmission of HIV has been the main route of transmission in developing nations. In the UK, this distinction has disappeared and heterosexual transmission of HIV has been the main route of transmission since 2000.

The human immunodeficiency virus can also be transmitted during pregnancy and delivery from an infected mother to the child. Implementation of antenatal screening programmes has significantly reduced the rate of HIV mother-to-child transmission.

Sharing of injection equipment between intravenous drug users (IVDU) is another identified route of HIV transmission. Transmission via infected blood products can also lead to HIV transmission.

### Clinical features

Acute infection with HIV may present with non-specific flu-like symptoms (maculopapular rash, pharyngitis, myalgia, lymphadenopathy, headache or, rarely, aseptic meningitis) and lasts for 12 weeks. After that period, patients remain asymptomatic for an average of 8 years (latency period of HIV infection). At the end of this period, HIV viral load starts to increase, whilst patients' CD4 count starts to decline. Unless treated with antiretroviral agents, patients become immunocompromised and at risk of developing acquired immunodeficiency syndrome (AIDS)-defining illnesses. AIDS-defining illnesses (Table I5.10) are infections and malignancies strongly associated with immunocompromised HIV-infected patients. It is important to ensure that patients with any AIDS-defining illnesses are tested for HIV.

### Laboratory diagnosis

Serology including immunoassays for HIV antigen and antibody. There is an interval between infection and development of detectable amounts of anti-HIV antibodies during which HIV-infected patients may test antibody negative (window period). The duration of the window period is 3–4 weeks with the new HIV assays.

### Treatment

Antiretroviral therapy is the most effective treatment for medium- and long-term survival for patients with any of the AIDS-defining illnesses.

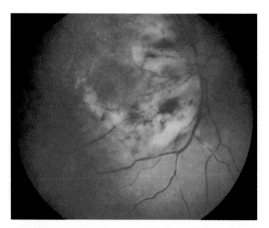

**Figure I5.89** Cytomegalovirus retinitis: 'scrambled egg and tomato sauce' appearance.

**Table I5.10** AIDS-defining illnesses

| | |
|---|---|
| Bacterial infections | *Mycobacterium avium* complex<br>Disseminated tuberculosis<br>Disseminated or extrapulmonary mycobacterial infection<br>Recurrent *Salmonella* septicaemia<br>*Notes*<br>• Any person with any form of mycobacterial infection must be tested for HIV. Not everyone with mycobacterial infection will be HIV infected<br>• Mycobacterial (tuberculosis or non-tuberculosis) infections commonly cause long-standing fever, weight loss, lymphadenopathy. Patients may also present with cough, anaemia and hepatosplenomegaly<br>• Treatment of non-tuberculosis mycobacterial infections is complex and depends on the antibiotic sensitivity of the species. All mycobacterial infections require combined anti-TB therapy for several months |
| Fungal infections | *Pneumocystis jiroveci* pneumonia (formerly *Pneumocystis carinii*)<br>• Most often presenting with shortness of breath, fever and dry cough.<br>• Treatment is with high-dose co-trimoxazole. Patients with severe hypoxia should also receive short-term steroids<br>Candidiasis of bronchi, trachea or lungs<br>Oesophageal candidiasis<br>Disseminated or extrapulmonary coccidioidomycosis<br>Extrapulmonary cryptococcosis, cryptococcal meningitis |
| Protozoal infections | Chronic intestinal cryptosporidiosis (for longer than 1 month)<br>Disseminated or extrapulmonary histoplasmosis<br>Toxoplasmosis of the brain<br>Chronic intestinal isosporiasis (for more than 1 month) |
| Viral infections | Cytomegalovirus disease (other than liver, spleen or lymph nodes)<br>• Most commonly involving retina and gastrointestinal tract<br>• Is mostly associated with severe immunosuppression (CD4 count <50 cells/mm$^3$)<br>Chronic ulcer(s) (for more than 1 month); bronchitis, pneumonitis or oesophagitis caused by herpes simplex virus<br>Progressive multifocal leucoencephalopathy<br>• Caused by JC virus, is associated with severe immunosuppression<br>• Presents with visual field defects, gait instability, and disrupted co-ordination |
| Malignancy | Invasive cervical cancer<br>Kaposi's sarcoma (KS)<br>• Caused by human herpes virus 8<br>• Can develop on skin and mucosa involving internal organs. Internal KS can affect lungs or gastrointestinal tract<br>• Antiretroviral therapy is the most effective treatment of local KS. Internal KS often requires chemotherapy as well<br>Non-Hodgkin's lymphoma<br>• Mostly presenting as anaemia, hepatosplenomegaly, lymphadenopathy and fever<br>• Strong association with Epstein–Barr virus and HIV infections; hence the need for testing patients for HIV<br>• Prognosis has significantly improved with antiretroviral therapy and combined chemotherapy regimes |
| Others/general | HIV-related encephalopathy<br>Recurrent pneumonia<br>• Patients with two episodes of pneumonia in 12 months must be tested for HIV infection<br>Wasting syndrome due to HIV |

# Case 21 | Normal fundus

**Frequency in survey for 3rd edition:** did not occur in the initial small survey of PACES Station 5,* Eyes.

The reasons why normal short cases may appear in PACES in Stations 1 and 3* have been discussed in Vol. 1, Station 1, Respiratory, Case 24, Abdominal, Case 11 and Station 3, Cardiovascular, Case 24. In the case of examination of the fundus, there is an additional reason and the College has particularly highlighted the possibility of using a normal fundus with its statement in the guide notes to examination centres: '. . . the inclusion of a normal optic fundus in Station 5 is permissible'. The reason for this is that the College has also recommended that in the case scenario, if the patient has diabetes, this may be stated. This is on the grounds that, in 'real life', when examining the fundi, it would be known whether or not the patient had diabetes. The College has accepted also that in 'real life', when the fundus of a person with diabetes is being examined, it is often normal.† Hence it wishes that some normal cases are included.

From the pre-PACES surveys, it was clear that the most common reason for finding no abnormality is missing the physical signs that are present (probably Anecdote in Vol. 1, Station 3, Cardiovascular, Case 24 and possibly Anecdote 2 in Vol. 1, Station 3, Cardiovascular, Case 11; see also Vol. 2, Section F, Experience 158). Other reasons for cases of 'normal' will be either because the physical signs are no longer present by the time the patient comes to the examination (see Anecdote in Vol. 1, Station 3, CNS, Case 28) or that the examiners and candidate disagree with the selectors of the cases about the presence of physical signs (this may have happened in the anecdote below; see also Vol. 2, Section F, Experience 198 and Vol. 2, Section F, Anecdote 303). The following anecdote is from the original, pre-PACES surveys.

## Anecdote

A candidate was asked to examine the fundi. He found no abnormality and diagnosed a normal fundus. He reports that the patient had multiple sclerosis and that he knows one of the examiners who has since confirmed that her fundi were considered to be normal. He passed the examination but he felt he would have failed if he had said 'bitemporal pallor'.

---

*It is unlikely that 'normal' would be a case in Station 5, Skin, Locomotor or Endocrine (except perhaps via 'Examine this patient's thyroid status' in the latter). If there were a shortage of patients in one subsection of Station 5 it seems more likely that patients from another subsection might be deployed. This may account for the cases where more than one from a subsection occurred in our survey; see Vol. 2, Section F, Experiences 20 and 36.

†It is worth remembering that in 'real life' patients with diabetes can have all the other possible fundal abnormalities; diabetes is common and people with diabetes are as prone to any of the other conditions which affect the eye as anybody else. Furthermore, since people with diabetes are the only ones having their fundi regularly checked, they are more likely to be found to have conditions such as myelinated nerve fibres or old choroiditis. Hence the instruction 'This patient has diabetes, please examine the fundus' could readily be associated with the finding of any retinal abnormality – as well as no abnormality!

# Station 5
# Other

| Short case | Checked and updated as necessary for this edition by |
|---|---|
| **1** Bilateral parotid enlargement/Mikulicz's syndrome | Dr Chris Fegan and Dr David Carruthers* |
| **2** Deep venous thrombosis (DVT)/Baker's cyst/cellulitis | Dr Chris Fegan and Dr David Carruthers* |
| **3** Peripheral vascular disease | Mr Phil Nichol* |
| **4** Osteogenesis imperfecta | Dr David Carruthers* |
| **5** Down's syndrome | Dr Bob Ryder |
| **6** Pernicious anaemia | Dr Chris Fegan* |
| **7** Klippel–Feil syndrome | Dr David Carruthers* |
| **8** Leg oedema | Dr Bob Ryder |

*All suggested changes by these specialty advisors were considered by Dr Bob Ryder and were either accepted, edited, added to or rejected with Dr Ryder making the final editorial decision in every case.

Dr Chris Fegan, Consultant Haematologist, University Hospital of Wales, Cardiff, UK
Dr David Carruthers, Consultant Rheumatologist, City Hospital, Birmingham, UK
Mr Phil Nichol, Consultant Vascular Surgeon, City Hospital, Birmingham, UK

# Case 1 | Bilateral parotid enlargement/ Mikulicz's syndrome

**Frequency in survey for 3rd edition:** 2% of attempts at MRCP short cases, in the original, pre-PACES, surveys.

**Survey note:** all patients with sicca symptoms (dry eyes and dry mouth) in our survey had parotid enlargement.

## Record

There is *bilateral parotid enlargement.** The conjunctivae are injected (the patient complains of *gritty eyes* – the dry eyes of keratoconjunctivitis sicca) and the tongue (touch it) is dry (or the patient complains of a *dry mouth*).†

This is Mikulicz's syndrome (diffuse swelling of lachrymal and salivary glands) which is most likely to be produced by:

1 Sarcoidosis (?lupus pernio, chest signs) but may also be caused by

2 Lymphoma (?lymph nodes, hepatosplenomegaly – both signs, of course, may also occur in sarcoid)

3 Leukaemia (?pallor, hepatosplenomegaly).

---

Reduction in tear secretion can be demonstrated with *Schirmer's test* in which a 5 mm wide strip of filter paper is folded 3 mm from one end and hooked into the lower conjunctival sac. Normal tear secretion moistens more than 15 mm of strip within 5 min.

**Secondary Sjögren's syndrome** (*Mikulicz's disease*) is the triad of dry mouth (xerostomia), keratoconjunctivitis sicca and a connective tissue disease, most commonly rheumatoid arthritis (50%) but also including autoimmune liver disease and fibrosing alveolitis. Bronchial, pancreatic and vaginal secretions may also be diminished. The lachrymal and salivary glands are not swollen as in *Mikulicz's syndrome* (the issue is complicated, though, by the fact that there is a high incidence of lymphoma in Sjögren's syndrome!).

**Primary Sjögren's syndrome** (30%) does not have the associated connective tissue disease. It is sometimes referred to as the *sicca syndrome*. Antinuclear antibody (ANA) is positive in 80% of patients. Antibodies to Ro (SS-A) and La (SS-B) should be looked for and identify patients at risk of extraglandular manifestations.

**Extraglandular manifestations of primary Sjögren's syndrome**

| | |
|---|---|
| Arthralgia/arthritis | 60% |
| Raynaud's phenomenon | 37% |
| Lymphadenopathy | 14% |
| Vasculitis | 11% |
| Kidney involvement | 9% |
| Liver involvement | 7% |
| Splenomegaly | 3% |
| Peripheral neuropathy | 2% |
| Myositis | 1% |

---

*Painless parotid enlargement can also occur in bulimia nervosa.
†Look for lack of a pool of saliva under the tongue. A helpful finding in the history is a positive *cracker test*: the patient reports difficulty chewing and swallowing a packet of crackers without fluids.

# Case 2 | Deep venous thrombosis (DVT)/ Baker's cyst/cellulitis

**Frequency in survey for 3rd edition**: 2% of attempts at MRCP short cases in the original, pre-PACES, surveys.

## Record 1

There is *unilateral* swelling of the R/L leg up to the knee joint which looks normal in appearance* (extension into the thigh suggests femoral or iliac vein thrombosis) associated with an erythematous or cyanotic hue to the skin, and (feel gently) tenderness to palpation in the calf. The affected calf feels indurated† and is *warmer than the other leg*. The patient has a deep venous thrombosis.‡

## Record 2

The R/L leg is *swollen, painful on movement* and *tender* on palpation. Both the knee joint and the upper, posterior compartment of the calf are swollen, and the normal contours of the joint are obscured by effusion (demonstrate the patellar tap; see Station 5, Locomotor, Case 19).§ A 'fullness' is (may be) palpable in the popliteal space. The diagnosis is a ruptured Baker's (popliteal) cyst (now check hands for rheumatoid arthritis; see Station 5, Locomotor, Case 1).¶

## Record 3

There is an *erythematous, warm swelling* of the R/L leg. There are (may be) vesicles/ bullae and crusts on the surface of the erythematous area (look for the portal of bacterial entry).** There is (may be) a puncture mark on the foot (say where exactly) perhaps caused by a thorn (or there may be fungal intertrigo of the feet with secondary bacterial infection). These features suggest cellulitis. There is (may be) *lymphangitis* (look for the reddish streaky lines running up the leg), and the inguinal lymph nodes are swollen and tender.

## Record 4

The skin on the R/L leg is *swollen* and *erythematous with a sharply demarcated, irregular border* which is tender to touch and has an 'orange-peel' epidermal surface. These features suggest erysipelas.††

---

*If there was associated swelling of the knee it would bring ruptured popliteal cyst and disease of the joint (infection, gout and pseudogout) into the differential diagnosis.

†The calf in DVT feels bulky and indurated and moves *en masse*, causing discomfort when gently swayed from side to side. This method is preferable to testing for the *Homan's sign* in which a sudden dorsiflexion of the corresponding foot can cause considerable pain. In the normal calf the muscle contours are clearly visible and a part of the muscle can be moved from side to side without pain or affecting the rest of the calf.

‡The definitive diagnosis can usually be made by Doppler ultrasonography which is non-invasive, quick and less expensive than venography, though the latter remains the gold standard.

§The popliteal cyst may rupture and dissect into the calf muscles, causing pain and acute swelling involving the upper part of the calf. The cyst may cause compression of the popliteal vein leading to oedema of the entire leg or a secondary DVT.

¶Ultrasound scanning has the advantage of being non-invasive but arthrography is the most definitive way to identify a popliteal cyst. The latter procedure also provides the opportunity for aspiration to rule out infection, gout and pseudogout.

**Group A streptococci and *Staphylococcus aureus* are the most commonly responsible organisms.

††Erysipelas is an acute infection of the skin and subcutaneous tissues caused by group A streptococci. It is most commonly seen on the face but may affect other parts of the body. The disease usually affects the two extremes of age.

The thrombophilia syndromes which predispose to deep vein thrombosis (DVT) include:

Antiphospholipid syndrome (?livedo reticularis; see Station 5, Skin, Case 29)

Factor V Leiden: 5% of the population

Prothrombin gene G20210A mutation: 2% of the population

Hyperhomocysteinaemia: 5–10% of the population

Deficiency of antithrombin III (up to 1 per 2000 of population)

Deficiency of protein C and protein S (vitamin K-dependent factors that act together to neutralize factors V and VIII).

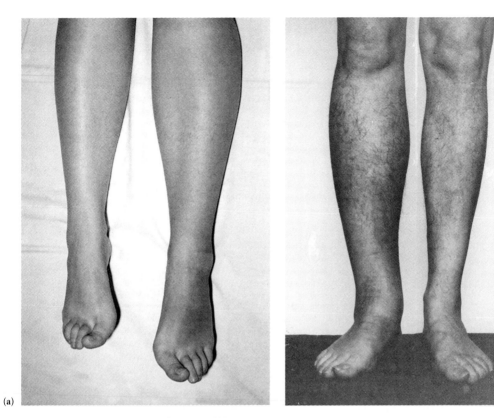

(a)

(b)

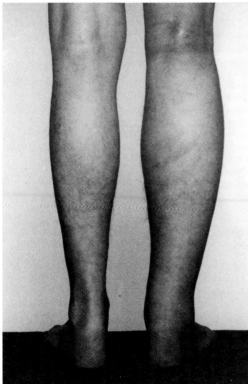

(c)

**Figure I5.90** (a) Left DVT. (b) Ruptured Baker's cyst; (c) posterior view.

# Case 3 | Peripheral vascular disease

**Frequency in survey for 3rd edition:** main focus of a short case in 0.8% of attempts at MRCP short cases in the original, pre-PACES, surveys. Additional feature in others.

## Record

The lower leg(s) are pale (pregangrenous areas may be pink), the toes bluish-red (there may be digital gangrene) and the *skin* is *atrophic* (may be stretched and *shiny*). There are *no pulses*\* palpable below the femorals (if allowed, listen for a bruit) and the lower legs and feet are *cold* to touch. There is often asymmetry of signs.

These signs suggest peripheral vascular disease (?arcus senilis, ?xanthelasma, ?tendon xanthomata, ?nicotine-stained fingers, ?diabetes,† history of ischaemic heart disease or cerebrovascular disease).

---

## Arteriosclerosis

This, the usual cause of peripheral vascular disease, is due to atheromatous plaques involving the intima of the arteries. As a rule there is superimposed thrombus formation. Degenerative changes occur in the media which frequently calcifies.† The superficial femoral artery is most commonly affected, leading to calf claudication. The next most common sites are the popliteal and aortic bifurcation, the latter leading to Leriche's syndrome.

*Leriche's syndrome* – claudication of low back, buttocks, thigh and calf; limb and buttock atrophy and pallor; impotence, weak or absent femoral pulses, systolic bruits over the lower abdomen and femorals; signs may be asymmetrical; may present as 'sciatica'.

## Buerger's postural test

When the legs are lifted to 45° above the horizontal plane, cadaveric pallor develops if the arterial supply is poor. If, while the clinician supports the legs, the patient flexes and extends the ankles to the point of mild fatigue, this enhances the sign. The patient now sits with his feet lowered to the ground for 2–3 min and an impaired arterial supply is indicated by a ruddy, cyanotic hue which spreads over the affected foot (*Buerger's sign*). This sequence indicates occlusion of a major lower limb artery.

**The ankle : brachial pressure index** uses a Doppler ultrasonic flow probe to determine the ratio of the peak systolic pressure at the ankle to that in the arm. Symptoms are unlikely to be due to arterial disease if the index is above 0.8. Measurements made immediately after exercise give a good index of disease but are more difficult to perform reliably. In diabetic patients with calcified arteries,† the test is unreliable as the pressure in the sphygmomanometer cuff may not reflect that in the artery.

## Takayasu's disease‡

This is an arteritis which affects chiefly, but not exclusively, young women from Japan and the Far East. It involves mainly the aortic arch and the large brachiocephalic arteries. Mononuclear cell infiltrates and fibrous proliferation produce progressive narrowing of the lumen and reduced flow in the upper extremities

---

\*The patient with intermittent claudication may have few signs other than reduced or absent pulses in the affected limb. As the atheromatous disease advances, signs of ischaemia appear: low skin temperature, pallor or cyanosis, trophic changes including dry, scaly and shiny skin; ischaemic damage may cause persistent reddish or reddish-blue discoloration; ischaemic ulcers and gangrene may develop.

†Peripheral vascular disease in diabetic patients is more progressive, with greater involvement of the more distal vessels which are of smaller calibre; medial calcification is twice as common. See also Station 5, Locomotor, Case 4.

‡There were one or two anecdotes in our surveys to suggest that this may have appeared on rare occasions in the MRCP short cases.

and to the brain. It develops slowly so that although the pulses gradually vanish (hence the alternative name – *pulseless disease*), collateral circulation opens up, allowing it to remain unnoticed for some time. Eventually the patient presents with symptoms such as fainting on turning the head suddenly or rising from supine to sitting, atrophy of the face, headaches, cataracts, optic atrophy, weakness and paraesthesiae of the upper extremities, hemiplegia and convulsions.

## Buerger's disease (thromboangiitis obliterans)

An obstructive arterial disease with segmental inflammation and proliferative lesions in medium and small arteries§ and veins of the limbs. Mostly affects young males aged 20–40 years, especially in Israel, the Orient and India. Patients are almost always moderate to heavy smokers; there may be an autoimmune mechanism triggered by tobacco products. Clinically the disease is characterized by ischaemia of the extremities§ and *migratory thrombophlebitis*. Raynaud's phenomenon (see Station 5, Skin, Case 22) is common. If the patient continues to smoke, the disease will progress with increasing ischaemia leading to gangrene and amputation of the extremities which is required in a high percentage of patients.

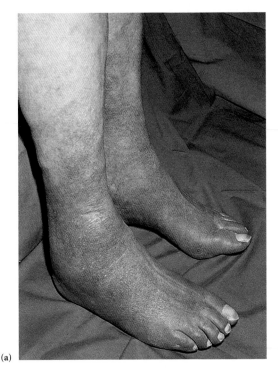

(a)

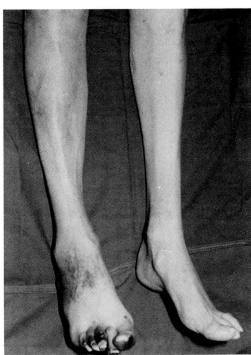

(b)

**Figure I5.91** (a) Peripheral vascular insufficiency. (b) Peripheral vascular disease with gangrenous toes.

§The features which distinguish this *thromboangiitis obliterans* from the common atheromatous arterial disease (*arteriosclerosis obliterans*) are the younger age of the patient, the relative sparing of larger arteries, the presence of migratory superficial thrombophlebitis, the increased involvement of the upper extremities, and more rapid progression. The diagnosis can be confirmed by biopsy of an early lesion showing a characteristic inflammatory and proliferative lesion on histology.

# Case 4 | Osteogenesis imperfecta

**Frequency in survey for 3rd edition:** main focus of a short case in 0.5% of attempts at MRCP short cases in the original, pre-PACES, surveys.

## *Record*

The *sclerae* are *slaty-blue*. (Look for evidence of *deformity* from poor fracture healing; ask the patient if he has been particularly prone to *fractures* in the past.) The diagnosis is osteogenesis imperfecta (the patient may be deaf due to *otosclerosis*).

---

Osteogenesis imperfecta is due to defects in type I collagen. In the adult the diagnosis is likely to be the milder tarda type* (usually dominant). In this type the sclerae are more likely to be blue and the fragile bones of childhood become stronger after adolescence though they remain abnormal. The blueness is due to the thin sclerae allowing choroid pigment to show through. Though blue sclerae are not always present, some patients manifest only blue sclerae or otosclerosis without clinical bone disease. Deafness from otosclerosis does not usually develop before the third decade and may occur even later still. Laxity of ligaments, hypotonia of muscles and muscle wasting (partly disuse atrophy) are other features which may occur. Serum alkaline and acid phosphatases are often elevated and the urine often contains hydroxyproline, pyrophosphate and glycosaminoglycans. Though no specific treatment is known, favourable responses to bisphosphonates offer promise, while bone marrow transplants remain experimental. Osteogenesis imperfecta may be confused with idiopathic juvenile osteoporosis but, in the latter condition, osteoporosis is typically confined to the vertebral column, there is no family history of fractures and the sclerae are normal in colour.

### Other conditions in which blue sclerae may occur

Marfan's syndrome (see Vol. 1, Station 3, Cardiovascular, Case 13)

Ehlers–Danlos syndrome (see Station 5, Skin, Case 28)

Pseudoxanthoma elasticum (see Station 5, Skin, Case 10)

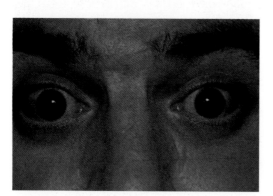

**Figure I5.92** Blue sclerae of osteogenesis imperfecta.

*Other types are:
1 The severe prenatal type which causes intrauterine death or life for only a few days after birth
2 The severe type in which the baby survives but is extremely susceptible to fractures. The bones are soft as well as brittle and may therefore bow. Deformities are common and walking may induce fractures. Blue sclerae are less common.

# Case 5 | Down's syndrome

**Frequency in survey for 3rd edition:** main focus of a short case in 0.5% of attempts at MRCP short cases in the original, pre-PACES, surveys. Additional feature in a further 0.6%.

## *Record*

This short-statured patient has *low-set ears*, a *flattened nasal bridge, slanting eyes, epicanthus*, white *'Brushfield spots'* in the iris and a small *mouth which hangs open*, revealing a large, heavily fissured tongue. There is an over-rolled helix of each ear. There is a single *transverse palmar crease* (not pathognomonic) and a short inward-curving little finger. The axial triradius is situated towards the centre of the palm (normally should be near the wrist). There is generalized hypotonia and hyperextensibility of the joints. The patient has Down's syndrome.

---

Trisomy 21 (occasionally translocation between 21 and 14). Increased incidence with increasing maternal age.

**Other features which may occur**
Congenital heart lesions (septal defects, Fallot's tetralogy)
Lenticular opacities
Mental retardation which varies from very mild (author of an autobiography) to very severe
Dementia of Alzheimer type
Haematological malignancies (in particular acute lymphoblastic leukaemia)
Decreased incidence of many common malignancies*
Hypothyroidism

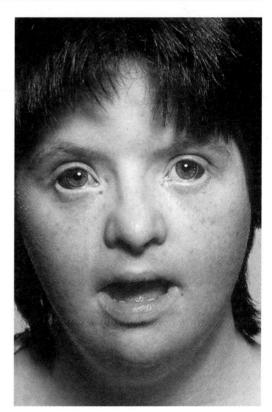

**Figure I5.93** Down's syndrome.

*Unclear whether this is due to tumour suppressor genes on chromosome 21 or reduced exposure to environmental risk factors.

# Case 6 | Pernicious anaemia

**Frequency in survey for 3rd edition:** 0.4% of attempts at MRCP short cases in the original, pre-PACES, surveys.

## Record

The patient has *pallor* (may be a pale lemon-yellow tinge), a *smooth tongue*\* and *angular stomatitis.*\* *Vitiligo*† is (may be) present. The likely diagnosis is pernicious anaemia (splenomegaly and pyrexia‡ may both occur).

---

### Other general clinical features of megaloblastic anaemias\*

Gastrointestinal symptoms
Weight loss
Hyperpigmentation
Infertility
Orthostatic hypotension.

### Haematological abnormalities associated with megaloblastic anaemias\*

Anaemia
Reticulocytopenia
Macrocytosis
Neutropenia
Thrombocytopenia
Neutrophil hypersegmentation
Poikilocytosis
Anisocytosis
Raised lactate dehydrogenase
Raised bilirubin
Raised serum iron
Decreased haptoglobin
Hypercellular bone marrow with megaloblastic morphology, giant bands and metamyelocytes

### Neuropsychiatric abnormalities associated with vitamin B12 deficiency

(See also Vol. 1, Station 3, CNS, Case 37)
Paraesthesiae
Peripheral neuropathy (absent ankle jerks; impaired touch and pain perception; impaired vibration sense and joint position sense [may be Romberg's positive] may also be due to dorsal column involvement)
Ataxia (posterior column involvement; ?joint position sense; ?Romberg's)
Decreased reflexes (peripheral neuropathy; see Vol. 1, Station 3, CNS, Case 1 and Case 37)
Increased reflexes (pyramidal tract involvement; see Vol. 1, Station 3, CNS, Case 6 and Case 37)
Spasticity (pyramidal tract involvement)
Weakness
Dementia (memory loss, disorientation, obtundation)
Incontinence (urinary or faecal)
Impotence
Optic atrophy
Abnormal smell or taste
Lhermitte's phenomenon (see Vol. 1, Station 3, CNS, Case 37)

---

\*Most patients with folate or vitamin B12 deficiency do not have many of the features listed. Even anaemia and raised mean corpuscular volume may be absent in a patient with otherwise severe folate or vitamin B12 deficiency; in one prospective study of patients with vitamin B12 deficiency, 44% did not have anaemia, 36% had a mean corpuscular volume equal to or less than 100, 86% had a normal white cell count, 79% a normal platelet count, 33% had a normal peripheral blood film, 43% had a normal lactate dehydrogenase and 83% a normal bilirubin.

†The cutaneous marker of organ-specific autoimmune diseases (see Station 5, Skin, Case 8) creates the suspicion of addisonian pernicious anaemia rather than any other cause of megaloblastic anaemia leading to pallor and a smooth tongue.
‡Why were you not previously aware that untreated pernicious anaemia may be associated with fever? Perhaps it should be called *hypo-cyanocobalaminic fever.* See Appendix 3).

Psychiatric abnormalities (depression, paranoia, list-lessness, acute confusional state, hallucinations, delusions, insomnia, apprehensiveness, psychosis, slow mentation, paraphrenia, mania, panic attacks, suicide)

## Causes of megaloblastic anaemia
### Vitamin B12 deficiency
Decreased ingestion (poor diet, lack of animal prod-ucts, strict vegetarianism)

Impaired absorption:

(a) failure of release of B12 from food protein (old age; partial gastrectomy)

(b) intrinsic factor deficiency (pernicious anaemia; total gastrectomy; destruction of gastric mucosa by caustics; congenital abnormality or absence of intrinsic factor)

(c) chronic pancreatic disease

(d) competitive parasites (bacteria in bowel diver-ticula, blind loops, fish tapeworm)

(e) intrinsic intestinal disease (ileal resection, Crohn's disease, radiation ileitis; tropical sprue, coeliac disease; infiltrative intestinal disease such as lymphoma or scleroderma; drug-induced malab-sorption; congenital selective malabsorption – Imerslund–Grasbeck syndrome)

Impaired utilization (congenital enzyme deficien-cies; lack of transcobalamin II; nitrous oxide administration)

### Folate deficiency
Decreased ingestion (poor diet, lack of vegetables; alco-holism; infancy)

Impaired absorption (intestinal short circuits; tropical sprue, coeliac disease; drugs such as anticonvulsants and sulphasalazine; congenital malabsorption)

Impaired utilization (folic acid antagonists such as methotrexate, triamterene, trimethoprim, pyrimeth-amine, ethanol; congenital enzyme deficiencies)

Increased requirement (pregnancy, infancy, hyperthy-roidism, chronic haemolytic disease, neoplastic disease, exfoliative skin disease)

Increased loss (haemodialysis)

### Drugs – metabolic inhibitors
Purine synthesis (methotrexate, 6-mercaptopurine, 6-thioguanine, azathioprine)

Pyrimidine synthesis (methotrexate, 5-fluorouracil)

Deoxyribonucleotide synthesis (hydroxyurea, cytosine arabinoside)

### Miscellaneous
Inborn errors (e.g. Lesch–Nyhan syndrome, hereditary orotic aciduria)

Unexplained disorders (pyridoxine-responsive mega-loblastic anaemia, thiamine-responsive megaloblas-tic anaemia, some cases of myelodysplastic syndrome, some cases of acute myelogenous leukaemia)

# Case 7 | Klippel–Feil syndrome

**Frequency in survey for 3rd edition:** 0.3% of attempts at MRCP short cases in the original, pre-PACES, surveys.

## Record

The patient has a *short neck*, with *limited rotation* of the head, a low hairline and a webbed neck.*

The limited rotation of the head suggests Klippel–Feil syndrome.

---

In Klippel–Feil syndrome, the number of cervical vertebrae is reduced and two or more may be fused. This bony deformity leads to shortening of the neck, but this does not in itself cause neurological symptoms. There may, however, be neurological complications from coexisting anomalies of the central nervous system (CNS). Basilar impression and syringomyelia (see Vol. 1, Station 3, CNS, Case 29) are problems which may be associated.

**Other problems which may be associated**

Hearing loss

Heart defects

Sprengel's deformity (upward displacement of the scapula)

Genitourinary anomalies (e.g. aplasia of the müllerian structures)

*Webbing of the neck is usually associated with Turner's syndrome (short stature, increased carrying angle, shield-like chest, short metacarpals, amenorrhoea, coarctation of the aorta) but is not pathognomonic. The limited rotation of the head is the pointer to the Klippel–Feil syndrome.

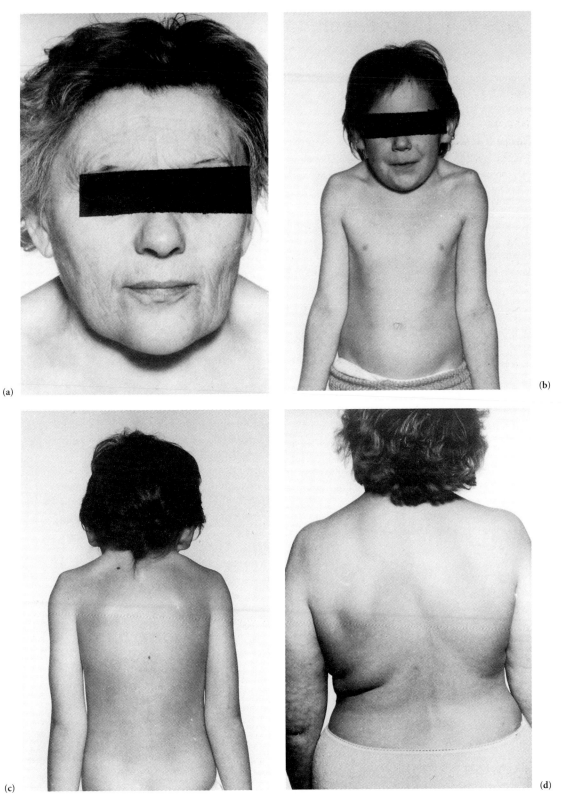

**Figure I5.94** Klippel-Feil syndrome. (a) Shortening of the neck demonstrated by a reduced ear lobe to shoulder distance. (b) Note webbed neck and (c) low hairline. (d) Scoliosis and low hairline resulting from deficiency of cervical vertebrae.

# Case 8 | Leg oedema

**Frequency in survey for 3rd edition:** main focus of a short case in 0.3% of attempts at MRCP short cases in the original, pre-PACES, surveys. Additional feature in many others.

## Record 1

There is *swelling* of the lower limbs which *pits on pressure*. The patient is (may be) breathless at rest, the *venous pressure* is *raised* and oscillating the ear lobe, and there is *sacral oedema*. These features suggest that the ankle oedema is due to congestive cardiac failure (now consider offering to extend the examination to look for features of cardiac and/or pulmonary disease and hepatomegaly).

## Record 2

This *elderly* female (or male) has bilateral lower limb oedema (check for pitting) up to the mid-calf (look for the presence of a walking aid, engorged jugular veins and, if allowed, sacral oedema). Her *Zimmer frame* suggests a degree of poor mobility and, in the absence of any other signs of cardiovascular disease, it is likely to be dependent oedema though the patient may be on some *salt-retaining drugs* such as steroids or non-steroidal anti-inflammatory drugs (NSAIDs).

---

## Causes of leg oedema

### Local causes

Dependent oedema

Venous disorders (chronic venous insufficiency) – pigmentation, induration and inflammation (lipodermatosclerosis)

Occlusion of a large vein:
  phlebothrombosis – *unilateral* (see Station 5, Other, Case 2)
  extrinsic compression

Popliteal (Baker's) cyst – *unilateral* (see Station 5, Other, Case 2)

Cellulitis – *unilateral* (see Station 5, Other, Case 2)

Lymphoedema – non-pitting, thickened and indurated skin ('pigskin'). May be idiopathic or secondary to proximal lymphatic obstruction (metastatic carcinoma, surgical removal of the regional lymph nodes, irradiation or chronic infection)

Gastrocnemius rupture – *unilateral* (swelling and ecchymosis around the ankle joint and foot)

Lipomatosis – in some cases of obesity the fat may be preferentially deposited in the lower limbs

### Systemic causes

Congestive cardiac failure

Hypoproteinaemia – nephrotic syndrome, liver cirrhosis, kwashiorkor, protein-losing enteropathy

Hypo- and hyperthyroidism

Drugs – corticosteroids, NSAIDs, vasodilators, calcium channel blockers, pioglitazone*

*Especially when used in combination with insulin.

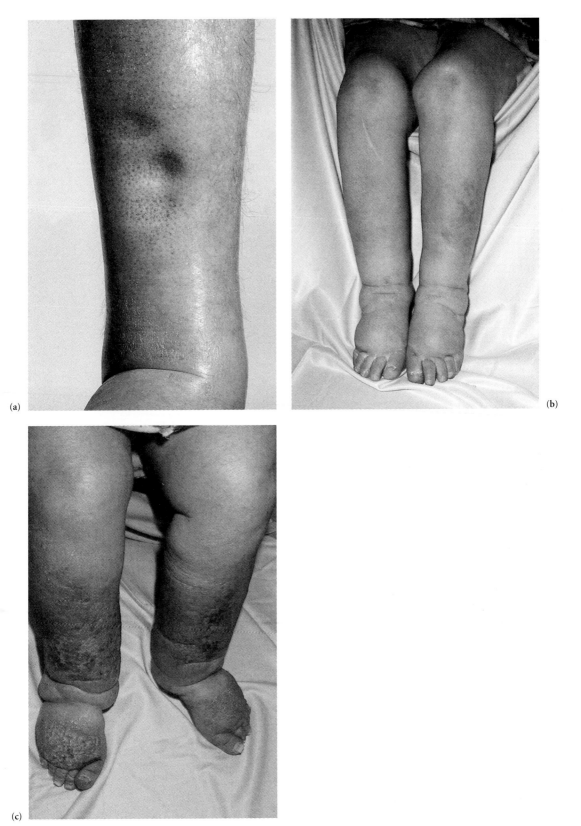

**Figure I5.95** (a) Oedema which has pitted with finger pressure. (b) Bilateral leg oedema in an elderly patient. (c) Lymphoedema of the legs.

# Appendices

These books exist as they are because of many previous candidates who, over the years, have completed our surveys and given us invaluable insight into the candidate experience. Please give something back by doing the same for the candidates of the future. For all of your sittings, whether they be a triumphant pass or a disastrous fail . . .

**Remember to fill in the survey at www.ryder-mrcp.org.uk**

THANK YOU

# 1 | Checklists

## 1 Pulse

### Observe

1 Face (malar flush, thyroid facies).
2 Neck (Corrigan's pulse, raised JVP, thyroidectomy scar, goitre) and chest (thoracotomy scar).

### Palpate and assess

3 Pulse.
4 Rate.
5 Rhythm (?slow atrial fibrillation).
6 Character (normal, collapsing, slow rising, jerky).
7 Carotid.
8 Opposite radial.
9 Radiofemoral delay.
10 All the other pulses.
11 Additional diagnostic features.

## 2 Heart

1 *Visual survey*:
  (a) breathlessness
  (b) *cyanosis*
  (c) pallor
  (d) *malar flush*
  (e) carotids
  (f) jugulars
  (g) *valvotomy scar*, midline scar
  (h) ankle oedema
  (i) clubbing; splinter haemorrhages.
2 Pulse (rate and rhythm).
3 Lift up the arm (?collapsing).
4 Radiofemoral delay.
5 Brachials and carotids (?slow rising).
6 Venous pressure.
7 Apex beat.
8 Tapping impulse.
9 Right ventricular lift.
10 Other pulsations, thrills, palpable sounds.
11 Auscultation (time heart sounds, etc.; turn patient onto left side; lean patient forwards).
12 Sacral oedema (?ankle oedema).
13 Lung bases.
14 Liver.
15 Blood pressure.

## 3 Chest

1 *Visual survey* – general appearance (cachexia, superior vena cava obstruction, systemic sclerosis, lupus pernio, kyphoscoliosis, *ankylosing spondylitis*).
2 Dyspnoea.
3 Lip pursing.
4 Cyanosis.
5 Accessory muscles.
6 Indrawing (intercostal muscles, supraclavicular fossae, lower ribs).
7 Chest wall (upward movement, asymmetry, scars, radiotherapy stigmata).
8 Clubbing (tobacco-staining, coal dust tattoos, rheumatoid deformity, systemic sclerosis).
9 Pulse (flapping tremor).
10 Venous pressure.
11 Trachea (deviation, tug, notch–cricoid distance).
12 Lymphadenopathy.
13 Apex beat.
14 Asymmetry.
15 Expansion.
16 Percussion (do not forget clavicles, axillae).
17 Tactile vocal fremitus.
18 Breath sounds.
19 Vocal resonance.
20 Repeat 14–19 on back of chest (feel for lymph nodes in the neck).

## 4 Abdomen

1 *Visual survey* (pallor, jaundice, spider naevi, etc.).
2 Pigmentation.
3 Hands (Dupuytren's contracture, clubbing, leuconychia, palmar erythema, flapping tremor).
4 Eyes (anaemia, icterus, xanthelasma).
5 Mouth (cyanosis, etc.).
6 Cervical lymph nodes.
7 Gynaecomastia.
8 Spider naevi.
9 Scratch marks.
10 Body hair.
11 Look at the abdomen (pulsation, distension, swelling, distended abdominal veins).

12 Palpation (light palpation, internal organs, inguinal lymph nodes).
13 Percussion.
14 Shifting dullness.
15 Auscultation.
16 Genitalia.
17 Rectal.

## 5 Visual fields
### Observe
1 *Visual survey* (acromegaly, hemiparesis, cerebellar signs).

### Test
2 Peripheral visual fields by confrontation.
3 Central scotoma with a red-headed hat pin.
4 Additional features.

## 6 Cranial nerves
1 Look.
2 Smell and taste (I, VII, IX).
3 Visual acuity (II).
4 Visual fields (II).
5 Eye movements (III, IV, VI).
6 Nystagmus (VIII, cerebellum and its connections).
7 Ptosis (III, sympathetic).
8 Pupils (light, accommodation – III).
9 Discs (II).
10 Facial movements (VII, V).
11 Palatal movement (IX, X).
12 Gag reflex (IX, X).
13 Tongue (XII).
14 Accessory nerve (XI).
15 Hearing (Weber, Rinné – VIII).
16 Facial sensation (including corneal reflex – V).

## 7 Arms
### Observe
1 Face (hemiplegia, nystagmus, wasting, Parkinson's, Horner's).
2 Neck (pseudoxanthoma elasticum, lymph nodes).
3 Elbows (psoriasis, rheumatoid nodules, scars, deformity).
4 Tremor.
5 Hands (joints, nails, skin).
6 Muscle bulk.
7 Fasciculation.

### Test
8 Tone.
9 Arms out in front (winging, myelopathy hand sign, sensory wandering).

10 Power:
  (a) arms out to the side (C5)
  (b) bend your elbows (C5,6)
  (c) push out straight (C7)
  (d) squeeze fingers (C8,T1)
  (e) hold the fingers out straight (radial nerve, C7)
  (f) spread fingers apart (ulnar nerve)
  (g) piece of paper between fingers (ulnar nerve)
  (h) thumb at ceiling (median nerve)
  (i) opposition (median nerve).
11 Coordination (rapid alternate motion, finger–nose).
12 Reflexes.
13 Sensation (light touch, pinprick, vibration, joint position).

## 8 Legs
### Observe
1 *Visual survey* (*Paget's disease*, hemiparesis, exophthalmos, nystagmus, thyroid acropachy, rheumatoid hands, nicotine-stained fingers, wasted hands, muscle fasciculation).
2 Obvious lesion (see group 1 diagnoses).
3 Bowing of the tibia.
4 Pes cavus.
5 One leg smaller than the other.
6 Muscle bulk.
7 Fasciculation.

### Test
8 Tone.
9 Power:
  (a) lift your leg up (L1,2)
  (b) bend your knee (L5,S1,2)
  (c) straighten your leg (L3,4)
  (d) bend your foot down (S1)
  (e) cock up your foot (L4,5).
10 Coordination (heel–shin).
11 Tendon reflexes (clonus).
12 Plantar response.
13 Sensation (light touch, pinprick, vibration, joint position).
14 Gait (ordinary walk, heel-to-toe, on toes, on heels).
15 Rombergism.

## 9 Legs and arms
As appropriate from *Checklists* 7 and 8.

## 10 Gait
1 *Visual survey* (cerebellar signs, Parkinson's, Charcot–Marie–Tooth, ankylosing spondylitis).

2 Check patient can walk.
3 Observe ordinary walk (ataxia, spastic, steppage, parkinsonian).
4 Arm swing (Parkinson's).
5 Turning (ataxia, Parkinson's).
6 Heel-to-toe (ataxia).
7 On toes (S1).
8 On heels (L5).
9 Romberg's test (sensory ataxia).
10 Gait with eyes closed.
11 Additional features.

## 11 Ask some questions

1 *Visual survey* (from top to toe, ?obvious diagnosis).
2 Specific questions (Raynaud's, systemic sclerosis/ CREST, hypo- or hyperthyroidism, Crohn's, nephrotic syndrome).
3 General questions (name, address).
4 Questions with long answers (last meal).
5 Articulation ('British Constitution', 'West Register Street', 'biblical criticism').
6 Repetition.
7 Additional signs.
8 Comprehension ('put out your tongue', 'shut your eyes', 'touch your nose').
9 Nominal dysphasia (keys).
10 Orofacial dyspraxia.
11 Higher mental function.

## 12 Fundi

*Observe*

1 *Visual survey* (Medic-Alert bracelet, etc.).

*Ophthalmoscopy*

2 Lens.
3 Vitreous.
4 Disc (optic atrophy, papillitis, papilloedema, myelinated nerve fibres, new vessels).
5 Arterioles and venules (silver wiring, AV nipping).
6 Each quadrant and macula (haemorrhages, microaneurysms, exudates, new vessels, photocoagulation scars, choroidoretinitis, retinitis pigmentosa, drusen).
7 Do not stop until you have finished and are ready.

## 13 Eyes

*Observe*

1 Face (e.g. myasthenic, tabetic, hemiparesis).
2 Eyes (exophthalmos, strabismus, ptosis, xanthelasma, arcus senilis).

3 Pupils (Argyll Robertson, Horner's, Holmes–Adie, IIIrd nerve).

*Test*

4 Visual acuity.
5 Visual fields.
6 Eye movements (ocular palsy, diplopia, nystagmus, lid lag).
7 Light reflex (direct, consensual).
8 Accommodation reflex.
9 Fundi.

## 14 Face

1 *Visual survey* of patient.
2 Scan the head and face.
3 Break down and scrutinize the parts of the face:
  (a) eyelids (ptosis, rash)
    eyelashes (scanty)
    cornea (arcus, interstitial keratitis)
    sclerae (icteric, congested)
    pupils (small, large, irregular, dislocated lens, cataracts)
    iris (iritis)
  (b) face (erythema, infiltrates)
    mouth (tight, shiny, adherent skin; pigmented patches, telangiectasia, cyanosis).
4 Additional features.

## 15 Hands

*Observe*

1 Face (*systemic sclerosis*, Cushing's, acromegaly, arcus senilis, icterus and spider naevi, exophthalmos).
2 Inspect the hands (rheumatoid, sclerodactyly, wasting, psoriasis, claw hand, clubbing).
3 Joints (swelling, deformity, Heberden's nodes).
4 Nails (pitting, onycholysis, clubbing, nail-fold infarcts).
5 Skin (colour, consistency, lesions).
6 Muscles (wasting, fasciculation).

*Palpate and test*

7 Hands (Dupuytren's contracture, nodules, calcinosis, xanthomata, Heberden's nodes, tophi).
8 Sensation (pinprick, light touch, vibration, joint position).
9 Tone.
10 Power.
11 Pulses.
12 Elbows.

## 16  Skin

1  *Visual survey* (regional associations: scalp, face, mouth, neck, trunk, axillae, elbows, hands, nails, genitalia, legs, feet).
2  Distribution (psoriasis on extensor areas, lichen planus in flexural areas, etc.).
3  Lesions – look for characteristic features (scaling, Wickham's striae, etc.).
4  Associated lesions (arthropathy, etc.).

## 17  Rash

1  *Visual survey* (scalp to sole).
2  Distribution.
3  Surrounding skin (?scratch marks).
4  Examine the lesion (colour, size, shape, surface, character, secondary features).
5  Additional features.

## 18  Neck

1  *Visual survey* of patient (eyes, face, legs).
2  Look at the neck (swallow).
3  Palpate the thyroid (swallow; size, consistency, etc.; pyramidal lobes, percuss over upper sternum).
4  Lymph nodes (supraclavicular, submandibular, postauricular, suboccipital, axillae, groins, spleen).
5  Auscultate the thyroid (distinguish from venous hum and conducted murmurs).
6  Assess thyroid status.

## 19  Thyroid status

1  *Visual survey* (exophthalmos, goitre, thyroid acropachy, pretibial myxoedema, myxoedematous facies).
2  Composure (fidgety, normal, immobile).
3  Pulse.
4  Ankle jerks.
5  Palms.
6  Tremor.
7  Eyes (lid retraction, lid lag).
8  Thyroid (look, palpate, auscultate).
9  Questions.

## 20  Knee

1  Observe (*rheumatoid, psoriasis,* gout).
2  Ask (pain).

3  Inspect (valgus, varus, flexion deformity, quadriceps, knee).
4  Palpate (temperature, tender).
5  Effusion (bulge sign, patellar tap).
6  Movement (flex knee).
7  Crepitus over the joint as flexion occurs.
8  Feel behind the knee for a Baker's cyst.
9  Instability (cruciate, McMurray's sign).
10  Other joints (psoriasis, inflammatory bowel disease, reactive arthritis, tophi).

## 21  Hip

1  Inspect (flexed, shortening, externally rotated, scars, rheumatoid).
2  Ask (pain).
3  Movement (flex, rotate, abduction, adduction, Thomas's test).
4  Straight leg raise (nerve root entrapment, neurological assessment).
5  Tenderness (trochanteric bursitis).
6  Length inequality.
7  Walk (antalgic gait, waddling gait).

## 22  'Spot' diagnosis

1  *Visual survey.*
2  Retrace the same ground more thoroughly:
   (a)  head (*Paget's, myotonic dystrophy*)
   (b)  face (*acromegaly, Parkinson's, hemiplegia,* myotonic dystrophy, tardive dyskinesia, hypopituitarism, Cushing's, hypothyroidism, systemic sclerosis)
   (c)  eyes (*jaundice, exophthalmos,* ptosis, Horner's, xanthelasma)
   (d)  neck (*goitre,* Turner's, spondylitis, torticollis)
   (e)  trunk (pigmentation, ascites, purpuric spots, spider naevi, wasting, pemphigus)
   (f)  arms (choreoathetosis, psoriasis, Addison's, spider naevi, *syringomyelia*)
   (g)  hands (acromegaly, *tremor,* clubbing, sclerodactyly, arachnodactyly, claw hand, etc.)
   (h)  legs (bowing, purpura, pretibial myxoedema, necrobiosis)
   (i)  feet (pes cavus).
3  Abnormal colouring (*pigmentation, icterus,* pallor).
4  Break down and scrutinize (especially face).
5  Additional features.

# 2 | Examination frequency of MRCP PACES short cases

The frequencies presented in the third edition of *An Aid the the MRCP PACES* are reproduced here, as we have not updated the figures due to the change in Station 5.

## Station 5, skin

| Short case | Main focus in PACES survey (%) | Predicted main focus in PACES from original surveys (%) | Predicted additional feature (%) |
|---|---|---|---|
| 1 Systemic sclerosis/CREST syndrome | 15 | 11 | 1 |
| 2 Neurofibromatosis (von Recklinghausen's disease) | 13 | 5 | 4 |
| 3 Osler–Weber–Rendu syndrome | 11 | 9 | — |
| 4 Psoriasis | 11 | 9 | 1 |
| 5 Rash of uncertain cause | 6 | 0 | — |
| 6 Dermatomyositis | 3 | 2 | — |
| 7 Xanthomata | 2 | 4 | 2 |
| 8 Vitiligo | 2 | 2 | — |
| 9 Adenoma sebaceum in tuberous sclerosis complex | 2 | 2 | — |
| 10 Pseudoxanthoma elasticum | 2 | 1 | — |
| 11 Lichen planus | 2 | 0.9 | — |
| 12 Yellow nail syndrome | 2 | 0.5 | — |
| 13 Gouty tophi | 2 | 0 | — |
| 14 Alopecia areata | 2 | 0 | — |
| 15 Eczema | 2 | 0 | — |
| 16 Pretibial myxoedema | 2 | 0 | — |
| 17 Clubbing | 2 | 4 | 14 |
| 18 Necrobiosis lipoidica diabeticorum | 2 | 5 | — |
| 19 Lupus pernio | 2 | 4 | — |
| 20 Tinea | 2 | 0 | — |
| 21 Koilonychia | 2 | 0 | — |
| 22 Raynaud's phenomenon | 0.5 | 0.9 | 2 |
| 23 Erythema nodosum | 0 | 5 | — |
| 24 Sturge–Weber syndrome | 0 | 5 | — |
| 25 Purpura | 0 | 4 | ? |
| 26 Peutz–Jeghers syndrome | 0 | 4 | — |
| 27 Vasculitis | 0 | 4 | ? |
| 28 Ehlers–Danlos syndrome | 0 | 2 | — |
| 29 Livedo reticularis | 0 | 2 | — |
| 30 Pemphigus/pemphigoid | 0 | 2 | — |
| 31 Radiation burn on the chest | 0 | 1 | ? |
| 32 Herpes zoster | 0 | 1 | — |
| 33 Henoch–Schönlein purpura | 0 | 1 | — |
| 34 Mycosis fungoides | 0 | 0.9 | — |
| 35 Morphoea | 0 | 0.9 | — |
| 36 Kaposi's sarcoma (AIDS) | 0 | 0.9 | — |

*(Continued)*

## Skin contd.

| Short case | Main focus in PACES survey (%) | Predicted main focus in PACES from original surveys (%) | Predicted additional feature (%) |
|---|---|---|---|
| 37 Porphyria | 0 | 0.9 | — |
| 38 Lupus vulgaris | 0 | 0.9 | — |
| 39 Dermatitis herpetiformis | 0 | 0.5 | — |
| 40 Urticaria pigmentosa (mastocytosis) | 0 | 0.5 | — |
| 41 Palmoplantar keratoderma (tylosis) | 0 | 0.5 | — |
| 42 Secondary syphilis | 0 | 0.5 | — |
| 43 Ectodermal dysplasia | 0 | 0.5 | — |
| 44 Partial lipodystrophy | 0 | 0.5 | — |
| 45 Fabry's disease | 0 | 0.5 | — |
| 46 Reiter's syndrome/reactive arthritis/keratoderma blennorrhagica | 0 | 0.5 | — |
| 47 Malignant melanoma | 0 | 0.5 | — |
| 48 Acanthosis nigricans | 0 | 0.5 | — |
| 49 Keratoacanthoma | 0 | 0.5 | — |
| 50 Pyoderma gangrenosum | 0 | 0.2 | — |
| 51 Psychogenic/factitious | 0 | 1 anecdote | — |

## Station 5, locomotor

| Short case | Main focus in PACES survey (%) | Predicted main focus in PACES from original surveys (%) | Predicted additional feature (%) |
|---|---|---|---|
| 1 Rheumatoid arthritis | 31 | 33 | 13 |
| 2 Psoriatic arthropathy | 12 | 12 | 1 |
| 3 Systemic sclerosis/CREST syndrome | 12 | 14 | 1 |
| 4 Diabetic foot/Charcot's joint | 7 | 0 | — |
| 5 Tophaceous gout | 6 | 2 | — |
| 6 Ankylosing spondylitis | 4 | 6 | — |
| 7 Paget's disease | 0 | 23 | — |
| 8 Osteoarthritis | 2 | 2 | — |
| 9 Marfan's syndrome | 2 | 2 | — |
| 10 Vasculitis | 2 | 0 | — |
| 11 Proximal myopathy | 2 | 0 | — |
| 12 One leg shorter and smaller than the other | 2 | 0 | — |
| 13 Radial nerve palsy | 1 | 0 | — |
| 14 Arthropathy associated with inflammatory bowel disease | 1 | 0 | — |
| 15 Polymyositis | 1 | 0 | — |
| 16 Systemic lupus erythematosus | 0 | 4 | — |
| 17 Old rickets | 0 | 0.6 | — |
| 18 Juvenile chronic arthritis | 0 | 0.6 | — |
| 19 Swollen knee | 0 | 2 | 3 |

## Station 5, endocrine

| Short case | Main focus in PACES survey (%) | Predicted main focus in PACES from original surveys (%) | Predicted additional feature (%) |
|---|---|---|---|
| 1 Exophthalmos | 26 | 23 | 19 |
| 2 Acromegaly | 24 | 17 | 3 |
| 3 Graves' disease | 9 | 17 | 9 |
| 4 Goitre | 7 | 15 | 6 |
| 5 Hypothyroidism | 6 | 11 | 1 |
| 6 Cushing's syndrome | 5 | 4 | 8 |
| 7 Addison's disease | 3 | 4 | — |
| 8 Hypopituitarism | 2 | 2 | 1 |
| 9 Pretibial myxoedema | 2 | 2 | 5 |
| 10 Gynaecomastia | 2 | 1 | 5 |
| 11 Turner's syndrome | 2 | 1 | — |
| 12 Klinefelter's syndrome/hypogonadism | 2 | 0.6 | — |
| 13 Bitemporal hemianopia | 2 | 0 | — |
| 14 Diabetic foot/Charcot's joint | 2 | 0 | — |
| 15 Necrobiosis lipoidica diabeticorum | 1 | 0 | — |
| 16 Short stature | 0.8 | 1 | — |
| 17 Pseudohypoparathyroidism | 0.4 | 1 | — |
| 18 Pendred's syndrome | 0 | 0.6 | — |

## Station 5, eyes

| Short case | Main focus in PACES survey (%) | Predicted main focus in PACES from original surveys (%) | Predicted additional feature (%) |
|---|---|---|---|
| 1 Diabetic retinopathy | 41 | 47 | — |
| 2 Retinitis pigmentosa | 16 | 8 | — |
| 3 Optic atrophy | 6 | 19 | 2 |
| 4 Ocular palsy | 6 | 0 | — |
| 5 Visual field defect | 4 | 0 | — |
| 6 Retinal vein occlusion | 2 | 3 | — |
| 7 Old choroiditis | 2 | 4 | — |
| 8 Papilloedema | 0 | 4 | — |
| 9 Cataracts | 2 | 1 | 8 |
| 10 Myasthenia gravis | 2 | 1 | — |
| 11 Albinism | 2 | 0 | — |
| 12 Exophthalmos | 2 | 0 | — |
| 13 Myelinated nerve fibres | 1 | 1 | — |
| 14 Hypertensive retinopathy | 1 | 8 | — |
| 15 Glaucoma/peripheral field loss | 1 | 0 | — |
| 16 Retinal artery occlusion | 0.5 | 1 | — |

*(Continued)*

## Eyes contd.

| Short case | Main focus in PACES survey (%) | Predicted main focus in PACES from original surveys (%) | Predicted additional feature (%) |
|---|---|---|---|
| 17 Asteroid hyalosis | 0 | 0.6 | — |
| 18 Drusen | 0 | 0.4 | — |
| 19 Laurence–Moon–Bardet–Biedl syndrome | 0 | 0.7 | — |
| 20 Cytomegalovirus choroidoretinitis (AIDS) | 0 | 0.1 | — |
| 21 Normal fundus | 0 | 0 | — |

## Station 5, other

| Short case | Main focus in PACES survey (%) | Predicted main focus in PACES from original surveys (%) | Predicted additional feature (%) |
|---|---|---|---|
| 1 Bilateral parotid enlargement/Mikulicz's syndrome | 0 | 2 | — |
| 2 Deep venous thrombosis/Baker's cyst/cellulitis | 0 | 2 | — |
| 3 Peripheral vascular disease | 0 | 0.8 | ? |
| 4 Osteogenesis imperfecta | 0 | 0.5 | — |
| 5 Down's syndrome | 0 | 0.5 | 0.6 |
| 6 Pernicious anaemia | 0 | 0.4 | — |
| 7 Klippel–Feil syndrome | 0 | 0.3 | — |
| 8 Leg oedema | 0 | 0.3 | ? |

# 3 | Texidor's twinge and related matters

The following excerpt from Richard Asher's book* is surely compulsory reading for all prospective members of the Royal College of Physicians. No physician's training is complete until the messages contained therein have been assimilated.

'It is pleasant to believe that the facts of medical science are there whether or not we name them; that the truth about clinical medicine exists quite independently of the names we bestow upon it. If that were so, our only responsibility would be to agree upon symbols or words for facts that already existed. That theoretical ideal is hardly ever fulfilled. A little patient thinking will soon convince the enquirer that it is not just a simple matter of finding words to fit the facts, but just as often of finding facts to fit the words. When christening a baby we wait for the child to be born and then we find a name for it. When christening a disease we sometimes wait for the name to be born and then we try to find a disease to suit it. With children we announce their names in the birth columns of The Times and with diseases we announce their names in the original articles of the medical journals. The only difference is that children's names have to be registered. There is no such procedure with medical terms. There is no Medical Registrar-General of Terminological Births and Deaths. Only medical dictionaries and the international list of classified diseases. These do not include every living medical term, and they list many that have died or that ought to be painlessly put away. There is something about a name, particularly an eponymous term, which brings into being things which never seemed to be there before. In creation the word may come first: the opening sentence of the Gospel of Saint John is – "In the beginning was the Word."

Take, for instance, Pel Ebstein fever. Every student and every doctor knows that cases of Hodgkin's disease may show a fever that is high for one week and low for the next week, and so on. Does this phenomenon really exist at all? If you collect the charts of 50 cases of Hodgkin's disease and compare them with the charts of 50 cases of disseminated malignant fever, do you really believe you could

pick out even one or two cases because of the characteristic fever? I think it is very unlikely indeed. Yet if, by the vagaries of chance, one case of Hodgkin's did run such a temperature, the news would soon travel round: "There's a good case of Hodgkin's disease in Galen Ward. You ought to have a look. It shows the typical Pel Ebstein fever very well".

The chart might be copied for teaching purposes, or even put in a book. The mere description and the naming of a mythical fever leads inevitably to its occurrence in textbooks. One popular textbook for nurses depicts particularly classical temperature charts, attributed to various fevers. I asked the author how many hospital notes she had combed before she found such beautiful examples: "Oh, there was no trouble about that," she replied, "I made them up out of my head".

I wonder whether any examples of Pel Ebstein and other fevers in textbooks have similar origins. It does not matter whether or not Pel Ebstein fever exists, my contention remains the same: the bestowal of a name upon a concept, whether real or imaginary, brings it into clinical existence.

Out of curiosity I looked up the original papers, and Dr Burrows kindly translated them for me. Both describe patients with chronic relapsing fever and splenomegaly but there is nothing in either paper to suggest any of them had Hodgkin's disease. Both describe cases of undulant fever and Ebstein suggested the name chronic relapsing fever, but it was very probably one of abortus fever.

An important example of the creation of a thing beginning with the word is gallstone colic. There is no such thing. Colic is a pain continuously waxing and waning, like the colonic cramps of food poisoning. Gallstone pain after its onset steadily climbs to an agonizing peak without any fluctuation, and then passes off. But the label colic has been so firmly stuck on to this pain that the pain is expected to be colic, assumed to be colic, believed to be colic and finally bullied into being colic, so that a man with gallstone pain will be described as having colicky pain, however steady it may be.

Contrariwise, if something has no individual descriptive term it has far less chance of clinical acceptance or clinical recognition. A rose without a name may smell as

*From the book *Talking Sense*, edited by Sir Francis Avery Jones (Pitman Medical, 1972).

sweet, but it has far less chance of being smelt. Supposing we take an unnamed fever and an unnamed pain to contrast with the examples I have given. In untreated pernicious anaemia there is often quite a high fever. Sixty per cent of cases with red cell counts under 1.5 million show a fever over 101°F. This invariably settles to normal levels within a week of one adequate injection of $B_{12}$. I make no assertion that this fever is of great importance. What I do assert is that had it been called the Addison–Castle fever or hypo-cyanocobalaminic fever there is not a medical student in the land who would not have heard of it, many doctors would be afraid to diagnose pernicious anaemia without its presence, and the proportion of patients showing the fever would rise sharply once the name got into nurses' textbooks (because if they did not show the fever they would have their thermometers put back in their mouths until they behaved themselves).

Now for a pain without a name. Have any of you ever had a very brief, sharp needle-like pain near the apex of the heart: acutely localized to one point seemingly inside the chest wall, but feeling as if something was adherent to it? Breathing sharpens it, so there is often a disinclination to take a deep breath while it lasts. It comes out of the blue, it passes off in a few minutes, and although acute it is not at all distressing.

Enquiries among my friends showed that quite a lot of them occasionally had this pain, but, till they knew other people had it too, they did not mention it; especially because it has no official name, and also because it did not bother them.

I circulated various doctors I knew, and also circularized 50 recently elected Fellows of the College of Physicians – to see if it was reasonably common. It was . . . So if any of you happen to have it, you are not branding yourselves as either grievously neurotic or grossly hypochondriacal if you admit to having it.

[In the second of the Lettsomian lectures, on which this essay is based, with the permission of the President of the Medical Society of London, Dr Asher asked his audience of medical men whether any of them had encountered anything closely resembling this pain in either themselves or their friends, and if they had, to raise their hands. Over a third of the audience held up their hands.]

There seems no doubt that this condition exists, yet, because it has no name, it has no official clinical existence. We cannot discuss it or investigate it or write about it. Whether or not the condition should be named I am unable to say.† Though the naming of disease is not in any way restricted or supervised it ought not to be undertaken lightly. A fertile medical author can easily beget a large number of clinical progeny by describing and naming them, but some of his youngsters may turn out to be illegitimate, and with others there may be much doubt about their paternity if others claim to have begotten them years ago.'

†In a foreword to *Sense and Sensibility* the author explained that the pain had been described and named 4 years previously by A.J. Miller and T.A. Texidor (1955) in the *Journal of the American Medical Association*, and that it might in future be known as Texidor's twinge.

# 4 | Abbreviations

| | |
|---|---|
| **ABG** | arterial blood gas |
| **ABPI** | Ankle Brachial Pressure Index |
| **ACE** | angiotensin-converting enzyme |
| **ACEI** | angiotensin-converting enzyme inhibitor |
| **ACTH** | adrenocorticotrophic hormone |
| **ADL** | activities of daily living |
| **AED** | antiepileptic drug |
| **AF** | atrial fibrillation |
| **AFB** | acid-fast bacilli |
| **AIDS** | acquired immunodeficiency syndrome |
| **ALT** | alanine aminotransferase |
| **AMT** | abbreviated mental test |
| **ANA** | antinuclear antibody |
| **ANCA** | antineutrophil cytoplasmic antibodies |
| **anti-GBM** | anti-glomerular basement membrane antibody |
| **APAS** | antiphospholipid antibody syndrome |
| **APTT** | activated partial thromboplastin time |
| **AS** | ankylosing spondylitis, aortic stenosis |
| **ASD** | atrial septal defect |
| **ATD** | antithyroid drug |
| **AV** | atrioventricular |
| | |
| **BMI** | Body Mass Index |
| **BP** | blood pressure |
| **BRAO** | branch retinal artery occlusion |
| | |
| **CABG** | coronary artery bypass graft |
| **CCF** | congestive cardiac failure |
| **CDAD** | *Clostridium difficile*-associated diarrhoea |
| **CK** | creatine kinase |
| **CLO (test)** | *Campylobacter*-like organism test |
| **CMO** | cystoid macular oedema |
| **CNS** | central nervous system, clinical nurse specialist |
| **COC** | combined oral contraceptive |
| **COMT** | catechol-omicron-methyltransferase |
| **COPD** | chronic obstructive pulmonary disease |
| **COX** | cyclo-oxygenase |
| **CPK** | creatine phosphokinase |
| **CRAO** | central retinal artery occlusion |
| **CRH** | corticotrophin-releasing hormone |
| **CRP** | C-reactive protein |

| | |
|---|---|
| **CRVO** | central retinal vein occlusion |
| **CSF** | cerebrospinal fluid |
| **CT** | computed tomography |
| **CTA** | computed tomography angiography |
| **CTCL** | cutaneous T-cell lymphoma |
| **CTPA** | computed tomography pulmonary angiogram |
| **CVA** | cardiovascular accident |
| **CVD** | cerebrovascular disease |
| **CVI** | Certificate of Visual Impairment |
| **CVP** | central venous pressure |
| **CVS** | cardiovascular system |
| **CWS** | cotton-wool spot |
| **CXR** | chest X-ray |
| | |
| **DD** | differential diagnosis, disc diameter |
| **DEXA** | dual-energy X-ray absorptiometry |
| **DIC** | disseminated intravascular coagulation |
| **DIDMOAD** | diabetes insipidus, diabetes mellitus, optic atrophy, deafness |
| **DIP** | distal interphalangeal |
| **DLBD** | diffuse Lewy body disease |
| **DM** | diabetes mellitus |
| **DMARD** | disease-modifying antirheumatic drug |
| **DRE** | digital rectal examination |
| **DVT** | deep vein thrombosis |
| **DWI** | diffusion-weighted imaging |
| | |
| **ECG** | electrocardiography |
| **ECHO** | echocardiography |
| **ED** | emergency department |
| **ELISA** | enzyme-linked immuno sorbent assay |
| **EMG** | electromyography |
| **ENT** | ear, nose and throat |
| **ERCP** | endoscopic retrograde cholangiopancreatography |
| **ESM** | ejection systolic murmur |
| **ESR** | erythrocyte sedimentation rate |
| **ETT** | exercise tolerance test |
| | |
| **FBC** | full blood count |
| **FNAC** | fine needle aspiration cytology |

| | | | | |
|---|---|---|---|
| FSH | follicle-stimulating hormone | INR | international normalized ratio |
| FT3 | free T3 | IRMA | intraretinal microvascular abnormality |
| FT4 | free T4 | ITP | idiopathic thrombocytopenic purpura |
| | | IUD | intrauterine device |
| GA | general anaesthetic | IVC | inferior vena cava |
| GBS | Guillain–Barré syndrome | | |
| GCA | giant cell arteritis | JCA | juvenile chronic arthritis |
| GCS | Glasgow Coma Score | JIA | juvenile idiopathic arthritis |
| G-CSF | granulocyte colony-stimulating factor | JVP | jugular venous pulse |
| GH | growth hormone | | |
| GHRH | growth hormone-releasing hormone | LAD | left anterior descending |
| GI | gastrointestinal | LBBB | left bundle branch block |
| GLP1 | glucagon-like peptide 1 | LDH | lactate dehydrogenase |
| GORD | gastro-oesophageal reflux disease | LDL | low-density lipoprotein |
| GRACE | global registry of acute coronary events | LFT | liver function test |
| GTN | glyceryl trinitrate | LH | luteinizing hormone |
| GUM | genitourinary medicine | LOC | loss of consciousness |
| | | LP | lumbar puncture |
| Hb | haemoglobin | LRTI | lower respiratory tract infection |
| HCC | hepatocellular carcinoma | LV | left ventricular |
| HCG | human chorionic gonadotrophin | LVH | left ventricular hypertrophy |
| HDL | high-density lipoprotein | | |
| HELLP | haemolysis elevated liver enzymes low platelets | MAHA | microangioathic haemolytic anaemia |
| | | MAO-B | monoamine oxidase type B |
| HFE | human haemochromatosis protein (gene) | MAP | mean arterial pressure |
| | | MAU | medical assessment unit |
| HHT | hereditary haemorrhagic telangiectasia | MCA | middle cerebral artery |
| HIV | human immunodeficiency virus | MCP | metacarpophalangeal |
| HOCM | hypertrophic obstructive cardiomyopathy | MCS | microscopy, culture and sensitivity |
| | | MCV | mean corpuscular volume |
| HPOA | hypertrophic pulmonary osteoarthropathy | MDT | multidisciplinary team |
| | | MEN | multiple endocrine neoplasia |
| HRCT | high-resolution computed tomography | MG | myasthenia gravis |
| HRT | hormone replacement therapy | MI | myocardial infarction |
| HTLV | human T-lymphotrophic virus | MLF | medial longitudinal fasciculus |
| HUS | haemolytic uraemic syndrome | MMSE | Mini Mental State Examination |
| | | MND | motor neurone disease |
| IA | intra-articular | MR | mitral regurgitation |
| IBD | inflammatory bowel disease | MRA | magnetic resonance angiography |
| IBS | irritable bowel syndrome | MRI | magnetic resonance imaging |
| ICD | implantable cardioverter defibrillator | MS | multiple sclerosis |
| ICE | ideas, concerns and expectations | MSSU | mid-stream sample of urine |
| ICP | intracranial pressure | MTP | metatarsophalangeal |
| ICU | intensive care unit | | |
| IGF | insulin-like growth factor | NAFLD | non-alcoholic fatty liver disease |
| IHD | ischaemic heart disease | NG | nasogastric |
| IL | interleukin | NSAID | non-steroidal anti-inflammatory drug |
| ILD | interstitial lung disease | NSTEMI | non-ST elevation myocardial infarction |
| IM | intramuscular | NVD | new vessels on disc |
| INO | internuclear ophthalmoplegia | NVE | new vessels elsewhere |

| | | | | |
|---|---|---|---|---|
| OA | osteoarthritis, optic atrophy | | SBE | subacute bacterial endocarditis |
| OCP | oral contraceptive pill | | SGLT2 | sodium/glucose co-transporter 2 |
| O&G | obstetrics and gynaecology | | SHO | senior house officer |
| OGD | oesophagogastroduodenoscopy | | SLE | systemic lupus erythematosus |
| OGTT | oral glucose tolerance test | | SOB | shortness of breath |
| OT | occupational therapy/therapist | | SOL | space-occupying lesion |
| | | | SPECT | single photon emission computed tomography |
| PA | posteroanterior | | | |
| PAF | paroxysmal atrial fibrillation | | SR | sinus rhythm |
| PBC | primary biliary cirrhosis | | SSc | systemic sclerosis |
| PBG | porphobilinogen | | SSRI | selective serotonin reuptake inhibitor |
| PD | Parkinson's disease | | STI | sexually transmissible infection |
| PE | pulmonary embolism | | SVC | superior vena cava |
| PEFR | peak expiratory flow rate | | SVT | supraventricular tachycardia |
| PFO | patent foramen ovale | | | |
| PIP | proximal interphalangeal | | TB | tuberculosis |
| PML | progressive multifocal leucoencephalopathy | | TED | thromboembolic disease |
| | | | TFT | thyroid function test |
| PMR | polymyalgia rheumatica | | TIA | transient ischaemic attack |
| PNS | peripheral nervous system | | TIMI | thrombolysis in myocardial infarction study group |
| po | *per os* | | | |
| PPI | proton pump inhibitor | | TLCO | transfer factor for the lung for carbon monoxide |
| PPK | palmoplantar keratoderma | | | |
| PR | *per rectum* | | TMJ | temporomandibular joint |
| PRP | panretinal photocoagulation | | TNF | tumour necrosis factor |
| PRV | polycythaemia rubra vera | | TPHA | *Treponema pallidum* haemagglutination |
| PSA | prostate-specific antigen | | TPO | thyroid peroxidise |
| PSP | progressive supranuclear palsy | | TR | tricuspid regurgitation |
| PT | prothrombin time | | TSH | thyroid-stimulating hormone |
| PTU | propylthiouracil | | TTG | tissue transglutaminase |
| PUVA | psoralen and UVA light | | TTP | thrombotic thrombocytopenic purpura |
| PV | *per vaginam* | | | |
| | | | UC | ulcerative colitis |
| RA | rheumatoid arthritis, right atrium/atrial | | U&E | urea and electrolytes |
| RAO | retinal artery occlusion | | URTI | upper respiratory tract infection |
| RAPD | relative afferent pupillary defect | | US | ultrasound |
| RCP | Royal College of Physicians | | UTI | urinary tract infection |
| RDT | rapid diagnostic testing | | UV | ultraviolet |
| RET | rearranged during transfection | | | |
| RIF | right iliac fossa | | VA | visual acuity |
| RMO | resident medical officer | | VEGF | vascular endothelial growth factor |
| ROM | range of motion | | VF | ventricular fibrillation |
| RP | retinitis pigmentosa | | VLDL | very low-density lipoprotein |
| RR | respiratory rate | | VT | ventricular tachycardia |
| RV | right ventricle/ventricular | | | |
| | | | WCC | white cell count |
| SACD | subacute combined degeneration of the cord | | WPW | Wolff–Parkinson–White |
| SAH | subarachnoid haemorrhage | | | |

# Index

# MRCP – it teaches more than it tests*

*'When you come out of the exam you realize that after months and months of hard work and swotting, the amount of knowledge you actually used could be written on a postage stamp!' (Vol. 2, Section F, Quotation 415)

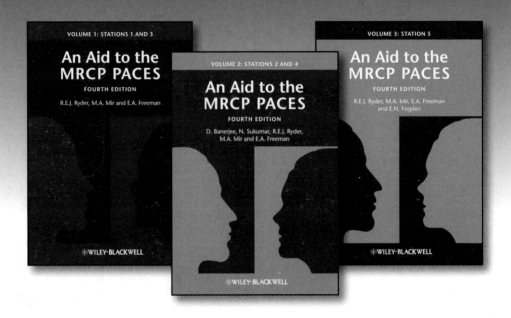